The Palgrave Handbook of Psychological Perspectives on Alcohol Consumption

Richard Cooke • Dominic Conroy
Emma Louise Davies
Martin S. Hagger • Richard O. de Visser
Editors

The Palgrave Handbook of Psychological Perspectives on Alcohol Consumption

palgrave
macmillan

Editors
Richard Cooke
Department of Psychology
University of Liverpool
Liverpool, UK

Liverpool Centre for Alcohol Research
Liverpool, UK

Emma Louise Davies
Department of Psychology, Health and
Professional Development
Oxford Brookes University
Oxford, UK

Richard O. de Visser
Brighton and Sussex Medical School
University of Sussex
Falmer, UK

Dominic Conroy
School of Psychology
University of East London
London, UK

Martin S. Hagger
Department of Psychological Sciences
University of California, Merced
Merced, CA, USA

Faculty of Sport and Health Sciences
University of Jyväskylä
Jyväskylä, Finland

ISBN 978-3-030-66940-9 ISBN 978-3-030-66941-6 (eBook)
https://doi.org/10.1007/978-3-030-66941-6

Cover illustration: eyepark/gettyimages

This Palgrave Macmillan imprint is published by the registered company Springer Nature Switzerland AG.
The registered company address is: Gewerbestrasse 11, 6330 Cham, Switzerland

Preface

Alcohol consumption is a behaviour with a long history. According to archaeologists, chemical traces of pottery jars from China (circa 7000 BC) contained residues of a fermented drink made from grapes, berries, honey and rice, and it has been claimed that wine was first produced in 5400 BC in Mesopotamia. In the present day, according to the World Health Organization's 2018 Global Status Report on alcohol and health, alcohol consumption continues to be a common activity in many societies worldwide. For example, in the Americas, European, and Western Pacific regions, more than 50% of the population describe themselves as current drinkers. However, alcohol consumption is less common elsewhere, with more than 50% of the population in African, Eastern Mediterranean, and South East Asian regions reporting to be abstinent.

Even within regions where alcohol consumption is common, people's consumption varies along several dimensions such as how frequently they drink (daily vs. weekly) and how much they drink on each occasion (one drink vs. multiple drinks). The combination of drinking quantity and frequency has been used to characterise an individual's drinking pattern. For instance, heavy episodic drinking is a drinking pattern that involves drinking above guideline limits during a single occasion; it can occur when drinking at home alone, at home with a partner after children have gone to bed (colloquially known as 'wine o'clock'), or while drinking at social events, like barbeques or parties. In contrast, low-risk drinking is a drinking pattern that involves drinking within guideline limits during drinking occasions, for instance having a glass of wine with a meal.

Because different drinking patterns have been shown to impact on what happens to individuals during, and after, the drinking occasion, psychologists have been keen to explore and understand why people drink the way they do. They hope that studying alcohol consumption will provide insight into important theoretical and applied issues. From a theoretical perspective, psychologists hope to discover the factors that determine drinking behaviour, by conducting tests of relations between individual and social factors advanced as putative predictors of alcohol consumption. Such tests can be used to evaluate theoretical accounts of drinking behaviour, as well as address applied issues such as to inform the design of interventions aimed at curbing potentially harmful drinking patterns; if determinants of alcohol consumption can be identified, it is possible to target these in interventions as a means to reduce drinking behaviour and the associated harms.

The overarching aim of the *Handbook of Psychological Perspectives on Alcohol Consumption* is to bring together psychological perspectives on alcohol consumption from across the globe to stimulate discussion and debate about issues related to alcohol consumption. Therefore, we invited a range of eminent researchers to contribute to this book, and they have delivered a collection of chapters that provide a comprehensive, detailed, and varied response to the important issues and questions on alcohol consumption. When considering who we wanted to invite to contribute to the Handbook, we sought to represent researchers from countries where much of the psychological research on alcohol has traditionally been conducted (i.e., Australia, New Zealand, the UK, the USA), as well as researchers based in countries with different patterns of alcohol consumption and varied cultures and histories with respect to alcohol, including Denmark, Italy, the Netherlands and Spain. The resulting Handbook, therefore, brings together a plurality of psychological perspectives on alcohol consumption in the best traditions of academic collaboration.

The book is divided into five distinct sections. In Section I, *Psychological Theories and Predictors* (Chaps. 2, 3, 4, and 5), contributors provide an overview of various models and theories of alcohol consumption which share the distinctively *psychological* quality of being focused on individual predictors of consumption. Psychology researchers have tended to test the utility of these theories by examining their constructs as correlates or predictors of alcohol consumption.

However, such correlational research is limited as a means to understand drinking behaviour. A key concern is that understanding drinking behaviour cannot be achieved by focusing exclusively on how individuals' beliefs, motives, or perceptions relate to their behaviour, because adopting this approach fails to account for the reality that alcohol consumption is an inherently *social* behaviour, which highlights the context or environment as an important determinant. For example, people generally consume alcohol in contexts that are inherently social, where they gather together to celebrate, chat, and relax. This means that an understanding of alcohol consumption needs to consider how it is shaped by external factors: the culture in which people live, the people with whom they drink, the location(s) where they drink, and the cues or prompts to drinking present in those locations. These issues are covered in Section II, *Social Contextual Factors* (Chaps. 6, 7, 8, 9, and 10).

Other psychological research focuses on how adolescents and young adults construct their drinking identities. This is important given the potential harms of excessive alcohol consumption in young people and also because patterns of drinking when young may relate to drinking patterns in adulthood. For example, it is normal for adolescents and young adults to construct and present their identities using social media channels. Their alcohol consumption, or their abstinence, is often a prominent feature of such activity. Studying alcohol often lends itself to qualitative methods where researchers adopt critical perspectives to explore these issues. Section III, *Drinking Identities* (Chaps. 11, 12, 13, and 14), covers a range of emerging issues in psychological research on alcohol including online drinking identities, sports teams' role in consumption, pre-drinking, and young people's drink refusal.

Relatively little research has been conducted with samples of children, but there has been a recent increase in interest in conducting studies with children to see how their beliefs about alcohol develop. Once children reach adolescence they become the focus of more psychological research. Three important issues relating to children and alcohol are covered in the Handbook: how parents discuss alcohol consumption with their adolescent children, how cultures affect adolescents' drinking, and the impact of school interventions on adolescent drinking behaviour and beliefs. These topics are covered in Section IV, *Developmental Trajectories for Alcohol Use* (Chaps. 15, 16, 17, and 18).

Psychological-informed interventions to promote safer drinking are covered in Section V, *Interventions to Reduce Alcohol Consumption* (Chaps. 18, 19, 20, 21, and 22). Interventions that are delivered at the population level (e.g., labels on alcoholic products) and the individual level (e.g., cognitive bias modification) are evaluated alongside approaches that have an explicit focus on psychological theories of alcohol consumption such as the social norms approach, which informs web-based personalised feedback interventions, or the model of action phases, which proposes that changing behaviours involves targeting change in both motivational and self-regulatory processes.

The final chapter of the Handbook, Chap. 23, provides a summary of key topics raised throughout the Handbook and presents a vision for future research studies. Specifically, the chapter discusses four themes—samples,

Bridgette M. Bewick is an associate professor at the University of Leeds. She seeks to understand how personalised feedback interventions can help intervene early with individuals who are drinking problematically. Bewick's contribution to research and practice in the addictions field was recognised in 2012 by her being awarded the 'SSA Fred Yates Prize Researcher of the Year'. She's an expert on the use of the Social Norms Approach and in developing ways for e-health solutions to support individuals to consider their own drinking behaviour and think through their potential to change.

Anna K. M. Blackwell is a senior research associate in the Tobacco and Alcohol Research Group at the University of Bristol, working as part of the Behaviour Change by Design programme team, funded by a Collaborative Award in Science from the Wellcome Trust (Behaviour Change by Design: 206853/Z/17/Z) awarded to Theresa Marteau, Paul Fletcher, Gareth Hollands and Marcus Munafò. Blackwell works on a number of projects that aim to generate evidence for the effectiveness of behaviour change interventions to reduce alcohol and tobacco related harm. Projects have included examining the impact of unit, calorie and health warning in alcohol labelling, altering the availability of alcohol-free drink options, reducing cigarette pack size and understanding the role of tobacco cigarette and e-cigarette cues on smoking craving and susceptibility.

Kim Bloomfield is a professor at the Centre for Alcohol and Drug Research, Aarhus University, Denmark. She is a guest professor at the Charité—University Medicine Berlin and at the Unit of Health Promotion Research, University of Southern Denmark, and associate researcher at the Alcohol Research Group, Emeryville, California, USA. Bloomfield is a social epidemiologist and has conducted several national general population surveys on alcohol and drugs in Denmark. She has been a co-investigator and multiple principal investigator of the international GENACIS and GENAHTO projects, respectively. Topics of interest include gender differences and social inequalities in health and alcohol use.

Lisa Buckley has focused on behaviour change research in efforts to reduce adolescent and young adult injury, primarily around the use of alcohol, experience of violence and road-related risk behaviours. Overall research expertise overlies health behaviour change programme development, implementation and evaluation where she has been a chief investigator with over $US8.5 million in research funding and publishing over 95 papers and reports. Her work takes a focus on promotive factors for well-being, particularly through supportive relationships with friends and parents and in schools. She has a strong interest in the way bystanders influence health behaviour.

Kim M. Caudwell is a sessional educator and a lecturer at CQUniversity, and a sessional academic at Curtin University. He has published research applying psychological theories to understand and predict various health behaviours, including alcohol consumption, tobacco use, and exercise. Caudwell's PhD programme of research culminated in the development and testing of an intervention to reduce pre-drinking alcohol consumption and related harm among undergraduates. His broad research interests include theoretical integration and application of dual system perspectives that may better explain why individuals pursue harmful health behaviours.

John D. Clapp is Professor of Social Work and Preventive Medicine at the University of Southern California. His work has largely focused on understanding drinking in situ. He has published numerous studies, and conceptual and methodological papers related to drinking events and the contexts of drinking.

Natasha Clarke is a research associate at the University of Cambridge. Clarke is interested in interventions that might reduce alcohol-related harm, with a particular focus on changing physical cues in the immediate drinking environment. Recent projects have explored the impact of alcohol labelling interventions, such as health warnings and unit information, on drink selection and consumption. She is also conducting studies that look at whether wine glass and bottle size can influence drinking behaviour as part of the Behaviour Change by Design programme.

Lester Coleman is an honorary senior research fellow at the University of Brighton. Coleman has led on a number of alcohol-related research projects, with grants from the South-East Regional Teenage Pregnancy Co-ordinator and the Drug Prevention Advisory Service, Joseph Rowntree Foundation, and the Alcohol Education and Research Council. Coleman helped to deliver recent research exploring parent-child conversations about alcohol on behalf of Drinkaware.

Dominic Conroy is Lecturer in Psychology at the University of East London. Conroy has published qualitative and quantitative research concerning health behaviour among young adults over the last decade. His qualitative, quantitative, and mixed methods research primarily concerns drinking practices among young adults. He is interested in exploring young adult drinking practices that illuminate issues of intimacy and social bonding underpinning alcohol use and developing understanding of flexible drinking styles and agency involved in young adults' alcohol use.

Megan Cook is a PhD student at the Centre for Alcohol Policy Research, La Trobe University in Melbourne. Her research investigates young children's knowledge about alcohol. Cook's research aims to understand how young children conceptualise alcohol in terms of how children define alcohol, what children believe happens when alcohol is consumed, and what perceptions children have of the normative role of alcohol within society. Her research interests also include age-appropriate assessment techniques (e.g. the revised Alcohol Expectancy Task and the use of qualitative interviews).

Richard Cooke is Senior Lecturer in Psychology at the University of Liverpool and a member of the Liverpool Centre for Alcohol Research. Cooke is interested in the utility of psychological theories to predict alcohol consumption in young adults. Recent projects have compared results across countries and used meta-analysis to synthesising research findings. Cooke is also interested in exploring how young adults interact with drinking guidelines and how the role of regret at the consequences of alcohol consumption informs future drinking.

Joel Crawford is a PhD student at the University of Liverpool. His PhD involves a mixed methods approach into developing knowledge of alcohol-related regret in young adults. His research interests include how psychological constructs interact with regret to influence alcohol consumption and how missing opportunities to consume alcohol socially lead to the experience of the missing out, colloquially known as the Fear of Missing Out (FoMO).

Helen F. Crosby is Lecturer in Psychology at Leeds Trinity University and an honorary lecturer at the University of Leeds. Crosby's background is in applied health, having worked in NHS mental health settings for over ten years. Her research has focused on developing and implementing effective therapies for people with substance use problems and for people who self-harm. Crosby's research is collaborative—working with academics, therapists and NHS staff, and people accessing treatment services.

Emma Louise Davies is Senior Lecturer in Psychology at Oxford Brookes University. Her research expertise is in the fields of health psychology and public health, specifically exploring alcohol use behaviours, and she has had a particular focus on applying behaviour change theories and developing interventions to improve health and well-being. Her recent key projects have explored the potential of using digital tools to reduce alcohol misuse in adolescents and young people. Davies is a member of the Global Drug Survey Core Research Team with lead responsibility for the alcohol section of the survey. She is also interested in exploring the meanings attached to drinking (and non-drinking) practices and experiences within different groups.

Robert C. Dempsey is Senior Lecturer in Psychology at Manchester Metropolitan University. Dempsey's research focuses on how an individual's perception of their social environment influences their physical and mental health, including work focusing on experiences of bipolar spectrum conditions, suicidality, and the role of perceived social norms in health-related behaviours (e.g. substance use, health protective behaviours). Dempsey collaborates with a range of stakeholders across his areas of research, including people with lived experience, public health and healthcare practitioners, voluntary sector organisations, as well as academics from a range of subject disciplines.

Matt Field is Professor of Psychology at the University of Sheffield. He conducts research into the psychological mechanisms that underlie alcohol problems and other substance addictions. He is particularly interested in the roles of decision-making and impulse control in addiction, recovery, and behaviour change more broadly. Recent projects include assessing the benefits of temporary alcohol restriction in heavy drinkers and examining the role of meaning of life and alcohol value in alcohol consumption.

Ian Goodwin is a senior lecturer in the School of English and Media Studies, Massey University, New Zealand. With a background in cultural studies Goodwin's research is wide ranging and often inter-disciplinary yet centres on understanding the societal changes associated with the rise of 'new' media technologies. Goodwin is interested in exploring intersections between contemporary media forms, popular culture, activism, citizenship, media policy, consumption, health and well-being, and space/place.

Martin S. Hagger is Professor of Health Psychology in the Department of Psychological Sciences at the University of California (UC), Merced, USA, and Professor of Research on Behavior Change in the Faculty of Sport and Health Sciences, University of Jyväskylä, Finland. He is the director of the Social and Health Psychology Applied Behavioral Research for Prevention and Promotion Lab at UC Merced. Hagger's research applies social psychological theory to predict, understand, and change health behaviours. A key focus of his research is to identify effects of psychological determinants, such as attitudes, intentions, self-efficacy, perceived control, self-control, planning, personality, and motives, of health behaviour, and help health professionals to use this information to promote health behaviour change through intervention. He is also interested in research synthesis, particularly testing predictions of psychological theory across multiple populations, contexts, and behaviours using meta-analysis.

Kyra Hamilton is an associate professor in the School of Applied Psychology and Menzies Health Institute Queensland at Griffith University, Australia. She has psychology and nursing qualifications and over 25 years of experience in the health field. She is founder and director of the Health and Psychology Innovations (HaPI) research laboratory. Hamilton's main areas of research are health psychology and behavioural medicine, and areas of expertise and innovation are health behaviour motivation, self-regulation, and change. Hamilton's research is applied widely to understand priority health- and risk-related behaviours in a wide range of population groups.

Derek Heim is Professor of Psychology and Director of Research at Edge Hill University. As a social psychologist with an interest in health behaviours, his primary research areas concern (a) addiction and substance use and (b) health and well-being. In these contexts, his work focuses on social, cultural and contextual influences, utilising both quantitative and qualitative research methods. He is Editor-in-Chief of *Addiction Research and Theory*, the leading outlet for contributions that view addictive behaviour as arising from psychological processes within the individual and social contexts, rather than the biological effects of the psychoactive substance. He served as a trustee of Alcohol Change (formerly Alcohol Research UK) between 2014 and 2020.

Manuel I. Ibáñez is Senior Lecturer in Psychology at the Universitat Jaume I and a researcher at the Centre for Biomedical Research Network on Mental Health (CIBERSAM) from the Instituto de Salud Carlos III. His main research interest is the role of personality on psychopathology. He has studied the interplay between personality and other risk factors in the development of alcohol use in adolescents and young adults from various countries. He is also examining other addictive behaviours in these populations.

Andrew Jones is a senior lecturer at the University of Liverpool. His research interests include the role of self-control and cognitive biases in the development and maintenance of alcohol (mis)use and overweight/obesity. He is also interested in the effectiveness of psychological treatments and evidence synthesis. Recent projects include randomised controlled trials of inhibitory control training for the reduction of heavy drinking and examining the compliance rates for mobile assessment protocols in substance users.

Emmanuel Kuntsche is Professor of Public Health at La Trobe University, Melbourne, and the Director of the Centre for Alcohol Policy Research. He is investigating the development and transformation of alcohol-related cognition from early childhood into adolescence and the role of parental alcohol socialisation. His research interests also include the measurement of both alcohol consumption (e.g. using ecological momentary assessment, smartphone apps and transdermal monitors) and related cognition (e.g. by means of the Alcohol Expectancy Task he developed).

Antonia Lyons is Professor of Health Psychology and Head of School at the School of Health, Victoria University of Wellington, New Zealand. She has researched widely on the social and cultural contexts of people's behaviours that are related to health and illness. One of her main research areas has been examining young people's drinking cultures and the role that social media play, including the impact of digital marketing.

Danielle R. Madden is Assistant Research Professor of Social Work at the University of Southern California. Her work examines contextual factors that impact substance use, risk behaviours of marginalized young adults with unstable housing, and product characteristics of e-cigarettes that influence abuse.

John McAlaney is an associate professor, chartered psychologist and chartered scientist at Bournemouth University. His research focuses on the psychological determinants of risk behaviours including substance use gambling, digital addiction and cybersecurity. McAlaney applies this research to real-world problems through his role as a Trustee of both the Gordon Moody Association, a residential service for problem gamblers, and Acts Fast, a charity which supports protective parents and family members of children who have been sexually abused.

Laura Mezquita is Senior Lecturer in Psychology at the Universitat Jaume I and a research collaborator at the Centre for Biomedical Research Network on Mental Health (CIBERSAM) from the Instituto de Salud Carlos III. Mezquita is interested in the influence of personality on the development of internalizing and externalizing psychopathology. Throughout the last decade she has focused on the externalizing spectrum. She has specifically studied the influence of personality in alcohol use and misuse, especially in young adults. She has published studies comparing young adults, from different countries, using risk models of alcohol and other drug use.

Kathryn L. Modecki studies how adolescents navigate the challenges of their teenage years and their pathways towards and away from problems (binge drinking, aggression, bullying, mental health problems). She maps adolescents' navigation of risk in the moment and over the long term, with a focus on youth living within disadvantaged settings. Modecki consults for organizations such as Outward Bound's At-Risk Programs, Florida Alliance of Boys & Girls Clubs, and the World Bank. She is situated in Menzies Health Institute Queensland and the School of Applied Psychology, Griffith University, Australia, and is a 2019/2020 Faculty Associate at the Berkman Klein Center for Internet & Society, Harvard University. Further information can be found at www.riskyadolescentpathways.com

Rebecca Monk is a social health psychologist and a senior lecturer at Edge Hill University. Her main research areas concern (i) the cognitive factors shaping health-related behaviour and (ii) investigating contextual influences on behaviour and cognition using a multi-methodological approach. Her research has focused primarily on the contextual variation in the peoples' substance use behaviours and associated beliefs. Specifically, she is interested in using advanced technology, for example smartphone applications, to gain real-time accounts, and to assess how these behaviours and beliefs may vary depending on one's location situational and social contexts.

Generós Ortet is Professor of Psychology at the Universitat Jaume I and a researcher at the Centre for Biomedical Research Network on Mental Health (CIBERSAM) from the Instituto de Salud Carlos III. His main research interests and publications are related to the study of personality traits and the assessment of individual differences. He has carried out longitudinal and cross-national studies on the influence of psychological factors on alcohol and substance use in both adolescents and young adults.

Elizabeth Partington is Senior Lecturer in Sport and Exercise Psychology at Northumbria University, and a member of the Department of Sport, Exercise and Rehabilitation's Informing policy and practice research group. Partington's research interests are focused around narrative psychology, athlete identity, athlete culture and athlete career transitions. Recent projects have included a longitudinal qualitative study of student athlete drinking motives and behaviours during and following the transition out of university. Partington is interested in exploring narrative interventions for different athlete career transitions. Partington is an HCPC registered practitioner and continues to provide sport psychology consultancy to elite athletes.

Sarah Partington is Principal Lecturer in Sport and Exercise Psychology at Northumbria University, and a member of the Department of Sport, Exercise and Rehabilitation's Informing policy and practice research group. Partington is a cultural sport psychologist, and her research interests are in narrative psychology, athlete mental health and well-being, and athlete crisis transitions. Recent projects have explored dominant narratives around student athlete drinking. Partington is interested in exploring narrative interventions for student athlete drinking and also for other athlete crisis transitions. Partington is an Health and Care Professions Council registered practitioner and regularly provides sport psychology support to elite athletes.

Emily Pechey is Research Assistant in the Behaviour Change by Design programme at the University of Cambridge. She previously worked as a research assistant at the Centre for Family Research, Cambridge, on studies of child development of executive function. She is now investigating the effectiveness of behaviour change interventions in promoting healthier lifestyles, including the impact of health warning labels on food- and alcohol-related attitudes, selection and consumption, as well as the mechanisms underlying these interventions.

Rachel Pechey is an epidemiologist at the University of Oxford. Pechey's research interests include exploring the effectiveness of different interventions that alter aspects of the physical micro-environment (sometimes referred to as 'choice architecture') to improve the healthiness and sustainability of diets, including reducing alcohol consumption. She is interested in understanding the mechanisms underlying the impact of such interventions and their potential impact on health inequalities.

Sara Rolando is a sociologist who works as a social researcher at Eclectica and is a contract professor at University of Torino. She completed her doctoral degree at the University of Helsinki, Finland, with a thesis comparing youth drinking cultures in different geographies. An expert in qualitative, web-based, and comparative methods, her main research interests are alcohol, gambling, drugs, and other addictive behaviours, which she has been investigating from different perspectives including cultures, careers, prevention, and policies.

Alexandra Sawyer is a senior research fellow at the University of Brighton and a chartered psychologist. Sawyer is a mixed methods researcher with a background in health psychology. Her recent projects have explored the conversations that parents have with their older children about alcohol, including the frequency, style, and content of conversations. This has been explored using in-depth interviews with parents and young people as well as analysing data from a large national survey.

Nigel Sherriff is Professor of Public Health and Health Promotion at the University of Brighton. He is a mixed methods researcher with interests in sexual health and HIV, health inequalities, and parenting. Much of his research has a focus on LGBTI and youth populations especially with an international/global focus. Recent projects have explored qualitatively and quantitatively the conversations parents have with their children about alcohol.

Koen Smit is a research officer with the Centre for Alcohol Policy Research, La Trobe University. He recently completed his doctorate which provided empirical evidence on alcohol involvement in early life (i.e., the role of alcohol exposure in the development of alcohol cognitions and the transition from expectancies to drinking motives to consumption patterns in early adolescence). Smit is extending this research line by further investigating alcohol cognitions among young children and the role of alcohol exposure (e.g. from siblings and peers) in alcohol use among adolescents. Other research interests include motives for pre-drinking in young adults and drinking motives among adults.

Jemma Todd is a clinical psychologist and Lecturer in Psychology at the University of Sydney, and also holds an adjunct research fellowship at the University of Western Australia. Todd uses quantitative research methods to explore the intersection of clinical and health psychology. Todd's research primarily focuses on the cognitive and emotional underpinnings of health behaviours such as binge drinking, as well as conditions such as chronic pain, sleep disorders, and anxiety. Her alcohol-related research has largely focused on health behaviour models.

Milica Vasiljevic is Assistant Professor in Social Psychology and the director of the MSc in Behavioural Science programme at Durham University. Vasiljevic investigates how cues in the environment impact health behaviours, and how this knowledge can be translated into effective behaviour change interventions to improve health and reduce inequalities. The bulk of her work to date has looked at how cues such as labelling and advertising affect people's decisions to eat (un)healthily, drink alcohol, and/or smoke tobacco. Some of her recent work has focused on how lower-strength alcohol labelling affects consumers' perceptions and alcohol consumption.

Richard O. de Visser is Reader in Psychology at the University of Sussex, where he teaches at the Brighton and Sussex Medical School. He is co-author of the textbook *Psychology for Medicine & Health Care* (3rd Edition, Sage). He uses quantitative, qualitative and mixed methods to explore social aspects of various health-related behaviours, with a particular focus on alcohol use.

Carmen Voogt is the project leader of the Alcohol Expertise Centre of the Trimbos Institute, which focuses on disseminating scientific insights about alcohol (prevention) and stimulating their application, thereby supporting professionals in their activities aimed at preventing and reducing alcohol-related harm. Her research focuses on the acquisition and development of children's alcohol knowledge as the basis for alcohol expectancies and transition from expectancies to drinking motives to consumption in early adolescence.

List of Figures

Fig. 2.1	The theory of planned behaviour overlaid with sample weighted average correlations for relationships reported in Cooke et al.'s (2016) meta-analysis of alcohol studies	35
Fig. 3.1	The Prototype Willingness Model. (Gerrard et al., 2008; Gibbons & Gerrard, 1995)	58
Fig. 4.1	Predictive factors on continua from fixed to unstable and distal to proximal	78
Fig. 5.1	Convergence between the most important models of normal personality traits and the UPPS impulsivity model	110
Fig. 5.2	Degree of influence (x-axis) of negative emotionality, positive emotionality, and disinhibition broad domains on the onset, use, and misuse of alcohol	116
Fig. 5.3	Etiological pathways to alcohol use and misuse	119
Fig. 7.1	Flowchart of study selection process	167
Fig. 8.1	Dynamic model of drinking events ('B' indicates balancing influences, 'R' indicates reinforcing influences)	190
Fig. 10.1	Percentage change (95% CI) in wine sales when wine is served in glasses varying in capacity (larger compared to smaller glasses)	238
Fig. 14.1	Information-motivation-behavioural skills model. (Adapted from Fisher et al., 2003)	328
Fig. 14.2	Health action process approach. (Retrieved from http://www.hapa-model.de)	341
Fig. 15.1	Scenario examples from the AET in relation to the Circumplex Model of Affect	356
Fig. 16.1	Alcohol recorded per capita consumption (L/year, pop. 15+). (Source: Global Information System on Alcohol and Health (GISAH), 2019)	379

Fig. 18.1	Contexts for adolescent intervention	429
Fig. 19.1	Existing health warnings from the US and UK	459
Fig. 21.1	Diagram of a basic model of a behaviour change mechanism of action (Hagger, 2019; Hagger, Moyers, et al., 2020). A behaviour change method or technique is proposed to relate to behaviour change through changes in modifiable theory-based determinants	502
Fig. 22.1	A schematic representing typical trials for different cognitive bias tasks	530
Fig. 22.2	The experimental medicine framework as applied to approach bias modification. (adapted from Sheeran, Klein, & Rothman, 2017)	534

List of Tables

Table 4.1 Correlations reported between psychological constructs and alcohol consumption 88
Table 13.1 Pre-drinking motive measures, their factors, and associations with DMQ-R subscales 309
Table 15.1 Age and alcohol-related cognitions 358

List of Boxes

Box 1.1	Definitions of Heavy Episodic Drinking	4
Box 1.2	Definitions of Low-Risk Drinking	5
Box 1.3	Phrases Used to Subjectively Describe Stages of Intoxication	9

1

Psychological Perspectives on Alcohol Consumption

Richard Cooke, Dominic Conroy, Emma Louise Davies, Martin S. Hagger, and Richard O. de Visser

Alcohol consumption can be considered from a variety of perspectives. For example, an epidemiological perspective would outline the prevalence of consumption, drinking patterns, and associated health conditions; a social policy perspective would emphasise the importance of evaluating the effectiveness of different alcohol control strategies; an economic perspective would highlight that alcohol consumption generates profits for businesses as well as costs for government agencies; a neuroscientific perspective would outline how alcohol affects the brain; and a sociological perspective would adopt a critical position on consumption and drinking practices.

To adopt a psychological perspective on alcohol consumption means, by comparison, to focus on individuals' consumption and the factors, issues, and

R. Cooke (✉)
Department of Psychology, University of Liverpool, Liverpool, UK

Liverpool Centre for Alcohol Research, Liverpool, UK
e-mail: cooker4@liverpool.ac.uk

D. Conroy
School of Psychology, University of East London, London, UK
e-mail: d.conroy@uel.ac.uk

E. L. Davies
Department of Psychology, Health and Professional Development, Oxford Brookes University, Oxford, UK
e-mail: edavies@brookes.ac.uk

R. Cooke et al. (eds.), *The Palgrave Handbook of Psychological Perspectives on Alcohol Consumption*, https://doi.org/10.1007/978-3-030-66941-6_1

narratives that are associated with drinking behaviour. For example, psychological research studies have addressed questions such as "how well do individuals' beliefs about alcohol predict their future drinking behaviour?"; "how does an individual's drinking behaviour (or abstinence) fit with their identity?"; and "how do individuals compare their drinking behaviour to other people's drinking behaviour?" It is assumed that individuals are attracted to alcohol given its potential to help them to achieve multiple desirable personal goals, such as socialising with friends, relaxing, or loosening inhibitions. Although individuals appear aware of the harms associated with alcohol, they tend not to dwell on them. Such findings challenge the paradigm directing much health-related research, which seeks to account for consumption in terms of population-level harm caused by individuals' behaviour and can help to steer debate towards a more nuanced, holistic understanding of the reasons for drinking, avoiding moral-based judgements. A key question guiding many psychological research studies about alcohol is: "Why do people drink alcohol?" A natural starting point, therefore, is a consideration of how psychologists have attempted to answer this question.

Why Do People Drink Alcohol?

Most people drink alcohol to achieve positive outcomes: to have fun, to increase their confidence, to lower their inhibitions in social settings, or to help them relax and forget their worries (Cooper, Kuntsche, Levitt, Barber, & Wolf, 2015; Kuntsche, Stewart, & Cooper, 2008). Thus, drinking alcohol can be seen to have positive effects both on the individual and on the people around them, marking it out as an inherently social behaviour that is as determined by external factors (culture, context, environment) as individual-level factors (see Section II).

Nevertheless, psychologists have typically focused on how individuals interact with alcohol consumption and have often adopted theory-driven, quantitative methods to understand why people drink alcohol. Such theories

M. S. Hagger
Department of Psychological Sciences, University of California, Merced, Merced, CA, USA

Faculty of Sport and Health Sciences, University of Jyväskylä, Jyväskylä, Finland
e-mail: mhagger@merced.edu

R. O. de Visser
Brighton and Sussex Medical School, University of Sussex, Falmer, UK
e-mail: r.o.devisser@bsms.ac.uk

have tended to adopt a deliberative, cognitive approach to explain drinking behaviour, focusing on the reasoned processing of available social information (see Section I). The individual is assumed to be a "reasoned actor", weighing up the pros (confidence, relaxation) and cons (negative affect, risk) to arrive at a decision whether or not to engage in a particular pattern of drinking (Cox & Klinger, 1988). From this perspective, therefore, decisions to drink (e.g., whether or not to drinking in a particular situation, how much to drink, when to stop) depend on an individual's consideration of the merits or demerits of what happens to *them* following consumption.

Although people often report drinking for the reasons outlined in psychological theories of alcohol consumption, it is less certain that people employ the same reasoning when deciding whether or not to drink; individuals are more likely to endorse positive motives for drinking (Cooper et al., 2015), making it debatable how much they genuinely reflect on the cons of drinking or weigh up the pros and cons of not drinking each time they arrive at the point of decision making. For example, Crawford, Jones, Rose, and Cooke (2020) found university students (i) reframed the cons of drinking in terms of the price to be paid to achieve social gains; (ii) failed to mention the pros of not drinking; and (iii) reported missing out on social drinking events to be aversive. Such results do not align with traditional theoretical accounts of drinking decisions.

Other qualitative studies have also provided evidence that drinkers report seeking to achieve positive emotional experiences wherein they maximise the pleasurable effects of consumption, drinking until they are "experiencing a buzz" (Beccaria, Petrilli, & Rolando, 2015) or reach a "sweet spot" (Graber et al., 2016), rather than focusing on losses that can follow drinking. Reaching this subjective stage of intoxication, drinkers perceive they obtain the full benefits of their drinking behaviour. For example, they report having fun, loosening up, or relaxing, while, crucially, remaining in control of themselves and their actions (Burgess, Cooke, & Davies, 2019). Because individuals vary in how much alcohol they can tolerate, phrases like the "sweet spot" necessarily refer to different amounts of alcohol consumption. This means that an "objective" definition of how much alcohol drinkers need to consume to reach the "sweet spot" is an elusive concept because the amount needed varies across drinkers. As discussed later in this chapter, subjective variation in alcohol tolerance represents a challenge for government and health agencies seeking to recommend universal low-risk guidelines. The discussion, thus far, has focused on why people drink alcohol. An equally important consideration is *how* people drink alcohol, that is, the different drinking patterns that people have adopted. A particular pattern of drinking that has been the focus of many psychological studies is heavy episodic drinking (HED), also known as binge drinking. This serves as a starting point for discussing how people consume alcohol.

How Is Heavy Episodic Drinking Defined?

Heavy episodic drinking (HED) is a phrase used to denote consuming more than a threshold number of drinks, or volume of alcohol, during a single drinking episode. Box 1.1 provides two definitions of HED.

Box 1.1 Definitions of Heavy Episodic Drinking

The National Institute for Alcohol Abuse and Alcoholism (NIAAA) defines heavy episodic (binge) drinking as follows:

> A 'binge' is a pattern of drinking alcohol that brings blood alcohol concentration (BAC) to 0.08 gram percent or above. For the typical adult, this pattern corresponds to consuming 5 or more drinks (male), or 4 or more drinks (female), in about 2 hours. Binge drinking is clearly dangerous for the drinker and society. (NIAAA, 2004, p. 3)
>
> The World Health Organization (WHO) defines heavy episodic drinking thus:
>
> Heavy episodic drinking (HED) is defined as 60 or more grams of pure alcohol on at least one occasion at least once per month. (World Health Organization, 2018, p. xiv)

enhancement > social > coping > conformity

There are limitations with both definitions shown in Box 1.1. For example, a limitation of the NIAAA definition is that what counts as a "standard drink" (i.e., in terms of alcohol-by-volume) varies between countries, while although the World Health Organization's (2018) can be difficult to operationalise. For example, 60 g equals slightly more than four "standard drinks" (56 g) in the USA, while in the UK, 60 g is equivalent to 3 and 3/4 standard servings of beer or wine (i.e., pints and 175 ml glasses, respectively). Such calculations make it difficult for individuals in the UK and USA to benchmark their consumption relative to this definition (see Kuntsche, Kuntsche, Thrul, & Gmel, 2017, for a detailed discussion of the issues with defining HED/binge drinking).

In the current text, this pattern of drinking will be referred to as *HED* rather than *binge drinking* for a number of reasons. One reason for using HED is that the phrase binge drinking may have a judgemental tone. There are also concerns about how precisely binge drinking is defined—an editorial by Ceballos and Babor (2017) noted that some alcohol journals have banned the use of binge drinking due to concerns about the validity of different definitions of the term. The term "binge drinking" also suffers from a colloquial and emotionally evocative association (e.g., the term is commonly used in the popular media).

Regardless of how HED is defined, it is a form of alcohol consumption that places considerable burdens on drinkers and society (Centers for Disease Control and Prevention, 2011; WHO, 2018). For example, Jones et al. (2008) noted that 26% of all deaths in 16- to 24-year-olds in the UK were alcohol related, resulting from accidents and alcohol poisoning, outcomes that are more likely when people engage in HED. Considering the costs to society associated with HED, various governments, government agencies, and health organisations have striven to encourage people to engage in what has often been labelled low-risk drinking, which is defined and discussed in the next section.

How Is Low-Risk Drinking Defined?

Low-risk drinking is a phrase used to define a pattern of alcohol consumption that when performed limits the likelihood of experiencing long-term (e.g., breast cancer, coronary heart disease, liver cirrhosis) and short-term (e.g., blackouts, hangover, nausea, vomiting) negative health outcomes. Box 1.2 presents two definitions of low-risk drinking. A key national difference between low-risk drinking guidelines is the timeframe specified for consumption, with definitions referring to either daily or weekly drinking. Different timeframes in guidelines mean that information is communicated about drinking occasions (daily) or a period of time where multiple drinking occasions can theoretically occur (weekly). Several countries—Canada, New Zealand, Poland, and the USA—publish both daily and weekly guidelines to capture different drinking patterns.

Box 1.2 Definitions of Low-Risk Drinking

Low-risk drinking is defined in terms of either the number of drink servings or the volume of alcoholic units one must drink less than on a daily, or weekly, basis to remain at low risk for these outcomes. Most countries propose a lower number of drinks/volume of alcohol for women relative to men. For example, the NIAAA define low-risk drinking for a man to be drinking four or fewer (USA) standard alcoholic drinks, whereas low-risk drinking for a woman is to drink three or fewer (USA) standard drinks.

The revised UK drinking guidelines (Department of Health, 2016) argue against gender differences for alcohol risk and instead propose that if men and women drink no more than 14 units,[1] over the course of a week, their lifetime likelihood of dying from an alcohol-related cause will be no more than 1%.

[1] A UK unit equals 8 g or 10 ml of pure alcohol and is the same as a single (25 ml) shot of spirits, approximately half a 175 ml glass of wine and approximately half a pint (568 ml) of beer, 1 cider, or lager.

Differences between countries in how alcohol is measured for sale, and the alcohol-by-volume of these measures, have led to a lack of consensus on what is considered low-risk drinking across countries (Furtwaengler & de Visser, 2013). The next section describes how governments disseminate low-risk guidelines and discuss how people respond to these guidelines.

How Do Governments Attempt to Encourage Low-Risk Drinking?

Low-risk drinking guidelines are an example of an *educational* alcohol control strategy—a policy designed to control the amount of alcohol consumed within a population, to educate and raise awareness among drinkers about guidelines by using mass media campaigns and labels on alcoholic products (see Chap. 19). Such an approach presupposes that increased awareness of guidelines will lead to reductions in individuals' consumption, which will also reduce the prevalence of alcohol-related harms at the population level. Because drinking guidelines assign responsibility for achieving low-risk drinking to individuals, psychologists have taken an active interest in how individuals interpret, respond to, and use these guidelines. Issues relating to how guidelines are interpreted and affect individuals' behaviour are discussed in the following sub-sections.

Are People Aware of Low-Risk Drinking Guidelines?

Young adults report a lack of awareness of guidelines (e.g., Cooke, French, & Sniehotta, 2010). One reason for this is that awareness of guidelines may fade over time, a suggestion supported by Holmes et al. (2016) in the UK and Livingston (2012) in Australia.

Do Low-Risk Drinking Guidelines Inform Alcohol Consumption?

Even when people are aware of guidelines, according to models of behaviour change, this is only the first step towards reducing consumption. Further steps include becoming motivated to act on guideline information and translating motivation into action (see Chaps. 14 and 21). Confirming the importance of these steps in bringing about behaviour change, studies conducted with young adults in Australia and the UK show that greater knowledge of guidelines does not translate into reduced consumption (Bowring et al., 2012; Cooke et al., 2010). There is also experimental evidence that increasing knowledge does not translate into drinking less (de Visser, Brown, Cooke, Cooper, & Memon, 2017).

Do People View Drinking Guidelines as Realistic?

Even when drinkers are aware of low-risk drinking guidelines, they may not use them for various reasons. For example, Lovatt et al. (2015, p. 1915) found that guidelines were judged to be unrealistic: "[t]heir too much is not our too much. According to that, their too much is like 'I've only just got started to be honest". If low-risk guidelines do not fit with drinking practices and notions of how much alcohol counts as "too much", people are unlikely to reduce their alcohol consumption in response to receiving them.

Educational strategies can be contrasted with *restrictive* alcohol control strategies such as raising the legal drinking age or changing the hours alcohol can be sold. Such strategies reduce consumption by restricting access to alcohol. Implementing restrictive policies would be an evidence-based approach to alcohol control; Anderson, Chisholm, and Fuhr's (2009) review of the literature on the effectiveness of alcohol policy identified restrictive policies as the best way to reduce alcohol harm at population level (Babor, 2010; Radaev, 2019).

However, findings from psychological research on restrictive policies suggest that introducing such policies would not be popular. de Visser et al. (2014) asked young people aged 16–25 from England to rate the *effectiveness* of eight alcohol control strategies. Participants rated the restrictive policy "raising the legal drinking age" as the least *effective* strategy and rated most other policies as not effective. The "most" effective policies were those related to policing the behaviour of others: "restricting service to drunk patrons" and "monitoring late night premises". Similar results have been found in samples recruited in the Netherlands and Norway (van der Sar et al., 2012) and suggest that the target audience for these policies, young adults, are unlikely to be receptive to such policies.

Taken together, results from psychological studies focused on alcohol control strategies are sobering. Educational approaches, which are more palatable to the general public, and the alcohol industry, have been shown to be ineffective in reducing consumption, partly because they assume that raising awareness of drinking guidelines is sufficient to change drinking behaviour, an approach which fails to acknowledge that theories of consumption (see Chaps. 2 and 3) and health behaviour change (see Chaps. 14 and 21) propose that additional steps are needed to translate awareness into action. Such approaches also fail to recognise how external factors shape consumption (see Section II).

Having shown how results from psychological studies of alcohol can be used to inform policy, the next section focuses on how psychologists define and measure alcohol consumption. Such discussion is warranted in this chapter of the Handbook because it is useful to consider these broader issues when reading later chapters. The discussion is intended to highlight issues of definition and methodology that apply to psychological research studies on alcohol.

How Do Psychologists Define Drinking Patterns in Research Studies?

Drinking patterns such as HED or low-risk drinking are labels used to describe consumption across several dimensions: (1) what *quantity* of alcohol is consumed?; (2) how *frequently* is alcohol consumed?; (3) over what *timeframe* is alcohol consumed?; (4) what *type* of alcohol (e.g., alcopops, beer, cider, lager, spirits, wine) is consumed?; (5) where is consumption *located*?. Drinking patterns can also be linked to the harms that occur following consumption. In psychological studies about consumption it is usually necessary to define a drinking pattern to ensure that participants know what they are being asked to consider.

A straightforward way to define drinking patterns is to refer to governments' or health organisations' definitions in the country in which the study is conducted. Such an approach has several advantages: participants should be somewhat aware of these guidelines, which have been developed with reference to local drink serving sizes and local health concerns. This strengthens their validity in terms of linking drinking patterns to population-level health outcomes.

An alternative way to define drinking patterns is to use cut-off scores from diagnostic tools such as the Alcohol Use Disorders Identification Test (AUDIT; Saunders, Aasland, Babor, de la Fuente, & Grant, 1993). For example, some studies have adopted a score of 8+ on the AUDIT as indicating a positive screen because scores of 8+ encompass the three AUDIT categorisations—hazardous (8–15), harmful (16–19), and probable dependence (20+)—linked to alcohol-related harms. An issue with using the AUDIT to assess drinking patterns is that it was not designed for this purpose—this is obvious given that only three of the AUDIT items assess consumption, with the remaining seven focused on harms. Measuring consumption using the AUDIT-C (i.e., completing the first three items) appears to be a more valid approach, although these items do not allow respondents to provide very detailed answers relative to other measures.

Another method for defining drinking patterns is to use subjective definitions like those shown in Box 1.3, which aim to capture subjective understanding of intoxication in a way that participants consider acceptable; Burgess et al.'s (2019) study was based on responses to open-ended questions at the end of a survey about alcohol. Participants wrote extremely detailed accounts of what it meant to them to approach and exceed the "tipping point". Such findings support qualitative studies that show drinkers can articulate their drinking "careers" in-depth and without difficulty.

Subjective definitions of stages of intoxication need to be carefully worded in surveys; otherwise there is a possibility that participants will misinterpret what they are being asked to report on. For instance, respondents to the *Global Drug Survey* (Barratt et al., 2017) are asked to report the number of times they got drunk in the past 12 months. Since getting drunk means different things to different people, this can affect how often people report it happening. In 2019, UK respondents reported getting drunk, on average, 51 times in the past year, while in 2020, the number of times people reported getting drunk an average of 33 times. An obvious difference between the surveys was that in 2019 the item about getting drunk did not define what this meant. By contrast, in the 2020 survey, the item provided a definition of what getting drunk involved: "we defined getting drunk as having drunk so much that your physical and mental facilities are impaired to the point your balance/speech may be effected, you are unable to focus clearly on things and that your conversation and behaviours are disinhibited" (Davies et al., 2020). How alcohol consumption patterns or behaviour is defined can affect how people report them.

Box 1.3 Phrases Used to Subjectively Describe Stages of Intoxication

- **"Feel the effects".** The amount of alcohol an individual reports that they must consume to feel it has had an effect on their mental or physical state (Davies, Cooke, Maier, Winstock, & Ferris, 2020)
- **The "sweet spot" (also known as "drunk as I want to be" or "experience a buzz").** The amount of alcohol an individual reports that they must consume to experience positive outcomes like relaxing and having fun while avoiding negative outcomes, for example, losing control, embarrassing yourself, feeling nauseous (Beccaria et al., 2015; Davies, Cooke, et al., 2020; Graber et al., 2016).
- **The "tipping point" (also known as "too much").** The amount of alcohol an individual reports that, when consumed, leads to, for example, a loss of control, embarrassing yourself, feeling nauseous, and may produce other unwanted health (blackout, hangover, vomiting) and social (arguments and fights) consequences (Davies, Cooke, et al., 2020; Davies, Puljevic, et al., 2020).

Discussion of how psychologists define drinking patterns also leads to consideration of how alcohol consumption is measured in research studies. Given the large number of studies that use survey methods to measure consumption—and the factors associated with it—the next section focuses on how consumption is measured in survey studies.

How Do Psychologists Measure Alcohol Consumption?

Self-Reported Measures of Consumption

Several self-report measures have been used by psychologists to measure alcohol consumption. For example, the popular timeline followback method (Sobell & Sobell, 1992) prompts participants to record their consumption over a defined period, such as the past 30 days. This method has shown good reliability and construct validity (Piano, Mazzuco, Kang, & Phillips, 2017). McKenna, Treanor, O'Reilly, and Donnelly (2018) provide a systematic review of the reliability and validity of self-report alcohol behavioural measures used in psychological research studies, using the COSMIN checklist to assess the psychometric properties of self-reported measures of drinking behaviour. Measures were coded into one of three types: *Short-term recall* measures, which ask respondents to recall all alcohol consumed within a defined timeframe; *Quantity-frequency* measures, which ask respondents about their usual drinking frequency and quantity; and *Graduated frequency* measures, which ask respondents to answer questions about drinks per occasion. Overall, McKenna (2018, p. 15) found there was heterogeneity in the psychometric properties reported by studies and concluded: "Currently, there is no gold standard for the measurement of alcohol consumption" (p. 15).

Beyond psychometric issues, there are several additional concerns with using self-report measures of consumption. First, there are concerns that participants will either over-estimate or under-estimate their responses (Heather et al., 2011), due to self-presentational concerns, despite data often being collected anonymously or being kept confidential. Second, there is evidence of measurement reactivity in consumption measures (McCambridge & Day, 2008). Third, consuming alcohol is known to affect memory and how this manifests itself when it comes to recalling the total number of drinks consumed during a drinking event is unclear. Fourth, some self-report measures ask participants to report consumption in terms of standard drink measures.

Because standard drink measures vary in alcohol-by-volume (e.g., wines vary in alcohol-by-volume between 11% and 14%) this means the units contained in the same size measure also vary; a UK 175 ml glass of wine contains 1.93 units if the wine is 11% volume and 2.45 units if wine is 14% volume. Each has the same measure size, but one has significantly more alcohol! Finally, assuming volume is accounted for, referencing standard measures is reasonable when considering drinking behaviour in licensed premises—where alcohol is sold in standard measures—but is highly questionable when asking people to record their drinking outside of licensed premises, that is, when asking people about how much they drink at home. There is evidence that when drinkers pour themselves a drink these measures tend to contain more alcohol than standard measures (de Beukelaar, Janse, Sierksma, Feskens, & de Vries, 2019; De Visser & Birch, 2012). Having covered issues around self-reported consumption, the final section presents a brief discussion of biological measures of consumption and observational methods.

Biological Measures of Consumption

A reliable and valid biomarker for alcohol consumption does not exist (see Piano et al., 2017), meaning alternative options are needed to obtain an objective measure of consumption. Breathalysers, which provide a measure of blood alcohol content, have been used in both survey (Riordan, Flett, Cody, Conner, & Scarf, 2019) and intervention studies (see Chap. 22) to measure consumption. Although they can provide an accurate measurement of individuals' alcohol consumption, several issues prevent widespread use in research: the costs of buying, maintaining, and (potentially) replacing devices; there is potential for missing data due to device failure or participants failing to provide a recording; and the measure is only able to capture alcohol consumption over a relatively brief prior period.

Transdermal sensors, worn either around the ankle (SCRAM) or wrist (e.g., WrisTAS), allow researchers to record consumption levels during a drinking event unobtrusively without the need to burden participants by asking them to provide breathalyser readings. SCRAM anklets measure the sweat expressed by the wearer to determine the presence, or absence, of biochemical markers of alcohol consumption and are the most commonly used transdermal sensors in alcohol studies (van Egmond, Wright, Livingston, & Kuntsche, 2020). However, further research is needed to establish the reliability of transdermal sensors; van Egmond et al.'s (2020) systematic review found, for example, that because SCRAM sensors were designed to measure HED in individuals in the criminal justice system, they are insensitive to low or moderate consumption. Additionally, wrist-wearable devices, like the WrisTAS, have a high failure rate for recording consumption, which calls into question their suitability for research.

Observational Methods of Consumption

Several researchers have sought to observe performance of alcohol consumption *in situ* in an attempt to capture the contextual, environmental, and social factors that influence drinking. These studies involve researchers assimilating themselves within drinking events and observing what happens (see Clapp et al., 2007, for a review). One advantage of using an observational approach is that contextual factors can be recorded, such as the presence of alcoholic drinks, others drinking, food, music, drinking games, and so on. Obviously, there are ethical concerns about conducting observational studies, in particular, over lack of consent to record individuals' consumption, which means the use of such methods is unlikely to replace less invasive methods in the immediate future. Having covered how psychologists define and measure drinking behaviour, the final two sections outline the global aims of this Handbook and an overview of its content.

What Is the Purpose of the Handbook?

Whilst there already exist a number of academic books on alcohol consumption, these have either adopted a focus on alcohol policy (Babor, 2010) or have tended to discuss application of models of addiction to the treatment of individuals with problematic drinking (Davis, Patton, & Jackson, 2017; Moss & Dyer, 2010; Svanberg, 2018). Books that focus on alcohol consumption at an everyday, general population level are less common. A recent exception is Conroy and Measham's (2020) collection which has provided a cross-disciplinary approach and has included discussion of research on alcohol using quantitative and qualitative methodologies. Missing from the field is a focused collection dedicated to covering the diversity and breadth of international psychological research on alcohol consumption to help identify how the field can be developed in the future to maximise its impact on people's lives.

Bringing together findings that employ different methods, perspectives, and theories is important because psychological research on alcohol consumption has suffered from a silo mentality, with researchers often seemingly unaware of relevant research conducted following different theoretical traditions, or that has adopted a different methodological perspective. Given the sheer diversity of methods that have been used in this field this is perhaps understandable, but it is time for researchers to work together to acknowledge the limitations of their own approaches and seek out approaches that provide a more nuanced, holistic understanding of alcohol use. Providing such an understanding of alcohol use is important given the large number of people who identify as current drinkers but who do not view their drinking behaviour as problematic.

It is important to focus on current drinkers for a number of reasons. A key reason is that there is potential to reduce their consumption using psychologically informed interventions (see Section V), which are less likely to be a safe option for problematic drinkers who often require detoxification or treatment programmes to reduce their consumption safely.

Another reason is that most current drinkers would not describe their drinking behaviour as problematic, even when it exceeds government guidelines (Davies, Cooke, et al., 2020). These drinkers construct their drinking identity as one of enjoying the effects of drinking, and only seeing themselves as having a problem if they have to seek treatment. By choosing to focus on current drinkers, this Handbook aims to foster discussion about what "normal" drinking looks like for this group: how it happens, what motivates it, how to prevent it from becoming problematic.

By bringing together research applying psychological approaches to alcohol, the goal is to help develop understanding of "normal" drinking for most current drinkers and provide constructive criticism to government agencies, health organisations, and other stakeholders about the reality of current drinkers' alcohol consumption. This criticism is intended to help identify limitations with the approaches that are often adopted when seeking to reduce population-level consumption and associated harms but also to propose alternative approaches that can overcome these limitations. The recent examples of temporary abstinence programmes like "Dry January" or "Hello Sunday Morning" show that innovative approaches can produce encouraging results (de Visser & Nicholls, 2020).

It is also important to note that this Handbook does not focus on models of addiction applied to alcohol. There are many books that focus on alcohol dependency and addition from multiple perspectives (Davis et al., 2017; Moss & Dyer, 2010; Svanberg, 2018). The current perspective is a unique one as it focuses on the factors, issues, and narratives surrounding psychological explanations of alcohol consumption, which has not previously been subject to comprehensive treatment in a single volume.

Overview of the Handbook

The Handbook is divided into five distinct sections. In Section I, Psychological Theories and Predictors (Chaps. 2, 3, 4, and 5) contributors provide an overview of various models and theories of alcohol consumption which share the distinctly *psychological* quality of being focused on individual-difference predictors of consumption. Psychologists assess the utility of these models using tests of association, such as correlating consumption with predictors or regressing consumption on predictors.

In the first section of the Handbook, evidence for the prediction of alcohol consumption using psychological theories and constructs is presented. In Chap. 2, Richard Cooke provides an overview of the evidence that several commonly used psychological theories of alcohol consumption and human motivation predict alcohol consumption. These models propose that individuals are reasoned actors who weigh the pros and cons of drinking versus not drinking. Such reasoned approaches are contrasted with more automatic, reactive, paths to consumption in Chap. 3, written by Emma Davies and Jemma Todd. The authors detail how dual-processing models can be applied to alcohol use, with a particular focus on the prototype willingness model. Having outlined and discussed multiple theories of alcohol consumption, the remaining chapters in this section discuss individual-difference predictors of consumption. In Chap. 4, Richard Cooke and Joel Crawford review the evidence for a range of psychological predictors of alcohol consumption including alcohol expectancies, drinking motives, intentions, and prototypes. In Chap. 5, Laura Mezquita, Generós Ortet, and Manuel Ibáñez outline the history of research using personality traits to predict alcohol use before reviewing the evidence base for traits as predictor variables.

Evidence presented in Section I provides only a limited understanding of drinking behaviour, due to its focus on internal drivers of alcohol consumption, which fails to acknowledge the reality that alcohol consumption is an inherently *social* behaviour—bringing people together to celebrate, chat, and relax. This means it is critical to consider how consumption is shaped by external factors: the culture people live in; the people they drink with; the location(s) where they drink; and the cues to drinking present in those locations. These issues are covered in Section II, Social Contextual Factors (Chaps. 6, 7, 8, 9, and 10).

In the second section of the Handbook evidence is presented to show how macro- and micro-social factors influence alcohol consumption. In Chap. 6, Richard O. de Visser argues that whereas psychology typically takes an individualistic approach to alcohol use—focusing on individual beliefs, motives, and intentions—alcohol consumption is for the most part a shared social behaviour: whether people drink with others or alone, their alcohol consumption is shaped by social and cultural factors. In Chap. 7, Giovanni Aresi and Kim Bloomfield pick up on this theme and provide a systematic review of studies of drinking cultures. They also consider the utility of the concept of national drinking cultures and efforts to group countries according to similarities and differences in drinking cultures. Their informative review is preceded by a helpful overview of the concept of culture and the methods used to study cultures. In Chap. 8, John D. Clapp and Danielle R. Madden explore event-level studies of alcohol consumption. They start with the important task of defining what is meant by an "event" and then go on to explore how the behaviour of individuals during a single event is related to environmental factors, group influences, and physiological processes. Their review addresses not only how people may conceptualise the components of events, but also how they can use portable and wearable technology to monitor these components and how and when it might be viable to intervene to reduce alcohol-related harm. Rebecca Monk and Derek Heim continue the focus on contextual influence on alcohol use in Chap. 9. They show that drinking may be influenced by contextual cues such as the location, the music being played, the gender composition of drinking groups, the day of the week, and affective states. Like Clapp and Madden, they make a strong case for more research to be conducted in semi-naturalistic settings and in real-life settings. In Chap. 10, Miki Vasiljevic and Rachel Pechey provide an overview of work that addresses some of the issues raised in Chaps. 8 and 9. They address how specific contextual factors may be manipulated to effect change in alcohol intake through their overview of two types of interventions. Their synthesis of studies illustrates how alcohol intake may be influenced by changing labels that indicate alcohol strength and by changing the size and/or shape of glasses. Together, these chapters show that a range of contextual features—ranging from the broad social context, through to the specific drinking context and the characteristics of a specific serving of alcohol—can influence individuals' alcohol consumption.

Beyond predicting alcohol use using internal and external factors, other psychological research focuses on how adolescents and young adults construct their drinking identities. It is normal for adolescents and young adults to construct and present their identities using social media channels. Their alcohol consumption, or increasingly their abstinence, is often a prominent feature of such activity. Studying identity naturally lends itself to qualitative methodologies where researchers adopt critical perspectives to explore these issues, which are collected together in Section III, Drinking Identities (Chaps. 11, 12, 13, and 14). This section covers a range of emerging issues in psychological research on alcohol including online drinking identities, sports teams' role in consumption, pre-drinking and the topic of young people's drink refusal.

In the third section of the Handbook, authors consider the interplay between different identities and alcohol consumption. In Chap. 11, Antonia Lyons and Ian Goodwin consider how alcohol consumption is presented online using social media channels. This chapter outlines how individuals use technology for impression formation—making their consumption seem to be a mostly positive experience. In Chap. 12, Liz Partington and Sarah Partington focus on the alcohol-sport paradox—the notion that although student athletes are generally healthier than student non-athletes, their alcohol consumption can be viewed as risky. In Chap. 13, Kim Caudwell and Martin S. Hagger discuss pre-drinking (also known as pre-loading), explaining how and why young people engage in this particular form of heavy episodic drinking, and the determinants of pre-drinking and different measures used to capture this drinking pattern. Section III ends with a timely chapter by Dominic Conroy and Richard O. de Visser, Chap. 14, about *not* drinking. In the past decade there has a been a trend among adolescents and young adults to eschew the norm of alcohol consumption in favour of drinking either small amounts of alcohol or avoiding alcohol altogether. Such changing patterns in behaviour are discussed in light of recent findings in this area.

Relatively little research has been conducted with samples of children, but there has been a recent increasing interest in conducting studies with children to understand how their beliefs about alcohol develop. Once children reach adolescence they become the focus of more psychological research. As a result, three youth-related issues are covered in this Handbook: how parents discuss alcohol consumption with their adolescent children and how cultures affect adolescents' drinking and the impact of schools' interventions on adolescent drinking behaviour and beliefs. These topics are covered in Section IV, Developmental Trajectories for Alcohol Use (Chaps. 15, 16, 17, and 18).

In Chap. 15, Megan Cook, Koen Smit, Carmen Voogt, and Emmanuel Kuntsche explore alcohol cognitions in the formative years, from age 2 to 12, including those learned from observing parental behaviour, and reinforced in role play activities such as shopping for groceries. The authors implore researchers to treat alcohol-related knowledge and behaviour in the same way that they would treat the acquisition of any other knowledge, as a critical factor in their later performance of a behaviour. In Chap. 16, Sara Rolando and Franca Beccaria contrast the perceptions of Finnish and Italian adolescents, through the discussion of qualitative studies conducted in the two countries. In this chapter the value of comparative qualitative studies in highlighting nuances in drinking cultures and experiences is evident. In Chap. 17, Alexandra Sawyer, Nigel Sherriff, and Lester Coleman discuss the influence of parental communication about alcohol on young people's drinking behaviours. Openness and honesty are required when young people have already developed a wide range of knowledge about alcohol when parents first consider that it is time to have a serious talk with their children. Finally, in Chap. 18, Kathryn L. Modecki, Lisa Buckley, and Kyra Hamilton consider a wide range of external factors that influence adolescent drinking, including identities, peers, norms, and the school environment, illustrating that even with the best communication skills, parents should not feel too bad if their child has a negative experience with drinking.

Psychologically informed interventions to promote safer drinking are covered in Section V, "Interventions to Reduce Alcohol Consumption" (Chaps. 18, 19, 20, 21, and 22). Interventions that are delivered at the population (e.g., labels on alcoholic products) and individual (e.g., cognitive bias modification) levels are evaluated alongside approaches that have an explicit focus on psychological theories of alcohol consumption. The latter include the social norms approach, which informs web-based personalised feedback interventions, and the model of action phases, which proposes that changing behaviours involves targeting change in both motivational and self-regulatory processes.

In Chap. 19, Anna K. M. Blackwell, Natasha Clarke, Emily Pechey, and Angela S. Attwood describe how the labelling of alcoholic products has been implemented in different countries and the strengths and weaknesses of this approach as a technique to reduce consumption. In Chap. 20, Bridgette Bewick, Robert Dempsey, John McAlaney, and Helen Crosby outline the components of web-based personalised feedback interventions and review the evidence that such approaches produce changes in drinking behaviour. In Chap. 21, Richard Cooke, Dominic Conroy, and Martin S. Hagger compare and contrast motivational and self-regulatory interventions that have been used to target reductions in alcohol consumption. In Chap. 22, Andy Jones and Matt Field provide a critical overview of research on cognitive bias modification, an intervention technique that aims to rewire the brain to disrupt implicit processes that often prompt excessive drinking.

The final chapter of the Handbook, Chap. 23, provides a summary of discussion throughout the Handbook and suggestions for future research. Specifically, the chapter discusses four emerging themes from the Handbook under the headings of samples, methods, theories, and applications. The chapter outlines current knowledge and developments in the theories and predictors of alcohol consumption; the social contextual factors, drinking identities; the developmental trajectories of alcohol consumption; and the development, application, and effectiveness of alcohol interventions. The chapter also highlights key limitations of current research including the preponderance of studies on student samples and studies with cross-sectional and correlational designs; a fixation on a narrow set of individual-based theories with a lack of integration; and the lack of translational work and engagement of key stakeholders in the research itself and disseminating findings to the groups most like to benefit from them.

The chapter concludes by highlighting the high value of research in the field, but also identified key research gaps and limitations to current knowledge and sets out a clear agenda for researchers applying psychological theory and methods to predict and explain social alcohol behaviour. There is a need to recruit research participants from a more diverse range of groups and populations and to use a more diverse range of methodologies in these studies. It is also important to encourage theoretical integration to afford a more comprehensive understanding of psychological determinants of alcohol consumption helping to ensure greater impact of psychological research including stakeholder engagement and working translational activities into research projects from the development stage.

References

Anderson, P., Chisholm, D., & Fuhr, D. C. (2009). Effectiveness and cost-effectiveness of policies and programmes to reduce the harm caused by alcohol. *Lancet (London, England), 373*(9682), 2234–2246. https://doi.org/10.1016/S0140-6736(09)60744-3

Babor, T. (Ed.). (2010). *Alcohol: No ordinary commodity: Research and public policy.* Oxford, UK: Oxford University Press.

Barratt, M. J., Ferris, J. A., Zahnow, R., Palamar, J. J., Maier, L. J., & Winstock, A. R. (2017). Moving on from representativeness: Testing the utility of the global drug survey. *Substance Abuse: Research and Treatment, 11*, 117822181771639. https://doi.org/10.1177/1178221817716391

Beccaria, F., Petrilli, E., & Rolando, S. (2015). Binge drinking vs. drunkenness. The questionable threshold of excess for young Italians. *Journal of Youth Studies, 18*(7), 823–838. https://doi.org/10.1080/13676261.2014.992321

Bowring, A. L., Gold, J., Dietze, P., Gouillou, M., Van Gemert, C., & Hellard, M. E. (2012). Know your limits: Awareness of the 2009 Australian alcohol guidelines among young people: Alcohol guidelines:

Awareness and risk. *Drug and Alcohol Review, 31*(2), 213–223. https://doi.org/10.1111/j.1465-3362.2011.00409.x

Burgess, M., Cooke, R., & Davies, E. L. (2019). *My own personal hell*: Approaching and exceeding thresholds of too much alcohol. *Psychology & Health, 34*, 1451–1469. https://doi.org/10.1080/08870446.2019.1616087

Ceballos, N., & Babor, T. F. (2017). Editor's corner: Binge drinking and the evolving language of alcohol research. *Journal of Studies on Alcohol and Drugs, 78*(4), 488–490. https://doi.org/10.15288/jsad.2017.78.488

Centers for Disease Control and Prevention. (2011). *Fact sheets: Binge drinking*. http://www.cdc.gov/alcohol/fact-sheets/bingedrinking.htm

Clapp, J. D., Holmes, M. R., Reed, M. B., Shillington, A. M., Freisthler, B., & Lange, J. E. (2007). Measuring college students' alcohol consumption in natural drinking environments: Field methodologies for bars and parties. *Evaluation Review, 31*(5), 469–489. https://doi.org/10.1177/0193841X07303582

Conroy, D., & Measham, F. (2020). *Young adult drinking styles: Current perspectives on research, policy and practice*. Palgrave Macmillan US: https://public.ebookcentral.proquest.com/choice/publicfullrecord.aspx?p=5987650

Cooke, R., French, D. P., & Sniehotta, F. F. (2010). Wide variation in understanding about what constitutes 'binge-drinking'. *Drugs: Education, Prevention and Policy, 17*(6), 762–775. https://doi.org/10.3109/09687630903246457

Cooper, M. L., Kuntsche, E., Levitt, A., Barber, L. L., & Wolf, S. (2015). Motivational models of substance use: A review of theory and research on motives for using alcohol, marijuana, and tobacco. In K. J. Sher (Ed.), *The Oxford handbook of substance use disorders* (Vol. 1). Oxford, UK: Oxford University Press. https://doi.org/10.1093/oxfordhb/9780199381678.013.017

Cox, W. M., & Klinger, E. (1988). A motivational model of alcohol use. *Journal of Abnormal Psychology, 97*(2), 168–180.

Crawford, J., Jones, A., Rose, A., & Cooke, R. (2020). 'You see the pictures the morning after and you're like I wish I was in them': an interpretative phenomenological analysis of university student's alcohol-related regrets. *Psychology & Health*. https://doi.org/10.1080/08870446.2020.1867728

Davies, E. L., Cooke, R., Maier, L. J., Winstock, A. R., & Ferris, J. A. (2020). Drinking to excess and the tipping point: An international study of alcohol intoxication in 61,000 people. *International Journal of Drug Policy, 83*, 102867. https://doi.org/10.1016/j.drugpo.2020.102867

Davies, E. L., Puljevic, C., Connolly, D., Zhuparris, A., Ferris, J. A., & Winstock, A. R. (2020). The world's favourite drug: What we have Learned about alcohol from over 500,000 respondents to the global drug survey. In D. Frings & I. P. Albery (Eds.), *Alcohol handbook: From synapse to society*. Cambridge, MA: Academic Press.

Davis, P., Patton, R., & Jackson, S. (Eds.). (2017). *Addiction: Psychology and treatment*. Hoboken, NJ: John Wiley & Sons.

de Beukelaar, M. F., Janse, M. L., Sierksma, A., Feskens, E. J., & de Vries, J. H. (2019). How full is your glass? Portion sizes of wine, fortified wine and straight spirits at home in the Netherlands. *Public Health Nutrition, 22*(10), 1727–1734. https://doi.org/10.1017/S1368980019000442

de Visser, R., Brown, C., Cooke, R., Cooper, G., & Memon, A. (2017). Using alcohol unit-marked glasses enhances capacity to monitor intake: Evidence from a mixed-method intervention trial. *Alcohol and Alcoholism, 52*, 206–212. https://doi.org/10.1093/alcalc/agw084

de Visser, R. O., & Birch, J. D. (2012). My cup runneth over: Young people's lack of knowledge of low-risk drinking guidelines: Young people's knowledge of alcohol guidelines. *Drug and Alcohol Review, 31*(2), 206–212. https://doi.org/10.1111/j.1465-3362.2011.00371.x

de Visser, R. O., Hart, A., Abraham, C., Memon, A., Graber, R., & Scanlon, T. (2014). Which alcohol control strategies do young people think are effective?: Alcohol policies. *Drug and Alcohol Review, 33*(2), 144–151. https://doi.org/10.1111/dar.12109

de Visser, R. O., & Nicholls, J. (2020). Temporary abstinence during Dry January: Predictors of success; impact on well-being and self-efficacy. *Psychology & Health, 35*, 1293–1305. https://doi.org/10.1080/08870446.2020.1743840

Department of Health. (2016). *UK chief medical officers' alcohol guidelines review summary of the proposed new guidelines.* https://www.gov.uk/government/uploads/sys-tem/uploads/attachment_data/file/489795/summary.pdf

Furtwaengler, N. A. F. F., & de Visser, R. O. (2013). Lack of international consensus in low-risk drinking guidelines. *Drug and Alcohol Review, 32*(1), 11–18. https://doi.org/10.1111/j.1465-3362.2012.00475.x

Graber, R., de Visser, R., Abraham, C., Memon, A., Hart, A., & Hunt, K. (2016). Staying in the 'sweet spot': A resilience-based analysis of the lived experience of low-risk drinking and abstention among British youth. *Psychology & Health, 31*(1), 79–99. https://doi.org/10.1080/08870446.2015.1070852

Heather, N., Partington, S., Partington, E., Longstaff, F., Allsop, S., Jankowski, M., … St Clair Gibson, A. (2011). Alcohol use disorders and hazardous drinking among undergraduates at English universities. *Alcohol and Alcoholism (Oxford, Oxfordshire), 46*(3), 270–277. https://doi.org/10.1093/alcalc/agr024

Holmes, J., Brown, J., Meier, P., Beard, E., Michie, S., & Buykx, P. (2016). Short-term effects of announcing revised lower risk national drinking guidelines on related awareness and knowledge: A trend analysis of monthly survey data in England. *BMJ Open, 6*(12), e013804. https://doi.org/10.1136/bmjopen-2016-013804

Jones, L., Bellis, M. A., Dedman, D., Sumnall, H., & Tocque, K. (2008). *Alcohol attributable fractions for England: Alcohol attributable mortality and hospital admissions.* North West Public Health Observatory and Department of Health.

Kuntsche, E., Kuntsche, S., Thrul, J., & Gmel, G. (2017). Bing drinking: Health impact, prevalence, correlates and interventions. *Psychology & Health, 32*, 976–1017. https://doi.org/10.1080/08870446.2017.1325889

Kuntsche, E., Stewart, S. H., & Cooper, M. L. (2008). How stable is the motive–alcohol use link? A cross-national validation of the drinking motives questionnaire revised among adolescents from Switzerland, Canada, and the United States. *Journal of Studies on Alcohol and Drugs, 69*(3), 388–396. https://doi.org/10.15288/jsad.2008.69.388

Livingston, M. (2012). Perceptions of low-risk drinking levels among Australians during a period of change in the official drinking guidelines: Perceptions of low-risk drinking. *Drug and Alcohol Review, 31*(2), 224–230. https://doi.org/10.1111/j.1465-3362.2011.00414.x

Lovatt, M., Eadie, D., Meier, P. S., Li, J., Bauld, L., Hastings, G., & Holmes, J. (2015). Lay epidemiology and the interpretation of low-risk drinking guidelines by adults in the United Kingdom: Lay epidemiology and the interpretation of low-risk drinking guidelines. *Addiction, 110*(12), 1912–1919. https://doi.org/10.1111/add.13072

McCambridge, J., & Day, M. (2008). Randomized controlled trial of the effects of completing the Alcohol Use Disorders Identification Test questionnaire on self-reported hazardous drinking. *Addiction, 103*(2), 241–248. https://doi.org/10.1111/j.1360-0443.2007.02080.x

McKenna, H., Treanor, C., O'Reilly, D., & Donnelly, M. (2018). Evaluation of the psychometric properties of self-reported measures of alcohol consumption: A COSMIN systematic review. *Substance Abuse Treatment, Prevention, and Policy, 13*(1), 6. https://doi.org/10.1186/s13011-018-0143-8

Moss, A. C., & Dyer, K. R. (2010). *Psychology of addictive behaviour*. Basingstoke, UK: Palgrave Macmillan.

National Institute on Alcohol Abuse and Alcoholism (NIAAA). (2004). NIAAA approves definition of binge drinking. *NIAAA Newsletter, 3*(Winter) https://pubs.niaaa.nih.gov/publications/Newsletter/winter2004/Newsletter_Number3.pdf

Piano, M. R., Mazzuco, A., Kang, M., & Phillips, S. A. (2017). Binge drinking episodes in young adults: How should we measure them in a research setting? *Journal of Studies on Alcohol and Drugs, 78*(4), 502–511. https://doi.org/10.15288/jsad.2017.78.502

Radaev, V. (2019). Making sense of alcohol consumption among Russian young adults in the context of post-2009 policy initiatives. In D. Conroy & F. Measham (Eds.), *Young adult drinking styles* (pp. 313–332). Cham, Switzerland: Palgrave Macmillan.

Riordan, B. C., Flett, J. A. M., Cody, L. M., Conner, T. S., & Scarf, D. (2019). The Fear of Missing Out (FoMO) and event-specific drinking: The relationship between FoMO and alcohol use, harm and breath alcohol concentration during orientation week. *Current Psychology*. https://doi.org/10.1007/s12144-019-00318-6

Saunders, J. B., Aasland, O. G., Babor, T. F., de la Fuente, J. R., & Grant, M. (1993). Development of the Alcohol Use Disorders Identification Test (AUDIT): WHO collaborative project on early detection of persons with harmful alcohol consumption--II. *Addiction (Abingdon, England), 88*(6), 791–804.

Sobell, L. C., & Sobell, M. B. (1992). Timeline follow-back: A technique for assessing self-reported alcohol consumption. In R. Z. Litten & J. P. Allen (Eds.), *Measuring alcohol consumption* (pp. 41–72). Totowa, NJ: Humana Press.

Svanberg, J. (2018). *The psychology of addiction*. London/Washington, DC: Routledge/ Taylor & Francis Group.

van der Sar, R., Storvoll, E. E., Brouwers, E. P. M., van de Goor, L. A. M., Rise, J., & Garretsen, H. F. L. (2012). Dutch and Norwegian support of alcohol policy measures to prevent young people from problematic drinking: A cross-national comparison. *Alcohol and Alcoholism, 47*(4), 479–485. https://doi.org/10.1093/ alcalc/ags032

van Egmond, K., J.C Wright, Livingston, M., & Kuntsche, E. (2020). Wearable transdermal alcohol monitors: A systematic review of detection validity, relationship between transdermal and breath alcohol concentration and influencing factors. *Alcoholism: Clinical and Experimental Research*, acer.14432. doi:https:// doi.org/10.1111/acer.14432

World Health Organization. (2018). *Global status report on alcohol and health 2018*. Geneva, Switzerland: World Health Organization.

Section I

Psychological Theories and Predictors

2

Psychological Theories of Alcohol Consumption

Richard Cooke

Introduction

Psychological theories are a way of making sense of the world around us. They propose explanations for psychological phenomena such as why one person engages in heavy episodic drinking (HED; see Chap. 1), while another does not. Psychological theories of alcohol consumption, such as alcohol expectancy theory (Oei & Baldwin, 1994), the cognitive model of binge drinking (Oei & Morawska, 2004), and the incentive motivation model (Cox & Klinger, 1988), and theories of human motivation like the Theories of Reasoned Action (TRA; Ajzen & Fishbein, 1973) and Planned Behaviour (Ajzen, 1991) that have been used to predict consumption, all assume that we act after careful consideration of the pros and cons of an action. According to these theories, an individual's decision to drink alcohol (or not) is driven by *psychological* variables, their beliefs, expectancies, intentions, and motives about drinking alcohol, which are used to inform a careful consideration of the pros and cons of drinking behaviour. These theories all propose that psychological variables act as key determinants of drinking behaviour. The present chapter focuses on theories that characterise humans as rational actors, rather than dual process or implicit models, which attempt to account for

R. Cooke (✉)
Department of Psychology, University of Liverpool, Liverpool, UK

Liverpool Centre for Alcohol Research, Liverpool, UK
e-mail: cooker4@liverpool.ac.uk

R. Cooke et al. (eds.), *The Palgrave Handbook of Psychological Perspectives on Alcohol Consumption*, https://doi.org/10.1007/978-3-030-66941-6_2

unplanned or spontaneous behaviours (see Chap. 3 for a discussion of such models). The chapter begins by providing a brief outline of each theory before reviewing existing evidence that theories account for drinking behaviour. Next, the chapter compares and contrasts theories in terms of conceptual overlap and research evidence, before discussing methodological issues with research in this field. Finally, the chapter draws together the results of this discussion.

Alcohol Expectancy Theory

Alcohol Expectancy Theory (Oei & Baldwin, 1994) stems from Bandura's Social Learning Theory (Bandura, 1977) and proposes that we (i) learn about alcohol consumption by observing others (see Chaps. 15 and 16) and (ii) internalise expectancies (beliefs) about alcohol consumption. Two types of expectancies are referenced in alcohol expectancy theory: outcome expectancies (i.e., what we expect will happen when we drink alcohol—labelled Alcohol Expectancies) and efficacy expectancies (i.e., how confident we are that we can refuse alcohol—labelled Drinking Refusal Self-Efficacy).

Alcohol Expectancies seek to capture expectancies people hold about consumption; does an individual expect that drinking alcohol will make them happy or sad? Will it relax or impair them? Will it increase their attractiveness to members of the opposite sex? Alcohol expectancies reflect a range of different positive or negative outcomes that are expected to follow consumption. Scales used to assess alcohol expectancies, like the Alcohol Outcomes Expectancies Scale (Leigh & Stacy, 1993), contain several sub-scales: Social Positive; Fun; Sex; Tension Reduction; Social Negative; Cognitive; Emotional; Physical. Individuals who score high on alcohol expectancies sub-scales are assumed to drink more alcohol, showing a positive relationship between expectancies and consumption.

Drinking refusal self-efficacy aims to capture the extent to which an individual feels confident (i.e., high in self-efficacy) they can refuse the offer of an alcoholic drink (see Chap. 14 for more on this issue). Those who score high on drinking refusal self-efficacy are assumed to drink less alcohol, because they have refused drink offers, so, researchers expect to find a negative relationship between drinking refusal self-efficacy scores and consumption. Instruments such as the Drinking Refusal Self-Efficacy Questionnaire (Young & Oei, 1990) are used to tap the construct. Scale items can either be summed into an overall score or used as three sub-scales representing emotional relief (e.g., 'when I am angry'), opportunistic drinking (e.g., 'when I am watching TV'), and social pressure (e.g., 'when my friends are drinking').

As noted by Cook et al. in Chap. 15, even young children report alcohol expectancies, based on observations of others' (e.g., their parents) drinking. This shows that alcohol expectancies can exist prior to experience of alcohol consumption. According to Oei and Morawska (2004), most research studies testing alcohol expectancy theory focused on alcohol expectancies as the main determinant of alcohol consumption, rather than testing both constructs as predictor variables, which makes it hard to evaluate claims for the theory; while researchers have continued to test the effects of alcohol expectancies and drinking refusal self-efficacy as predictors of consumption, reflection on the sufficiency of the theory is lacking. Reflection on alcohol expectancy theory did, however, inspire the creation of the cognitive model of binge drinking, described in the next section.

The Cognitive Model of Binge Drinking

The cognitive model of binge drinking (Oei & Morawska, 2004) is an application of Alcohol Expectancy Theory to predict a drinking pattern, binge drinking, which has been defined as consuming more than a threshold number of drinks, or volume of alcohol, during a single drinking episode (e.g., HED, see Chap. 1). Like Alcohol Expectancy Theory, the model comprises alcohol expectancies and drinking refusal self-efficacy. Where this model differs is that Oei and Morawska (2004) apply the theoretical underpinnings of Alcohol Expectancy Theory to address two key issues related to binge drinking.

First, the cognitive model of binge drinking has been used to underpin a drinking typology using scores from model variables (i.e., expectancies and refusal self-efficacy). At one extreme, non-drinkers are expected to possess both low alcohol expectancies (i.e., they do not expect alcohol consumption will lead to desirable outcomes) and high drinking refusal self-efficacy (i.e., they find it easy to refuse drinks; see Chap. 14 for more). At the other extreme, alcoholics are expected to hold both high alcohol expectancies (i.e., they expect alcohol consumption will lead to desirable outcomes) and low drinking refusal self-efficacy (i.e., they find it hard to refuse drinks). Between these extremes other drinker types—binge drinkers, social drinkers, and problematic drinkers—are located, with drinker types varying in terms of either their alcohol expectancies or their drinking refusal self-efficacy. For example, binge drinkers are argued to possess higher alcohol expectancies than social drinkers; they anticipate more desirable outcomes from drinking. However, both binge and social drinkers are assumed to possess higher drinking refusal self-efficacy than problematic drinkers, who share binge drinkers' high expectancies about alcohol consumption but also possess low drinking refusal self-efficacy. Morawska and Oei (2005) provided evidence for this typology in a sample of Australian university students. They showed that binge drinkers reported more positive alcohol expectancies than social drinkers and that both drinker types reported similar drinking refusal self-efficacy scores that were higher than scores reported by problematic drinkers.

Second, the model has been used to predict alcohol consumption. For example, Oei and Jardim (2007) tested the predictive utility of the model for alcohol consumption among self-defined Asian Australian and white Australian university students. Separate regression analyses were conducted to predict consumption in these samples. For Asian students, the model accounted for 19% of the variance in consumption, with drinking refusal self-efficacy a significant predictor, but with no other significant effects; variation in drinking refusal self-efficacy may be all that matters when predicting drinking among Asian students. In contrast, the model accounted for 37% of the variance in consumption among white students with significant effects for both predictors. In addition, entry of the interaction term between the two predictors added 7% variance to the model and reduced alcohol expectancies to non-significance. Decomposing this interaction showed that when drinking refusal self-efficacy was high, there was no difference in consumption regardless of alcohol expectancies. However, when drinking refusal self-efficacy was low, individuals with positive expectancies drank more.

One interpretation of these results is that white students who are high in drinking refusal self-efficacy behave in the same way as Asian students do in that their alcohol expectancies do not predict their consumption. In contrast, alcohol expectancies predict consumption for white students low in drinking refusal self-efficacy. This study shows that drinking refusal self-efficacy was the most important predictor of alcohol consumption for both groups and that alcohol expectancies were only important for white university students *low* in drinking refusal self-efficacy.

Oei and Jardim noted that Asian students had significantly higher average drinking refusal self-efficacy scores than white students. Thus, it is possible that alcohol expectancies are unimportant in this sample because they *only* matter when drinking refusal self-efficacy is low, which was not the case in this sample of Asian students. This study suggests that there are cultural differences in alcohol expectancies, a proposal backed up by group comparisons which show that white students reported higher positive expectancies on several sub-scales (confidence, sexual interest, tension reduction) compared to Asian students and that Asian students reported higher negative expectancies.

If Asian students score higher for negative expectancies, then they may focus more on drinking refusal self-efficacy rather when considering drinking. A paper by Oh and Kim (2014) tested the importance of drinking refusal self-efficacy in a sample of Korean university students. They used the three sub-scales of drinking refusal self-efficacy (Social Pressure, Opportunistic Drinking, Emotional Relief) to predict frequency and quantity of alcohol consumption. All three sub-scales were significant predictors of consumption, with models accounting for 39% of the variance in drinking frequency and 37% of the variance in drinking quantity. These results support Oei and Jardim's findings that drinking refusal self-efficacy predicts consumption in Asian students; however, because the authors did not measure alcohol expectancies, we cannot make any claims about the cognitive model of binge drinking.

Finally, a study by Newton, Barrett, Swaffield, and Teesson (2014) used a longitudinal design to provide a test of the effects of the model in a sample of Australian adolescents; follow-up data was collected on three occasions: 6 months later; 12 months later; 18 months later. Alcohol expectancies and drinking refusal self-efficacy both predicted consumption over time, with a one unit increase in alcohol expectancies being associated with a 51% increase in binge drinking, while a one unit increase in drinking refusal self-efficacy was associated with a 27% decrease in binge drinking over the study duration. Such results support the proposals of the cognitive model of binge drinking and using a longitudinal design increases confidence in findings. Findings are also interesting because they come from an adolescent sample who are experiencing a developmental trajectory for drinking, as discussed in Chaps. 16 and 17.

Augmenting the Cognitive Model of Binge Drinking with Other Variables

Other studies have sought to augment the cognitive model of binge drinking by measuring additional constructs, like measures of mental health. For example, Goldsmith, Thompson, Black, Tran, and Smith (2012) included a measure of generalised anxiety disorder alongside measures of drinking refusal self-efficacy and tension reduction alcohol expectancies in a model to predict consumption in a sample of US university students. This model accounted for 35% of the variance in consumption with main effects for all predictors and a significant three-way interaction.

Decomposing the interaction showed that at *high* levels of drinking refusal self-efficacy there was little difference in rates of alcohol consumption depending on the combination of generalised anxiety disorder and tension reduction alcohol expectancies. Conversely, when drinking refusal self-efficacy was *low*, individuals who also reported low anxiety scores showed the highest alcohol consumption, regardless of tension reduction expectancies; the combination of low ability to refuse a drink and low anxiety = high alcohol consumption. Among individuals with low drinking refusal self-efficacy who also had high anxiety scores, tension reduction expectancies helped to determine consumption; students who scored high on tension reduction expectancies (i.e., believing that alcohol consumption reduces tension) drank more alcohol than those who scored low. Indeed, students who scored low for all three variables reported the lowest levels of alcohol consumption. This study's results show that when drinking refusal self-efficacy is high, other factors do not predict consumption. When drinking refusal self-efficacy is low, other factors have a role to play in prediction, a result that mirrors what Oei and Jardim (2007) found.

Alternatively, Hasking, Boyes, and Mullan (2015) proposed a sequence of action where cognitive model constructs are consequent on other predictors; the sequence of action that leads to drinking alcohol begins with sensitivity to reward and sensitivity to punishment from Reinforcement Sensitivity Theory (Gray, 1970, see Chap. 5), which informs alcohol expectancies. These expectancies inform drinking refusal self-efficacy, which ultimately predicts drinking. Hasking et al. tested their model in a sample of drinkers (44% were university students) with a *cross-sectional* design, where alcohol consumption was measured using the Alcohol Use Disorders Identification Test (AUDIT; see Chap. 1). Fifty-two percent of the variance in AUDIT scores was accounted for by the model, providing support for the proposed sequence of action: sensitivity to reward had a positive relationship with alcohol expectancies (confidence) and sensitivity to punishment had a positive relationship with negative alcohol expectancies. Higher confidence was associated with lower social pressure drinking refusal self-efficacy, and more negative expectancies were linked to reduced belief in emotional relief drinking refusal self-efficacy. Both sub-scales negatively predicted consumption.

While this paper provides a useful example of how to integrate theories when predicting alcohol consumption, the use of a cross-sectional design undermines confidence in results (see Study Design Issues below) and could explain why the variance accounted for by this model is quite high. Further tests of this model using prospective designs are needed to increase confidence in this sequence of action.

A key issue with the cognitive model of binge drinking is that it is rarely referenced by researchers testing the model; a search of the Web of Science database yielded only two hits (Oei & Jardim, 2007; Oei & Morawska, 2004) and yet other papers discussed in the chapter have tested the model. Given the promising results found for drinking refusal self-efficacy as a predictor of consumption in general, and for alcohol expectancies among those with low self-efficacy, researchers need to reference the model more often when they use it. Two other methodological issues with the cognitive model are that (1) studies have used cross-sectional designs to test the cognitive model of binge drinking, which limit the conclusions one can draw about the model in predictive terms, and (2) researchers do not always use the same measures to assess constructs, with drinking refusal self-efficacy measured in a variety of ways, some of which lack construct validity. For example, Hasking et al. (2015) created their own measure rather than using a validated scale. It is challenging to advance knowledge if constructs are not measured consistently.

In some ways, the cognitive model of binge drinking remains overshadowed by the Alcohol Expectancy Theory literature it emerged from, which is a shame because results to date show that drinking refusal self-efficacy, rather than alcohol expectancies, is the better predictor of consumption. Overall, results suggest that constructs from the cognitive model of binge drinking can predict alcohol consumption but more research is needed to confirm the theoretical underpinnings of the model.

Incentive Motivation Model

Cox and Klinger's (1988) incentive motivation model proposes that humans are motivated to pursue positive incentives and avoid negative incentives. When applied to alcohol, Cox and Klinger state:

> [A] person's motivation to use alcohol is intertwined with his or her incentive motivation in this and other life areas and the affective change that results from that motivation. (p. 169)

The authors go on to note that affective change—a change in affect from its current state—occurs as a result of pursuing positive incentives or avoiding negative incentives. After acknowledging the pharmacological effects of alcohol on affective change, and noting there are situational drivers of alcohol consumption, including whether a person is alone or with other people, and if with other people, the degree to which they encourage or discourage drinking, as well as the availability of alcohol in the immediate situation (see Sect. 2), this model focuses primarily on the motivational effects of alcohol consumption, with a particular emphasis on weighing up the positive affective outcomes one would anticipate following from drinking alcohol against the positive affective outcomes one would anticipate following from *not* drinking alcohol.

Overall, the incentive motivation model positions the individual as the main agent of their drinking behaviour, although the authors make the point that while they view drinking initiation as a conscious weighing of pros and cons, subsequent drinking might be driven by habitual or implicit processes (see Chaps. 3 and 22).

Alcohol researchers who have followed Cox and Klinger's theorising have tended to focus on two tenets of the model. First, outcomes sought from substance use can be done for internal (i.e., am I drinking because I want to) or external reasons (i.e., am I drinking in response to other people). Second, if drinking alcohol is perceived to lead to an 'approach positive' goal (i.e., feel more confident) or an 'avoid negative' goal (i.e., stop feeling stressed), then it is likely that alcohol consumption will follow; in both situations the incentive to drink outweighs the incentive to not drink. Alternatively, if drinking alcohol is perceived to lead to an 'approach negative' goal (i.e., feel sick) or an 'avoid positive' goal (i.e., act embarrassingly in front of a date), it is *unlikely* that alcohol consumption will follow; in both situations the incentive to not drink outweighs the incentive to drink.

Cooper (1994) proposed crossing these two dimensions to provide four motives for alcohol consumption: conformity (external, negative); coping (internal, negative); enhancement (internal, positive); and social (external, positive). She developed the Drinking Motives Questionnaire-Revised (DMQ-R) to measure these motives. The DMQ-R has been used to assess the predictive relationships between motives and alcohol consumption as well as being used to determine which motive is the most important driver of an individual's drinking.

A recent literature review by Cooper, Kuntsche, Levitt, Barber, and Wolf (2015) provides evidence that drinking motives are linked to both alcohol use and HED enhancement motives had, on average, a medium-sized correlation with consumption ($r = 0.49$) and a large-sized correlation with HED ($r = 0.51$); social motives had medium-sized relationships with consumption ($r = 0.42$) and HED ($r = 0.40$); coping motives had medium-sized links with consumption ($r = 0.30$) and HED ($r = 0.36$); and conformity motives had small-sized relationships with consumption ($r = 0.09$) and HED ($r = 0.15$). See Chap. 4 for more on the individual drinking motives.

Cooper et al. also reported that when the four motives were simultaneously regressed on consumption, the hierarchy of

enhancement > social > coping > conformity

was found. In contrast, when the same regression analysis was run for HED, coping motives were shown to be more important than social motives, suggesting that internal motives (enhancement and coping) are key predictors of HED. A key limitation with these analyses, however, is that most of the studies used cross-sectional designs, which means they were predicting consumption and HED that had already occurred.

Nevertheless, they do match results reported when prospective designs were used (Cooper, 1994; Cooper et al., 2008; Kuntsche & Cooper, 2010). Kuntsche and Cooper (2010) asked a sample of young adults, who had completed baseline measures of drinking and the DMQ-R, to respond to text messages sent at 1 pm on four consecutive Saturdays and Sundays. These messages asked them to indicate their consumption in the past 24 hours, to capture Friday night and Saturday night drinking, respectively. Kuntsche and Cooper found that after controlling for past drinking, gender, age, and weekend day (i.e., Friday vs. Saturday), enhancement motives significantly predicted alcohol consumption. In another study, Cooper et al. (2008) showed that coping and enhancement motives predicted alcohol consumption 15 years after they were measured in a sample of US adolescents aged 13–19 years. This is impressive evidence that internal motives for drinking are a stable guide to future alcohol consumption.

In sum, there is evidence that enhancement and coping motives predict consumption and HED. Such results imply that internal motives are more important drivers of consumption than external motives. The lack of evidence that conformity motives predict consumption undermines the model to a degree.

Having outlined theories of alcohol consumption, two theories of human motivation that have used to predict alcohol use—the Theories of Reasoned Action and Planned Behaviour—are considered.

The Theories of Reasoned Action and Planned Behaviour

The Theory of Reasoned Action (TRA; Ajzen & Fishbein, 1973) proposes that a person's intention to act is the most proximal predictor of their action. Intentions are assessed by asking individuals how strongly they agree with items like 'I intend to drink alcohol in the next week' on a Likert scale from

Strongly Disagree to Strongly Agree. Individuals who strongly agree with such items are assumed to be more likely to consume alcohol compared to individuals who strongly disagree. Intentions are based on two constructs: attitudes (i.e., positive or negative evaluations of behavioural performance) and subjective norms (i.e., perceptions of important others' approval or disapproval of behavioural performance). The TRA assumes that behavioural performance is mostly under one's control, an assumption that is especially problematic for alcohol consumption, where people admit to it being outside of their control at least on occasion (Norman, Bennett, & Lewis, 1998). Schlegel, DAvernas, Zanna, DeCourville, and Manske (1992) illustrated the importance of this issue by comparing prediction of alcohol consumption among problem and non-problem drinkers in a 12-year longitudinal study. They found that while intentions predicted alcohol consumption among both drinker types, a measure of *perceived behavioural control* over drinking also predicted consumption among problem drinkers.

Ajzen's (1991) Theory of Planned Behaviour (TPB) is an extension of the TRA with the main difference between the models being that the TPB includes an additional variable, perceived behavioural control, to account for the fact that many behaviours are not fully under an individual's control. This is important in applying the models to consumption as it is widely recognised that consumption is not always fully under one's control (see Sect. 2).

In the TPB, intentions are based on three constructs: attitudes, subjective norms, and perceived behavioural control (i.e., perceptions of control over behavioural performance). Ajzen conceptualised perceived behavioural control as a combination of two constructs: self-efficacy (i.e., one's confidence that they can perform a behaviour; Bandura, 1977) and perceived control (i.e., how much control over behavioural performance an individual has; Ajzen, 2002). Perceived behavioural control is also viewed as a predictor of behaviour to the extent that responses reflect *actual* control over behavioural performance; if perceptions are not accurate, then perceived behavioural control will not predict behaviour (Ajzen, 2002).

A meta-analysis published by Cooke, Dahdah, Norman, and French (2016) provides a statistical review of TPB relationships for alcohol studies (see Fig. 2.1). They included 40 studies that tested cross-sectional relationships between intentions, attitudes, subjective norms, and perceived behavioural control and 19 studies that prospectively tested consumption relationships with intentions and perceived behavioural control. Cooke et al. found a large-sized, sample-weighted, average correlation between attitudes and intentions ($r_+ = 0.62$) and a medium-sized, sample-weighted, average correlation between subjective norms and intentions ($r_+ = 0.47$). These results support Ajzen's

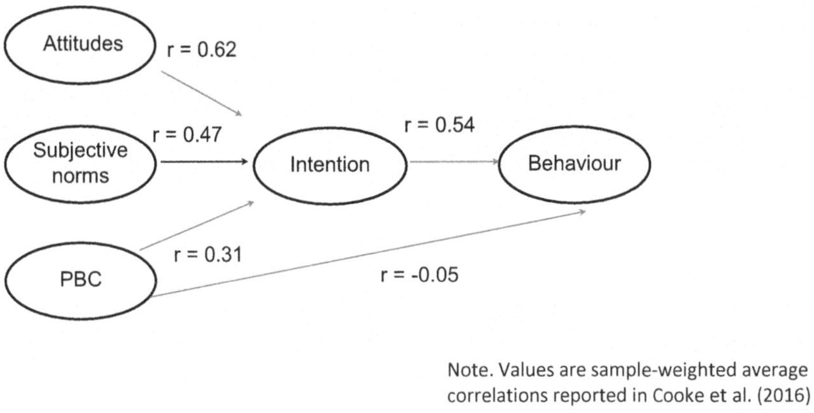

Fig. 2.1 The theory of planned behaviour overlaid with sample weighted average correlations for relationships reported in Cooke et al.'s (2016) meta-analysis of alcohol studies

claim that attitudes and subjective norms are related to drinking intentions. There was also a large-sized sample-weighted average correlation between intentions and consumption ($r_+ = 0.54$), supporting the proposal that intentions predict alcohol consumption prospectively.

By contrast, results from Cooke et al.'s meta-analysis provide limited support for the pathways between perceived behavioural control and intentions. While there was a medium-sized, sample-weighted, average correlation between perceived behavioural control and intentions ($r_+ = 0.31$), inspection of the forest plot showed that several studies reported negative correlations—this means that higher intentions to drink alcohol were associated with *lower* perceived behavioural control. This pattern did not occur in equivalent forest plots for the attitude-intention and subjective norm-intention relationships and is not consistent with model tenets. In addition, the perceived behavioural control-consumption pathway was null and negative ($r_+ = -0.05$); because the confidence intervals included zero it is possible that the 'true' correlation between consumption and perceived behavioural control is zero. Several of the correlations were negative showing that *low* perceived behavioural control was related to *high* consumption, which while making intuitive sense, goes against the model's tenets.

Cooke et al. offered three explanations for the effects found for perceived behavioural control. First, they suggested that when completing measures, participants may overestimate how much control they actually have over consumption, leading to inaccurate responses. Second, participants may misinterpret what is meant by control when answering items; a think aloud study by French, Cooke, Mclean, Williams, and Sutton (2007) found that while answering perceived behavioural control items, some participants discussed control over behaviour that follows drinking (i.e., running around naked, acting embarrassingly) rather than control over *drinking* itself. Misinterpreting items in this way is likely to generate inaccurate responses which attenuate the size of relationships. Finally, Cooke et al. suggested that some individuals might wish to attribute a lack of control over their behaviour; sub-group analyses showed that while perceived behavioural control had a negative relationship with studies that focused on 'getting drunk,' its relation with light drinking (i.e., low risk; see Chap. 1) was positive. This means that individuals appear happier to attribute being in control when thinking about low-risk drinking patterns, but don't want to admit to being in control (or acknowledge that they are not in control) over more harmful patterns of consumption.

Burgess, Cooke, and Davies's (2019) recent paper offers an alternative view on how control links to consumption. In this study, drinkers were asked to describe in their own words how they feel as they approach their 'tipping point' (i.e., the point at which they have drunk too much; see Chap. 1). Two common patterns were reported. The first pattern was of anxiety, fear, and worry about losing control and not wanting to reach the 'tipping point.' The second pattern consisted of generally positive feelings resulting from drinking, such as enjoyment and relaxation. These findings provide a further explanation for the negative perceived behavioural control-behaviour relationship reported in Cooke et al.'s meta-analysis. Perhaps participants recruited into studies where a negative perceived behavioural control-behaviour relationship was found either (1) maintained high levels of control by drinking low amounts of alcohol and/or (2) wanted to lose control and did so by drinking high amounts of alcohol (Norman et al., 1998). In both groups there is a negative relationship. Alternatively, because Burgess et al.'s data shows that people in a sample can drink to achieve opposing goals, this has the potential to reduce the size of the correlations between perceived behavioural control, intention, and consumption, because scores are averaged across the whole sample.

Due to concerns about the size of the perceived behavioural control relationships, Cooke et al. also reported results for studies which measured the sub-components: perceived control and self-efficacy, separately. These analyses show that self-efficacy had medium-sized relationships with intentions ($r_+ = 0.48$) and consumption ($r_+ = 0.41$), while perceived control had null relationships with both intentions ($r_+ = -0.10$) and consumption ($r_+ = -0.13$). It should be noted that there were only eight self-efficacy studies and five perceived control studies, so, caution should be used when interpreting these effect sizes. Several limitations of Cooke et al.'s meta-analysis should be acknowledged. Most of the samples were drawn from university student populations and almost all included studies had majority female samples.

Notwithstanding these issues, this meta-analysis provides evidence to support several TPB pathways including those from attitudes, and subjective norms, to intentions and from intentions to consumption. In contrast, the perceived behavioural control pathways varied in both size and direction, with some studies reporting that no relationship exists. Overall, there is evidence to support the claim that the TPB can predict alcohol consumption and intentions. This section ends by providing some observations about the theories covered in depth.

Observations About Theories Covered in the Chapter

A systematic review of studies testing alcohol expectancy theory or the cognitive model of binge drinking would help clarify the evidence base for these theories, establish the extent to which drinking refusal self-efficacy predicts alcohol consumption, and the role of alcohol expectancies in predicting consumption. Given that alcohol expectancies rarely predict consumption when included alongside drinking refusal self-efficacy in regression models, consideration should be given to reframing the role of alcohol expectancies in these theories. One option would be to propose alcohol expectancies as a moderator of the relationship between drinking refusal self-efficacy and consumption. Evidence that alcohol expectancies moderates the relationship between drinking refusal self-efficacy and alcohol consumption has been shown in several studies (e.g., Goldsmith et al., 2012; Oei & Jardim, 2007).

Alternatively, consideration should also be given to Oei and Burrow's (2000) suggestion that drinking refusal-self-efficacy mediates the effects of alcohol expectancies on drinking. These authors made this claim after showing that entering alcohol expectancies *after* drinking refusal self-efficacy into a regression model indicated expectancies had no predictive effect on consumption. In contrast, entering expectancies *before* drinking refusal self-efficacy showed expectancies predicted consumption. Unfortunately, as this is not a formal test of mediation further tests are required. However, conducting such tests in future studies would be worthwhile because research shows that young children with no personal experience of drinking alcohol report alcohol expectancies based on their perceptions of older children and adults (see Chap. 15). Such expectancies may inform perceptions of drinking refusal self-efficacy, which are likely to develop at a later age because it relates to refusing a drink and one has to be offered a drink to be able to demonstrate confidence in refusing it (see Chap. 14).

Considering the incentive motivation model, Cooper et al.'s (2015) review of the drinking motives literature found that enhancement motives were the strongest predictor of both alcohol consumption and HED and that conformity motives were the weakest predictor of both outcomes. Social motives predicted alcohol consumption better than HED and, vice versa, coping motives better predicted HED than consumption. Based on this evidence, it would seem that (i) enhancement motives should always be measured in alcohol studies as they have been repeatedly shown to predict alcohol consumption and HED, (ii) conformity motives should only be measured when there is a clear justification for doing so, such as to test the idea that conformity motives predict light drinking patterns (Cooper et al., 2015), and (iii) researchers should consider measuring social motives if they are interested in alcohol consumption and coping motives if the focus is on HED.

An additional point to make is to consider the factor structure of the four-factor model. Fernandes-Jesus et al. (2016) used confirmatory factor analysis to test the factor structure of the model and found that an 18-item version of the DMQ-R had better psychometric properties than the 20-item version. One of the two items that loaded sub-optimally in this study, the coping item 'Because you feel more self-confident and sure of yourself,' also had a low factor loading in the original paper by Cooper (1994) and a study conducted by Hauck-Filho, Teixeira, and Cooper (2012). Given that Kuntsche et al. have now developed and validated a short-form version of the DMQ-R that has 12 items, it appears that future studies are needed to confirm the psychometric properties of the original and new scales.

The biggest challenge to the TPB as a model to predict alcohol consumption is the lack of evidence for the path from perceived behaviour control to consumption. While an obvious option would be to return to using the TRA, as outlined earlier, research has shown that perceptions of control can predict alcohol consumption, with this relationship stronger for problem drinkers (Schlegel et al., 1992). An alternative approach would be to replace perceived behaviour control with self-efficacy; Cooke et al. (2016) found that self-efficacy had medium-sized relationships with both consumption and intentions, albeit based on data from only eight studies, so, including self-efficacy instead of perceived behavioural control would produce a TPB which is similar to the shibboleths of the theory but replaces a predictor variable that has an inconsistent relationship with consumption and intentions with one that appears to have a stronger relationship.

However, a potentially more useful approach would be to replace perceived behavioural control with drinking refusal self-efficacy; Foster, Dukes, and Sartor (2016) found that drinking refusal self-efficacy predicted consumption alongside intentions. Including drinking refusal self-efficacy has the potential to change the focus of TPB alcohol studies from seeing if the theory predicts alcohol consumption (i.e., the more one intends to drink, the more one should drink) to seeing if the theory predicts limiting or reducing consumption (i.e., the more one intends to *limit* one's drinking, the less they should drink; cf., Ajzen & Sheikh, 2013; Cooke, Sniehotta, & Schuz, 2007). Changing the focus from control or self-efficacy over drinking to control or self-efficacy over drink *refusal* may further encourage researchers to consider how the TPB could be used to inform interventions to reduce alcohol consumption (see Chap. 21) and would be a welcome example of theoretical integration.

A final point is that few studies have used longitudinal designs to test the predictive utility of the TPB as a model of alcohol consumption. This is in contrast to the other theories covered in this chapter. Given that much TPB research in this area is done with university samples there are challenges to using longitudinal designs, however, researchers are encouraged to employ these designs where possible to provide tests of prediction over longer time-frames. Now the theories have been considered individually, the next section compares and contrasts results across theories.

Conceptual Overlap in Psychological Theories of Alcohol Consumption

Several theories covered in this chapter include similar constructs. For example, alcohol expectancies are alcohol-specific outcome expectancies, which according to Ajzen, are one of the two beliefs that underpin attitudes. Similarly, drinking refusal self-efficacy is the opposite of self-efficacy that is sometimes measured in TPB alcohol studies (Norman & Conner, 2006). Inspection of the items used to assess alcohol expectancies and drinking motives shows that there is some overlap between items tapping positive alcohol expectancies and enhancement motives, but little overlap between negative alcohol expectancies and motive items. There is no obvious overlap between drinking motives and TPB constructs. Thus, drinking motives appear to be relatively independent of constructs in other theories.

Competition Between Theories to Predict Alcohol Consumption

One way to compare prediction of theories used to predict alcohol consumption is to examine results from studies that have measured variables from two or more theories. Doing so allows researchers to determine which variables remain significant predictors of consumption after accounting for the effects of variables from competitor theories. For example, Foster et al. (2016) reported the results of a study that compared prediction of consumption using alcohol expectancies, drinking refusal self-efficacy, and intentions—directly testing the cognitive model of binge drinking and the TPB. Results provided support for both theories as drinking refusal self-efficacy and intentions predicted alcohol consumption, while alcohol expectancies did not predict consumption.

Additionally, Atwell, Abraham, and Duka (2011) sought to develop a parsimonious model of alcohol consumption. After reviewing the literature they noted a multitude of competing predictor variables and decided to measure as many predictors as possible, to control for the effects of competing predictors. In total, they included 30 predictor variables, including variables from the cognitive model of binge drinking, the incentive motivation model, and the TPB, in a regression analysis predicting AUDIT scores (see Chap. 1). A model containing six predictors—age of onset; descriptive norm frequency; descriptive norm quantity; self-efficacy; sensation seeking; social motives—accounted for 58% of the variance in AUDIT scores. These results provide support for the incentive motivation model, because social motives were a significant predictor, and some support for the TPB, which sometimes contains a measure of self-efficacy, but no support for the cognitive model of binge drinking. It should be noted that Atwell et al. did not measure drinking refusal self-efficacy and used a cross-sectional design.

Finally, Cooke et al.'s (2021) study was inspired by Atwell et al.'s paper, while noting that a cross-sectional design limits the conclusions one can make. They measured a large set of predictors at baseline and then used a longitudinal design with follow-up consumption measured six months later. In addition, university students were recruited from six different European countries, providing a rare example of a cross-cultural sample. Included in the set of predictors were variables from all of the models covered in this chapter—alcohol expectancies, drinking motives, drinking refusal self-efficacy, intentions, and perceived behavioural control—along with baseline measures of past consumption, demographic variables, personality variables including sensation seeking (see Chap. 5) and prototypes (see Chap. 3). Cooke et al. found that similarity to prototypical abstinent drinker predicted quantity of alcohol consumption while having lower drinking refusal self-efficacy, and higher conformity motives, predicted frequency of alcohol consumption. However, none of the psychological predictors drawn from the models described in this chapter predicted HED. These results provide some support for the cognitive model of binge drinking and incentive motivation model, but no support for the TPB as neither intentions nor perceived behavioural control predicted consumption or HED after controlling for the effects of other predictors.

Cooke et al.'s (2021) study has a number of limitations, including a medium-term follow-up—longer than most studies testing predictive relationships for theories—that might have been too stringent a test of prediction—predictor variables might have changed between baseline and follow-up six months later—and a sample that mainly reported light drinking patterns. The sample also overrepresented women and white participants. Nevertheless, Cooke et al. (2021) provide a comprehensive test of the predictive power of variables from different theories and will hopefully encourage other researchers to conduct similar studies to provide direct tests of the claims of theories.

Cooke et al.'s (2021) results for HED might reflect the fact that most participants reported light drinking patterns; over 60% of the sample scored in the low-risk category on the AUDIT (Cooke et al., 2019). Alternatively, a recent paper by Cooke, Bailey, Jennings, Yuen, and Gardner (2020) found that the only predictor of HED was scores on the self-report habit index (Gardner, de Bruijn, & Lally, 2012), with psychological variables like intentions and perceived behavioural control not predicting HED. While it should be acknowledged that this study has a small sample size, and a two-week follow-up, these results suggest it is possible that heavier patterns of drinking are better predicted by habitual processes. These are measured in relatively few studies that test theories, although when they are they often add to prediction (Gardner et al., 2012; Norman, 2011; see Chap. 4 for more on this topic).

Theoretical Integration

Atwell et al. (2011), Cooke et al. (2021), and Foster et al.'s (2016) studies allow researchers to directly test competing theoretical accounts of consumption which have the potential to suggest revisions to theories. For example, one interpretation of Foster et al.'s findings is that alcohol expectancies may be antecedent to other predictors (cf. Hasking et al., 2015). This idea was examined in a novel paper by Urbán, Kökönyei, and Demetrovics (2008) where they tested the following logic model in a sample of Hungarian adolescents:

sensation seeking → expectancies → drinking motives → alcohol consumption

Urban et al.'s hypothesis was that those with higher levels of sensation seeking (see Chap. 5) will form more positive alcohol expectancies, which produce more positive drinking motives, and these positive motives lead to increased consumption. Path analysis provided support for the hypothesised sequence of action although there are two caveats.

First, based on a principal components analysis the authors determined that there was only one factor that accounted for the drinking motives items. Thus, in contrast to Cooper's (1994) recommendations, they created a composite item reflecting all 20 items, rather than keeping the four motives separate. This means we do not know the size of the relationships between the four motives and consumption. Second, despite measuring alcohol consumption 30 days after assessing psychological variables the authors created a composite variable based on 30-day consumption and six indices all based on past consumption. This means we cannot be sure that this model predicts future consumption. Notwithstanding these caveats, Urban et al. provide a welcome addition to theorising because by attempting to integrate theories together (see Chap. 13 for more on theoretical integration). Having compared theories, the next section considers methodological issues with theoretical research studies.

Methodological Issues with Theoretical Research on Alcohol Consumption

Selective Testing of Variables

Selective testing of variables, for instance, testing constructs from one theory while accounting for demographic predictors, limits understanding of which theories predict alcohol consumption. If you only test one theory, then you cannot know if results will remain the same when you test constructs from other theories in your analysis. Taken to extremes, the research literature becomes a set of disconnected papers each claiming to show that the variables they measured are the 'best' predictor(s) of consumption, while neglecting to mention that they may only be the 'best' predictor because they have not been compared to other 'best' predictors! Studies that have tested two or more models—Atwell et al. (2011), Cooke et al. (2020), Foster et al. (2016)—are more useful than any number of studies testing only one model because they allow researchers to compare competing theoretical accounts for consumption.

Study Design Issues

There is an over-reliance on cross-sectional study designs in the alcohol literature. For example, Cooper et al. (2015) noted this issue as a limitation of their review of the drinking motives literature. The main issue with cross-sectional designs is that studies are not predicting alcohol consumption—consumption has already taken place. As a result, cross-sectional designs are unable to tell us if a set of variables predict consumption in the future.

When researchers do use prospective designs they typically use short-term follow-ups for a number of reasons ranging from a desire to minimise the time between measurement of predictors and measurement of behaviour because of concerns that predictors might change (Ajzen, 1996) to concerns over attrition associated with longer-term follow-ups, an issue that has been highlighted in the literature testing alcohol interventions (Radtke, Ostergaard, Cooke, & Scholz, 2017). There is also consideration of the timeframe that participants are asked to report their behaviour over—it is easier for you to recall what you did in the past week compared to the past two weeks, month, three months, and so on. Unfortunately, while these are all sound reasons for minimising the gap between measurement of predictors and behaviour, this does mean that research, to date, has provided favourable conditions for predictor variables to account for variance in alcohol consumption. Because predictors are unlikely to change one week after they have been measured, then this can create an impression that predictors will remain effective at predicting alcohol consumption over longer time periods.

Cooke et al. (2021) show this phenomenon to be a potential illusion. In most studies, past drinking behaviour has a large-sized correlation with future drinking behaviour. In Cooke et al.'s study, they showed that the correlation between baseline HED drinking and HED measured six months later was $r = 0.35$, much smaller than you normally find when the gap between measurements is shorter. Such results should encourage tests of prediction over longer timeframes to confirm that predictive effects persist over time.

A related issue is that there are relatively few longitudinal designs testing prediction of alcohol consumption using psychological theories. Such studies provide a useful insight into how scores on predictor variables measured at one time can predict alcohol consumption in the future. For example, Cooper et al. (2008) found that adolescents' scores on coping and enhancement motives predicted alcohol consumption 15 years later, suggesting they are viable targets for interventions aimed at adolescents. Obviously, such studies are resource intensive and can require co-ordination with organisations that run cohort or longitudinal surveys, so they are not the default option for future research studies testing psychological theories. Nevertheless, such studies are now needed to test the competing claims of theories. Studies are routinely done to monitor trends in consumption over time, we need similar studies to monitor trends in *prediction* of consumption over time. Such studies would allow us to more fully test the claims of psychological theories of alcohol consumption.

Experimental Evidence for Alcohol Theories

There is the lack of experimental research conducted to test theoretical claims about alcohol consumption; if we modify alcohol expectancies or increase drinking refusal self-efficacy, using an intervention, does this change subsequent consumption? If theories are a valid description of why people drink, successfully modifying the variables in the theories in an intervention should bring about changes in consumption (see Chap. 21). As an example, the TPB has been used for this purpose (Cameron et al., 2015; Epton et al., 2014; Norman et al., 2018) with interventions targeting the antecedents to intentions (attitudes, subjective norms, perceived behavioural control) using persuasive communications. While results for these interventions have been mixed, they do provide a test of the TPB's claims that changing beliefs that underpin intentions brings about changes in intentions that, ultimately, lead to changes in consumption. Indeed, Norman et al. (2018) found in their intervention study that changes in intentions mediated the effects of the intervention on consumption six months later (see Chap. 21 for more on this study). There is a dearth of equivalent interventions studies based on alcohol expectancy theory/cognitive model of binge drinking or the incentive motivation model. One recent study by Fearnow-Kenny et al. (Fearnow-Kenney et al., 2016) targeted alcohol expectancies among college-student athletes, however, the intervention failed to produce changes in expectancies in the intervention group.

Non-University Samples

Few studies cited in this chapter recruited samples of non-university students; Cooke et al. (2016) noted that 33 of the 40 studies included in their TPB meta-analysis recruited such samples. While this pattern is not so apparent for the other theories covered in this chapter, there is still a preponderance of theory-testing taking place with university samples, with adolescents the next most commonly sampled population. What is lacking is research testing theories in older populations, such as those who had graduated and are now working, those who are parents, and those who are retired. There is also an absence of studies with young adult populations not recruited from university settings. We know very little about the utility of psychological theories to predict alcohol consumption reported by samples who have left school and entered the workforce without attending university. For theories to provide general accounts of alcohol consumption, there is a need to recruit samples who have not entered higher education or training upon reaching adulthood.

Future Research Directions for Psychological Theories of Alcohol Consumption

Following Atwell et al.'s (2011) example researchers are encouraged to test predictors from multiple theories in future studies. This research is needed to test the competing claims of different theories of alcohol consumption. There is also a need for more theoretical integration to synthesise ideas from different theories; because there is not unequivocal evidence to support any of the theories covered in this chapter—alcohol expectancies do not predict consumption in the presence of drinking refusal self-efficacy; conformity motives rarely predict consumption; perceived behavioural control has an inconsistent relationship with consumption—now is the time to propose new theories of alcohol consumption that draw together insights across theoretical traditions. Researchers should consider creating theories that contain constructs shown to predict consumption from different theories: drinking refusal self-efficacy, enhancement motives, and intentions. Because most tests of theories have focused on only one theory, existing evidence for constructs from different theories is largely independent of evidence for competing theories and constructs within them. Thought should be given to how these hybrid theories—containing constructs from different theories—would fit together to influence consumption and each other. In addition, when creating new theories, there is also a need to incorporates measures of implicit or automatic processes (e.g., habits, prototypes, willingness; see Chaps. 3 and 4) to capture these influences that are generally overlooked by theories of consumption and human motivation covered in this chapter. While such a theory may still focus on individual action, it is important to acknowledge the role of external/cultural/contextual/environmental/social influences on consumption in a manner that is mostly lacking from the existing literature on theories of alcohol consumption.

Conclusions

This chapter has outlined and reviewed the evidence for three frequently tested psychological theories of alcohol consumption: the cognitive model of binge drinking, the incentive motivation model, and the TPB. In general, research evidence supports some of the predictions made by these theories. However, a range of methodological issues, including an over-reliance on cross-sectional study designs and over-sampling of university students, means that caution should be exercised before making definitive claims about the utility of these theories. There is also an urgent need for studies comparing prediction *between* theories. Such studies will extend existing findings and improve our understanding of which theories provide the best account of alcohol consumption and allow for the possibility of theoretical integration, especially there is more evidence for particular predictor variables than theories as a whole at the present time.

References

Ajzen, I. (1991). The theory of planned behavior. *Organizational Behavior and Human Decision Processes, 50,* 179–211. https://doi.org/10.1016/0749-5978(91)90020-T

Ajzen, I. (1996). The directive influence of attitudes on behavior. In P. M. Gollwitzer & J. A. Bargh (Eds.), *Psychology of action* (pp. 385–403). New York, NY: Guildford Press.

Ajzen, I. (2002). Perceived behavioral control, self-efficacy, locus of control, and the theory of planned behavior. *Journal of Applied Social Psychology, 32*, 665–683.

Ajzen, I., & Fishbein, M. (1973). Attitudinal and normative variables as predictors of specific behaviors. *Journal of Personality and Social Psychology, 27*, 41–57.

Ajzen, I., & Sheikh, S. (2013). Action versus inaction: Anticipated affect in the theory of planned behavior: Anticipated affect. *Journal of Applied Social Psychology, 43*(1), 155–162. https://doi.org/10.1111/j.1559-1816.2012.00989.x

Atwell, K., Abraham, C., & Duka, T. (2011). A parsimonious, integrative model of key psychological correlates of UK university students' alcohol consumption. *Alcohol and Alcoholism (Oxford, Oxfordshire), 46*(3), 253–260. https://doi.org/10.1093/alcalc/agr016

Bandura, A. (1977). Self-efficacy: Toward a unifying theory of behavioral change. *Psychological Review, 84*(2), 191–215.

Burgess, M., Cooke, R., & Davies, E. L. (2019). *My own personal hell*: Approaching and exceeding thresholds of too much alcohol. *Psychology & Health, 34*(12), 1451–1469. https://doi.org/10.1080/08870446.2019.1616087

Cameron, D., Epton, T., Norman, P., Sheeran, P., Harris, P. R., Webb, T. L., … Shah, I. (2015). A theory-based online health behaviour intervention for new university students (U@Uni:LifeGuide): Results from a repeat randomized controlled trial. *Trials, 16*. https://doi.org/10.1186/s13063-015-1092-4

Cooke, R., Bailey, O., Jennings, J., Yuen, C., & Gardner, B. (2020). Do preparatory behaviours predict alcohol consumption among UK university students? *British Journal of Health Psychology*, https://doi.org/10.1111/bjhp.12489

Cooke, R., Beccaria, F., Demant, J., Fernandes-Jesus, M., Fleig, L., Negreiros, J., Scholz, U., & de Visser, R. (2019). Patterns of alcohol consumption and alcohol-related harm among European university students. *European Journal of Public Health*, ckz067. https://doi.org/10.1093/eurpub/ckz067.

Cooke, R., Beccaria, F., Demant, J., Fernandes-Jesus, M., Fleig, L., Scholz, U., & de Visser, R. O. (2021). Predicting alcohol consumption among European university students using data from the CALIBRATE study. *Unpublished manuscript*

Cooke, R., Dahdah, M., Norman, P., & French, D. P. (2016). How well does the theory of planned behaviour predict alcohol consumption? A systematic review and meta-analysis. *Health Psychology Review, 10*, 148–167. https://doi.org/10.1080/17437199.2014.947547

Cooke, R., Sniehotta, F., & Schuz, B. (2007). Predicting binge-drinking behaviour using an extended TPB: Examining the impact of anticipated regret and descriptive norms. *Alcohol and Alcoholism, 42*(2), 84–91. https://doi.org/10.1093/alcalc/agl115

Cooper, M. L. (1994). Motivations for alcohol use among adolescents: Development and validation of a four-factor model. *Psychological Assessment, 6*(2), 117–128. https://doi.org/10.1037/1040-3590.6.2.117

Cooper, M. L., Krull, J. L., Agocha, V. B., Flanagan, M. E., Orcutt, H. K., Grabe, S., … Jackson, M. (2008). Motivational pathways to alcohol use and abuse among Black and White adolescents. *Journal of Abnormal Psychology, 117*(3), 485–501. https://doi.org/10.1037/a0012592

Cooper, M. L., Kuntsche, E., Levitt, A., Barber, L. L., & Wolf, S. (2015). Motivational models of substance use: A review of theory and research on motives for using alcohol, marijuana, and tobacco. In K. J. Sher (Ed.), *The Oxford handbook of substance use disorders* (Vol. 1). Oxford, England: Oxford University Press. https://doi.org/10.1093/oxfordhb/9780199381678.013.017

Cox, W. M., & Klinger, E. (1988). A motivational model of alcohol use. *Journal of Abnormal Psychology, 97*(2), 168–180.

Epton, T., Norman, P., Dadzie, A.-S., Harris, P. R., Webb, T. L., Sheeran, P., … Shah, I. (2014). A theory-based online health behaviour intervention for new university students (U@Uni): Results from a randomised controlled trial. *BMC Public Health, 14*. https://doi.org/10.1186/1471-2458-14-563

Fearnow-Kenney, M., Wyrick, D. L., Milroy, J. J., Reifsteck, E. J., Day, T., & Kelly, S. E. (2016). The effects of a web-based alcohol prevention program on social norms, expectancies, and intentions to prevent harm among college student-athletes. *The Sport Psychologist, 30*, 113–122.

Fernandes-Jesus, M., Beccaria, F., Demant, J., Fleig, L., Menezes, I., Scholz, U., … Cooke, R. (2016). Validation of the drinking motives questionnaire—Revised in six European countries. *Addictive Behaviors, 62*, 91–98. https://doi.org/10.1016/j.addbeh.2016.06.010

Foster, D. W., Dukes, K., & Sartor, C. E. (2016). The road to drink is paved with high intentions: Expectancies, refusal self-efficacy, and intentions among heavy drinking college students. *Alcohol, 50*, 65–71. https://doi.org/10.1016/j.alcohol.2015.11.004

French, D. P., Cooke, R., Mclean, N., Williams, M., & Sutton, S. (2007). What do people think about when they answer theory of planned behaviour questionnaires?: A 'think aloud' study. *Journal of Health Psychology, 12*(4), 672–687. https://doi.org/10.1177/1359105307078174

Gardner, B., de Bruijn, G.-J., & Lally, P. (2012). Habit, identity, and repetitive action: A prospective study of binge-drinking in UK students: Habit, identity, and repetitive action. *British Journal of Health Psychology, 17*(3), 565–581. https://doi.org/10.1111/j.2044-8287.2011.02056.x

Goldsmith, A. A., Thompson, R. D., Black, J. J., Tran, G. Q., & Smith, J. P. (2012). Drinking refusal self-efficacy and tension-reduction alcohol expectancies moderating the relationship between generalized anxiety and drinking behaviors in young adult drinkers. *Psychology of Addictive Behaviors, 26*(1), 59–67. https://doi.org/10.1037/a0024766

Gray, J. A. (1970). The psychophysiological basis of introversion-extraversion. *Behavior Research and Therapy, 8*, 249–266.

Hasking, P., Boyes, M., & Mullan, B. (2015). Reward and cognition: Integrating reinforcement sensitivity theory and social cognitive theory to predict drinking behavior. *Substance Use & Misuse, 50*(10), 1316–1324. https://doi.org/10.3109/10826084.2015.1005315

Hauck-Filho, N., Teixeira, M. A. P., & Cooper, M. L. (2012). Confirmatory factor analysis of the Brazilian version of the Drinking Motives Questionnaire-Revised

(DMQ-R). *Addictive Behaviors, 37*(4), 524–527. https://doi.org/10.1016/j.addbeh.2011.11.023

Kuntsche, E., & Cooper, M. L. (2010). Drinking to have fun and to get drunk: Motives as predictors of weekend drinking over and above usual drinking habits. *Drug and Alcohol Dependence, 110*(3), 259–262. https://doi.org/10.1016/j.drugalcdep.2010.02.021

Leigh, B. C., & Stacy, A. W. (1993). Alcohol outcome expectancies: Scale construction and predictive utility in higher order confirmatory models. *Psychological Assessment, 5*(2), 216–229. https://doi.org/10.1037/1040-3590.5.2.216

Morawska, A., & Oei, T. P. S. (2005). Binge drinking in university students: A test of the cognitive model. *Addictive Behaviors, 30*(2), 203–218. https://doi.org/10.1016/j.addbeh.2004.05.011

Newton, N. C., Barrett, E. L., Swaffield, L., & Teesson, M. (2014). Risky cognitions associated with adolescent alcohol misuse: Moral disengagement, alcohol expectancies and perceived self-regulatory efficacy. *Addictive Behaviors, 39*(1), 165–172. https://doi.org/10.1016/j.addbeh.2013.09.030

Norman, P. (2011). The theory of planned behavior and binge drinking among undergraduate students: Assessing the impact of habit strength. *Addictive Behaviors, 36*(5), 502–507. https://doi.org/10.1016/j.addbeh.2011.01.025

Norman, P., Bennett, P., & Lewis, H. (1998). Understanding binge drinking among young people: An application of the theory of planned behaviour. *Health Education Research, 13*(2), 163–169. https://doi.org/10.1093/her/13.2.163-a

Norman, P., Cameron, D., Epton, T., Webb, T. L., Harris, P. R., Millings, A., & Sheeran, P. (2018). A randomized controlled trial of a brief online intervention to reduce alcohol consumption in new university students: Combining self-affirmation, theory of planned behaviour messages, and implementation intentions. *British Journal of Health Psychology, 23*(1), 108–127. https://doi.org/10.1111/bjhp.12277

Norman, P., & Conner, M. (2006). The theory of planned behaviour and binge drinking: Assessing the moderating role of past behaviour within the theory of planned behaviour. *British Journal of Health Psychology, 11*(1), 55–70. https://doi.org/10.1348/135910705X43741

Oei, T. P. S., & Baldwin, A. R. (1994). Expectancy theory: A two-process model of alcohol use and abuse. *Journal of Studies on Alcohol, 55*(5), 525–534. https://doi.org/10.15288/jsa.1994.55.525

Oei, T. P. S., & Burrow, T. (2000). Alcohol expectancy and drinking refusal self-efficacy: A test of specificity theory. *Addictive Behaviors, 25*(4), 499–507. https://doi.org/10.1016/s0306-4603(99)00044-1

Oei, T. P. S., & Jardim, C. L. (2007). Alcohol expectancies, drinking refusal self-efficacy and drinking behaviour in Asian and Australian students. *Drug and Alcohol Dependence, 87*(2–3), 281–287. https://doi.org/10.1016/j.drugalcdep.2006.08.019

Oei, T. P. S., & Morawska, A. (2004). A cognitive model of binge drinking: The influence of alcohol expectancies and drinking refusal self-efficacy. *Addictive Behaviors, 29*(1), 159–179. https://doi.org/10.1016/S0306-4603(03)00076-5

Oh, H., & Kim, Y. (2014). Drinking behavior and drinking refusal self-efficacy in Korean college students. *Psychological Reports, 115*(3), 872–883. https://doi.org/10.2466/21.18.PR0.115c31z2

Radtke, T., Ostergaard, M., Cooke, R., & Scholz, U. (2017). Web-based alcohol intervention: Study of systematic attrition of heavy drinkers. *Journal of Medical Internet Research, 19*(6), e217. https://doi.org/10.2196/jmir.6780

Schlegel, R. P., D'Avernas, J. R., Zanna, M. P., DeCourville, N. H., & Manske, S. R. (1992). Problem drinking: A problem for the theory of reasoned action? *Journal of Applied Social Psychology, 22*(5), 358–385. https://doi.org/10.1111/j.1559-1816.1992.tb01545.x

Urbán, R., Kökönyei, G., & Demetrovics, Z. (2008). Alcohol outcome expectancies and drinking motives mediate the association between sensation seeking and alcohol use among adolescents. *Addictive Behaviors, 33*(10), 1344–1352. https://doi.org/10.1016/j.addbeh.2008.06.006

Young, R., & Oei, T. P. S. (1990). *Drinking Expectancy Profile: A manual.* University of Queensland.

3

Drinking beyond intentions: The prototype willingness model and alcohol consumption

Emma Louise Davies and Jemma Todd

Introduction

This chapter focuses on dual process models from social psychology that have been applied to predict alcohol consumption, with a specific focus on the Prototype Willingness Model (PWM). Before outlining research evidence about the application of dual process theories to alcohol use and misuse, this chapter will consider why such an approach may be beneficial when compared to theories of behaviour that assume alcohol consumption is always under conscious control. Then, the chapter will take an in-depth look at the PWM, a dual process theory that has been applied to understanding alcohol consumption in primarily, but not limited to, adolescent and young adult populations. Interventions to reduce alcohol consumption using the PWM will then be discussed and critically appraised. The chapter ends by looking at the challenge of measuring the reactive constructs within dual process models such as the PWM, as well as highlighting avenues for future research.

E. L. Davies (✉)
Department of Psychology, Health and Professional Development, Oxford Brookes University, Oxford, UK
e-mail: edavies@brookes.ac.uk

J. Todd
School of Psychology, University of Sydney, Sydney, NSW, Australia

School of Psychological Science, University of Western Australia, Sydney, NSW, Australia

R. Cooke et al. (eds.), *The Palgrave Handbook of Psychological Perspectives on Alcohol Consumption*, https://doi.org/10.1007/978-3-030-66941-6_3

Limitations of Models Based on Intentions

A large number of social psychological theories and models have been proposed to explain and predict alcohol consumption with varying degrees of success (see Chap. 2). These include the Major Theorists Model (Fishbein et al., 2001), the Theory of Reasoned Action (Fishbein & Ajzen, 1975), Theory of Planned Behaviour (TPB; Ajzen, 1991), the Integrative Behavioural Model (Kasprzyk, Montaño, & Fishbein, 1998), and the Integrative Model of reasoned action (IM; Fishbein, 2008), which have been influential in the study of alcohol consumption and many other health behaviours (Hagger & Hamilton, 2020). According to these models, intentions are the most important predictor of behaviour and the stronger the intention to carry out the behaviour, the more likely it is to be performed. These models assume that intentions are formed through conscious deliberation of personal outcomes and feelings (attitudes), beliefs about what others think (subjective norms), and in the TPB and IM the consideration of belief in ability to carry out the behaviour (perceived behavioural control; PBC; Ajzen, 1991).

Whilst the TPB has been integral to much of the health behaviour research to date, meta-analyses indicate that intentions predict, on average, 28% of the variance in behaviour across a wide range of behavioural domains (Sheeran, 2002). Whilst this goes some way in accounting for behaviour, a large proportion of the variance remains unexplained, as there is often a discrepancy between what people intend to do and what they actually do (Orbell & Sheeran, 1998; Rhodes & de Bruijn, 2013; Sheeran, 2002). This intention-behaviour gap is particularly problematic in predicting and explaining alcohol consumption (Pomery, Gibbons, Reis-Bergan, & Gerrard, 2009), as alcohol consumption, like other risk behaviours, can sometimes be a goal-directed behaviour but can also occur in response to environmental cues (Crossley, 2001; Thaler & Sunstein, 2009). Thus, there is a renewed focus on understanding the social and 'automatic' nature of some health (risk) behaviours, such as alcohol consumption (Avishai-Yitshak & Sheeran, 2016; Hollands, Marteau, & Fletcher, 2016; Marteau, Fletcher, Hollands, & Munafo, 2020) in addition to planned elements of these behaviours.

Dual Process Models

Dual process models assume that there are two different systems underlying behavioural decision making (see Evans & Stanovich, 2013, for a review). One involves a reasoned and planned consideration of the costs, benefits, and outcomes of undertaking a particular behaviour, and this reasoned system requires cognitive effort and attention (Kahneman, 2011; Strack & Deutsch, 2004). This system is often what underlies the assumed processes that determine behaviour in social cognition and motivational models and theories that have been frequently applied to predict health behaviours, including alcohol consumption (see Chap. 2). The other system is faster and activated by associations in the physical or social environment. This more reactive system needs little cognitive effort and attention and may occur outside of conscious awareness (Deutsch & Strack, 2020; Strack & Deutsch, 2004). Hofmann, Friese, and Strack (2009) distinguish between the two processes by describing a 'battle' between individuals' self-control and their impulses. They define self-control as the ability to override impulsive behaviours in order to achieve a higher-order goal and as something that requires attention and effort. Alcohol use is often an impulsive behaviour, driven by cues in both the physical and social environment (Yarmush, Manchery, Luehring-Jones, & Erblich, 2016), and people often report drinking more than they plan to (Fairlie, Cadigan, Patrick, Larimer, & Lee, 2019). Thus, dual process models may offer a useful way to explain and predict alcohol consumption (Gerrard, Gibbons, Houlihan, Stock, & Pomery, 2008).

There are a range of different ways in which dual processes have been conceptualised within dual process theories. For example, Strack and Deutsch (2004) proposed an influential dual processing theory, the Reflective-Impulsive Model (RIM), in an attempt to explain social behaviours. Within the reflective system of this model, knowledge about the potential consequences of a particular course of behaviour activates intentional behaviour. The pros and cons of a particular course of action are evaluated before a decision is made about how to act. Within the impulsive system, behaviour is activated by perceptual inputs such as cues in the environment: this system does not require as much cognitive effort as the reflective system and thus can guide behaviour when an individual is highly distracted, or when the reflective system is undertaking other tasks (Deutsch & Strack, 2020; Strack & Deutsch, 2004). Hofmann, Friese, and Wiers (2008) have extended the RIM to include not only a reflective system and impulsive system, but also situational or dispositional boundary conditions which may shift processing from one system to the other system. These conditions can include habit, cognitive load, substance effects, working memory and executive function, and mood.

Kahneman (2011), like many other theorists, made a similar distinction to Strack and Deutsch in his book about human decision making; 'Thinking, fast and slow'. He called the two processes 'System 1' and 'System 2'. System 1 is the faster, automatic system, whereas System 2 requires thought and effort. Kahneman described the effortful system as lazy and suggests that we rely on system 1 as it is easier to do so. If necessary we can switch between the two systems in order to solve a problem or to complete a more challenging task, but it requires more resources, leaving us depleted of energy (Kahneman, 2011).

It is also acknowledged within dual process models of behaviour that the two methods of decision-making can occur simultaneously (Gerrard et al., 2008). Fuzzy-trace theory, for example, suggests that the automatic system is more sophisticated than the effortful system and requires better developed decision-making skills (Reyna & Brainerd, 1995). It is cognitively less effort to use the impulsive system and so this is preferred for analysing complex real-world situations, rather than using the more effortful reflective system. However, in an unfamiliar or stressful situation the effortful system may still be activated alongside habitual, or cued, sets of behaviours (Ouellette & Wood, 1998). Thus, it is possible to override the automatic system when situations might be dangerous or risky. This sophisticated dual decision-making system starts to develop during childhood, but it may not become fully developed until adulthood. Thus, adolescents, who are cognitively less advanced than adults, may be susceptible to bypassing important cues and information, leading to increased risk behaviours (Boyer, 2006).

Dual Process Models and Alcohol Use/Misuse

When considering drinking behaviour, dual process models have high face validity, in that it seems intuitive that whilst sometimes alcohol consumption is in part governed by intentions to drink (reasoned pathway), there are likely to be strong social (see Chap. 6) and environmental (see Chap. 8) influences (social reaction pathway). Drinking behaviours may occur because of a learned association between social or environmental cues and the behaviour. For example, over time one may learn to associate being in the pub with drinking alcohol or feeling stressed with drinking alcohol to relieve such feelings. Risky behaviour may also occur reactively as a result of being in a social situation where there is an opportunity to engage in the behaviour and strong social influences (Gibbons, Gerrard, & Lane, 2003; Gibbons, Kingsbury, Gerrard, & Wills, 2011). There is no specific alcohol use-based dual process model; however, the Prototype Willingness Model was designed to account for health-risk behaviours, including alcohol consumption, and therefore comes the closest to being a dual process model of alcohol consumption. The rest of this chapter therefore focuses on the Prototype Willingness Model as an example of a dual process model applied to alcohol consumption.

Introducing the Prototype Willingness Model

The Prototype Willingness Model (PWM; Gerrard et al., 2008; Gibbons & Gerrard, 1995) extends the reasoned action approach with the addition of a social reaction pathway to behaviour. It was originally proposed to account for adolescent health risk-taking on the basis that this type of behaviour is often driven by social reactions to risk-conducive situations. This focus, however, makes it highly applicable to alcohol consumption, particularly in young people, who often find themselves in such situations. The PWM is composed of two key constructs: prototypes and willingness.

Prototypes

Prototypes are assumed to be highly distinctive images of a certain 'type' of person, and they may have both positive and negative characteristics associated with them (see also Chap. 4, this volume). For example, adolescents often have a clear idea about the typical person their age who drinks, and might describe this typical person as self-confident, popular, attractive, or careless. This image is assumed to be widely recognised and that most young people will tend to agree on what a particular risk taker is like (Gerrard et al., 2006). According to the PWM, it is these clear and powerful images that motivate the decision to engage in risk behaviour by a process of social comparison. If the image is evaluated in a positive light (prototype evaluation) and is perceived to be more similar to oneself (prototype similarity), the individual is more likely to engage in that risk behaviour (Gibbons & Gerrard, 1995). Conversely, if the image is evaluated in a negative light and is inconsistent with self-image, the individual is less likely to engage in the risk behaviour (Gerrard et al., 2006). Engaging in risk behaviour thus has social consequences; by performing the risk behaviour, the individual could become more similar to the 'type of person' (i.e. prototype) who engages in that behaviour and will assume the characteristics associated with the prototype, whether positive or negative. Gaining aspects of the associated prototype is an important social consequence for adolescents whose self-image is still under construction (Gibbons & Gerrard, 1995). The more favourable the prototype, the more likely an individual will want to gain the associated characteristics. Prototype perceptions may be influenced by peers (Ouellette, Gerrard, Gibbons, & Reis-Bergan, 1999), as well as parental rules about alcohol (Cleveland, Turrisi, Gibbons, Gerrard, & Marzell, 2018).

Some researchers have also made distinctions between types of prototypes, such as those associated with engaging in the target behaviour (actors) or not engaging in the behaviour (abstainers). For example, within the alcohol consumption literature, Gerrard et al. (2002) assessed the PWM within a large sample of adolescents and found that abstainer prototypes were sometimes seen as goal states by non-drinkers; however, actor prototypes were sometimes seen as more negative than their self-image. Rivis, Sheeran, and Armitage (2006) explored a range of health risk and health protective behaviours in a sample of adolescents and found that abstainer prototypes were just as relevant as actor prototypes and argued that both should be considered as potentially independent predictors of behaviour. Rivis et al. (2006) also considered the valence of the prototype and found that this did not necessarily match onto health risk behaviours having consistently positive or negative prototypes. For example, they found that whilst drinker prototypes were evaluated more positively and more similar to the self, 'fatty food eater' prototypes were evaluated more negatively (Rivis et al., 2006), providing further evidence that researchers need to consider a nuanced approach to understanding which prototypes are relevant to each specific behaviour and sample.

Willingness

The second key construct within the social reaction pathway is willingness (see also Chap. 4). Within the PWM, the effect of prototype perceptions on behaviour is mediated by behavioural willingness, the extent to which someone is prepared to engage in a risk behaviour in a given risk-conducive situation. Willingness can also be described as 'openness' to risk opportunity and rests on the assumption that although someone may have no intention or expectation about undertaking certain behaviours, they do have an idea about how they might react if certain situations arise (Gibbons et al., 2003). Intentions require effortful consideration of the implications of engaging in certain behaviours and how that might impact upon a person's goals. In contrast with intention, willingness is assumed to operate with little thought given to any consequences of engaging in a behaviour. It is assumed that those who may be willing but not intending to engage in risk behaviours rarely seek out opportune situations and so simply asking about their intentions will not offer any insight into their actual behaviours. However, given the right set of social circumstances, those who show a willingness to engage in the health risk behaviour may be likely to do so (Gibbons, Gerrard, Ouellette, & Burzette, 2000). Many adolescents, for example, are unlikely to report that they intend to get drunk, but may be willing to do so if they find themselves in certain situations, for example, at a house party where their friends are drinking alcohol (Gerrard et al., 2008).

Gibbons et al. (2000) also argue that individuals who are intending to drink alcohol might be more accepting of the consequences (such as a hangover), whereas individuals who are willing to drink will not have considered any adverse outcomes. This lack of forethought means that unplanned behaviour could be more harmful to young people, as they do not consider themselves to be personally vulnerable to risks (Gibbons, Gerrard, Ouellette, & Burzette, 1998). As individuals gain more experience with a behaviour there may be a shift from willingness-based to intention-based decision-making. For example, once a young person has been to a number of parties and consumed alcohol they may associate parties with drinking and plan to do so when they next attend a party. Evidence for a developmental shift from reactive to planned behaviour from early to middle adolescence was found in research conducted in the United States (Pomery et al., 2009). In early adolescence (12–13 years old), willingness was the strongest predictor of substance use, smoking, and class skipping behaviour. However, by middle adolescence (15 years old), behavioural intention or expectation tended to be stronger predictors. Further, for young people aged 11–17 years with prior experience of smoking, measures of intentions to smoke were more predictive of smoking behaviour than measures of willingness to smoke, whilst willingness was more predictive for those with no prior smoking experience (Pomery et al., 2009). Supporting this shift from unplanned to planned behaviour, Davies, Paltoglou, and Foxcroft (2017) found that drinking behaviour in adolescents aged 11–17 years was predicted by willingness, whereas young adult drinking (aged 18 +) was better predicted by intentions.

Prototype Willingness Model Pathways

In common with other dual process models, there are two routes to behaviour within the PWM: a conscious, planned route via attitudes, subjective norms, and intentions and a reactive pathway that is a faster, more spontaneous route, operating outside of conscious control (Gerrard et al., 2008). The reactive pathway takes into account that for young people, risky behaviours tend to occur in a social context and are often unplanned. Within this pathway the prototypes that young people have about typical people their age who drink, or abstain from drinking, are influential to their own willingness to consume alcohol, due to the importance of self-image and social comparison in

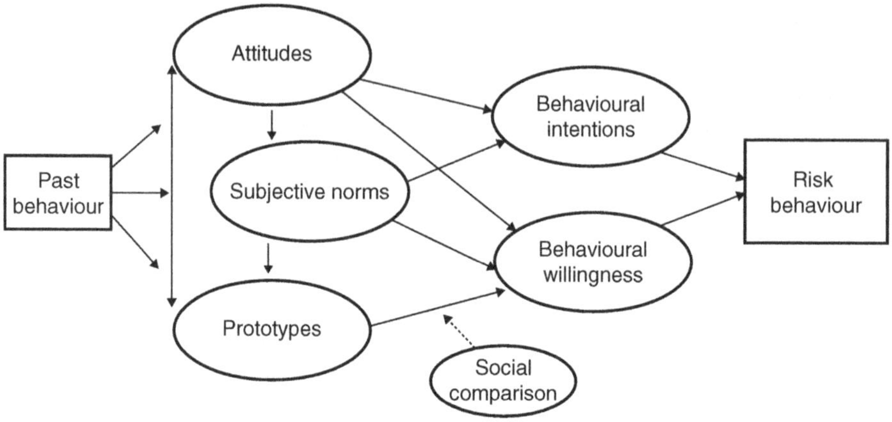

Fig. 3.1 The Prototype Willingness Model. (Gerrard et al., 2008; Gibbons & Gerrard, 1995)

adolescence (see Fig. 3.1). When prototypes for drinkers and drinking are more favourable, then young people will be more willing to drink (and therefore gain some of the associated prototype characteristics). As Fig. 3.1 illustrates, past behaviour is important in the PWM and may influence current behaviour through attitudes and intentions or prototypes and willingness.

Prototype Willingness Model and Alcohol Use

Two meta-analyses have been conducted to determine whether the PWM enhanced prediction of health behaviours above intentions and the theory of planned behaviour (Todd, Kothe, Mullan, & Monds, 2016; van Lettow, de Vries, Burdorf, & van Empelen, 2016; see also Chap. 4). Whilst these meta-analyses included a similar number of studies (81 articles reporting on 90 studies from 1990 to 2014 and 69 articles reporting on 80 studies from 1990 to 2013, respectively), their objectives differed, and each offers a unique perspective on social reactivity in health risk. The broad findings of these meta-analyses will be considered, alongside research conducted since, drawing specifically on findings in relation to alcohol consumption and risky drinking. Note that when considering effect sizes, Cohen's (1992) guidelines for small ($0.1 \leq r < 0.3$), medium ($0.3 \leq r < 0.5$), and large ($r > 0.5$) correlation effect sizes have been applied.

van Lettow et al. (2016) provided an in-depth focus on prototype similarity and prototype favourability and their roles in explaining health risk and health protective behaviours. Overall, the weighted correlations indicated that prototype similarity ($r+ = 0.27$) and prototype favourability ($r+ = 0.20$) were associated with behaviour (representing small effect sizes) and also interacted to predict behaviour ($r+ = 0.32$; medium effect size). Todd et al. (2016) found PWM constructs explained 20.5% of the variance in behaviour. These findings provide evidence for the PWM, in which unplanned, socially reactive decisions to engage in health (risk) behaviour are considered important to account for (Gerrard et al., 2008).

Interestingly, van Lettow et al. (2016) found that both prototype similarity ($r+ = 0.26$) and favourability ($r+ = 0.22$) had similar sized associations with health risk behaviours (small effect sizes); however, prototype similarity was more strongly correlated ($r+ = 0.43$; medium effect size) with health risk willingness than prototype favourability was ($r+ = 0.28$; small effect size). For health protective behaviours, prototype similarity ($r+ = 0.34$; medium effect size) was a stronger predictor of health protective behaviour than prototype favourability ($r+ = 0.15$; small effect size). Similarly, Todd et al. (2016) found a stronger association between prototype similarity and willingness ($r = 0.406$), intention ($r = 0.466$), and behaviour ($r = 0.408$; all medium effect sizes) than was found for prototype favourability (willingness, $r = 0.313$, medium effect size; intention, $r = 0.227$, small effect size; behaviour, $r = 0.286$, small effect size).

When looking at research conducted since these meta-analyses, researchers have found evidence for the role of prototypes in predicting alcohol related behaviour, although studies vary on whether it is prototype similarity or favourability (or both) that predicts behaviour. For example, Dillard, Ferrer, Bulthuis, and Klein (2018) conducted a longitudinal study of drinking prototypes in 340 college students and found that holding more positive prototypes of excessive drinkers predicted alcohol consumption the following year. Willingness and TPB constructs were not included, so the full model was not tested. On the other hand, in a cross-sectional study, Litt, Lewis, Fairlie, and Head-Corliss (2018) found prototype similarity but not favourability was associated with alcohol-related cognitions and consumption behaviour in a sample of 294 young adults.

In their commentary, Gibbons and Gerrard (2016) suggested that prototype similarity may in part be accounted for by perceptions of similarity to one's own past behaviour, potentially accounting for stronger prototype similarity towards engaging in health protective behaviours. They encouraged further exploration of where prototype similarity and prototype favourability are inconsistent, as this may indicate a change. For example, if an individual held favourable prototypes towards alcohol drinkers, but low perceived similarity, this could potentially indicate a risk of commencing drinking. Todd and van

Lettow (2016) expanded on this notion further, suggesting that favourability may depend more on social context, whilst similarity may rely on an internal self-perception of one's own image.

Whilst van Lettow et al. (2016) looked at health risk behaviour and health promoting behaviour categories separately, they did not look at specific behaviours. However, this was a focus of Todd et al. (2016)'s meta-analysis. Todd et al. (2016) included 29 studies investigating alcohol use, representing the largest behaviour category. As the studies were separated by behaviour, we are able to look at these alcohol use studies specifically.

Of all the included behaviours, Todd et al. (2016) found that the PWM was best at predicting alcohol use, explaining 42.5% of the variance in behaviour. There was a medium-effect-sized correlation between prototype and willingness ($r = 0.440$) and prototype and alcohol consumption behaviour ($r = 0.376$) and a large-effect-sized correlation between willingness and alcohol consumption behaviour ($r = 0.535$). Todd et al. did not however investigate prototype favourability and prototype similarity separately for alcohol use. Based on the overall findings of these 29 studies, the PWM seems a good model to explain alcohol consumption.

It is worth noting that Todd et al. (2016) made a comparison between the reasoned pathway (i.e. attitudes, subjective norms, and intention drawn from the TPB) and social reactive pathway (i.e. PWM-specific constructs of prototypes and willingness). When the impact of intention on behaviour was controlled for, behavioural willingness only explained an additional 1.4% of variance in alcohol use behaviour. It therefore appears that whilst the PWM can be used to explain health-risk behaviours such as alcohol consumption, other models that focus on reasoned decision-making appear to also explain such behaviours equally well overall.

Ajzen (1991) has argued that willingness, along with intentions, are facets of behavioural expectations and therefore are unlikely to make unique contributions to the prediction of behaviour. Consistent with this premise, Todd et al. (2016)'s meta-analysis, willingness, and intention were highly correlated (averaged weighted $r = 0.749$; large effect size), suggesting an overlap in constructs. One possible explanation for this finding is that the present measurement of willingness and intention constructs does not adequately capture the differential reasoned and social reactive pathways. Hofmann et al. (2008) have noted that willingness does not preclude conscious consideration of the scenario; it can incorporate reasoned aspects and therefore might not adequately capture non-cognitive, implicit, impulsive processes. Future research could explore whether there are better measurement techniques for assessing these constructs to further delineate how reasoned versus socially reactive aspects of decision-making differ. Alternatively, the reasoned and reactive pathways may be synchronous for some contexts or behaviours. For example, people may intend to drink alcohol at a party, and at the same time, their drinking pattern could be influenced unconsciously by the drinking behaviours of others around them. Whilst Todd et al. (2016)'s meta-analysis provides some insights into how these models differ across different behaviours and samples, a more targeted approach is needed to determine when intention- and motivation-based decision-making aligns with socially influenced or impulsive health behaviour.

Further, that prototypes explained a small but similar amount of additional variance in behaviour (1.1%) as willingness, above intentions, suggests that the optimal placement of constructs within the PWM may not be as originally specified. Whilst willingness might mediate the prototype-behaviour relationship, the prototype similarity and favourability constructs are likely to, at least in part, have a direct influence on behaviour.

In addition to considering alternative ways to measure the PWM constructs, it is also important to consider what kinds of images are most relevant to certain health (risk) behaviours. To date research has largely focused on actor and abstainer prototypes, that is, prototypes of those who engage in the target behaviour and those who do not (Rivis et al., 2006). However, some researchers have expanded the range of prototypes investigated and also the specific behaviours. The distinction between an 'actor' verses an 'abstainer' prototype may particularly oversimplify drinking behaviours in cultures where regular drinking is the norm (Davies, Martin, & Foxcroft, 2013). To improve on this, researchers have begun to explore a broader range of drinker prototypes. For example, in the Netherlands, researchers have identified different dimensions of drinker prototypes such as 'tipsy', 'moderate', and 'heavy' drinkers (van Lettow, Vermunt, de Vries, Burdorf, & van Empele, 2013). In a naturalistic bar lab setting, other researchers have explored the influence of abstainer and social and heavy drinker prototype perceptions on observed alcohol use (Spijkerman, Larsen, Gibbons, & Engels, 2010). In this case favourable perceptions of the heavy drinker prototype were associated with increased consumption of alcoholic drinks. Using more nuanced prototypes may help to improve the prediction of behaviour as individuals may find it easier to call to mind these specific prototypes, increasing access to perceived similarity or favourability of such images.

Davies (2019) conducted a prospective study looking at the prediction of three alcohol-related behaviour measures: AUDIT-C risky alcohol use scores, alcohol-related harms, and unplanned drinking a month later. Rather than merely using a standard 'drinker prototype', Davies investigated three different drinker prototypes: heavy drinker, social drinker, and non-drinker. Consistent with Todd et al. (2016)'s meta-analysis, intention ($r = 0.599$; large effect size) was a stronger correlate of drinking behaviour than willingness was ($r = 0.450$; medium effect size). Also consistent with the meta-analytic findings, but not with the PWM, Davies (2019) found evidence for a direct prediction of behaviour from prototype perceptions. Support was found for different types of drinker prototypes, particularly perceived similarity towards images of heavy drinkers ($r = 0.368$; medium effect size) and (lack of) perceived similarity towards images of non-drinkers ($r = -0.391$; medium effect size), in predicting alcohol consumption. Davies' research therefore provides further impetus for a revised PWM including a direct pathway from prototype perceptions to behaviour and for the inclusion of specific prototype images that are relevant to the behaviour in question. A further recent study has also found that prototype perceptions mediate the relationship between prior drinking behaviour and future drinking intentions, suggesting that prototypes may also feed into reasoned action, warranting further consideration (Rhodes, Loiewski, Potocki, & Ralston, 2017).

Intervention Applications of the PWM

As the meta-analytic evidence has shown, the PWM can explain and predict consumption. A number of studies have now also shown that it may offer a suitable basis for an intervention to change behaviours. Work has been undertaken to develop interventions in a number of behavioural domains. Related to alcohol consumption specifically, there have been a number of studies that have tested whether targeting PWM constructs can bring about reductions in alcohol consumption.

Gerrard et al. (2006) conducted a longitudinal intervention called the Strong African American Families Programme, which was designed to delay and reduce the uptake of health risk behaviours in low-income African American children nearing adolescence. Whilst this intervention consisted of many components, part of it was influenced by the PWM and involved challenging the prototypes that adolescents have of people their age who drink. Activities included learning to recognise similarities and differences between oneself and people one's age who drink, being provided with information about the prevalence of drinking and being shown videos of older adolescents dealing with high-risk situations (Brody et al., 2004). Overall the programme was successful in delaying the onset of alcohol use, and those who took part in the programme rated drinker prototypes less favourably. Intervention effects were even maintained at five-year follow-up (Brody, Chen, Kogan, Murry, & Brown, 2010). However, it is not clear what the specific impact of the prototype aspect of the intervention was in this multi-component intervention.

Several smaller scale experimental studies have manipulated prototypes towards health risk behaviours. For example, Blanton et al. (2001) constructed a fake newspaper article reporting that people who did not use condoms were perceived in a negative way by their peers. Participants who read this article reported higher levels of willingness to use condoms themselves. Drawing on this study, Todd and Mullan (2011) employed a fake newspaper article reporting the results of a survey of other same aged students that presented a negative image of binge drinkers. However, this aspect of the study was not successful in reducing binge drinking in female students. One explanation could be that this information was not perceived as credible by the student participants, who experienced heavy drinking as normal behaviour.

Building on the idea of using a broader range of prototypes, van Lettow, de Vries, Burdorf, Boon, and van Empelen (2015) used prototype alteration as an additional strategy within 'Drinktest', a digital intervention based on personalised feedback about drinking and cue reminders. Within this intervention, participants were encouraged to think about characteristics that they would like to use to describe themselves. Positive descriptions, such as 'social' and 'spontaneous', were used as descriptors of drinking in moderation, and participants were advised that their peers valued such positive characteristics. Excessive drinking, on the other hand, was framed as annoying, uncontrolled, volatile, and insecure. The addition of this feature to the Drinktest intervention produced greater reductions in alcohol consumption compared to a version of the intervention that did not include personal characteristics, possibly due to participants' desire to distance themselves from the negative prototype descriptions (van Lettow et al., 2015).

Theory-based interventions are often more effective than those not based on theory, but only if the theory is appropriately targeted and operationalised within the intervention (Prestwich et al., 2014). Thus, it is important that theoretical constructs within the PWM are operationalised in an appropriate way to bring about the desired changes in behaviour. Whilst the Drinktest intervention by van Lettow et al. (2015) was successful in attempting to make prototype images more personally relevant, the authors highlighted the need to also tailor prototypical characteristics to individual preferences. Exploration of relevant prototype descriptions within specific target groups is therefore needed at the intervention development stage.

Whilst the PWM interventions to date targeting alcohol consumption show promise, they have also exposed numerous ways in which the PWM or interventions arising from the model need further development. Recent research has suggested that high-risk drinkers might inaccurately identify with low-risk prototype descriptions (Pettigrew, Jongenelis, Pratt, Slevin, & Chikritzhs, 2017), and thus if researchers do not adequately assess both PWM constructs and drinking behaviour prior to intervention development, interventions risk being ineffective or potentially even having unintended consequences. Furthermore, there is at present still a lack of agreement in the literature about modifying prototypes (Davies, Martin, & Foxcroft, 2016). There is still only a relatively small evidence base for interventions based on the PWM even outside of alcohol consumption and in other behavioural domains. Most of these interventions are similar to those described here and attempt to alter people's perceptions of prototypes. Davies et al. (2016) found that expert participants were sceptical about the use of fake survey data to present desirable/undesirable prototypes, as it may not resonate with the experiences of young people and could raise ethical issues about the use of manipulative information. Because of this, it could be preferable to focus on ways to resist social pressures to drink and target willingness more explicitly. This could be achieved through the use of implementation intentions, that is, plans to link contexts with outcomes (see Chap. 21). For example, this could include plans to refuse an extra drink when peers are encouraging someone to drink or plans to replace an alcoholic drink with a soft drink (Davies, 2016). Whether interventions target prototypes or willingness, more research is needed to determine the optimal way of achieving either goal within interventions.

Davies and colleagues have designed an intervention to reduce alcohol misuse in adolescents based on the PWM. After formative work to derive age and culturally relevant prototype descriptions (Davies et al., 2013), they conducted a Delphi study to develop the intervention with feedback from a panel of experts (Davies et al., 2016) and from young people in the target age group of 13–15 years old (Davies, Martin, & Foxcroft, 2015). They then identified key behaviour change techniques that mapped onto the specific PWM constructs. In the next step, Davies (2016) conducted a qualitative project to gain feedback around the proposed content of the intervention, named the 'Alcohol Smart Quiz', from adolescents and their teachers. In this way, Davies was able to ensure that the prototype constructs and the proposed intervention were relevant to the specific target sample. This intervention is yet to be implemented and so it is not yet possible to say whether this systematic approach to developing intervention content was effective.

Looking beyond the PWM, there is a dearth of interventions based on other dual process models that target alcohol consumption. Friese, Hofmann, and Wiers (2011) reviewed developments in health behaviour intervention techniques and provided a framework for intervention development. They classified intervention techniques according to dual process distinctions, that is, targeting impulsive structures versus targeting reflective structures. They also went one step further by distinguishing a third category of intervention strategies; those targeting self-control, which they suggest play a role in the relative impact of reflective versus impulsive systems on behaviour. Friese et al.'s framework is drawn largely from Hofmann et al's (2008) dual process model of health behaviour, and the inclusion of self-control is consistent with other health behaviour models such as self-control theory (Baumeister & Heatherton, 1996), temporal self-regulation theory (Hall & Fong, 2007), and integrated self-control theory (Hoffman, Dohle, & Diel, 2020). Friese et al. (2011) reviewed a number of individual strategies that have successfully targeted alcohol consumption, such as modifying the impulsive system by changing automatic associations or changing attentional biases. However, Friese et al.'s review focused on intervention strategies to target specific constructs that could be classified as belonging to one or the other dual pathway, rather than on interventions that test a complete dual process model. Nonetheless, their framework may prove useful to future dual process intervention design.

Further Directions of Measurement Within Dual Process Models

As we have shown already in this chapter, there is sufficient evidence to suggest that the PWM can predict alcohol consumption and emerging evidence that it can be a useful basis for interventions. However, the PWM constructs are generally assessed with self-report measures and generally these measures are completed in non-drinking contexts (for an exception see Spijkerman et al., 2010). Issues with self-report have been discussed in Chap. 1 and the effect of context on how participants answer questionnaire items is discussed in Chap. 2. Using questionnaire measures to record heuristic and socially reactive constructs such as prototypes and willingness may not fully capture these constructs, if they are truly unplanned and context-driven. It could be argued that traditional explicit measures require conscious deliberation on the part of participants (Fishbein, 2008). For example, when asking young people how 'willing' they are to act in a certain way, questionnaire measures allow them to consider their response in a way that may not capture their propensity to act without much forethought in a social situation.

Some researchers have attempted to address these issues by exploring new ways to measure constructs in the PWM. Reaction time tasks offer the possibility of capturing the kind of decision-making that might occur in drinking contexts. When one is offered an alcoholic drink, there is rarely the time to fully weigh up the pros and cons of taking that drink. Comello and Slater (2011) asked participants to read a scenario about drinking and then respond quickly either 'yes' or 'no' to indicate whether they would engage in risky action. This task produced dichotomous responses, which it could be argued are much more representative of real-life decision-making (because someone either drinks or does not drink) than the Likert scale measures used to measure willingness in other studies. However, they did not measure actual drinking behaviour in this study, and it would be informative to explore whether this particular reaction time measure could predict more variance in drinking behaviour than a typical questionnaire item.

Another way in which researchers have attempted to more accurately measure the reactive processes of the PWM and other dual process models has been via the Implicit Attitude Test (IAT). The IAT is a widely used measure of implicit attitudes and involves the pairing of words and categories (Greenwald, McGhee, & Schwartz, 1998). In a standard IAT procedure as applied to alcohol, participants categorise alcohol words and non-alcohol-related words with positive and negative attributes. The difference in reaction time to categorise alcohol and positive compared to alcohol and negative indicate whether the participant has a positive or negative implicit attitude towards alcohol (Greenwald et al., 1998). Ratliff and Howell (2015) compared implicit measures with traditional questionnaire-based measures of prototypes in the prediction of sun protection behaviours and found implicit measures were better predictors of behaviour. They argued that using implicit measures rather than explicit questionnaire measures to assess constructs that are conceptualised as automatic is likely to improve the explanatory power of models such as the PWM. A further study employed this method to examine implicit prototypes of feminists, which were found to predict both willingness to engage in and actual feminist behaviours (Redford, Howell, Meijs, & Ratliff, 2016). In another study on risky behaviours, a combination of implicit and explicit measures were used to evaluate how athletes perceived performance enhancing substance (PES) user prototypes (Whitaker, Petroczi, Backhouse, Long, & Nepusz, 2016). For explicit prototype measures, athletes generally appeared to hold more favourable images of non-PES users than PES users, whereas implicit measures revealed that PES users held a slightly stronger association between PES user images and 'good', compared to 'bad' (Whitaker et al., 2016), suggesting a role for including implicit measures in prototype assessments.

Whilst implicit measures of prototype and willingness have not yet been explored in the context of alcohol use, Davies et al. (2017) have investigated implicit attitudes towards alcohol consumption and their relationship with PWM constructs. There is a substantial body of research which implicates a role for implicit attitudes in the prediction and explanation of alcohol use in young people (Goodall & Slater, 2010; Houben, Havermans, & Wiers, 2010; Pieters, van der Vorst, Engels, & Wiers, 2010; Thush et al., 2007; Thush & Wiers, 2007). In Davies et al.'s (2017) study of 501 young people, implicit alcohol attitudes were only weakly related to some of the explicit measures in the study and were not able to add to the prediction of willingness to drink over and above prototype perceptions. However, when comparing younger (school pupils) and older (university students) participants, implicit alcohol attitudes added to the prediction of behaviour, over and above intentions and willingness, for the older sample. On the other hand, willingness was the better predictor of behaviour for the younger sample. These findings suggested that for those with less experience of alcohol consumption, the usual measure of willingness was sufficient to capture their propensity to act in a social situation, supporting its utility and the assumptions of the PWM. However, for those with more experience of alcohol consumption, implicit attitudes were able to capture additional variance in behaviour over and above standard willingness and intention measures.

Whilst implicit measures confer many advantages, like questionnaire measures, implicit measures can also be influenced by context. This is particularly relevant in alcohol-related research, where research tends to be conducted in environments far removed from drinking contexts. For example, in one IAT study, respondents who completed measures in a pub environment were more likely to link alcohol with positive expectancies than those who completed the same measures in a lecture theatre (Monk, Pennington, Campbell, Price, & Heim, 2016). One way to address this limitation would be to measure implicit prototypes or willingness to drink in situ. There is a growing body of research where ecological momentary assessment (EMA) tools are used to gather real-time information from participants, via their mobile phones (Heron & Smyth, 2010), including in alcohol-related research (Shiffman, 2009). There has been preliminary research incorporating EMA into PWM alcohol research, although it is alcohol consumption rather than PWM that tends to be measured through EMA (e.g. Teunissen, Spijkerman, Kuntsche, Engels, &

Scholte, 2017). Recently, Slavish, Scaglione, Hultgren, and Turrisi (2019) measured willingness and intentions to drink as well as alcohol consumption through EMA, with promising findings, although they did not incorporate measures of prototypes. This is an exciting direction for better understanding alcohol consumption through contextually relevant PWM assessments.

It is worth noting that the authors who originally proposed the PWM have argued that the social reaction pathway is not always necessarily automatic and that implicit measures are not sufficiently capable of measuring impulse (Gibbons et al., 2011). Further work is therefore needed to explore the measure of implicit alcohol prototypes within the PWM framework, as well as continuing to explore an appropriate way to capture willingness to drink, without recourse to questionnaire measures. Such measurement issues are likely to be relevant to other dual process models of behaviour as well as the PWM.

Future Directions

So, where to from here for dual process models such as the PWM, when applied to alcohol consumption? One such angle is to extend the developmental focus to look at alcohol consumption within older adults (Gibbons & Gerrard, 2016). The PWM was originally developed to explain adolescent health risk behaviour, and it is unclear whether socially reactive elements still play a role in alcohol consumption by older adulthood. It is also worth considering potential cross-cultural differences (or similarities) in understanding alcohol use. Cross-cultural differences in the PWM constructs have been found for health risk behaviours such as smoking and unprotected sexual intercourse (Gibbons, Helweg-Larsen, & Gerrard, 1995) and healthy eating (Ohtomo, Hirose, & Midden, 2011), and whilst some studies exploring alcohol use have been conducted within different cultural groups outside the United States (e.g. Hukkelberg & Dykstra, 2009; Jaigarun et al., 2018), no studies have made direct cultural or cross-national comparisons of the explanatory ability of the PWM for alcohol consumption. These extensions will help to provide a more comprehensive picture of the role of reasoned and reactive processes in alcohol-related behaviours across different populations and contexts, in order to better understand and reduce alcohol consumption.

Conclusions

This chapter explored dual process models of alcohol use and misuse as a way to remedy the intention-behaviour gap often found within reasoned models of health behaviour such as the TPB. The chapter focused on PWM as a specific example of a dual process model, in which alcohol consumption is proposed to be influenced by a reasoned, planned pathway derived from the TPB and also a socially reactive, impulsive, and sometimes sub-conscious pathway. This chapter has also presented ways in which the PWM has or could be extended. For example, some research has found a direct relationship between prototypes and behaviour, which does not exist in the original conceptualisation. Other researchers have argued that in order to truly assess the reactive pathway in dual process models, measurement tools that capture the sub-conscious processes better than self-report questionnaires, such as reaction-time measures, are more appropriate. Further, other dual process models have included 'boundary conditions' such as motivation and self-control to better explain how reasoned or reactive pathways might be activated (Hofmann et al., 2008; Friese et al., 2011; Strack & Deutsch, 2004) and may be worth considering within the PWM framework. This chapter also reviewed PWM and dual process interventions for alcohol misuse, of which there is a small but growing literature base. One possible limiting factor in designing PWM interventions is how to best target the constructs of prototypes and willingness, and where PWM interventions are successful, how to identify the specific mechanisms of change. The expanding fields of intervention mapping and behaviour change technique taxonomies may therefore be of use to more specifically target certain theoretical constructs, in order to develop dual process interventions to target alcohol consumption that are both theory-driven and evidence-based.

References

Ajzen, I. (1991). The theory of planned behavior. *Organizational Behavior and Human Decision Processes, 50*(2), 179–211. https://doi.org/10.1016/0749-5978(91)90020-T

Avishai-Yitshak, A., & Sheeran, P. (2016). Implicit processes and health behavior change. In K. Sweeny & M. Robbins (Eds.), *Wiley Encyclopedia of health psychology*. New York, NY: Wiley.

Baumeister, R. F., & Heatherton, T. F. (1996). Self-regulation failure: An overview. *Psychological Inquiry, 7*(1), 1–15. https://doi.org/10.1207/s15327965pli0701_1

Blanton, H., Vanden Eijnden, R., Buunk, B. P., Gibbons, F. X., Gerrard, M., & Bakker, A. (2001). Accentuate the negative: Social images in the prediction and promotion of condom use. *Journal of Applied Social Psychology, 31*(2), 274–295. https://doi.org/10.1111/j.1559-1816.2001.tb00197.x

Boyer, T. W. (2006). The development of risk-taking: A multi-perspective review. *Developmental Review, 26*(3), 291–345. https://doi.org/10.1016/j.dr.2006.05.002

Brody, G. H., Chen, Y. F., Kogan, S. M., Murry, V. M., & Brown, A. C. (2010). Long-term effects of the strong African American families program on youths' alcohol use. *Journal of Consulting and Clinical Psychology, 78*(2), 281–285. https://doi.org/10.1037/a0018552

Brody, G. H., Murry, V. M., Gerrard, M., Gibbons, F. X., Molgaard, V., McNair, L., … Neubaum-Carlan, E. (2004). The strong African American families program: Translating research into prevention programming. *Child Development, 75*(3), 900–917. https://doi.org/10.1111/j.1467-8624.2004.00713.x

Cleveland, M. J., Turrisi, R., Gibbons, F. X., Gerrard, M., & Marzell, M. (2018). The effects of mothers' protective parenting and alcohol use on emerging adults' alcohol use: Testing indirect effects through prototype favorability among African American youth. *Alcoholism-Clinical and Experimental Research, 42*(7), 1291–1303. https://doi.org/10.1111/acer.13775

Cohen, J. (1992). A power primer. *Psychological Bulletin, 112*, 155–159. https://doi.org/10.1037/0033-2909.112.1.155

Comello, M. L. G., & Slater, M. D. (2011). Effects of adverts from a drug and alcohol prevention campaign on willingness to engage in alcohol-related risky behaviors. *Journal of Health Psychology, 16*(8). https://doi.org/10.1177/1359105311406153

Crossley, M. L. (2001). Rethinking psychological approaches towards health promotion. *Psychology & Health, 16*(2), 161–177. https://doi.org/10.1080/08870440108405497

Davies, E. L. (2016). Feasibility of the prototype willingness model as the basis for school-delivered alcohol misuse prevention: A qualitative think aloud study to explore acceptability of 'The Alcohol Smart Quiz' with adolescents and teachers. *Journal of Health Psychology.* https://doi.org/10.1177/1359105316648481

Davies, E. L. (2019). Similarity to prototypical heavy drinkers and non-drinkers predicts AUDIT-C and risky drinking in young adults: Prospective study. *Psychology & Health*, 1–19. https://doi.org/10.1080/08870446.2018.1532510

Davies, E. L., Martin, J., & Foxcroft, D. R. (2013). Young people talking about alcohol: Focus groups exploring constructs in the prototype willingness model. *Drugs: Education, Prevention and Policy, 20*(4), 269–277. https://doi.org/10.3109/09687637.2012.726662

Davies, E. L., Martin, J., & Foxcroft, D. R. (2015). Development and acceptability of a co-produced online intervention to prevent alcohol misuse in adolescents: A think aloud study. *JMIR Human Factors, 2*(2), e13. https://doi.org/10.2196/humanfactors.4452

Davies, E. L., Martin, J., & Foxcroft, D. R. (2016). Development of an adolescent alcohol misuse intervention based on the prototype willingness model: A Delphi study. *Health Education, 116*(3). https://doi.org/10.1108/HE-01-2015-0006

Davies, E. L., Paltoglou, A. E., & Foxcroft, D. R. (2017). Implicit alcohol attitudes predict drinking behaviour over and above intentions and willingness in young adults but willingness is more important in adolescents: Implications for the prototype willingness model. *British Journal of Health Psychology, 22*(2), 238–253. https://doi.org/10.1111/bjhp.12225

Deutsch, R., & Strack, F. (2020). Changing behavior using the reflective-impulsive model. In M. Hagger, L. D. Cameron, K. Hamilton, N. Hankonen, & T. Lintonen (Eds.), *Handbook of behavior change* (pp. 164–177). New York, NY: Cambridge University Press.

Dillard, A. J., Ferrer, R. A., Bulthuis, K. R. K., & Klein, W. M. P. (2018). Positive excessive drinker prototypes predict greater drinking and alcohol problems. *British Journal of Health Psychology, 23*(4), 1000–1020. https://doi.org/10.1111/bjhp.12335

Evans, J. S. B. T., & Stanovich, K. E. (2013). Dual-process theories of higher cognition: Advancing the debate. *Perspectives on Psychological Science, 8*(3), 223–241. https://doi.org/10.1177/1745691612460685

Fairlie, A. M., Cadigan, J. M., Patrick, M. E., Larimer, M. E., & Lee, C. M. (2019). Unplanned heavy episodic and high-intensity drinking: Daily-level associations with mood, context, and negative consequences. *Journal of Studies on Alcohol and Drugs, 80*(3), 331–339. https://doi.org/10.15288/jsad.2019.80.331

Fishbein, M. (2008). A reasoned action approach to health promotion. *Medical Decision Making, 28*(6), 834–844. https://doi.org/10.1177/0272989x08326092

Fishbein, M., & Ajzen, I. (1975). *Belief, attitude, intention and behavior: An introduction to theory and research*. Reading, MA: Addison-Wesley.

Fishbein, M., Triandis, H. C., Kanfer, F. H., Becker, M., Middlestadt, S. E., & Eichler, A. (2001). Factors influencing behavior and behavior change. In A. Baum, T. A. Revenson, & J. E. Singer (Eds.), *Handbook of health psychology* (pp. 3–17). Mahwah, NJ: Lawrence Erlbaum.

Friese, M., Hofmann, W., & Wiers, R. W. (2011). On taming horses and strengthening riders: Recent developments in research on interventions to improve self-control in health behaviors. *Self and Identity, 10*(3), 336–351. https://doi.org/10.1080/15298868.2010.536417

Gerrard, M., Gibbons, F. X., Brody, G. H., Murry, V. M., Cleveland, M. J., & Wills, T. A. (2006). A theory-based dual-focus alcohol intervention for preadolescents: The strong African American families program. *Psychology of Addictive Behaviors, 20*(2), 185–195. https://doi.org/10.1037/0893-164x.20.2.185

Gerrard, M., Gibbons, F. X., Houlihan, A. E., Stock, M. L., & Pomery, E. A. (2008). A dual-process approach to health risk decision making: The prototype willingness model. *Developmental Review, 28*(1), 29–61. https://doi.org/10.1016/j.dr.2007.10.001

Gerrard, M., Gibbons, F. X., Reis-Bergan, M., Trudeau, L., Vande Lune, L. S., & Buunk, B. (2002). Inhibitory effects of drinker and nondrinker prototypes on adolescent alcohol consumption. *Health Psychology, 21*(6), 601–609. https://doi.org/10.1037//0278-6133.21.6.601

Gibbons, F. X., & Gerrard, M. (1995). Predicting young-adults health risk behavior. *Journal of Personality and Social Psychology, 69*(3), 505–517. https://doi.org/10.1037/0022-3514.69.3.505

Gibbons, F. X., & Gerrard, M. (2016). Reactions to the meta-analyses of the prototype willingness model. *Health Psychology Review, 10*(1), 44–46. https://doi.org/10.1080/17437199.2015.1116020

Gibbons, F. X., Gerrard, M., & Lane, D. J. (2003). A social reaction model of adolesc ent health risk. In J. Sulls & K. A. Wallston (Eds.), *Social psychological foundations of health and illness* (pp. 107–136). Oxford, UK: Blackwell.

Gibbons, F. X., Gerrard, M., Ouellette, J. A., & Burzette, R. (1998). Cognitive antecedents to adolescent health risk: Discriminating between behavioral intention and behavioral willingness. *Psychology & Health, 13*(2), 319–339.

Gibbons, F. X., Gerrard, M., Ouellette, J. A., & Burzette, R. (2000). Discriminating between behavioural intention and behavioural willingness: Cognitive antecedents to adolescent health risk. In P. Norman, C. Abrabam, & M. Conner (Eds.), *Understanding and changing health behaviour: From health beliefs to self-regulation* (pp. 137–161). Amsterdam, Netherlands: Harwood Academic.

Gibbons, F. X., Helweg-Larsen, M., & Gerrard, M. (1995). Prevalence estimates an adolescent risk behaviour – Cross-cultural differences in social-influence. *Journal of Applied Psychology, 80*(1), 107–121. https://doi.org/10.1037/0021-9010.80.1.107

Gibbons, F. X., Kingsbury, J. H., Gerrard, M., & Wills, T. A. (2011). Two ways of thinking about dual processing: A response to Hofmann, Friese and Wiers (2008). *Health Psychology Review, 5*(2), 158–161. https://doi.org/10.1080/17437199.2010.541823

Goodall, C. E., & Slater, M. D. (2010). Automatically activated attitudes as mechanisms for message effects: The case of alcohol advertisements. *Communication Research, 37*(5), 620–643. https://doi.org/10.1177/0093650210374011

Greenwald, A. G., McGhee, D. E., & Schwartz, J. L. K. (1998). Measuring individual differences in implicit cognition: The implicit association test. *Journal of Personality and Social Psychology, 74*(6), 1464–1480. https://doi.org/10.1037/0022-3514.74.6.1464

Hagger, M., & Hamilton, K. (2020). Changing behavior using integrated theories. In M. Hagger, L. D. Cameron, K. Hamilton, N. Hankonen, & T. Lintonen (Eds.), *The handbook of behavior change* (pp. 208–224). New York, NY: Cambridge University Press.

Hall, P. A., & Fong, G. T. (2007). Temporal self-regulation theory: A model for individual health behavior. *Health Psychology Review, 1*(1), 6–52. https://doi.org/10.1080/17437190701492437

Heron, K. E., & Smyth, J. M. (2010). Ecological momentary interventions: Incorporating mobile technology into psychosocial and health behaviour treatments. *British Journal of Health Psychology, 15*, 1–39. https://doi.org/10.1348/135910709x466063

Hoffman, W., Dohle, S., & Diel, K. (2020). Changing behavior using integrated self-control theory. In M. Hagger, L. D. Cameron, K. Hamilton, N. Hankonen, & T. Lintonen (Eds.), *Handbook of Behavior Change* (pp. 150–163). New York, NY: Cambridge University Press.

Hofmann, W., Friese, M., & Strack, F. (2009). Impulse and self-control from a dual-systems perspective. *Perspectives on Psychological Science, 4*(2), 162–176. https://doi.org/10.1111/j.1745-6924.2009.01116.x

Hofmann, W., Friese, M., & Wiers, R. W. (2008). Impulsive versus reflective influences on health behavior: A theoretical framework and empirical review. *Health Psychology Review, 2*(2), 111–137. https://doi.org/10.1080/17437190802617668

Hollands, G. J., Marteau, T. M., & Fletcher, P. C. (2016). Non-conscious processes in changing health-related behaviour: A conceptual analysis and framework. *Health Psychology Review*, 1–14. https://doi.org/10.1080/17437199.2015.1138093

Houben, K., Havermans, R. C., & Wiers, R. W. (2010). Learning to dislike alcohol: Conditioning negative implicit attitudes toward alcohol and its effect on drinking behavior. *Psychopharmacology, 211*(1), 79–86. https://doi.org/10.1007/s00213-010-1872-1

Hukkelberg, S. S., & Dykstra, J. L. (2009). Using the prototype/willingness model to predict smoking behaviour among Norwegian adolescents. *Addictive Behaviors, 34*(3), 270–276. https://doi.org/10.1016/j.addbeh.2008.10.024

Jaigarun, P., Corte, C., McCreary, L. L., Finnegan, L., Hughes, T. L., & Thorkildsen, T. (2018). Attributes of the drinker prototype among Thai adolescents. *Cogent Psychology, 5*(1), 1–10. https://doi.org/10.1080/23311908.2018.1502501

Kahneman, D. (2011). *Thinking, fast and slow*. London, UK: Penguin.

Kasprzyk, D., Montaño, D. E., & Fishbein, M. (1998). Application of an integrated Behavioral model to predict condom use: A prospective study among high HIV risk Groups1. *Journal of Applied Social Psychology, 28*(17), 1557–1583. https://doi.org/10.1111/j.1559-1816.1998.tb01690.x

Litt, D. M., Lewis, M. A., Fairlie, A. M., & Head-Corliss, M. K. (2018). An examination of the relative associations of prototype favorability, similarity, and their interaction with alcohol and alcohol-related risky sexual cognitions and behavior. *Emerging Adulthood*, 2167696818790827. https://doi.org/10.1177/2167696818790827

Marteau, T., Fletcher, P. C., Hollands, G. J., & Munafo, M. (2020). Changing behavior by changing environments. In M. Hagger, L. D. Cameron, K. Hamilton, N. Hankonen, & T. Lintonen (Eds.), *Handbook of behavior change*. New York, NY: Cambridge University Press.

Monk, R. L., Pennington, C. R., Campbell, C., Price, A., & Heim, D. (2016). Implicit alcohol-related expectancies and the effect of context. *Journal of Studies on Alcohol and Drugs, 77*(5), 819–827. https://doi.org/10.15288/jsad.2016.77.819

Ohtomo, S., Hirose, Y., & Midden, C. J. H. (2011). Cultural differences of a dual-motivation model on health risk behaviour. *Journal of Risk Research, 14*(1), 85–96. https://doi.org/10.1080/13669877.2010.503936

Orbell, S., & Sheeran, P. (1998). 'Inclined abstainers': A problem for predicting health-related behaviour. *British Journal of Social Psychology, 37*(2), 151–165. https://doi.org/10.1111/j.2044-8309.1998.tb01162.x

Ouellette, J. A., Gerrard, M., Gibbons, F. X., & Reis-Bergan, M. (1999). Parents, peers, and prototypes: Antecedents of adolescent alcohol expectancies, alcohol consumption, and alcohol-related life problems in rural youth. *Psychology of Addictive Behaviors, 13*(3), 183–197. https://doi.org/10.1037/0893-164X.13.3.183

Ouellette, J. A., & Wood, W. (1998). Habit and intention in everyday life: The multiple processes by which past behavior predicts future behavior. *Psychological Bulletin, 124*(1), 54–74. https://doi.org/10.1037/0033-2909.124.1.54

Pettigrew, S., Jongenelis, M. I., Pratt, I. S., Slevin, T., & Chikritzhs, T. (2017). Drinkers' identification with varying alcohol consumption prototypes. *Drug and Alcohol Review*, n/a-n/a. https://doi.org/10.1111/dar.12466

Pieters, S., van der Vorst, H., Engels, R., & Wiers, R. W. (2010). Implicit and explicit: Cognitions related to alcohol use in children. *Addictive Behaviors, 35*(5), 471–478. https://doi.org/10.1016/j.addbeh.2009.12.022

Pomery, E. A., Gibbons, F. X., Reis-Bergan, M., & Gerrard, M. (2009). From willingness to intention: Experience moderates the shift from reactive to reasoned behavior. *Personality and Social Psychology Bulletin, 35*(7), 894–908. https://doi.org/10.1177/0146167209335166

Prestwich, A., Sniehotta, F. F., Whittington, C., Dombrowski, S. U., Rogers, L., & Michie, S. (2014). Does theory influence the effectiveness of health behavior interventions? Meta-analysis. *Health Psychology, 33*(5), 465–474. https://doi.org/10.1037/a0032853

Ratliff, K. A., & Howell, J. L. (2015). Implicit Prototypes Predict Risky Sun Behavior. *Health Psychology, 34*(3), 231–242. https://doi.org/10.1037/hea0000117

Redford, L., Howell, J. L., Meijs, M. H. J., & Ratliff, K. A. (2016). Implicit and explicit evaluations of feminist prototypes predict feminist identity and behavior. *Group Processes and Intergroup Relations, Online first*, 1–16. https://doi.org/10.1177/1368430216630193

Reyna, V. F., & Brainerd, C. J. (1995). Fuzzy-trace theory – An interim synthesis. *Learning and Individual Differences, 7*(1), 1–75. https://doi.org/10.1016/1041-6080(95)90031-4

Rhodes, N., Loiewski, C., Potocki, B., & Ralston, R. (2017). Prototypes of drinkers and accessibility of injunctive norms predict college drinking. *Journal of Health Psychology.*, 1359105316683240. https://doi.org/10.1177/1359105316683240

Rhodes, R. E., & de Bruijn, G.-J. (2013). How big is the physical activity intention–behaviour gap? A meta-analysis using the action control framework. *British Journal of Health Psychology, 18*(2), 296–309. https://doi.org/10.1111/bjhp.12032

Rivis, A., Sheeran, P., & Armitage, C. J. (2006). Augmenting the theory of planned behaviour with the prototype/willingness model: Predictive validity of actor versus abstainer prototypes for adolescents' health-protective and health-risk intentions. *British Journal of Health Psychology, 11*, 483–500. https://doi.org/10.1348/135910705x70327

Sheeran, P. (2002). Intention-behavior relations: A conceptual and empirical review. In M. Hewstone & W. Stroebe (Eds.), *European review of social psychology* (Vol. 12, pp. 1–36). Chichester, UK: John Wiley & Sons.

Shiffman, S. (2009). Ecological momentary assessment (EMA) in studies of substance use. *Psychological Assessment, 21*(4), 486–497. https://doi.org/10.1037/a0017074

Slavish, D. C., Scaglione, N. M., Hultgren, B. A., & Turrisi, R. (2019). An ecological momentary assessment of affect, mental health symptoms, and decisions to drink among first-year college women: A pilot study. *Prevention Science, 20*(5), 753–764. https://doi.org/10.1007/s11121-018-0966-6

Spijkerman, R., Larsen, H., Gibbons, F. X., & Engels, R. (2010). Students' drinker prototypes and alcohol use in a naturalistic setting. *Alcoholism-Clinical and Experimental Research, 34*(1), 64–71. https://doi.org/10.1111/j.1530-0277.2009.01067.x

Strack, F., & Deutsch, R. (2004). Reflective and impulsive determinants of social behavior. *Personality and Social Psychology Review, 8*(3), 220–247. https://doi.org/10.1207/s15327957pspr0803_1

Teunissen, H. A., Spijkerman, R., Kuntsche, E., Engels, R. C. M. E., & Scholte, R. H. J. (2017). Cool or fool? The association between drinker prototypes and alcohol consumption using multiple time-point diary assessments in adolescent males. *Substance Use & Misuse, 52*(5), 656–665. https://doi.org/10.1080/10826084.2016.1253743

Thaler, R. H., & Sunstein, C. R. (2009). *Nudge: Improving decisions about health, wealth and happiness*. New York, NY: Penguin.

Thush, C., & Wiers, R. W. (2007). Explicit and implicit alcohol-related cognitions and the prediction of future drinking in adolescents. *Addictive Behaviors, 32*(7), 1367–1383. https://doi.org/10.1016/j.addbeh.2006.09.011

Thush, C., Wiers, R. W., Ames, S. L., Grenard, J. L., Sussman, S., & Stacy, A. W. (2007). Apples and oranges? Comparing indirect measures of alcohol-related cognition predicting alcohol use in at-risk adolescents. *Psychology of Addictive Behaviors, 21*(4), 587–591. https://doi.org/10.1037/0893-164x.21.4.587

Todd, J., Kothe, E., Mullan, B., & Monds, L. (2016). Reasoned versus reactive prediction of behaviour: A meta-analysis of the prototype willingness model. *Health Psychology Review, 10*(1), 1–24. https://doi.org/10.1080/17437199.2014.922895

Todd, J., & Mullan, B. (2011). Using the theory of planned behaviour and prototype willingness model to target binge drinking in female undergraduate university students. *Addictive Behaviors, 36*(10), 980–986. https://doi.org/10.1016/j.addbeh.2011.05.010

Todd, J., & van Lettow, B. (2016). A closer look at prototypes: Similarity, favourability, and the prototype willingness model. A response to the commentary of Gibbons and Gerrard. *Health Psychology Review, 10*(1), 47–49. https://doi.org/10.1080/17437199.2016.1138872

van Lettow, B., de Vries, H., Burdorf, A., Boon, B., & van Empelen, P. (2015). Drinker prototype alteration and cue reminders as strategies in a tailored web-based intervention reducing adults' alcohol consumption: Randomized controlled trial. *Journal of Medical Internet Research, 17*(2), 3–20. https://doi.org/10.2196/jmir.3551

van Lettow, B., de Vries, H., Burdorf, A., & van Empelen, P. (2016). Quantifying the strength of the associations of prototype perceptions with behaviour, behavioural willingness and intentions: A meta-analysis. *Health Psychology Review, 10*(1), 25–43. https://doi.org/10.1080/17437199.2014.941997

van Lettow, B., Vermunt, J. K., de Vries, H., Burdorf, A., & van Empele, P. (2013). Clustering of drinker prototype characteristics: What characterizes the typical drinker? *British Journal of Psychology, 104*(3), 382–389. https://doi.org/10.1111/bjop.12000

Whitaker, L., Petroczi, A., Backhouse, S. H., Long, J., & Nepusz, T. (2016). The role of the self in assessing doping cognition: Implicit and explicit measures of athletes' doping-related prototype perceptions. *Psychology of Sport and Exercise, 24*, 159–167. https://doi.org/10.1016/j.psychsport.2016.02.005

Yarmush, D. E., Manchery, L., Luehring-Jones, P., & Erblich, J. (2016). Gender and impulsivity: Effects on cue-induced alcohol craving. *Alcoholism: Clinical and Experimental Research, 40*(5), 1052–1057. https://doi.org/10.1111/acer.13030

4

Psychological Predictors of Alcohol Consumption

Richard Cooke and Joel Crawford

Introduction

Numerous psychological constructs have been proposed to predict alcohol consumption. Identification of these predictors is aimed at providing a better understanding of drinking behaviour in theoretical terms but also from an applied perspective; identifying constructs that predict consumption can inform the development of effective interventions to reduce the prevalence of heavy episodic drinking (HED; see Chap. 1) and reduce experience of the negative health and social consequences that can follow. To date, the literature describing the predictive effects of psychological constructs on alcohol consumption has usually been framed in the context of theoretical accounts of consumption, such as those covered in Chaps. 2 and 3. As a result, it can be challenging to evaluate effects of specific constructs on consumption. The present chapter aims to accomplish this task. It begins by outlining reasons for focusing on psychological constructs as predictors of consumption before defining constructs and reviewing the available evidence. The chapter goes on

R. Cooke (✉)
Department of Psychology, University of Liverpool, Liverpool, UK

Liverpool Centre for Alcohol Research, Liverpool, UK
e-mail: cooker4@liverpool.ac.uk

J. Crawford
Department of Psychology, University of Liverpool, Liverpool, UK
e-mail: j.crawford3@liverpool.ac.uk

R. Cooke et al. (eds.), *The Palgrave Handbook of Psychological Perspectives on Alcohol Consumption*, https://doi.org/10.1007/978-3-030-66941-6_4

to summarise the evidence for these constructs, before outlining a number of common methodological issues with studies testing predictive effects. The chapter concludes with suggestions for future research.

Why Focus on Psychological Constructs as Predictors of Alcohol Consumption?

Factors used to predict alcohol consumption can be classified on various continua, for example, from stable to unstable (see Fig. 4.1). Stable (fixed) factors, including demographic factors like ethnic group, gender, or nationality, do not change over time. Further along this continuum can be found factors such as habits and personality traits, for example, impulsivity or sensation seeking (see Chap. 5), that can be considered relatively stable; habits develop in response to repeated experiences of behavioural performance, while traits develop over time. At the other end of this continuum are unstable (variable) factors like the psychological constructs covered in this chapter, for example, drinking intentions, drinking motives, drinking refusal self-efficacy, and willingness.

Factors can also be considered on a continua from distal to proximal (see Fig. 4.1). Distal factors are assumed to exert less influence on alcohol consumption relative to proximal factors; when both types of factors are entered into a regression model to predict drinking behaviour, we should expect that proximal factors will be significant, whereas distal factors are expected to be

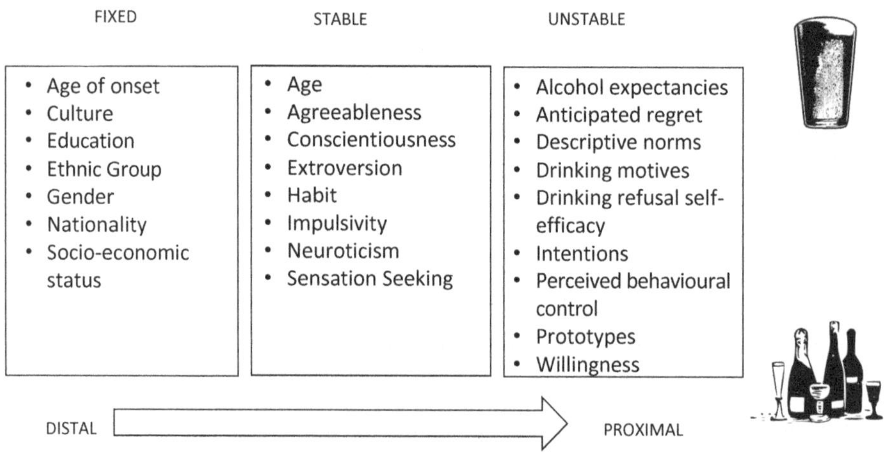

Fig. 4.1 Predictive factors on continua from fixed to unstable and distal to proximal

non-significant. This claim has been demonstrated in studies where demographic factors and psychological constructs are entered into a regression model; in many cases, demographic factors cease to predict consumption, whereas psychological constructs emerge as significant predictors (Godin et al., 2010; Hagger & Hamilton, 2020).

The stability/instability of a factor is thought to covary with its status as a distal/proximal predictor of consumption. Hence, stable (fixed) factors are considered to act as distal influences on consumption—they are assumed to have relatively weak predictive utility once the effects of other variables are controlled for. Conversely, unstable (variable) factors are usually labelled as proximal influences on behaviour, meaning they are assumed to retain predictive utility even after controlling for the effects of distal factors. According to different theoretical accounts, drinking intentions, drinking motives, drinking refusal self-efficacy, and willingness have all been posited to be the *most* proximal determinant(s) of consumption, that is, the most important factor when predicting drinking (see Chap. 2).

Why should proximal factors provide better prediction of alcohol consumption? One reason is that because they are relatively unstable (variable) they reflect individuals' current circumstances, for example, having more or less responsibility, more or less income, dealing with health issues (or not), in a manner that is not possible with fixed or more stable factors. This responsiveness is important because alcohol consumption is not always stable over time (Bewick et al., 2008; Ferrer, Dillard, & Klein, 2011; Giese, Stok, & Renner, 2019; Vik, Cellucci, & Ivers, 2003). Thus, the capacity of psychological constructs to reflect the situation that individuals' currently find themselves in should allow them to be more closely linked to current consumption patterns.

In the next section, the evidence that frequently used psychological constructs predict alcohol consumption is summarised. Most of the constructs come from theories described in Chaps. 2 and 3. However, as the aim of the present chapter is to review the evidence for individual constructs, the focus is on specific constructs rather than theories and models per se (see Chaps. 2 and 3 for discussion of theories). All of the constructs included in this chapter have been shown to have non-trivial correlations with consumption in multiple studies and most have been shown to have independent predictive effects on drinking when included in regression models that control for the effects of other constructs.

Psychological Constructs Proposed to Predict Alcohol Consumption

Alcohol Expectancies

Alcohol expectancies are an alcohol-specific form of outcome expectancies, as described in Bandura's (1977) Social Cognitive Theory. Alcohol expectancies are people's beliefs about how an outcome—in this case alcohol consumption—will affect them (e.g., "My alcohol consumption negatively affects my school grades"). Some individuals believe that alcohol consumption has positive effects such as reducing their tension levels (Marlatt, 1987) or increasing their self-confidence (Niaura et al., 1988). Other individuals believe that consumption has negative consequences such as impairing their thoughts or heightening their emotional distress. Alcohol expectancies are usually assessed using validated questionnaires (Leigh & Stacy, 1993; Young & Oei, 1990).

Early studies testing the predictive effects of alcohol expectancies (Brown, 1985; Christiansen & Goldman, 1983; Oei, Foley, & Young, 1990) did not typically measure other psychological constructs, meaning their unique effect independent of other psychological constructs could not be established. However, later studies tested the predictive utility of alcohol expectancies in conjunction with other psychological constructs in order to examine their independent effects. For example, Baldwin, Oei, and Young (1993) compared prediction of frequency and quantity of alcohol consumption in a sample of Australian university students using their alcohol expectancies and drinking refusal self-efficacy, that is, an individual's stated confidence in their ability refuse drinking alcohol, such as declining offers of drinks (see below). Results showed that alcohol expectancies predicted quantity of consumption while drinking refusal self-efficacy predicted frequency of consumption. Later research found that alcohol expectancies do not always predict consumption when controlling for the effects of other constructs. For example, Oei and Jardim (2007) found that alcohol expectancies did not predict the consumption in a sample of Asian Australian university students, although they did predict white Australian students' drinking. Overall, results show that alcohol expectancies do not always predict consumption.

Anticipated Regret

Anticipated regret is the expectation that regret, the negative emotion experienced when one recognises their present situation would be different had they taken a different course of action, will be experienced if a behaviour is performed (Richard, van der Pligt, & de Vries, 1995). People can experience such regret from proposed *actions* (i.e., engaging in HED) and *inactions* (i.e., abstaining from HED; see Brewer, DeFrank, & Gilkey, 2016, for a review). In predictive studies, regret is usually measured using one or two Likert scale items.

Brewer et al.'s (2016) meta-analysis estimated that anticipated regret has a small-sized average relationship ($r_+ = 0.29$) with health behaviours across studies. In the alcohol literature, most researchers have focused on *action* anticipated regret (e.g., Cooke, Sniehotta, & Schuz, 2007). While action anticipated regret is typically significantly correlated with consumption, when it is entered into a regression model alongside other constructs, it seldom accounts for unique variance in consumption (Cooke et al., 2007; Jones, Crawford, Rose, Christiansen, & Cooke, 2020). To date, Riordan, Conner, Flett, and Scarf (2015) conducted the only study to have examined the relationship between consumption and *inaction* anticipated regret, also known as 'the fear of missing out.' They found inaction anticipated regret had a significant relationship with quantity of consumption in a single session in a sample of New Zealand university students but did not correlate with either weekly alcohol consumption or frequency of consumption. Recent qualitative work suggests that inaction anticipated regret may be an important driver of alcohol consumption, especially during the early weeks of university life, as newly enrolled students are highly focused on forming new social relationships (Crawford, Jones, Rose, & Cooke, 2020). At present, there is little evidence that anticipated regret predicts consumption.

Descriptive Norms

Descriptive norms reflect individuals' perceptions of other people's behaviour, such as friends and family, for example, "How many of your friends engage in HED?" They are differentiated from injunctive (subjective) norms (see Chap. 2) by their focus on others' *behaviour* as opposed to others' perceptions of *your* behaviour. For example, asking "Do your friends engage in HED?" measures descriptive norms, whereas asking "Do your friends approve of you engaging in HED?" measures injunctive norms (Manning, 2009). Descriptive norms capture the extent to which salient others' typical behaviour reflect a norm with which an individual is more likely to comply because the views of salient others are probably highly influential. Questionnaire measures of descriptive norms are usually measured using two Likert scale items. In some studies, items ask about men and women separately (Campo et al., 2003; Cooke et al., 2007); in others, items ask about frequency and quantity of peers' consumption (Atwell et al., 2011).

Manning's (2009) meta-analysis reported descriptive norms had a medium-sized average relationship ($r_+ = 0.34$) with behaviour across studies. In the alcohol literature, the most common application of descriptive norms is to inform interventions based on the 'social norms' approach (Perkins & Berkowitz, 1986, see Chap. 20), with few studies assessing the size of the relationship between descriptive norms and consumption. A study by Campo et al. (2003) showed that university students who reported higher descriptive norms for drinking were more likely to report drinking themselves. However, this study did not measure other variables shown to predict drinking, and other studies have found that descriptive norms do not predict consumption when entered into regression models alongside other constructs (Cooke et al., 2007; Elliott & Ainsworth, 2012; Zhang et al., 2018). Existing evidence suggests that descriptive norms do not consistently predict consumption.

Drinking Motives

Drinking motives are reasons reported by individuals for why they drink alcohol, predicated on the premise that motives likely determine behaviour. Research on these variables is based on Cox and Klinger's (1988) incentive motivation model and in particular the contention that all substance use behaviours can be categorised on two dimensions. First, is a substance used to achieve an approach goal (i.e., feel more confident) or to achieve an avoidance goal (i.e., stop feeling stressed)? These can be thought of as positive and negative motives for substance use. Second, are the outcomes sought from substance use done for internal or external reasons (e.g., "Am I drinking because I want to or am I drinking in response to other people?"). Crossing these two dimensions provides four drinking motives: conformity (negative, external); coping (negative, internal); enhancement (positive, internal); and social (positive, external). Cooper's (1994) Drinking Motives Questionnaire-Revised is a validated scale used to assess these motives (Cooper, 1994). More recently, a short form of this questionnaire has been developed and validated (Kuntsche & Kuntsche, 2009).

Cooper, Kuntsche, Levitt, Barber, and Wolf's (2015) recent review of the drinking motives literature showed that enhancement motives had a medium-sized *sample-weighted* relationship with consumption. Social and coping motives also had medium-sized sample-weighted relationships with consumption, while conformity motives had a small-sized sample-weighted relationship with consumption. Cooper et al. noted that conformity motives are the least strongly endorsed motive for drinking, which might explain the small relationship. The authors also reported *sample-weighted* beta coefficients for each motive as a predictor of consumption in models that controlled for the effects of the other three motives. Results showed that enhancement motives were the strongest, and conformity motives the weakest, predictors of consumption when the effects of other motives were controlled for. There are a number of limitations with this review (see below) with one being that most of the included studies used cross-sectional designs (see Chap. 2, for more on this issue), limiting inferences about predicting future consumption using motives. Nevertheless, other studies using prospective designs have shown enhancement motives predict consumption (Kuntsche & Cooper, 2010) and coping and enhancement motives have been shown to predict consumption 15 years later (Cooper et al., 2008). In sum, enhancement motives appear to be a significant predictor of consumption but the evidence for the other motives as predictors of consumption is less clear cut.

Drinking Refusal Self-Efficacy

Drinking refusal self-efficacy (Oei & Baldwin, 1994) is the confidence one possesses that they can refuse the offer of an alcoholic drink. Higher scores indicate greater confidence in refusing an alcoholic drink which means there should be a negative relationship with consumption. Several questionnaires have been developed to tap drinking refusal self-efficacy, such as the Drinking Refusal Self-Efficacy Questionnaire-Revised (Oei, Hasking, & Young, 2005). The items can either be summed into an overall scale or used as three subscales representing emotional relief (e.g., "when I am angry"), opportunistic drinking (e.g., "when I am watching TV"), and social pressure (e.g., "when my friends are drinking").

In general, research has shown that drinking refusal self-efficacy has a medium-sized negative correlation with consumption (Ehret, Ghaidarov, & LaBrie, 2013; Foster, Dukes, & Sartor, 2016; Lee, Oei, & Greeley, 1999; Morawska & Oei, 2005; Oei & Jardim, 2007; Oh & Kim, 2014). Beyond these results, there is also evidence that it can predict consumption. Oei and Jardim (2007) reported that in a sample of Australian university students, separated into Asian and white sub-groups, overall drinking refusal self-efficacy score predicted consumption in both groups. Relatedly, Oh and Kim (2014) showed the three drinking refusal self-efficacy sub-scales all predicted drinking frequency in a sample of Korean university students and that the social pressure and emotional relief sub-scales also predicted drinking volume. It should be noted that no other psychological constructs were included in these analyses. Finally, Foster et al. (2016) compared prediction of drinks consumed per week by alcohol expectancies, drinking refusal self-efficacy, and intentions (see next section). They found that drinking refusal self-efficacy and intentions both predicted weekly drinking, while alcohol expectancies did not. Overall, results suggest that drinking refusal self-efficacy may predict consumption even after controlling for the effects of other variables. More tests of this claim are required.

Intentions

An individual's intentions are their plan to perform a given behaviour (e.g., "I intend to engage in HED), and it is assumed that the stronger one's intentions are the more likely behavioural performance will follow (Ajzen, 1991). Researchers usually measure intentions using multiple Likert scale items. In the alcohol literature, intentions have been shown to have large correlations with alcohol consumption. Two meta-analyses (Cooke, Dahdah, Norman, & French, 2016; Todd, Kothe, Mullan, & Monds, 2016) independently reported that intentions had large-sized averaged relationships with consumption. Primary studies typically report that intentions prospectively predict consumption when tested alongside additional constructs such as beliefs, attitudes, and motives (French & Cooke, 2012; Norman, 2011; Norman & Conner, 2006; Norman, Conner, & Stride, 2012).

A recent longitudinal experience-sampling study by Labhart, Anderson, and Kuntsche (2017) provides a more ecologically valid test of the intention-alcohol consumption relationship. They sent prompts to participants' smartphones to assess their drinking intentions at 5 pm and then sent further prompts to ask participants to report their alcohol consumption at 8 pm that evening and 10 am the next day. Labhart et al. reported large-sized correlations between intentions and consumption for men ($r = 0.70$) and women ($r = 0.54$). This study confirms the predictive utility of intentions, while highlighting the use of technology to access reports of consumption in real time (see Chaps. 8 and 9, for more on this topic).

A small number of studies have examined prediction of alcohol consumption by intentions to limit or avoid consumption. These studies provide evidence that intentions to limit consumption also predict consumption, albeit in a negative manner. For example, Cooke et al. (2007) showed that intentions to limit HED significantly predicted consumption (i.e., higher intentions to *limit* drinking were associated with lower reported drinking). In sum, intentions can be considered one of the best psychological predictors of consumption.

Perceived Behavioural Control

Perceived behavioural control is a variable that reflects perceptions of internal and external control over behavioural performance. The internal aspects of perceived behavioural control are similar to Bandura's (1977) construct self-efficacy (i.e., "I am confident I can engage in HED"), and researchers have measured self-efficacy alongside perceived behavioural control in several studies (Norman, Armitage, & Quigley, 2007; Norman & Conner, 2006). The external aspect of perceived behavioural control is intended to capture control over behavioural performance (i.e., "HED is completely under my control") and can be thought of as perceived control. A discussion of the different conceptions of perceived behavioural control in the context of alcohol consumption can be found in Cooke et al. (2016). Perceived behavioural control is usually measured using between two and six Likert scale items.

Cooke et al.'s (2016) meta-analysis synthesised evidence for perceived behavioural control as a correlate of alcohol consumption. Due to heterogeneity in measurement of perceived behavioural control, results were presented for three constructs: perceived behavioural control (as composed of items measuring self-efficacy and perceived control, e.g., Conner, Warren, Close, & Sparks, 1999); self-efficacy (items only measuring self-efficacy, e.g., Norman & Conner, 2006); and perceived control (items only measuring perceived control, e.g., Elliott & Ainsworth, 2012). Self-efficacy had a positive, medium-sized, average correlation ($r+ = .41$) with self-reported consumption; individuals who were more confident reported drinking more alcohol. In contrast, there was a negative, null, correlation between consumption and perceived behavioural control ($r+ = -.05$) and a negative, small-sized, correlation between consumption and perceived control ($r+ = -13$). Examining predictive results from primary studies shows that when the effects of other psychological constructs are controlled for, perceived behavioural control rarely predicts consumption (Elliott & Ainsworth, 2012; Norman, 2011; Norman & Conner, 2006) although Norman et al. (2012) did report a significant predictive effect. These results suggest that perceived behavioural control does not reliably predict consumption.

Prototype Evaluation and Prototype Similarity

Prototypes represent people's mental representations or 'image' of a typical binge drinker or abstinent individual. There are two prototype constructs: prototype evaluation (i.e., one's positive or negative evaluation of the image) and prototype similarity (i.e., one's view of oneself as similar or dissimilar to the image). Prototypes are typically assessed using visual analogue scales, where participants are asked to report agreement on a 100-point scale.

Research has shown that both kinds of prototypes can predict alcohol consumption (Davies, 2019; Norman et al., 2007; Rivis & Sheeran, 2013). For example, Rivis and Sheeran (2013) found prototype evaluation predicted consumption in a sample of English university students after controlling for the effects of intentions and perceived behavioural control, although they could not replicate this effect in a second study. Alternatively, Norman et al. (2007) found that prototype similarity predicted consumption after controlling for intentions and self-efficacy in a sample of English university students.

Two recent meta-analyses (Todd et al., 2016; van Lettow, de Vries, Burdorf, & van Empelen, 2016) provide evidence that prototypes are associated with consumption. Todd et al. (2016) reported a medium-sized average correlation ($r+$ = 0.38) between prototypes and consumption. van Lettow et al. (2016) reported that prototype evaluation ($r+$ = 0.22) and prototype similarity ($r+$ = 0.26) both had small-sized average correlations with health behaviours. Each meta-analysis has limitations: van Lettow et al.'s results were not specifically on alcohol consumption, while Todd et al. combined results across both prototype variables to ensure sufficient numbers of effect sizes to conduct the analysis.

One reason for this lack of studies is that most studies measuring prototypes are designed to test the proposals of Gibbons and Gerrard's (1995) Prototype Willingness Model (see Chap. 3), which states that the effects of prototypes on behaviour are mediated by willingness (see next section). As a result, researchers using this model to predict consumption have not always reported the correlation between prototypes and consumption. This means it is uncertain how consistent the effects of prototypes are. Based on the studies that have tested the direct effect of prototypes on consumption, they appear to be worthy of inclusion in future tests of psychological constructs of drinking.

Willingness

Willingness aims to capture the fact that while young people may not intend to engage in risky behaviours, they might be *willing* to do so given the right circumstances. For example, consider a teenager going to a house party with the firm intention of drinking only non-alcoholic beverages. When they arrive, they find that everyone else is drinking and decide to go with the flow and drink alcoholic beverages. Researchers measure willingness by asking participants to imagine how they would react when facing such scenarios.

Todd et al.'s (2016) meta-analysis reported a large-sized sample-weighted relationship between willingness and consumption ($r+ = .54$). Studies typically find that willingness predicts consumption even in the presence of competitor constructs (Davies, 2019; Davies, Paltoglou, & Foxcroft, 2017; Zimmermann & Sieverding, 2011). For example, Davies et al. (2017) reported that willingness and intentions both predicted consumption in a sample of adolescents, while Zimmermann and Sieverding (2011) found that willingness added to the prediction of men's alcohol consumption after controlling for the effects of intentions. Nevertheless, both studies also noted that willingness did not predict consumption for all populations; Davies et al. found willingness did not predict consumption in a majority female sample of university students and, similarly, Zimmermann and Sieverding found that willingness did not predict women's alcohol consumption. It should also be noted that willingness and intentions are often highly correlated (see below). In sum, willingness appears to be able to predict consumption in samples that typically consume more alcohol (i.e., adolescents, men) but is less effective at predicting consumption among samples that tend to consume less alcohol (i.e., women; for more see Chap. 3).

Summary of Evidence for Psychological Constructs of Alcohol Consumption

Table 4.1 summarises the correlations between consumption and each of the psychological constructs covered in this chapter. Consumption has large-sized relationships with intentions and willingness, medium-sized relationships with enhancement motives, social motives, and prototypes, while other constructs show more variability in the size of the correlations. It should be noted that the quality of evidence for each predictor varies considerably. For some constructs, there are meta-analyses that provide precise estimates of the

Table 4.1 Correlations reported between psychological constructs and alcohol consumption

Variable	Example papers	Correlation with alcohol consumption
Anticipated regret	Cooke et al. (2007); Riordan et al. (2015)	Range = 0.15 to 0.34
Alcohol expectancies	Foster et al. (2016); Lee et al. (1999)	Negative expectancies range = 0.14 to 0.51 Positive expectancies range = 0.08 to 0.27
Descriptive norms	Cooke et al. (2007); Elliott and Ainsworth (2012)	Range = 0.19 to 0.44
Drinking motives	Atwell et al. (2011); Studer et al. (2014)	Coping weighted mean = 0.30 Conformity weighted mean = 0.09 Enhancement weighted mean = 0.49 Social weighted mean = 0.42
Drinking refusal self-efficacy	Foster et al. (2016); Lee et al. (1999)	Range = −0.27 to −0.49
Intentions	French and Cooke (2012); Norman and Conner (2006)	Sample-weighted average correlations = 0.54 and 0.64
Perceived behavioural control	Norman and Conner (2006); Norman et al. (2007)	Sample-weighted average correlation = −0.05
Prototypes	Norman et al. (2007); Zimmermann and Sieverding (2011)	Sample-weighted average correlation = 0.38[a]
Willingness	Davies et al. (2017); Zimmermann and Sieverding (2011)	Sample-weighted average correlations = 0.54

Note. [a]Value reflects correlations between consumption and either prototype evaluation or prototype similarity

sample-weighted average correlation between the predictor and consumption across studies based on multiple studies. For other constructs, weighted effect sizes have been computed. For all other constructs, because such summary statistics are not available, the range of correlations is presented. Next, we critically evaluate the results for the constructs, acknowledging that it is challenging to compare results across constructs summarised in such different ways.

We begin our critical evaluation of the evidence for psychological constructs as predictors of alcohol consumption by reviewing the meta-analytic evidence reported in two meta-analyses (Cooke et al., 2016; Todd et al., 2016). In both meta-analyses, the relationship between intentions and consumption was found to be large in size, providing evidence that these variables are related to one another. In addition, path analyses reported by Todd et al. (2016) estimate intentions account for around 40% of the variance in consumption. Todd et al.'s meta-analysis also shows that consumption has a large-sized relationship with willingness and a medium-sized relationship with prototypes, while Cooke et al. report a null relationship between perceived behavioural control and consumption. Based on such results, researchers wanting to predict alcohol consumption should measure intentions, prototypes, and willingness.

Cooper et al.'s (2015) review of the drinking motives literature reports *sample-weighted* average correlations between consumption and each of the four motives as well as sample-weighted average beta values for studies that regressed consumption on models containing the four motives. Inspection of sample-weighted correlations shows that enhancement motives have the biggest relationship with consumption, followed by social and coping motives, but conformity motives do not appear to correlate with consumption. The beta values replicate this pattern while also showing that the effects are relatively small.

There are a number of limitations with Cooper et al.'s review which mean caution should be exercised in interpreting results. First, because the review was not reported systematically there is a possibility of selection bias regarding included studies. Second, the authors note that most studies used cross-sectional designs, meaning that researchers were 'predicting' something that had already happened. Despite concerns with the review, evidence from prospective studies (Cooper et al., 2008; Kuntsche & Cooper, 2010) corroborates the review's findings and researchers are encouraged to measure enhancement motives in future studies.

While the evidence base for the other motive variables as predictors of consumption is inconsistent at present, until studies are conducted that measure drinking motives alongside other variables consistently shown to predict consumption—for example, intentions, prototypes, and willingness—we will not know the true effect sizes for motives as predictors of consumption.

Summary statistics for the relationships between consumption and the other predictor variables covered in this chapter—anticipated regret, alcohol expectancies, descriptive norms, drinking refusal self-efficacy—are not available. Consequently, the only way to evaluate the claims that these variables are associated with consumption is to focus on correlation and regression results reported in primary studies. We begin by considering correlational evidence.

As Table 4.1 shows, correlations with consumption for these variables are mainly small-sized and vary between studies. Of this set of constructs, drinking refusal self-efficacy has the most consistent set of results, with mostly medium-sized correlations with consumption. Because there is also evidence that drinking refusal self-efficacy predicts consumption after controlling for other psychological constructs (Foster et al., 2016), we suggest that drinking refusal self-efficacy is worthy of further tests as a predictor of consumption.

At the present time, there is no evidence that alcohol expectancies, anticipated regret, or descriptive norms predict consumption after controlling for the effects of other psychological constructs. For example, Foster et al. (2016) found alcohol expectancies did not significantly predict consumption after controlling for the effects of drinking refusal self-efficacy and intentions. Similarly, Cooke et al. (2007) found that neither anticipated regret nor descriptive norms predicted consumption after the effects of intentions and other variables were controlled for. Given that meta-analyses, using data drawn from a range of behaviours, have found that the sample-weighted average correlations between behaviour and anticipated regret (Brewer et al., 2016), and descriptive norms (Manning, 2009), are small-sized and medium-sized, respectively, such findings should perhaps not be seen as too surprising.

Both variables appear to be distal rather than proximal predictors of drinking behaviour and might be better viewed as antecedent to constructs that have shown to possess stronger predictive effects, such as enhancement motives, intentions, prototypes, and/or willingness. Consistent with this idea, anticipated regret has been shown to predict intentions in some studies (Barratt & Cooke, 2018; Cooke et al., 2007). For example, Barratt and Cooke found that anticipated regret was the only predictor of English first year university students' intentions and that regret was one of three predictors of final year students' intentions. Conversely, studies have consistently shown that descriptive norms do not predict alcohol intentions (Cooke et al., 2007; Elliott & Ainsworth, 2012; Zhang et al., 2018), so, their effects on consumption might not be antecedent to other psychological constructs.

It is important to note, however, that showing alcohol expectancies, anticipated regret, or descriptive norms predict intentions in a regression model does not provide evidence that they have an indirect effect on consumption via intentions. Formal tests of mediation (Hayes, 2018; Preacher & Hayes, 2004) are required to establish this mechanism of action. Such tests would allow researchers to explore the idea that psychological constructs can affect consumption indirectly. For example, Davies (2019) tested the ability of intentions and willingness to mediate the relationship between six prototype measures and consumption. She found that while both variables mediated relationships between prototypes and consumption, the effect of intention was stronger than willingness for three of the six variables, suggesting intentions are a more effective mediator of these relationships than willingness (see Chap. 3).

Alternatively, researchers should also consider the possibility that psychological constructs moderate predictive relationships between other constructs and consumption. For instance, Oei and Jardim (2007) found in their sample of white Australian university students that those who reported low drinking refusal self-efficacy and high alcohol expectancies consumed more alcohol than students with low drinking refusal self-efficacy who held low alcohol expectancies; finding it hard to refuse the offer of an alcoholic drink only led to higher consumption *if* students also held positive expectancies about how alcohol would affect them. Such moderation tests tend to be restricted to control or background variables—Norman and Conner (2006) showed that past behaviour moderated the intention-behaviour relationship—but additional tests of moderation would be welcome. In the next section, we consider several methodological issues in research studies focused on predicting alcohol consumption. It is important to address these issues because they can undermine the generalisability of results.

Methodological Issues Concerning Predictive Research on Alcohol Consumption

Selective Testing of Variables

There are practical limits to the number of variables that can be measured in any given study. If participants are asked too many questions, there is risk they will fail to complete the study or neglect to respond with due care. However, if too few variables are measured in a study, or the set of measures is restricted in some way (e.g., selectively testing variables drawn from one theory), confirmation bias is possible; study findings may show that the *selected* set of variables predict drinking, but such results fail to rule out the possibility that other constructs also contribute to prediction of consumption. As Campo et al. (2003) note with regard to the social norms literature:

> few (studies) actually control for the effects of other variables that would allow for a better understanding of which variables actually are directly related to drinking behaviour. (Campo et al., 2003, p. 485)

An example of such selective testing of constructs is provided by Cooke et al. (2007), a study prospectively testing prediction of English university students' HED using several psychological predictors—anticipated regret, descriptive norms, intentions, perceived behavioural control—covered in this chapter. Students were asked to complete a survey containing measures of these constructs plus a measure of their past HED as a control variable. A regression model containing these variables showed that intentions and past HED were the only significant predictors of consumption. Thus, it was claimed that intentions predicted consumption after controlling for the effects of past HED and the other predictors.

Although a reasonable claim, it is unclear from this study if *unmeasured* variables might also have predicted HED either (i) alongside intentions and past consumption or (ii) in place of these variables. It is entirely possible that other variables, like drinking refusal self-efficacy, enhancement motives, prototypes, or willingness, would have predicted HED in this sample. Because they were not measured we do not know.

Unfortunately, selective testing of a small set of variables to predict alcohol consumption is seemingly the default way to conduct research in this field. Additionally, researchers apparently work without awareness of constructs from other models, as if these other variables do not exist. Such an approach can lead to claims such as "(drinking) motives provide the final common pathway to substance use through which influences of more distal variables are mediated" (Cooper et al., 2015, p. 32). Such a sweeping claim cannot be verified *until* researchers compare predictive effects of drinking motives against predictive effects for other variables, as well as conducting formal tests of mediation of the effects of other constructs by motives.

Cooke et al. (2021) provide one of the first studies to address the issue of selective testing in the prediction of alcohol consumption. They measured most of the variables covered in this chapter: alcohol expectancies, anticipated regret, descriptive norms, drinking refusal self-efficacy, drinking motives, intentions, perceived behavioural control, prototype evaluation, and prototype similarity, and recruited a large sample of participants ($N > 1200$) to provide sufficient power to include all variables in the model. They predicted three alcohol outcomes: drinking quantity; drinking frequency; and HED frequency. Follow-up data was collected six months after baseline measures of constructs and outcomes were reported. Baseline outcomes were controlled for in each model because they are often the best predictor of follow-up outcomes.

Results indicated that along with baseline outcomes, prototype similarity to abstinent drinkers was the only psychological predictor of drinking quantity at follow-up, while drinking frequency was predicted by prototype similarity to abstinent drinkers, drinking refusal self-efficacy and conformity motives. No psychological variables predicted total HED frequency, although the baseline measure did. Cooke et al. (2021) provide a stringent test of the predictive utility of psychological variables because (i) predictor variables from competing theories were included in the regression models and (ii) consumption was measured six months later. Such studies allow researchers to see what variables remain significant when the predictive effects of other variables are controlled for. They show that prototypes predicted quantity and frequency of consumption and that frequency of drinking was predicted by drinking refusal self-efficacy, as has been shown in previous studies (Baldwin et al., 1993). The results for conformity motives show that they can predict frequency of consumption in samples that drink relatively infrequently (Cooper et al., 2015).

Future studies directly comparing sets of constructs most likely to predict variance in alcohol consumption based on extant research are now needed to identify the most viable correlates of consumption. For example, drinking refusal self-efficacy has been shown to be a better predictor of alcohol consumption than alcohol expectancies, so, more tests are needed that compare predictive effects for drinking refusal self-efficacy with effects for variables like intentions, also shown to predict consumption (Foster et al., 2016). By narrowing down researchers' focus to these most viable constructs, more accurate comparisons between theories will be provided, which should prompt theory development (see Chap. 2) and lead to better interventions—by working out which variables actually predict consumption, when controlling for competitors, it is more likely we will identify targets for intervention that, if modified, will bring about changes in consumption.

Independence of Constructs

One issue with including multiple constructs in regression models is that they should be independent of one another because including variables that correlate too highly reduces the variance that the model accounts for. Correlations greater than 0.80 are considered collinear and researchers are advised to avoid including both variables in models (Field, 2018).

Within the alcohol literature, there are examples of variables that correlate highly enough to raise concerns about collinearity. For example, Fernandes-Jesus et al.'s (2016) confirmatory factor analysis showed that enhancement and social motives correlated above 0.79 in a large sample of university students. Alternatively, Todd et al.'s (2016) meta-analysis reported that the sample-weighted average correlation between intentions and willingness, in alcohol consumption studies, was 0.75. Despite these high correlations, researchers have included enhancement and social motives (Studer et al., 2014) and intentions and willingness (Davies et al., 2017), in regression models potentially reducing the variance explained by the model because scores on both constructs overlap to such an extent. If both constructs are so highly correlated it does not matter which one is included in the model because the extra variance gained from including both is likely to be low. In addition, collinearity between constructs included in a model can mean that the variance explained in the outcome variable can be misleading. Of course, care needs to be taken in determining when to measure variables. Davies et al. (2017) showed that while willingness did not predict drinking among university students, it did among adolescents. The best solution to this issue is for researchers to consider carefully which variables to include when designing the study.

Context

Most predictive studies of alcohol consumption require participants to complete measures of psychological constructs in a non-drinking context like a laboratory, lecture theatre, or library. This is despite evidence that context can affect responses (Cooke & French, 2011; Monk & Heim, 2013). For example, Cooke and French (2011) recruited a sample of English university students to complete a survey measuring constructs from the theory of planned behaviour (Ajzen, 1991, Chap. 2) in either a drinking context (bar) or a non-drinking context (library). The authors noted that because most previous alcohol studies using this theory had collected data in non-drinking contexts, where environmental (i.e., alcoholic beverages) and social (i.e., people consuming alcoholic beverages) cues to alcohol consumption were absent, they believed that the absence of such cues might have led studies to underestimate the size of the subjective norm-intention relationship (see section "Descriptive Norms" for a definition of subjective norms).

Cooke and French (2011) found that context moderated the size of the subjective norm-intention relationship; subjective norms, measured in the bar, had a stronger relationship with intentions compared to subjective norms measured in the library. Similar context effects were reported by Monk and Heim (2013). They found that when participants were exposed to alcohol-related visual cues in a laboratory setting they reported more positive consequences of consumption compared to when they were exposed to neutral cues. A limitation of both studies is that because independent groups designed were used, meaning participants only completed measures in one context, it is possible that differences between participants recruited into each context account for the differences in scores. A recent replication study by Cooke (2020) sought to test the effect of context on scores on psychological predictors using a repeated measures design, thereby overcoming this limitation. Cooke found that the context effects remained, with significantly higher scores for predictors in the drinking context versus the non-drinking context, and also, that while scores from the drinking context were able to predict self-reported consumption (measured the following day) scores from the non-drinking context did not predict consumption. Chapters 8 and 9 provide further detail about how contextual factors influence both consumption and predictors of consumption.

Timeframe

Ajzen (1996) has claimed that the key to optimising prediction of behaviour is to measure predictor variables as close as possible to the performance of behaviour: by doing so, the chances that constructs will change before the behaviour is performed is minimised, thus increasing the chance that they will predict behaviour. Despite this principle, measuring constructs and behaviour during the same evening or within a 24-hour span is relatively uncommon in the alcohol literature (see Cooke, 2020; French & Cooke, 2012; Jones et al., 2020; Labhart et al., 2017, for exceptions). Researchers tend to use follow-up periods of between one week (Cooke et al., 2007) and one month (Hagger, Lonsdale, & Chatzisarantis, 2012). The main disadvantage of this approach is that it assumes alcohol consumption is a static phenomenon. Giese et al. (2019) noted sizable fluctuations in alcohol consumption over the semester when comparing consumption reported on a fortnightly basis. University students drank more at the start of the semester, when responsibilities were presumably lower, than near to the end of the semester when assessments were due.

This is important because if researchers find a set of factors predict behaviour over the short term (e.g., a week later), they may suggest these are key factors to target in intervention. For example, intentions may emerge as a key predictor of alcohol consumption one week later, so time and resources are invested in developing an intervention targeting intentions which, when evaluated in a trial, does not work. There may be several reasons why the intervention did not work, but an obvious one is maybe the effect found in the predictive study only holds under very specific circumstances, perhaps even only during that time of year in that sample of students (see Chap. 22 for more on how results from laboratory studies do not always translate into the real world). Until studies are conducted that vary the follow-up timeframe, only limited data will be available on how the prediction of consumption by psychological variables varies over time.

Targeting Psychological Constructs in Alcohol Reduction Interventions

From an intervention perspective, it makes sense to create interventions that seek to modify psychological determinants of alcohol consumption because such constructs are relatively unstable (variable) they should be easier to modify than more stable (fixed) factors; trying to make someone less impulsive is going to be harder than changing the beliefs that underpin their intentions (see Oei & Morawska, 2004; Chaps. 5 and 21). Interventions have begun to adopt such approaches with some success (van Lettow, de Vries, Burdorf, Boon, & van Empelen, 2015; Chap. 3), but there is a need for further studies that target a wider range of predictors, as certain constructs, for example, alcohol expectancies, drinking motives, and drinking refusal self-efficacy, have rarely been the focus of interventions (see Chap. 2).

Samples Recruited in Predictive Studies

The vast majority of samples used to test predictive relationships between consumption and psychological variables are recruited from university populations. Samples also tend to be predominantly female and white. While it is reasonable to recruit university samples given that this group represent a high-risk population known to engage in alcohol consumption more than their non-university peers (Bewick et al., 2008; Davoren, Demant, Shiely, & Perry, 2016), it does mean that researchers know less about psychological drivers of consumption in other populations. For example, few studies have used tested the predictive utility of constructs covered in this chapter regarding consumption in older populations or populations who did not attend university. Given recent trends showing an increase in alcohol consumption in middle-aged groups (Health Survey for England, 2016), it is imperative that such studies are conducted.

Future Research Directions

In several studies, researchers have tested the effect of self-reported experience of habit on HED (Cooke, Bailey, Jennings, Yuen, & Gardner, (2020); Gardner, de Bruijn, & Lally, 2012; Murray & Mullan, 2019; Norman, 2011). For example, Norman (2011) found habit predicted HED after controlling for intentions and perceived behavioural control. Also, Gardner et al. (2012) found habit, intentions, and the interaction between them, all predicted HED. Decomposing the interaction showed that individuals with high intentions and high habits engaged in HED more than individuals with high intentions and low habits. Finally, Cooke et al. (2020) found that habits were the only predictor of HED. More research on habits, including investigating how they develop, is strongly advocated.

Cross-cultural studies comparing prediction of consumption would help to establish if results from one country generalise to other countries. This is important because there are clear cultural (e.g., light drinking most days vs. heavy drinking on a few days of the week) and legislative (e.g., access and availability of alcohol, legal drinking age) differences between countries (see Chaps. 7 and 16). These cultural differences may affect prediction of consumption using psychological constructs.

In addition, more studies conducted using ecological momentary assessment methods to capture fluctuation in psychological variables over time would be welcome. Such studies could be used to explore whether or not beliefs change in response to negative alcohol experiences. It would also be worthwhile to conduct more studies in situ, during drinking events. For example, to see whether psychological variables measured at the outset of a drinking event (see Chap. 8) change during the course of consuming alcoholic drinks.

Conclusions

Based on a review of existing evidence several psychological constructs—enhancement motives, intentions, prototypes, and willingness—show promise as predictors of alcohol consumption. Drinking refusal self-efficacy is another variable that has been shown to predict consumption, but further tests of this claim are needed. Researchers need to conduct more studies that compare prediction using a wider range of variables, utilising alternative study designs (e.g., cross-lagged panel designs, ecological momentary assessment, longitudinal designs) and analytic techniques (mediation and moderated regression models, multi-level modelling). Such tests will provide clearer evidence about which constructs predict alcohol consumption that would make an important contribution to knowledge and aid the development of more effective interventions to reduce alcohol consumption.

References

Ajzen, I. (1991). *The theory of planned behavior. Organizational Behavior and Human Decision Processes, 50*, 179–211. https://doi.org/10.1016/0749-5978(91)90020-T

Ajzen, I. (1996). The directive influence of attitudes on behavior. In P. M. Gollwitzer & J. A. Bargh (Eds.), *Psychology of action* (pp. 385–403). New York, NY: Guildford Press.

Atwell, K., Abraham, C., & Duka, T. (2011). A parsimonious, integrative model of key psychological correlates of UK university students' alcohol consumption. *Alcohol and Alcoholism (Oxford, Oxfordshire), 46*(3), 253–260. https://doi.org/10.1093/alcalc/agr016

Baldwin, A. R., Oei, T. P. S., & Young, R. (1993). To drink or not to drink: The differential role of alcohol expectancies and drinking refusal self-efficacy in quantity and frequency of alcohol consumption. *Cognitive Therapy and Research, 17*(6), 511–530. https://doi.org/10.1007/BF01176076

Bandura, A. (1977). Self-efficacy: Toward a unifying theory of behavioral change. *Psychological Review, 84*(2), 191–215.

Barratt, J. M., & Cooke, R. (2018). Do gender and year of study affect the ability of the theory of planned behaviour to predict binge-drinking intentions and episodes? *Drugs: Education, Prevention and Policy, 25*(2), 181–188. https://doi.org/10.1080/09687637.2016.1257564

Bewick, B. M., Mulhern, B., Barkham, M., Trusler, K., Hill, A. J., & Stiles, W. B. (2008). Changes in undergraduate student alcohol consumption as they progress through university. *BMC Public Health, 8*, 163. https://doi.org/10.1186/1471-2458-8-163

Brewer, N. T., DeFrank, J. T., & Gilkey, M. B. (2016). Anticipated regret and health behavior: A meta-analysis. *Health Psychology, 35*(11), 1264–1275. https://doi.org/10.1037/hea0000294

Brown, S. A. (1985). Expectancies versus background in the prediction of college drinking patterns. *Journal of Consulting and Clinical Psychology, 53*(1), 123–130. https://doi.org/10.1037/0022-006X.53.1.123

Campo, S., Brossard, D., Frazer, M. S., Marchell, T., Lewis, D., & Talbot, J. (2003). Are social norms Campaigns really magic bullets? Assessing the effects of students' misperceptions on drinking behavior. *Health Communication, 15*(4), 481–497. https://doi.org/10.1207/S15327027HC1504_06

Christiansen, B. A., & Goldman, M. S. (1983). Alcohol-related expectancies versus demographic/background variables in the prediction of adolescent drinking. *Journal of Consulting and Clinical Psychology, 51*(2), 249–257. https://doi.org/10.1037/0022-006X.51.2.249

Conner, M., Warren, R., Close, S., & Sparks, P. (1999). Alcohol consumption and the theory of planned behavior: An examination of the cognitive mediation of past behaviorid. *Journal of Applied Social Psychology, 29*(8), 1676–1704. https://doi.org/10.1111/j.1559-1816.1999.tb02046.x

Cooke, R. (2020). *How does context affect psychological predictors of alcohol consumption?* [Poster Presentation]. UK Society for Behavioural Medicine, Bath, UK.

Cooke, R., Bailey, O., Jennings, J., Yuen, C., & Gardner, B. (2020). Do preparatory behaviours predict alcohol consumption among UK university students? *British Journal of Health Psychology*. https://doi.org/10.1111/bjhp.12489

Cooke, R., Beccaria, F., Demant, J., Fernandes-Jesus, M., Fleig, L., Scholz, U., & de Visser, R. O. (2021). *Predicting alcohol consumption among European university students using data from the CALIBRATE study* [Manuscript in preparation]. Department of Psychology, University of Liverpool.

Cooke, R., Dahdah, M., Norman, P., & French, D. P. (2016). How well does the theory of planned behaviour predict alcohol consumption? A systematic review and meta-analysis. *Health Psychology Review, 10*, 148–167. https://doi.org/10.1080/17437199.2014.947547

Cooke, R., & French, D. P. (2011). The role of context and timeframe in moderating relationships within the theory of planned behaviour. *Psychology & Health, 26*(9), 1225–1240. https://doi.org/10.1080/08870446.2011.572260

Cooke, R., Sniehotta, F., & Schuz, B. (2007). Predicting binge-drinking behaviour using an extended TPB: Examining the impact of anticipated regret and descriptive norms. *Alcohol and Alcoholism, 42*(2), 84–91. https://doi.org/10.1093/alcalc/agl115

Cooper, M. L. (1994). Motivations for alcohol use among adolescents: Development and validation of a four-factor model. *Psychological Assessment, 6*(2), 117–128. https://doi.org/10.1037/1040-3590.6.2.117

Cooper, M. L., Krull, J. L., Agocha, V. B., Flanagan, M. E., Orcutt, H. K., Grabe, S., … Jackson, M. (2008). Motivational pathways to alcohol use and abuse among Black and White adolescents. *Journal of Abnormal Psychology, 117*(3), 485–501. https://doi.org/10.1037/a0012592

Cooper, M. L., Kuntsche, E., Levitt, A., Barber, L. L., & Wolf, S. (2015). Motivational models of substance use: A review of theory and research on motives for using alcohol, Marijuana, and Tobacco. In K. J. Sher (Ed.), *The Oxford handbook of substance use disorders* (Vol. 1). Oxford, UK: Oxford University Press. https://doi.org/10.1093/oxfordhb/9780199381678.013.017

Cox, W. M., & Klinger, E. (1988). A motivational model of alcohol use. *Journal of Abnormal Psychology, 97*(2), 168–180.

Crawford, J., Jones, A., Rose, A., & Cooke, R. (2020). 'You see the pictures the morning after and you're like I wish I was in them': an interpretative phenomenological analysis of university student's alcohol-related regrets. *Psychology & Health.* https://doi.org/10.1080/08870446.2020.1867728

Davies, E. L. (2019). Similarity to prototypical heavy drinkers and non-drinkers predicts AUDIT-C and risky drinking in young adults: Prospective study. *Psychology & Health, 34*(4), 403–421. https://doi.org/10.1080/08870446.2018.1532510

Davies, E. L., Paltoglou, A. E., & Foxcroft, D. R. (2017). Implicit alcohol attitudes predict drinking behaviour over and above intentions and willingness in young adults but willingness is more important in adolescents: Implications for the Prototype Willingness Model. *British Journal of Health Psychology, 22*(2), 238–253. https://doi.org/10.1111/bjhp.12225

Davoren, M. P., Demant, J., Shiely, F., & Perry, I. J. (2016). Alcohol consumption among university students in Ireland and the United Kingdom from 2002 to 2014: A systematic review. *BMC Public Health, 16*, 173. https://doi.org/10.1186/s12889-016-2843-1

Ehret, P. J., Ghaidarov, T. M., & LaBrie, J. W. (2013). Can you say no? Examining the relationship between drinking refusal self-efficacy and protective behavioral strategy use on alcohol outcomes. *Addictive Behaviors, 38*(4), 1898–1904. https://doi.org/10.1016/j.addbeh.2012.12.022

Elliott, M. A., & Ainsworth, K. (2012). Predicting university undergraduates' binge-drinking behavior: A comparative test of the one- and two-component theories of planned behavior. *Addictive Behaviors, 37*(1), 92–101. https://doi.org/10.1016/j.addbeh.2011.09.005

Fernandes-Jesus, M., Beccaria, F., Demant, J., Fleig, L., Menezes, I., Scholz, U., … Cooke, R. (2016). Validation of the drinking motives questionnaire—Revised in six European countries. *Addictive Behaviors, 62*, 91–98. https://doi.org/10.1016/j.addbeh.2016.06.010ssss

Ferrer, R. A., Dillard, A. J., & Klein, W. M. P. (2011). Projection, conformity and deviance regulation: A prospective study of alcohol use. *Psychology & Health*, 1–16. https://doi.org/10.1080/08870446.2011.620106

Field, A. (2018). *Discovering statistics using IBM SPSS statistics* (5th ed.). London, UK: SAGE.

Foster, D. W., Dukes, K., & Sartor, C. E. (2016). The road to drink is paved with high intentions: Expectancies, refusal self-efficacy, and intentions among heavy drinking college students. *Alcohol, 50*, 65–71. https://doi.org/10.1016/j.alcohol.2015.11.004

French, D. P., & Cooke, R. (2012). Using the theory of planned behaviour to understand binge drinking: The importance of beliefs for developing interventions. *British Journal of Health Psychology, 17*(1), 1–17. https://doi.org/10.1111/j.2044-8287.2010.02010.x

Gardner, B., de Bruijn, G.-J., & Lally, P. (2012). Habit, identity, and repetitive action: A prospective study of binge-drinking in UK students: Habit, identity, and repetitive action. *British Journal of Health Psychology, 17*(3), 565–581. https://doi.org/10.1111/j.2044-8287.2011.02056.x

Gibbons, F. X., & Gerrard, M. (1995). Predicting young adults' health risk behavior. *Journal of Personality and Social Psychology, 69*(3), 505–517.

Giese, H., Stok, F. M., & Renner, B. (2019). Perceiving college peers' alcohol consumption: Temporal patterns and individual differences in overestimation. *Psychology & Health, 34*(2), 147–161. https://doi.org/10.1080/08870446.2018.1514118

Godin, G., Sheeran, P., Conner, M., Bélanger-Gravel, A., Gallani, M. C. B. J., & Nolin, B. (2010). Social structure, social cognition, and physical activity: A test of four models. *British Journal of Health Psychology, 15*(1), 79–95. https://doi.org/10.1348/135910709X429901

Hagger, M. S., & Hamilton, K. (2020). *Effects of socio-demographic factors in the theory of planned behavior: A mediation model in multiple samples and behaviors* [Preprint]. PsyArXiv https://doi.org/10.31234/osf.io/rfx9d

Hagger, M. S., Lonsdale, A., & Chatzisarantis, N. L. D. (2012). A theory-based intervention to reduce alcohol drinking in excess of guideline limits among undergraduate students: Undergraduate alcohol intervention. *British Journal of Health Psychology, 17*, 18–43. https://doi.org/10.1111/j.2044-8287.2010.02011.x

Hayes, A. F. (2018). *Introduction to mediation, moderation, and conditional process analysis: A regression-based approach (Second edition)*. New York, NY: Guilford Press.

Health Survey for England. (2016). *Health survey for England*. London, UK: NATCEN Social Research.

Jones, A., Crawford, J., Rose, A., Christiansen, P., & Cooke, R. (2020). Regret me not: Examining the relationship between alcohol consumption and regrettable experiences. *Substance Use & Misuse, 55*, 2379-2388. https://doi.org/10.1080/10826084.2020.1817084

Kuntsche, E., & Cooper, M. L. (2010). Drinking to have fun and to get drunk: Motives as predictors of weekend drinking over and above usual drinking habits. *Drug and Alcohol Dependence, 110*(3), 259–262. https://doi.org/10.1016/j.drugalcdep.2010.02.021

Kuntsche, E., & Kuntsche, S. (2009). Development and validation of the drinking motive questionnaire revised short form (DMQ–R SF). *Journal of Clinical Child & Adolescent Psychology, 38*(6), 899–908. https://doi.org/10.1080/15374410903258967

Labhart, F., Anderson, K. G., & Kuntsche, E. (2017). The spirit is willing, but the flesh is weak: Why young people drink more than intended on weekend nights-an event-level study. *Alcoholism: Clinical and Experimental Research, 41*(11), 1961–1969. https://doi.org/10.1111/acer.13490

Lee, N. K., Oei, T. P. S., & Greeley, J. D. (1999). The interaction of alcohol expectancies and drinking refusal self-efficacy in high and low risk drinkers. *Addiction Research, 7*(2), 91–102. https://doi.org/10.3109/16066359909004377

Leigh, B. C., & Stacy, A. W. (1993). Alcohol outcome expectancies: Scale construction and predictive utility in higher order confirmatory models. *Psychological Assessment, 5*(2), 216–229. https://doi.org/10.1037/1040-3590.5.2.216

Manning, M. (2009). The effects of subjective norms on behaviour in the theory of planned behaviour: A meta-analysis. *British Journal of Social Psychology, 48*(4), 649–705. https://doi.org/10.1348/014466608X393136

Marlatt, G. A. (1987). Alcohol, the magic elixir: Stress, expectancy, and the transformation of emotional states. In E. Gottheil, K. A. Druly, S. Pshko, & S. P. Weinstein (Eds.), *Stress and addiction* (pp. 302–322). New York, NY: Brunner/Mazel.

Monk, R. L., & Heim, D. (2013). Environmental context effects on alcohol-related outcome expectancies, efficacy, and norms: A field study. *Psychology of Addictive Behaviors, 27*(3), 814–818. https://doi.org/10.1037/a0033948

Morawska, A., & Oei, T. P. S. (2005). Binge drinking in university students: A test of the cognitive model. *Addictive Behaviors, 30*(2), 203–218. https://doi.org/10.1016/j.addbeh.2004.05.011

Murray, K. S., & Mullan, B. (2019). Can temporal self-regulation theory and 'sensitivity to reward' predict binge drinking amongst university students in Australia? *Addictive Behaviors, 99*, 106069. https://doi.org/10.1016/j.addbeh.2019.106069

Niaura, R. S., Rohsenow, D. J., Binkoff, J. A., Monti, P. M., Pedraza, M., & Abrams, D. B. (1988). Relevance of cue reactivity to understanding alcohol and smoking relapse. *Journal of Abnormal Psychology, 97*, 133–152.

Norman, P. (2011). The theory of planned behavior and binge drinking among undergraduate students: Assessing the impact of habit strength. *Addictive Behaviors, 36*(5), 502–507. https://doi.org/10.1016/j.addbeh.2011.01.025

Norman, P., Armitage, C. J., & Quigley, C. (2007). The theory of planned behavior and binge drinking: Assessing the impact of binge drinker prototypes. *Addictive Behaviors, 32*(9), 1753–1768. https://doi.org/10.1016/j.addbeh.2006.12.009

Norman, P., & Conner, M. (2006). The theory of planned behaviour and binge drinking: Assessing the moderating role of past behaviour within the theory of planned behaviour. *British Journal of Health Psychology, 11*(Pt 1), 55–70. https://doi.org/10.1348/135910705X43741

Norman, P., Conner, M. T., & Stride, C. B. (2012). Reasons for binge drinking among undergraduate students: An application of behavioural reasoning theory: Reasons for binge drinking. *British Journal of Health Psychology, 17*(4), 682–698. https://doi.org/10.1111/j.2044-8287.2012.02065.x

Oei, T. P. S., & Baldwin, A. R. (1994). Expectancy theory: A two-process model of alcohol use and abuse. *Journal of Studies on Alcohol, 55*(5), 525–534. https://doi.org/10.15288/jsa.1994.55.525

Oei, T. P. S., Foley, J., & Young, R. M. D. (1990). The in vivo manipulation of alcohol-related beliefs in male social drinkers in a naturalistic setting. *British Journal of Medical Psychology, 63*(3), 279–286. https://doi.org/10.1111/j.2044-8341.1990.tb01620.x

Oei, T. P. S., Hasking, P. A., & Young, R. M. (2005). Drinking refusal self-efficacy questionnaire-revised (DRSEQ-R): A new factor structure with confirmatory factor analysis. *Drug and Alcohol Dependence, 78*(3), 297–307. https://doi.org/10.1016/j.drugalcdep.2004.11.010

Oei, T. P. S., & Jardim, C. L. (2007). Alcohol expectancies, drinking refusal self-efficacy and drinking behaviour in Asian and Australian students. *Drug and Alcohol Dependence, 87*(2–3), 281–287. https://doi.org/10.1016/j.drugalcdep.2006.08.019

Oei, T. P. S., & Morawska, A. (2004). A cognitive model of binge drinking: The influence of alcohol expectancies and drinking refusal self-efficacy. *Addictive Behaviors, 29*(1), 159–179. https://doi.org/10.1016/S0306-4603(03)00076-5

Oh, H., & Kim, Y. (2014). Drinking behavior and drinking refusal self-efficacy in Korean college students. *Psychological Reports, 115*(3), 872–883. https://doi.org/10.2466/21.18.PR0.115c31z2

Perkins, H. W., & Berkowitz, A. D. (1986). Perceiving the community norms of alcohol use among students: Some research implications for campus alcohol education programming. *The International Journal of the Addictions, 21*(9–10), 961–976. https://doi.org/10.3109/10826088609077249

Preacher, K. J., & Hayes, A. F. (2004). SPSS and SAS procedures for estimating indirect effects in simple mediation models. *Behavior Research Methods, Instruments, & Computers, 36*(4), 717–731. https://doi.org/10.3758/BF03206553

Richard, R., van der Pligt, J., & de Vries, N. (1995). Anticipated affective reactions and prevention of AIDS. *The British Journal of Social Psychology, 34*(*Pt 1*), 9–21.

Riordan, B. C., Conner, T. S., Flett, J. A. M., & Scarf, D. (2015). A brief orientation week ecological momentary intervention to reduce university student alcohol consumption. *Journal of Studies on Alcohol and Drugs, 76*(4), 525–529. https://doi.org/10.15288/jsad.2015.76.525

Rivis, A., & Sheeran, P. (2013). Automatic risk behavior: Direct effects of binge drinker stereotypes on drinking behavior. *Health Psychology, 32*(5), 571–580. https://doi.org/10.1037/a0029859

Studer, J., Baggio, S., Mohler-Kuo, M., Dermota, P., Daeppen, J.-B., & Gmel, G. (2014). Differential association of drinking motives with alcohol use on weekdays and weekends. *Psychology of Addictive Behaviors, 28*(3), 651–658. https://doi.org/10.1037/a0035668

Todd, J., Kothe, E., Mullan, B., & Monds, L. (2016). Reasoned versus reactive prediction of behaviour: A meta-analysis of the prototype willingness model. *Health Psychology Review, 10*(1), 1–24. https://doi.org/10.1080/17437199.2014.922895

van Lettow, B., de Vries, H., Burdorf, A., Boon, B., & van Empelen, P. (2015). Drinker prototype alteration and cue reminders as strategies in a tailored web-based intervention reducing adults' alcohol consumption: Randomized controlled trial. *Journal of Medical Internet Research, 17*(2), e35. https://doi.org/10.2196/jmir.3551

van Lettow, B., de Vries, H., Burdorf, A., & van Empelen, P. (2016). Quantifying the strength of the associations of prototype perceptions with behaviour, behavioural willingness and intentions: A meta-analysis. *Health Psychology Review, 10*(1), 25–43. https://doi.org/10.1080/17437199.2014.941997

Vik, P. W., Cellucci, T., & Ivers, H. (2003). Natural reduction of binge drinking among college students. *Addictive Behaviors, 28*(4), 643–655. https://doi.org/10.1016/S0306-4603(01)00281-7

Young, R., & Oei, T. P. S. (1990). *Drinking expectancy profile: A manual.* St Lucia, QLD: University of Queensland.

Zhang, J., Jemmott, J. B., Icard, L. D., Heeren, G. A., Ngwane, Z., Makiwane, M., & O'Leary, A. (2018). Predictors and psychological pathways for binge drinking among South African men. *Psychology & Health, 33*(6), 810–826. https://doi.org/10.1080/08870446.2018.1429613

Zimmermann, F., & Sieverding, M. (2011). Young adults' images of abstaining and drinking: Prototype dimensions, correlates and assessment methods. *Journal of Health Psychology, 16*(3), 410–420. https://doi.org/10.1177/1359105310373412

5

Personality Traits and Alcohol Use and Misuse

Laura Mezquita, Generós Ortet, and Manuel I. Ibáñez

Introduction

There are multiple biological, psychological, and social variables that can influence alcohol use and misuse (Engel, 1977). This chapter focuses on the review of the association of distal and nonspecific psychological variables that have been related to alcohol consumption and alcohol use disorders (AUDs), i.e. personality traits. In addition, the role of other proximal and specific psychological variables on alcohol consumption such as drinking motives will be proposed as possible mediators that may help to understand these complex associations. The better understanding of the different etiological pathways to alcohol use and misuse, in which personality is involved, is useful to design personality-targeted prevention/intervention programmes to reduce alcohol consumption and alcohol-related problems and other externalizing behaviours. The effectiveness of such interventions will be also discussed along this chapter.

L. Mezquita (✉) • G. Ortet • M. I. Ibáñez
Department of Basic and Clinical Psychology and Psychobiology, Universitat Jaume I, Castelló de la Plana, Spain

Centre for Biomedical Research Network on Mental Health (CIBERSAM), Instituto de Salud Carlos III, Castellón de la Plana, Spain
e-mail: lmezquit@uji.es

R. Cooke et al. (eds.), *The Palgrave Handbook of Psychological Perspectives on Alcohol Consumption*, https://doi.org/10.1007/978-3-030-66941-6_5

Throughout the chapter, the term "alcohol use" is employed to describe alcohol drinking patterns, such as frequency or quantity, and does not necessarily involve problematic alcohol use, whereas "alcohol misuse" refers to alcohol-related negative consequences or alcohol use disorders (also referred to as alcoholism in less modern classifications).

A Brief History of Personality-Based Alcoholism Typologies

Since the first attempts made to describe "alcoholic typologies" in the mid-nineteenth century, and despite some first simplistic proposals of "alcoholic personality", several personality traits have been consistently related to different patterns of alcohol use and misuse. Thus, reviewing the earlier alcoholism typologies and those personality traits that characterized each one may be a good starting point to know how this research field has evolved.

In the mid-nineteenth century, alienists (i.e., former term for psychiatrists or psychologists) began proposing different alcoholism typologies based on observing distinct use patterns in alcoholic patients from asylums for the insane (e.g., acute, periodic, and chronic oniomania or wine mania). One example is Carpenter (1850), famous for their text on the subject "*On the use and abuse of alcoholic liquors in health and disease*". A few years later, new emerging typologies also began to include other characteristics to classify pathological drinkers, such as family history of alcoholism, comorbid psychopathology, and negative consequences related to alcohol use and personality. In 1889, French alienist LeGrain differentiated between "morally insane alcoholics" who do everything in excess due to a poorly developed moral sense and "weak-willed alcoholics" who possess an adequate moral sense, but who lack willpower and drink either because they like the taste or from habit, and "dipsomaniacs", who are impulsive drinkers whose willpower dissolves in alcohol.

A few years later, Cimbal proposed four alcoholic types based on the personality descriptions of hundreds of problematic drinkers: "Decadent drinkers" are too tired to respond to anything that requires selective effort. They become adventurers, gamblers, cocainists, and diverse sexual perverts. "Impassioned drinkers" are unable to inhibit their libidinal drives and are passionate, discordant, and mentally and emotionally immature. "Spineless drinkers" take to alcohol because it is the cheapest and easiest form of social interaction, present low intelligence, and are incapable of gauging the consequences of their acts. "Self-aggrandizing drinkers" not only strive beyond their ability, but also lack the energy to materialize their ambitions. They also crave power and domination (see Babor, 1996).

In the mid-twentieth century, based on a review of 24 prior typologies, Bowman and Jellinek (1941) produced a comprehensive alcoholism typology in which they identified four major alcoholic subtypes. These types included primary or "true" alcoholics, characterized by their inability to abstain, their immediate liking for alcohol's effects and the rapid development of an uncontrollable need for alcohol. Two further types—steady endogenous symptomatic drinkers and intermittent endogenous symptomatic drinkers—develop alcoholism as a result of major psychiatric disorders. Finally, stammtisch alcoholics develop alcoholism by exogenous causes (e.g., environmental causes) and were social drinkers and easy-going alcoholics who used alcohol on a daily basis around the tables set aside for regular customers in cafes, bars, or restaurants. However, this classification attracted little attention until Jellinek reviewed the typology with attention to etiologic elements (e.g., psychosocial and physiological vulnerability), alcoholic processes (e.g., nature of dependence), and damage elements in the physical, mental, and socio-economic fields (Babor, 1996). The updated typology included five alcoholism subtypes: alpha, beta, epsilon, delta, and gamma. According to Jellinek, only gamma and delta exhibit sufficient evidence for alcohol dependence to represent true disease entities. Gamma alcoholics drink because of psychological vulnerability and exhibit loss of control, whereas delta alcoholics drink owing to social and economic influences and show an inability to abstain from alcohol consumption (Babor, 1996). For two decades, the gamma-delta alcoholism typology was the most well-accepted classification system, and the notion of an "addictive personality" was so influential that the DSM first and second editions classified alcoholism and drug addiction as types of "sociopathic personality disturbances", and later in a broader category of "personality disorders" (Ball, 2005). In these neologies, personality characteristics, such as failure to self-control and sociopathic behaviour, were considered core traits for developing alcoholism.

The early 1980s witnessed efforts to overcome the old and less systematic typologies which arguably reflected the social stigma/biases of the times. Researchers began to formulate new typologies that incorporated greater complexity to fit better with available empirical data. These included Zucker's developmental model, which proposed four alcoholism subtypes: antisocial alcoholism, developmentally limited alcoholism, negative-affect alcoholism, and primary alcoholism (Zucker, 1994). There was also Babor's typology, which proposed type A and B alcoholisms (Babor et al., 1992). However, the most influential alcoholism typologies were probably Cloninger's Type I and Type II alcoholisms (Cloninger, Sigvardsson, & Bohman, 1996). Cloninger's Type I alcoholism develops as a result of years of excessive alcohol consumption and can take a minor or severe form. It affects both men and women and shows both genetic and environmental influences. This alcoholism type is characterized by motivation to reduce tension and reflects anxiety-related personality traits. Alcoholism Type II begins in adolescence and early adulthood and is associated with antisocial behaviour. The related personality traits are novelty seeking and impulsivity, and motivation to drink is caused by alcohol reinforcement properties (Babor, 1996; Leggio, Kenna, Fenton, Bonenfant, & Swift, 2009). See Chap. 2 for more on models that propose negative and positive reasons for drinking. It is worth emphasizing that Babor and Zucker's models present a high degree of convergence with Cloninger's typology. Types I and II closely resemble Babor's Type A and B alcoholisms. Furthermore, Type I alcoholism would be the equivalent to Zucker's negative-affect alcoholism, while Type II alcoholism would be related to Zucker's antisocial and developmentally limited alcoholism.

At the present time, methodological and statistical techniques have been employed to replicate and find new alcoholism typologies. For example, cluster analysis allows a set of participants to be grouped in such a way that the participants in the same group (called a cluster) are more similar (in some sense) to one another than to those in other groups. Using this technique, different research studies have identified between two and five subtypes of alcoholism (Leggio et al., 2009). The difference in the number of clusters obtained across studies could be due, in part, to the different number of variables included in the analysis (i.e., illness curse, motivation, personality, severity, among others) and also to variability in the samples used (e.g., youngsters, chronic patients). Despite these differences, many similarities have emerged among some of the obtained typologies, and personality characteristics seem relevant in many of them. For example, Lesch's model identifies the "anxiety or conflict" and "depression" subtypes that describe alcoholics to self-medicate with alcohol for its sedative and antidepressant effects, respectively. Similarly, Del Boca and Hesselbrock proposed the "internalizing typology" in which alcoholics are characterized by high anxiety and depression, and drink to relieve boredom and anxiety. Moreover, parallel characteristics were described in other typologies, such as the "anxiopathic" and "timophatic" subtypes of Cardoso, or the "negative affect" subtype of Windle and Scheldt (Leggio et al., 2009). All these clusters are related to anxiety/negative-affect personality characteristics and coping drinking motivations. Moreover, in the same studies, the following subtypes have been identified: "adaptation", "externalizing", "sociopathic," and "chronic/antisocial personality" (Leggio et al., 2009), all of which are related to aggressive behaviour and impulsivity. These models highlight the relevant role of personality traits (i.e., negative emotionality and disinhibition/impulsivity) in the development of alcohol disorders.

From the above discussion, it is apparent that there is a long-standing tradition of psychological research intended to help explain links between personality and alcohol use and misuse. Initial attempts were driven, in part, by a desire to explain the apparent heterogeneity among alcoholics, and "personality" became a key theoretical device in this project. However, a more consistent type of approach has predominated since the early twentieth century after the "trait approach" to personality emerged. This perspective has allowed specific personality characteristics to be associated with different alcohol outcomes, such as drinking onset, drinking frequency, drinking quantity, and alcohol use disorders. However, before reviewing the associations of personality traits with the different patterns of alcohol use and misuse it is essential to know and understand the most well-accepted bio dispositional personality models and the similarities/discrepancies between them.

Personality Trait Models

Bio dispositional models assume that the core of personality refers to a limited number of basic traits or behavioural dispositions which are relatively stable and consistent over time which are the product of the complex interaction between genes and environmental factors (Boyle, Matthews, & Saklofske, 2008). Figure 5.1 summarizes the most well-accepted bio dispositional personality models with the aim of facilitating the reading and the understanding of later sections.

In addition, we can differentiate between two distinct approaches to theorizing personality. One approach, evident in explanatory or "bottom-up" models, refers to efforts to demonstrate how specific biological systems underpin different personality traits which they themselves underpin (and, therefore, help explain) patterns of behaviour. Examples of these models are the personality models of Gray (1991) and Cloninger (1998). Specifically, Gray (1991) proposed the existence of diverse biological systems (i.e., the Behavioral Inhibition System [BIS], the Behavioral Activation System [BAS] and the Fight Flight Freeze System [FFFS]) (Corr & McNaughton, 2012). Whereas punishment sensitivity or negative emotionality traits would be related to the BIS, extraversion would be related to the BAS (Segarra, Poy, López, & Moltó,

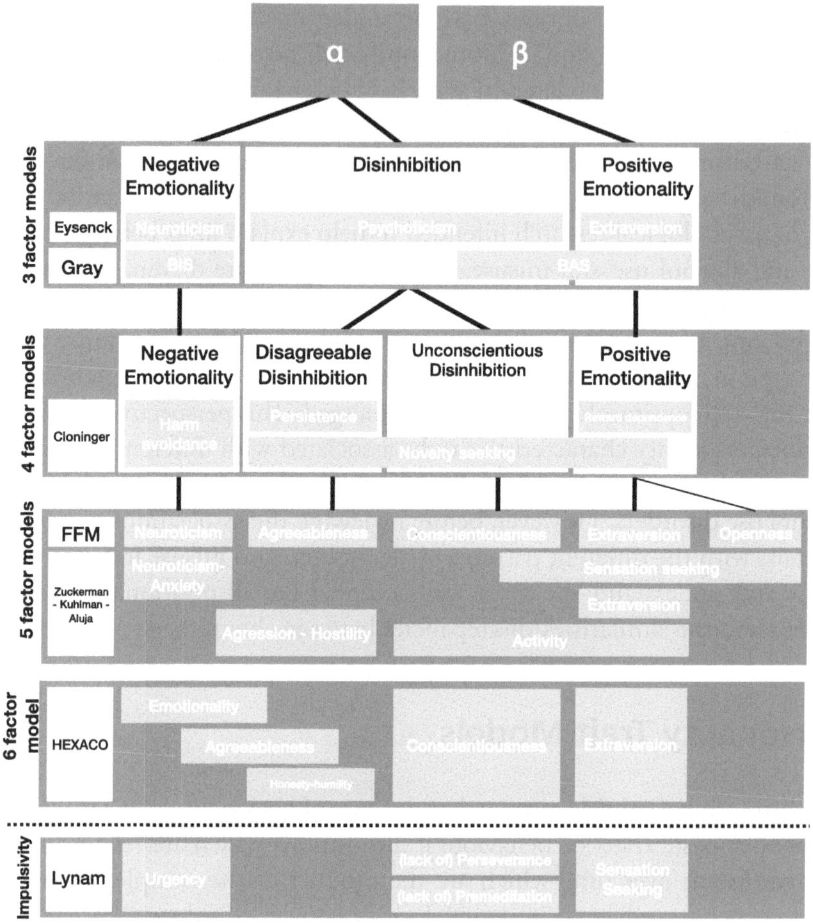

Fig. 5.1 Convergence between the most important models of normal personality traits and the UPPS impulsivity model

2014; Smillie, 2008; Smillie, Loxton, & Avery, 2013; Smillie, Pickering, & Jackson, 2006). Based on Gray's model, Cloninger (1998) proposed the existence of four personality factors: two related to sensitivity to aversive and appetitive stimuli (similarly to the BIS and the BAS, respectively), namely, *harm avoidance* and *novelty seeking*; a third one related to the acquisition of conditioned signals of reward, namely, *reward dependence*; a fourth one characterized by resistance to extinction due to intermittent reinforcement, namely, *persistence*.

On the other hand, in descriptive or "top-down" models, having obtained the main personality narrow traits and broad domains, the authors attempted to link those traits to neurological architecture and physiological systems. The development of these models was possible due to devising mathematical bases to evaluate latent constructs (the well-known Classical Test Theory) and the development of factor analysis. Thus, it is possible to test if there is shared variance between different reported traits (or adjectives/terms), and if they form part of the same personality broad trait. Examples of "top-down" models are the Eysenck's model (Eysenck, 1990), the Zuckerman model (Zuckerman, 2005), or the Big Five (Goldberg, 1993; John, Naumann, & Soto, 2008). Among them, the efforts to link traits to biological processes are most apparent in Eysenck's and Zuckerman work. On the one hand, Eysenck proposed the existence of three basic personality dimensions: psychoticism, extraversion, and neuroticism in an attempt to link psychological disorders to normal personality (Eysenck, 1990). The psychological mechanism of extraversion and neuroticism would be the need for stimulation and emotional reactivity, respectively. The biological mechanism underlying psychoticism is not well established (Eysenck, 1990). On the other hand, Zuckerman (2005) proposed the existence of five domains based on the results of two studies in which they performed a factor analysis of 46 and 33 personality questionnaires, respectively, by assessing temperamental and biological aspects of personality. The resulting domains from the factor analysis were named: neuroticism-anxiety, extraversion/sociability, aggression-hostility, impulsive sensation seeking and activity.

However, one of the most frequently used bio dispositional models of personality is the Big Five (a.k.a. the Five-Factor Model) (John et al., 2008). The origins of the Big Five lies in the lexical hypothesis, which considers natural language to be the source of dispositional attributes for a scientific taxonomy of personality. The origin of the lexical hypothesis was initially recognized by authors like Galton, who defended that "the most important individual differences in human transactions will come to be encoded as single terms in some or all of the world's languages". Other authors, like Allport or Cattell, also contributed to lexical hypothesis research by drawing up lists of those terms/adjectives or developing and performing the first exploratory factor analyses of those terms/adjectives (Goldberg, 1993). Nowadays, the most replicated structure following these procedures suggests the existence of five broad traits named neuroticism, extraversion, openness, agreeableness, and conscientiousness. The neuroticism and extraversion domains would encompass predispositions to negative and positive emotional states, respectively. Openness to experience refers to curiosity. Individuals with high levels of openness wish to participate in new ideas and hold unconventional values. Agreeableness would characterize people who are altruistic, compassionate, and willing to help.

Finally, conscientiousness characterizes people who care about achieving goals are scrupulous, reliable, and not very impulsive (McCrae & Costa, 2008).

A more recent model that stems from a similar procedure to the Big Five is HEXACO (Ashton & Lee, 2007). HEXACO consists of six factors (honesty-humility, emotionality, extraversion, agreeableness, conscientiousness, and openness) derived from factor analyses of English and non-English language personality questionnaires. The biggest difference between the Big Five and HEXACO is the addition of the honesty-humility factor. However, this factor does not represent an "addition" to the Big Five but characterizes the repartitioning of the variance of neuroticism and agreeableness into HEXACO agreeableness, emotionality, and honesty-humility (Anglim & O'Connor, 2019).

In addition, some models also focus on specific facets/narrow traits of personality, rather than on broad domains, which would be studied for their relevance to understand alcohol use and misuse. One of them is the impulsivity model of Whiteside and Lynam (2001), which describes four traits of impulsiveness: Urgency, (lack of) Perseverance, (lack of) Premeditation, and Sensation seeking (UPPS model). Previous studies that have related the UPPS model with the Big Five found that urgency was associated with neuroticism, sensation seeking was linked to extraversion, and (lack of) perseverance and (lack of) premeditation were related to low conscientiousness (Whiteside & Lynam, 2001). In a later revision of the model, the urgency facet was divided into positive urgency and negative urgency (Cyders et al., 2007). Although it was assumed that positive urgency would be related mainly to extraversion and negative urgency to neuroticism, both showed the closest associations with neuroticism (Ibáñez et al., 2016).

As we have seen, although different models attempt to describe personality using broad domains, the content of the proposed domains resemble one another well. In addition, the factor analysis results suggest that rather than these models being incompatible proposals, they analyse the domain structure at different levels (Markon, Krueger, & Watson, 2005). That is, the personality structure would be hierarchical not only at the lower traits level, but also at the broad traits level. As shown in previous studies, when a variety of personality questionnaires from different personality models were included, the factor analysis results showed that two factors of the highest order emerged and resembled those proposed by Digman (1997): alpha and beta factors. At the three-factor level, negative emotionality, disinhibition (grouped into the alpha factor), and positive emotionality (under the beta factor) would be located. Disinhibition would be divided into unconscientious and disagreeable disinhibitions at the four-factor level. Whereas the former was related to (low) conscientiousness, the latter would be associated with (low) agreeableness. Finally, at the five-factor level, positive emotionality would be differentiated into an extraversion factor, which would be more linked to characteristics of sociability and activity, and another of openness (Markon et al., 2005; Mezquita, Ibáñez, Moya, Villa, & Ortet, 2014). If we bear in mind the convergence, similarities, and specificities of the most broadly used bio dispositional personality models, it could help to easily understand the results of alcohol-personality studies, regardless of the personality model/questionnaire employed in each specific study. In the next section we will mainly focus on the associations of personality and alcohol outcomes from the Five-Factor Model approach, and we also present results that employ other measures that could be easily integrated given the convergence between nomenclatures exposed in this section.

Approaches to Understanding Links Between Personality and Alcohol Use

There are different approaches to study the role of personality in alcohol use and misuse. On the one hand, we can examine the simple associations between both variables, that is, if personality and alcohol outcomes are correlated. This approach includes mainly cross-sectional studies, but also longitudinal studies (see Chaps. 2 and 4 for more on design issues in predictive studies). The latter refers to prospective designs when personality is assessed only at baseline and alcohol use only in the follow-up (e.g., Mezquita et al., 2014). But also longitudinal studies in which the correlations of personality and alcohol outcomes change (i.e., growth models) have been explored (e.g., Littlefield, Sher, & Wood, 2009). However, if we intend to disentangle the reciprocal relationship between personality and alcohol use and misuse (e.g., how personality influences alcohol use; but also how alcohol use influences personality), more complex, longitudinal designs are required. These kinds of studies involve assessment of both personality and alcohol use at two (or more) time points. This section aims to present the main findings about the associations of personality and different alcohol outcomes from both kinds of studies.

As mentioned in the previous section, the Big Five is one of the most widely used models of personality traits in basic and applied psychology. Not surprisingly, many studies have demonstrated links between the Big Five personality traits with alcohol use (John et al., 2008; Soto, 2019). Based on the results of systematic reviews and meta-analyses, neuroticism, low agreeableness, and low conscientiousness are the broad domains that relate most to substance use disorders (Kotov, Gamez, Schmidt, & Watson, 2010; Malouff, Thorsteinsson, Rooke, & Schutte, 2007; Ruiz, Pincus, & Schinka, 2008). A similar pattern has been observed for alcohol use disorders. While high neuroticism and low conscientiousness have been related to alcohol use disorders both cross-sectionally and longitudinally, associations with low agreeableness have been found only cross-sectionally (Bogg & Roberts, 2004; Malouff et al., 2007). The Big Five domains are also associated with drinking frequency, drinking quantity, and HED (see Chap. 1 for a definition) and negative alcohol-related consequences. Higher extraversion levels are associated with more frequent drinking and greater volume of consumption, especially among adolescents and young adults. High neuroticism is associated mainly with alcohol-related problems, suggesting that drinking acts as coping motive (see Chap. 4). Low conscientiousness is linked to both higher levels of alcohol use and alcohol-related problems (Ibáñez et al., 2015; Mezquita et al., 2018; Ortet, Martínez, Mezquita, Morizot, & Ibáñez, 2017). Moreover, a meta-analysis has also shown that all three domains are related to HED (Adan, Forero, & Navarro, 2017). "Binge" drinkers are more likely to be extroverts, neurotic, or lack conscientiousness.

Similar results have been found when other personality models are employed. Thus psychoticism and, to a lesser extent, extraversion (from Eysenck's model), sensitivity to reward (from Gray's model), sociability, aggression-hostility, impulsive sensation seeking (from Zuckerman's model), novelty seeking, and low persistence (from Cloninger's model) have also been associated with many alcohol-related outcomes, while neuroticism (from Eysenck's model) and harm avoidance (from Cloninger's model) have been related to alcohol use disorders and difficulties to stop drinking (Aluja, Lucas, Blanch, & Blanco, 2019; Sher & Trull, 1994). Regarding the existing link between specific impulsivity facets and different alcohol-related outcomes, two meta-analyses have suggested that the impulsivity facets associated with extraversion (i.e., sensation seeking and positive urgency) are also related to alcohol consumption in adolescence. The same studies conclude that those impulsivity facets close to neuroticism (i.e., urgency) are associated with problematic alcohol use, drinking problems, and alcohol dependence in older adolescents and adults. Finally, facets linked to low conscientiousness (i.e., lack of perseverance and lack of premeditation) are related to alcohol use and alcohol dependence in adults (Coskunpinar, Dir, & Cyders, 2013; Stautz & Cooper, 2013).

In addition, from a developmental perspective, different researchers have studied how changes in personality are related to modifications in alcohol use and misuse along with how alcohol use and misuse development are related to personality changes. Most of these studies have explored the interrelationship of personality and alcohol outcomes during the transition from adolescence to adulthood partly because personality changes are more pronounced during this life period (Roberts, Walton, & Viechtbauer, 2006). Specifically, in emerging adulthood (from 18 to 22 years of age), conscientiousness and emotional stability traits tend to increase (known as the "maturity principle"). This developmental period has also been referred to as "maturing out" because it has been linked to individuals playing adult roles, taking responsibilities and adopting a more conventional lifestyle (Roberts et al., 2006). Interestingly, alcohol use disorders show a pattern of onset, escalation, and decline in accordance with these personality changes, especially during this lifespan period (Hicks, Durbin, Blonigen, Iacono, & McGue, 2012; Littlefield et al., 2009). Indeed, those studies that have performed growth curve models show that changes in negative emotionality and disinhibition from adolescence to the mid-thirties covary with changes in alcohol use and problematic alcohol involvement (Littlefield et al., 2009; Littlefield, Sher, & Wood, 2010a; Quinn & Harden, 2013).

Overall, evidence from correlational studies suggests that high positive emotionality characteristics (e.g., high extraversion, high sensation seeking) are related to drinking onset, early stages of alcohol use, and specific alcohol use patterns like HED. High negative emotionality (e.g., high neuroticism, low emotional stability, high harm avoidance) is associated mainly with alcohol-related problems and alcohol disorders. Finally, high disinhibition (e.g., low conscientiousness, lack of perseverance) is associated with all the developmental stages of alcohol use and misuse (Ibáñez, Ruipérez, Villa, Moya, & Ortet, 2008; Malouff et al., 2007) (see Fig. 5.2).

Overall, evidence suggests that certain personality characteristics are associated with various alcohol outcomes and different stages of alcohol use and misuse. However, specifying the functional relationship between personality and alcohol use (i.e., if personality comes before consumption or consumption comes before personality) is less clear, particularly due to the lack of longitudinal studies that repeatedly measure variables over time which would allow the effects of each factor on the other factor to be disentangled. Different theoretical models have been postulated to explain how this relationship might work. The vulnerability/predisposition model implies that the personality profile puts individuals at increased risk for alcohol use. This means that impulsive individuals would be at more risk of developing alcohol-related problems. Alternatively, the scar/complication model proposes that alcohol use influences personality changes, so persons with problematic alcohol use

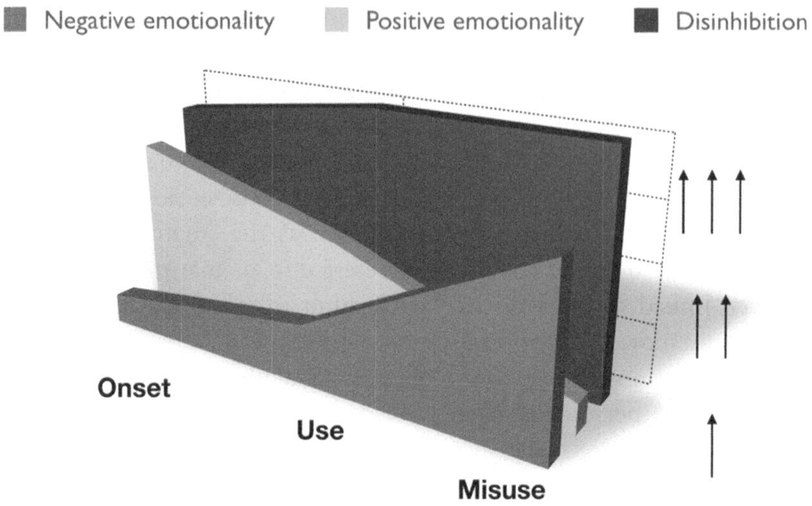

Fig. 5.2 Degree of influence (x-axis) of negative emotionality, positive emotionality, and disinhibition broad domains on the onset, use, and misuse of alcohol

experience increased impulsivity. Another approach is outlined by the transactional model, which represents a combination of the first two models, and defends the notion that bidirectional processes exist between personality and alcohol involvement. Finally, the common cause model proposes that a third variable is responsible for personality-alcohol covariation. For example, the same genetic factors might be responsible for disinhibition personality characteristics and alcohol misuse (Littlefield, Vergés, Wood, & Sher, 2012; Samek et al., 2018).

Quinn, Stappenbeck, and Fromme (2011) have provided evidence for transactional relationships in college students assessed once per year from the freshman year to the senior year. They showed that impulsivity and sensation seeking traits predicted increases in heavy drinking over time, but also heavy drinking predicted increases in sensation seeking and impulsivity over time. Littlefield et al. (2012) also found that across colleges, there was some evidence to suggest that heavy drinking predicted higher scores for novelty seeking. When examined over a longer period (freshman, sophomore and senior year vs. freshman year, senior year and post-college), heavy drinking did not significantly predict changes in personality, but personality predicted changes in heavy drinking. These findings, together with the fact that the authors found reliable evidence for the correlated changes between personality and alcohol use, especially in emerging adulthood, led to the conclusion that the impact of alcohol involvement on personality change may be limited to shorter intervals within specific developmental timeframes. Consequently, they suggested that the relation between changes in personality and alcohol involvement could be best viewed from a non-causal perspective. Further tests of these findings, using similar longitudinal designs, but recruiting non-university samples would help to confirm this claim.

Samek et al. (2018) reported the results of a twin study which tested the common cause model alongside other theoretical models in a single study. Twin studies allow researchers to explore the impact of genetic similarity on personality-alcohol use relationships. The authors found that during the transition from adolescence (17 years) to young adulthood (24 years), low constraint (which is similar to low conscientiousness) and aggressive under control (which is related to low agreeableness) predicted increases in Alcohol Use Disorder (AUD) symptoms, which supports the vulnerability/predisposition model by suggesting the personality is antecedent to consumption. From young adulthood (24 years) to later adulthood (29 years), low constraint and aggressive under control also predicted increases in AUD symptoms, but AUD symptoms were also related to low constraint and higher aggressive under control five years later, which supports the transactional model—meaning that personality and alcohol use influence one another. These results suggest that at earlier ages, personality influences alcohol use, possibly because personality is more stable than alcohol use, whereas once alcohol use had become stable, the transactional model has stronger explanatory power, showing bidirectional effects. Moreover, shared additive genetics accounted for the prospective associations between personality and the alcohol symptoms of AUD, which supports the common cause model. In other words, a third variable—genetic variation—mediated the relationship between personality and alcohol use.

Taken together, research results suggest that the interrelation between personality and alcohol use appears bidirectional, and there is evidence that various models—vulnerability, transactional, common cause—can account for the different types of association between personality and alcohol use and misuse. While vulnerability models might be more plausible in earlier life stages (pre-adolescence to adolescence or early adulthood), transactional models seem well-suited to later stages, but only when short time intervals are considered. When long assessment periods are taken into account, it seems that personality-alcohol outcome associations are better understood as non-causal and that a common cause model (e.g., genetics) is more plausible. However, as very few studies are available, along with major differences in the timeframes and measures employed by authors, more research is needed in this field to draw firm conclusions about the functional relations between personality traits and alcohol outcomes throughout someone's lifetime.

Etiological Pathways for Alcohol Use and Misuse

Although the association between personality and alcohol use and alcohol misuse needs further examination, it is clear that different personality domains are associated with distinct patterns of alcohol use and misuse. These associations can be explained by various etiological pathways; different interrelated etiological pathways have been developed to explain personality-alcohol associations: (1) positive-affect regulation; (2) negative-affect regulation; (3) deviance proneness pathway (Ibáñez et al., 2008; Sher, Grekin, & Williams, 2005). To test the plausibility of these complex models, additional variables are included in the theoretical/empirical models, in addition to personality and alcohol outcomes. That is, if we know how personality is related to an alcohol use-related third factor (i.e., mediating variable) which is, in turn, related to alcohol outcomes, we can better understand the associations of personality with drinking.

The positive-affect regulation pathway refers to drinking to experience positive alcohol reinforcement effects. In this case, motivation to consume could be attributable to the psychobiological effects of alcohol in the brain areas related to appetitive motivation (Ibáñez et al., 2008). To support this idea, enhancement drinking motives (i.e., "to get a high" or "because it's fun") have been associated with different alcohol-related outcomes, such as drinking quantity and frequency (Mezquita, Stewart, Kuntsche, & Grant, 2016), weekend drinking (Mezquita et al., 2014; Studer et al., 2014), and HED (White, Anderson, Ray, & Mun, 2016). Cross-sectional (Mezquita et al., 2018) and longitudinal (Vernig & Orsillo, 2015) studies have related enhancement motives with alcohol-related problems, even though these associations seem largely mediated by alcohol use (Merrill, Wardell, & Read, 2014; Mezquita et al., 2018). Thus, enhancement drinking motives could facilitate drinkers consuming larger quantities of alcohol and presenting higher heavy drinking patterns which, in turn, could facilitate more problems developing with alcohol use (e.g., missed a day at work, went to work drunk, had withdrawal symptoms). Enhancement motives have also shown a mediational effect between personality traits of positive emotionality and unconscientious disinhibition (low conscientiousness) and different alcohol-related outcomes. Therefore, high extraversion and low conscientiousness traits would predispose to higher enhancement motives which, in turn, would be associated with heavier drinking and more serious alcohol-related problems. These results support the existence of a positive-affect regulation pathway (Mezquita et al., 2018) (see Fig. 5.3).

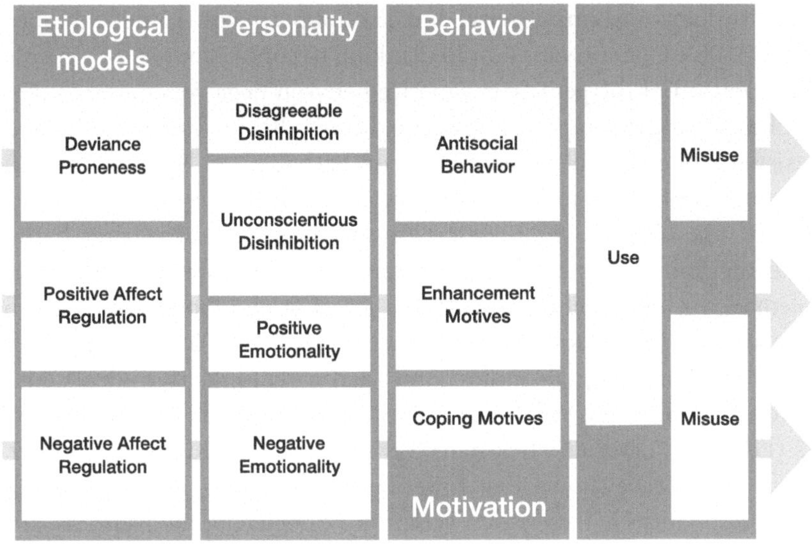

Fig. 5.3 Etiological pathways to alcohol use and misuse

The negative-affect regulation pathway, also known as the self-medication or internalizing pathway, refers to drinking alcohol to decrease distress (Ibáñez et al., 2008). According to the basis that alcohol reduces negative affective states, people may be specifically motivated to reduce anxiety and discomfort (i.e., "to forget my worries" or "to relax"). Coping drinking motives have been related to drinking alcohol at home, drinking alone, heavy drinking (Mohr et al., 2005; O'Hara et al., 2014), and mainly to alcohol-related problems in cross-sectional (Mezquita et al., 2018) and longitudinal studies (Merrill et al., 2014; Vernig & Orsillo, 2015). The relation between coping motives and alcohol-related problems remains significant, even when alcohol use is controlled for (Merrill et al., 2014; Mezquita et al., 2018), which supports the fact that drinking to cope is a particularly maladaptive behaviour (Cooper, Kuntsche, Levitt, Barber, & Wolf, 2016). Regarding the aetiology of this covariation, twin studies have revealed that associations between coping drinking motives and alcohol outcomes are explained by shared genetic factors (Young-Wolff, Kendler, & Prescott, 2012). Moreover, the associations of personality characteristics of negative emotionality with alcohol-related problems and alcohol use disorders, as reported in previous studies (Malouff et al., 2007; Ruiz, Pincus, & Dickinson, 2003), would be explained partly by their association with coping drinking motives (Blevins, Abrantes, & Stephens, 2016; Mezquita et al., 2018). There is also evidence to suggest that changes in coping motives specifically mediate the relation between changes in neuroticism (and also impulsivity) and alcohol problems (Littlefield, Sher, & Wood, 2010b). Genetic variation in drinking to cope accounts for a considerable proportion of the genetic covariance between negative emotionality and alcohol use disorder symptoms (Littlefield et al., 2011). These results support the existence of a negative-affect regulation pathway (see Fig. 5.3). See Chap. 4 for more on drinking motives as predictors of alcohol use.

Finally, the deviance proneness pathway, or the externalizing pathway, defends the notion that alcohol use forms part of a more general pattern of problematic or antisocial behaviour that starts in childhood and is attributable to deficits in the socialization process (Littlefield & Sher, 2016; Sher et al., 2005). Longitudinal studies conducted with adults (Kendler, Ohlsson, Edwards, Sundquist, & Sundquist, 2016; Mezquita et al., 2014) and adolescents (Edwards, Gardner, Hickman, & Kendler, 2015; Kendler, Gardner, & Prescott, 2011) have shown that suffering maltreatment, impulsive or disinhibited personality characteristics, symptoms of behavioural disorders, affiliation with drinkers or deviant peers, and permissive or negligent parental educational styles would predict long-term alcohol and drug use. Studies about the structure of psychopathology have also demonstrated that alcohol use and misuse converge with conduct disorders and other drug use outcomes in a suprafactor of externalizing psychopathology (Conway et al., 2019; Lahey, Krueger, Rathouz, Waldman, & Zald, 2017), while a common genetic factor apparently explains the covariance between antisocial behaviour and substance use disorders (Kendler & Myers, 2014). Antagonistic (low agreeableness) and unconscientious (low conscientiousness) personality traits are closely related to the externalizing spectrum (Lahey et al., 2017; Mezquita et al., 2015; Widiger et al., 2019). Twin studies suggest a significant genetic overlap between these disinhibition personality traits and the externalizing spectrum (Blonigen, Hicks, Krueger, Patrick, & Iacono, 2005; Krueger et al., 2002). Taken together, research results suggest the relevance of a specific deviance proneness pathway (see Fig. 5.3).

Overall, characteristics of positive emotionality and unconscientious disinhibition are related, at least partially, to alcohol use and misuse through enhancement motives, which suggests the existence of a positive-affect regulation pathway. Negative emotionality would be related mainly to alcohol misuse through coping motives, which indicates the existence of a negative-affect regulation pathway. Finally, disagreeable disinhibition and unconscientious disinhibition would be related to alcohol use and misuse, but also to antisocial behaviour, externalizing psychopathology and affiliation with deviant peers among others, which suggests the existence of a deviant proneness pathway to alcohol use and misuse in which alcohol use and abuse forms part of a more general deviant pattern of behaviour. Such knowledge about different personality etiological pathways to alcohol use and misuse, and the relevance of other variables implied in each pathway (e.g., motives, antisocial behaviour, affiliation with deviant peers), could help to design better prevention and intervention programmes to avoid or reduce alcohol consumption and alcohol-related problems and disorders.

Personality-Targeted Interventions to Prevent and Reduce Alcohol Use and Misuse

If some individuals were at risk of alcohol use and misuse based partly on their personality characteristics, would the interventions that focus on these features help to prevent and reduce alcohol drinking and alcohol-related problems? To answer this question, it is important to differentiate between universal and selective prevention/intervention programmes. Universal programmes target general populations, regardless of how individuals have been defined in alcohol use risk terms and are based on delivering generic intervention components (e.g., knowledge and skills) to participants or patients. Selective intervention programmes target potential people with high-risk factors for substance misuse (e.g., heavy drinkers) to reduce and prevent alcohol-related negative outcomes (Edalati, Afzali, Castellanos-Ryan, & Conrod, 2019). Meta-analytic studies suggest that universal programmes would be effective in reducing substance use in elementary schools and in the mid-adolescence life stage, while programmes that target high-risk students are promising from the mid-adolescence stage to later ages (Onrust, Otten, Lammers, & Smit, 2016).

Although programmes that target high-risk students (e.g., "binge" drinkers) for alcohol-related outcomes are promising, they cannot be extended to those adolescents who are at risk of developing problems with drugs, but who have not yet shown significant problems with its use (Conrod, Stewart, Comeau, & Maclean, 2006). In order to overcome the limitation of previous selective prevention/treatment programmes, the PreVenture Program was developed. In this case, participants were selected according to their risk personality profiles for substance use (Conrod et al., 2006). That is, the participants who score one standard deviation above the mean on the sensation-seeking and impulsivity scales (traits related to the positive-affect regulation pathway) and the hopelessness and anxiety sensitivity scales (traits related to the negative-affect regulation pathway), assessed with the Substance Use Risk Profile Scale (SURPS, Woicik, Stewart, Pihl, & Conrod, 2009), attend brief individual- or group-based intervention sessions that target their dominant personality profile. Interventions generally last between two and six sessions, and each session lasts 90 minutes. Intervention includes psychoeducational, motivational enhancement therapy and cognitive-behavioural therapy (Conrod, 2016). Specifically, participants are guided in a goal setting exercise, designed to enhance motivation to change behaviour. Psychoeducational strategies are used to teach participants about their target personality trait and associated problematic coping behaviours like avoidance, interpersonal dependence, aggression, risky behaviours and substance misuse. They are then introduced to the cognitive behavioural model and guided in breaking down personal experience according to the physical, cognitive, and behavioural components of an emotional response. A novel component to this intervention approach is the fact that all exercises discuss thoughts, emotions, and behaviours in a personality-specific way, for example, identifying situational triggers and cognitive distortions related to Sensation Seeking specifically. Then, participants are encouraged to identify and challenge personality-specific cognitive distortions that lead to problematic behaviours (Conrod, 2016; Newton, Teesson, Barrett, Slade, & Conrod, 2012).

A recent review has suggested that the PreVenture program can lower the rates of alcohol and illicit drug use and substance-related harm by approximately 50% in high-risk adolescents (i.e., $d = 0.47$), with effects lasting for up to 3 years (Conrod, 2016; Edalati & Conrod, 2019). These interventions have also been associated with a 25% reduction in the likelihood of transitioning to mental health problems, such as anxiety, depression, suicidal ideation, and conduct problems. Other studies have also shown that this programme is beneficial for all high-risk youths regardless of their socio-economic status or peer victimization experience (Edalati et al., 2019). However, it is important to note that most of these studies have been conducted with children and adolescents (Conrod, 2016), which means that research is needed to see if the PreVenture program is also effective for non-adolescent populations.

More recently, research efforts have focused on studying the competing effects of universal (i.e., Climate program), selective (i.e., PreVenture program), and combined programs (Climate and PreVenture, CAP) to reduce alcohol- and cannabis-related outcomes. Specifically, the Climate programme is based on the effective harm-minimization approach to prevention, and the participants learn about the short- and long-term effects of alcohol and cannabis, normative alcohol and cannabis use, drug refusal and harm-minimization skills, and tips on staying safe and first aid (Newton et al., 2012).

On the one hand, Teesson et al. (2017) found no advantage of the combined approach (CAP) over universal (Climate) or selective prevention alone

(PreVenture) in reducing alcohol-related outcomes. On the other hand, Newton et al. (2018) reported that the universal Climate and the combined CAP programmes were equally effective in increasing cannabis-related knowledge for up to two years. Evidence was inconclusive as to whether interventions reduced cannabis use and cannabis-related harm. These preliminary results suggest that combining both programme types is no more effective in reducing drug use. We should bear in mind that previous meta-analyses have shown that universal and selective programmes are effective for different age groups (Onrust et al., 2016). Therefore, staging interventions with the universal first, followed by selective interventions (for high-risk individuals) in later years, may have better effects (Newton et al., 2018). The greater effectiveness of personality-target intervention programmes compared to universal programmes needs to be further investigated, partly due to the high costs that derive from implementing programmes like PreVenture.

To summarize, personality-target interventions benefit from previous knowledge on personality traits and alcohol use and misuse associations. These programmes show a moderate effect on delaying consumption and reducing drinking frequency and quantity, HED, and alcohol-related problems in adolescents. They also provide promising results in clinical and adult populations. However, further research is needed to firmly conclude which types of prevention and treatment programmes, and even the combination of different types, are more effective and efficient in reducing alcohol-related outcomes in various alcohol use stages (onset, regular habit, alcohol use disorders) and populations (pre-adolescents, adolescents, adults, clinical populations).

Future Research Directions

Although much progress has been made in studying personality and its relation to drinking behaviour, future research should provide further evidence about the functional relationship between personality and alcohol use and misuse. Discussion should also explore how this empirical evidence may help improve existing prevention/intervention programmes (e.g., including psychoeducation about the reciprocal effects between alcohol use and personality). Finally, it is worth mentioning that the influence of personality on alcohol-related outcomes is relevant, but only explains a limited percentage of the variance of complex alcohol use and misuse behaviour. There are also other related biological (e.g., genetic factors), psychological (e.g., expectancies about alcohol's effects), and social variables (e.g., economic or demographic factors) that influence drinking behaviour and alcohol use disorders. These should be taken into account to explain alcohol consumptions and the alcohol use disorders.

Conclusions

Since the first propositions of alcoholism typologies, the question of how personality characteristics are linked to alcohol-related outcomes has proven compelling yet challenging for psychological researchers. The popular growth of the trait theory approach and the support of cumulative empirical evidence have helped delineate links between personality alcohol use and misuse. Characteristics of positive emotionality, disinhibition, and negative emotionality have been consistently related to different alcohol outcomes. To explain these associations, the existence of three personality aetiological pathways to alcohol use and misuse has been proposed. On the positive-affect regulation pathway, the personality characteristics of positive emotionality would predispose to drink because "it is fun" or because "I like the feeling" (i.e., enhancement drinking motives) which, in turn, predispose to higher alcohol use and more alcohol-related problems. On the negative-affect regulation pathway, negative emotionality would predispose to drink "to relax" or "to avoid my problems" which would, in turn, be related to more alcohol-related problems (e.g., stronger physical dependence, non-compliance at work, etc.). Finally, the association of disagreeable disinhibition or low agreeableness (in addition to unconscientious disinhibition or low conscientiousness) traits with alcohol outcomes would seem to be better conceptualized from a deviance proneness pathway, in which alcohol use and misuse would form part of a more general pattern of deviant behaviour. The findings about the associations between personality and alcohol outcomes have also influenced the development of useful personality-target interventions to prevent and treat alcohol abuse and alcohol-related problems.

Acknowledgements Preparation of this chapter was supported in part by grants from the Spanish Ministry of Science, Innovation and Universities (MICIU/FEDER RTI2018-099800-B-I00) and the Universitat Jaume I (Grants UJI-A2017-18, UJI-B2017-74 and UJI-A2019-08).

References

Adan, A., Forero, D. A., & Navarro, J. F. (2017). Personality traits related to binge drinking: A systematic review. *Frontiers in Psychiatry, 8*, 1–11. https://doi.org/10.3389/fpsyt.2017.00134

Aluja, A., Lucas, I., Blanch, A., & Blanco, E. (2019). Personality and disinhibitory psychopathology in alcohol consumption: A study from the biological-factorial personality models of Eysenck, Gray and Zuckerman. *Personality and Individual Differences, 142*, 159–165. https://doi.org/10.1016/j.paid.2019.01.030

Anglim, J., & O'Connor, P. (2019). Measurement and research using the big five, HEXACO, and narrow traits: A primer for researchers and practitioners. *Australian Journal of Psychology, 71*, 16–25. https://doi.org/10.1111/ajpy.12202

Ashton, M. C., & Lee, K. (2007). Empirical, theoretical, and practical advantages of the HEXACO model of personality structure. *Personality and Social Psychology Review, 11*, 150–166. https://doi.org/10.1177/1088868306294907

Babor, T. F. (1996). The classification of alcoholics typology theories from the 19th century to the present. *Alcohol Research and Health, 20*, 6–14.

Babor, T. F., Hofmann, M., DelBoca, F. K., Hesselbrock, V., Meyer, R. E., Dolinsky, Z. S., & Rounsaville, B. (1992). Types of alcoholics: I. Evidence for an empirically derived typology based on indicators of vulnerability and severity. *Archives of General Psychiatry, 49*(8), 599–608.

Ball, S. A. (2005). Personality traits, problems, and disorders: Clinical applications to substance use disorders. *Journal of Research in Personality, 39*, 84–102.

Blevins, C. E., Abrantes, A. M., & Stephens, R. S. (2016). Motivational pathways from antecedents of alcohol use to consequences: A structural model of using alcohol to cope with negative affect. *American Journal of Drug & Alcohol Abuse, 42*, 395–403. https://doi.org/10.3109/00952990.2016.1141915

Blonigen, D. M., Hicks, B. M., Krueger, R. F., Patrick, C. J., & Iacono, W. G. (2005). Psychopathic personality traits: Heritability and genetic overlap with internalizing and externalizing psychopathology. *Psychological Medicine, 35*, 637–648.

Bogg, T., & Roberts, B. W. (2004). Conscientiousness and health-related behaviors: A meta-analysis of the leading behavioral contributors to mortality. *Psychological Bulletin, 130*, 887–919. https://doi.org/10.1037/0033-2909.130.6.887

Bowman, K. M., & Jellinek, E. M. (1941). Alcohol addiction and its treatment. *Quarterly Journal of Studies on Alcohol, 2*, 98–176. https://doi.org/10.15288/qjsa.1941.2.98

Boyle, G. J., Matthews, G., & Saklofske, D. H. (Eds.). (2008). *The SAGE handbook of personality theory and assessment: Volume 1 — Personality theories and models*. Thousand Oaks, CA: Sage. https://doi.org/10.4135/9781849200462

Carpenter, W. B. (1850). *On the use and abuse of alcoholic liquors in health and disease*. Philadelphia, PA: Lea and Blanchard. https://doi.org/10.1037/12212-000

Cloninger, C. R. (1998). The genetics and psychobiology of the seven-factor model of personality. In K. R. Silk (Ed.), *Review of psychiatry series. Biology of personality disorders* (pp. 63–92). Arlington, VA: American Psychiatric Association.

Cloninger, C. R., Sigvardsson, S., & Bohman, M. (1996). Type I and type II alcoholism: An update. *Alcohol Health & Research World, 20*, 18–23.

Conrod, P. J. (2016). Personality-targeted interventions for substance use and misuse. *Current Addiction Reports, 3*, 426–436. https://doi.org/10.1007/s40429-016-0127-6

Conrod, P. J., Stewart, S. H., Comeau, N., & Maclean, M. (2006). Efficacy of cognitive-behavioral interventions targeting personality risk factors for youth alcohol misuse. *Journal of Clinical Child and Adolescent Psychology, 35*, 550–563. https://doi.org/10.1207/s15374424jccp3504_6

Conway, C. C., Forbes, M. K., Forbush, K. T., Fried, E. I., Hallquist, M. N., Kotov, R., … Eaton, N. R. (2019). A hierarchical taxonomy of psychopathology can transform mental health research. *Perspectives on Psychological Science, 14*, 419–436. https://doi.org/10.1177/1745691618810696

Cooper, M. L., Kuntsche, E., Levitt, A., Barber, L. L., & Wolf, S. (2016). Motivational models of substance use: A review of theory and research on motives for using alcohol, marijuana, and tobacco. In *The Oxford handbook of substance use and substance use disorders* (Vol. 1, pp. 375–421). New York, NY: Oxford University Press. https://doi.org/10.1093/oxfordhb/9780199381678.013.017

Corr, P. J., & McNaughton, N. (2012). Neuroscience and approach/avoidance personality traits: A two stage (valuation-motivation) approach. *Neuroscience and Biobehavioral Reviews, 36*, 2339–2354. https://doi.org/10.1016/j.neubiorev.2012.09.013

Coskunpinar, A., Dir, A. L., & Cyders, M. A. (2013). Multidimensionality in impulsivity and alcohol use: A meta-analysis using the UPPS model of impulsivity. *Alcoholism: Clinical and Experimental Research, 37*, 1441–1450. https://doi.org/10.1111/acer.12131

Cyders, M. A., Smith, G. T., Spillane, N. S., Fischer, S., Annus, A. M., & Peterson, C. (2007). Integration of impulsivity and positive mood to predict risky behavior: Development and validation of a measure of positive urgency. *Psychological Assessment, 19*, 107–118. https://doi.org/10.1037/1040-3590.19.1.107

Digman, J. M. (1997). Higher-order factors of the Big Five. *Journal of Personality and Social Psychology, 73*, 1246–1256.

Edalati, H., Afzali, M. H., Castellanos-Ryan, N., & Conrod, P. J. (2019). The effect of contextual risk factors on the effectiveness of brief personality-targeted interventions for adolescent alcohol use and misuse: A cluster-randomized trial. *Alcoholism: Clinical and Experimental Research, 43*, 997–1006. https://doi.org/10.1111/acer.14016

Edalati, H., & Conrod, P. J. (2019). A review of personality-targeted interventions for prevention of substance misuse and related harm in community samples of adolescents. *Frontiers in Psychiatry, 9*, 1–9. https://doi.org/10.3389/fpsyt.2018.00770

Edwards, A. C., Gardner, C. O., Hickman, M., & Kendler, K. S. (2015). A prospective longitudinal model predicting early adult alcohol problems: Evidence for a robust externalizing pathway. *Psychological Medicine, 46*, 957–968. https://doi.org/10.1017/S0033291715002457

Engel, G. L. (1977). The need for a new medical model: A challenge for biomedicine. *Science, 196*, 129–136.

Eysenck, H. J. (1990). Biological dimensions of personality. In *Handbook of personality: Theory and research* (pp. 244–276). New York, NY: Guilford.

Goldberg, L. R. (1993). The structure of phenotypic personality traits. *American Psychologist, 48*, 26–34. https://doi.org/10.1016/j.jrp.2008.04.002

Gray, J. A. (1991). The neuropsychology of temperament. In J. Strelau & A. Angleitner (Eds.), *Perspectives on individual differences. Explorations in temperament: International perspectives on theory and measurement* (pp. 105–128). New York, NY: Plenum Press.

Hicks, B. M., Durbin, C. E., Blonigen, D. M., Iacono, W. G., & McGue, M. (2012). Relationship between personality change and the onset and course of alcohol dependence in young adulthood. *Addiction, 107*, 540–548.

Ibáñez, M. I., Camacho, L., Mezquita, L., Villa, H., Moya-Higueras, J., & Ortet, G. (2015). Alcohol expectancies mediate and moderate the associations between Big Five personality traits and adolescent alcohol consumption and alcohol-related problems. *Frontiers in Psychology*, 6. https://doi.org/10.3389/fpsyg.2015.01838

Ibáñez, M. I., Ruipérez, M. A., Villa, H., Moya, J., & Ortet, G. (2008). Personality and alcohol use. In G. Boyle, G. Matthews, & D. Saklofske (Eds.), *The SAGE handbook of personality theory and assessment, Vol. 1: Personality theories and models* (pp. 677–697). Thousand Oaks, CA: Sage.

Ibáñez, M. I., Sabater-Grande, G., Barreda-Tarrazona, I., Mezquita, L., López-Ovejero, S., Villa, H., … Georgantzís, N. (2016). Take the money and run: Psychopathic behavior in the trust game. *Frontiers in Psychology, 7*. https://doi.org/10.3389/fpsyg.2016.01866

John, O. P., Naumann, L. P., & Soto, C. J. (2008). Paradigm shift to the integrative big-five trait taxonomy: History, measurement, and conceptual issues. In O. P. John, R. W. Robins, & L. A. Pervin (Eds.), *Handbook of personality: Theory and research* (3rd ed., pp. 114–153). New York, NY: Guilford Press.

Kendler, K. S., Gardner, C. O., & Prescott, C. A. (2011). Toward a comprehensive developmental model for alcohol use disorders in men. *Twin Research and Human Genetics, 14*, 1–15.

Kendler, K. S., & Myers, J. (2014). The boundaries of the internalizing and externalizing genetic spectra in men and women. *Psychological Medicine, 44*, 647–655. https://doi.org/10.1017/S0033291713000585

Kendler, K. S., Ohlsson, H., Edwards, A. C., Sundquist, J., & Sundquist, K. (2016). A developmental model for alcohol use disorders in Swedish men. *Psychological Medicine, 46*, 2759–2770. https://doi.org/10.1017/S0033291716001409

Kotov, R., Gamez, W., Schmidt, F., & Watson, D. (2010). Linking "big" personality traits to anxiety, depressive, and substance use disorders: A meta-analysis. *Psychological Bulletin, 136*, 768–821.

Krueger, R. F., Hicks, B. M., Patrick, C. J., Carlson, S. R., Iacono, W. G., & McGue, M. (2002). Etiologic connections among substance dependence, antisocial behavior and personality: Modeling the externalizing spectrum. *Journal of Abnormal Psychology, 111*, 411–424.

Lahey, B. B., Krueger, R. F., Rathouz, P. J., Waldman, I. D., & Zald, D. H. (2017). A hierarchical causal taxonomy of psychopathology across the life span. *Psychological Bulletin, 143*, 142–186. https://doi.org/10.1037/bul0000069

Leggio, L., Kenna, G. A., Fenton, M., Bonenfant, E., & Swift, R. M. (2009). Typologies of alcohol dependence. From Jellinek to genetics and beyond. *Neuropsychology Review, 19*, 115–129. https://doi.org/10.1007/s11065-008-9080-z

Littlefield, A. K., Agrawal, A., Ellingson, J. M., Kristjansson, S., Madden, P. A. F., Bucholz, K. K., … Sher, K. J. (2011). Does variance in drinking motives explain the genetic overlap between personality and alcohol use disorder symptoms? A twin study of young women. *Alcoholism: Clinical and Experimental Research, 35*, 2242–2250.

Littlefield, A. K., & Sher, K. J. (2016). Personality and substance use disorders. In K. J. Sher (Ed.), *The Oxford handbook of substance use and substance use disorders* (Vol. 1). Oxford University Press. https://doi.org/10.1093/oxfordhb/9780199381678.013.006

Littlefield, A. K., Sher, K. J., & Wood, P. K. (2009). A "maturing out" of problematic alcohol involvement related to personality change? *Journal of Abnormal Psychology, 118*, 360–374. https://doi.org/10.1037/a0015125

Littlefield, A. K., Sher, K. J., & Wood, P. K. (2010a). A personality-based description of maturing out of alcohol problems: Extension with a five-factor model and robustness to modeling challenges. *Addictive Behaviors, 35*, 948–954.

Littlefield, A. K., Sher, K. J., & Wood, P. K. (2010b). Do changes in drinking motives mediate the relation between personality change and "maturing out" of problem drinking? *Journal of Abnormal Psychology, 119*, 93–105. https://doi.org/10.1037/a0017512

Littlefield, A. K., Vergés, A., Wood, P. K., & Sher, K. J. (2012). Transactional models between personality and alcohol involvement: A further examination. *Journal of Abnormal Psychology, 121*, 778–783. https://doi.org/10.1037/a0026912

Malouff, J. M., Thorsteinsson, E. B., Rooke, S. E., & Schutte, N. S. (2007). Alcohol involvement and the Five-Factor Model of personality: A meta-analysis. *Journal of Drug Education, 37*, 277–294. https://doi.org/10.2190/DE.37.3.d

Markon, K., Krueger, R., & Watson, D. (2005). Delineating the structure of normal and abnormal personality: An integrative hierarchical approach. *Journal of Personality and Social Psychology, 88*, 139–157.

McCrae, R. R., & Costa, P. T. (2008). Empirical and theoretical status of the Five-Factor Model of personality traits. In G. J. Boyle, G. Matthews, & D. H. Saklofske (Eds.), *Personality theory and assessment. Personality theories and models* (Vol. 1, pp. 273–294). London, England: Sage.

Merrill, J. E., Wardell, J. D., & Read, J. P. (2014). Drinking motives in the prospective prediction of unique alcohol-related consequences in college students. *Journal of Studies on Alcohol and Drugs, 75*, 93–102.

Mezquita, L., Bravo, A. J., Ortet, G., Pilatti, A., Pearson, M. R., & Ibáñez, M. I. (2018). Cross-cultural examination of different personality pathways to alcohol use and misuse in emerging adulthood. *Drug and Alcohol Dependence, 192*, 193–200. https://doi.org/10.1016/j.drugalcdep.2018.08.004

Mezquita, L., Ibáñez, M. I., Moya, J., Villa, H., & Ortet, G. (2014). A longitudinal examination of different etiological pathways to alcohol use and misuse. *Alcoholism, Clinical and Experimental Research, 38*, 1770–1779. https://doi.org/10.1111/acer.12419

Mezquita, L., Ibáñez, M. I., Villa, H., Fañanás, L., Moya-higueras, J., & Ortet. (2015). Five-factor model and internalizing and externalizing syndromes: A 5-year prospective study. *Personality and Individual Differences, 79*, 98–103. https://doi.org/10.1016/j.paid.2015.02.002

Mezquita, L., Stewart, S. H., Kuntsche, E., & Grant, V. V. (2016). Cross-cultural examination of the five-factor model of drinking motives in Spanish and Canadian undergraduates. *Adicciones, 28*, 215–220. https://doi.org/10.20882/adicciones.822

Mohr, C. D., Tennen, H., Temple, M., Clark, J., Armeli, S., Todd, M., Carney, M. A., Tennen, H., Temple, M., Todd, M., Clark, J., & Carney, M. A. (2005). Moving beyond the keg party: A daily process study of college student drinking motivations. *Psychology of Addictive Behaviors, 19*, 392–403. https://doi.org/10.1037/0893-164X.19.4.392

Newton, N. C., Teesson, M., Barrett, E. L., Slade, T., & Conrod, P. J. (2012). The CAP study, evaluation of integrated universal and selective prevention strategies for youth alcohol misuse: Study protocol of a cluster randomized controlled trial. *BMC Psychiatry, 12*, 118. https://doi.org/10.1186/1471-244X-12-118

Newton, N. C., Teesson, M., Mather, M., Champion, K. E., Barrett, E. L., Stapinski, L., … Slade, T. (2018). Universal cannabis outcomes from the Climate and Preventure (CAP) study: A cluster randomised controlled trial. *Substance Abuse: Treatment, Prevention, and Policy, 13*, 1–13. https://doi.org/10.1186/s13011-018-0171-4

O'Hara, R. E., Boynton, M. H., Scott, D. M., Armeli, S., Tennen, H., Williams, C., & Covault, J. (2014). Drinking to cope among african american college students: An assessment of episode-specific motives. *Psychology of Addictive Behaviors, 28*, 671–681. https://doi.org/10.1037/a0036303

Onrust, S. A., Otten, R., Lammers, J., & Smit, F. (2016). School-based programmes to reduce and prevent substance use in different age groups: What works for whom? Systematic review and meta-regression analysis. *Clinical Psychology Review, 44*, 45–59. https://doi.org/10.1016/j.cpr.2015.11.002

Ortet, G., Martínez, T., Mezquita, L., Morizot, J., & Ibáñez, M. I. (2017). Big five personality trait short questionnaire: Preliminary validation with Spanish adults. *The Spanish Journal of Psychology, 20*, E7. https://doi.org/10.1017/sjp.2017.8

Quinn, P. D., & Harden, K. P. (2013). Differential changes in impulsivity and sensation seeking and the escalation of substance use from adolescence to early adulthood. *Development and Psychopathology, 25*, 223–239. https://doi.org/10.1017/S0954579412000284

Quinn, P. D., Stappenbeck, C. A., & Fromme, K. (2011). Collegiate heavy drinking prospectively predicts change in sensation seeking and impulsivity. *Journal of Abnormal Psychology, 120*, 543–556. https://doi.org/10.1037/a0023159

Roberts, B. W., Walton, K. E., & Viechtbauer, W. (2006). Patterns of mean-level change in personality traits across the life course: A meta-analysis of longitudinal studies. *Psychological Bulletin, 132*, 1–25. https://doi.org/10.1037/0033-2909.132.1.1

Ruiz, M. A., Pincus, A. L., & Dickinson, K. A. (2003). NEO PI-R predictors of alcohol use and alcohol-related problems. *Journal of Personality Assessment, 81*, 226–236.

Ruiz, M. A., Pincus, A. L., & Schinka, J. A. (2008). Externalizing pathology and the five-factor model: A meta-analysis of personality traits associated with antisocial personality disorder, substance use disorder, and their co-occurrence. *Journal of Personality Disorders, 22*, 365–388. https://doi.org/10.1521/pedi.2008.22.4.365

Samek, D. R., Hicks, B. M., Durbin, E., Hinnant, J. B., Iacono, W. G., & McGue, M. (2018). Codevelopment between key personality traits and alcohol use disorder from adolescence through young adulthood. *Journal of Personality, 86*, 261–282. https://doi.org/10.1111/jopy.12311

Segarra, P., Poy, R., López, R., & Moltó, J. (2014). Characterizing carver and White's BIS/BAS subscales using the five factor model of personality. *Personality and Individual Differences, 61–62*, 18–23. https://doi.org/10.1016/j.paid.2013.12.027

Sher, K. J., Grekin, E. R., & Williams, N. A. (2005). The development of alcohol use disorders. *Annual Review of Clinical Psychology, 1*, 493–523. https://doi.org/10.1146/annurev.clinpsy.1.102803.144107

Sher, K. J., & Trull, T. J. (1994). Personality and disinhibitory psychopathology: Alcoholism and antisocial personality disorder. *Journal of Abnormal Psychology, 103*, 92–102. https://doi.org/10.1037/0021-843X.103.1.92

Smillie, L. D. (2008). What is reinforcement sensitivity? Neuroscience paradigms for approach-avoidance process theories of personality. *European Journal of Personality, 22*, 359–384.

Smillie, L. D., Loxton, N. J., & Avery, R. E. (2013). Reinforcement sensitivity theory, research, applications, and future. In T. Chamorro-Premuzic, S. von Stumm, & A. Furnham (Eds.), *The Wiley-Blackwell handbook of individual differences* (pp. 101–131). Malden, MA: Wiley-Blackwell.

Smillie, L. D., Pickering, A. D., & Jackson, C. J. (2006). The new reinforcement sensitivity theory: Implications for personality measurement. *Personality and Social Psychology Review, 10*, 320–335.

Soto, C. J. (2019). How replicable are links between personality traits and consequential life outcomes? The life outcomes of personality replication project. *Psychological Science*. https://doi.org/10.1177/0956797619831612

Stautz, K., & Cooper, A. (2013). Impulsivity-related personality traits and adolescent alcohol use: A meta-analytic review. *Clinical Psychology Review, 33*, 574–592. https://doi.org/10.1016/j.cpr.2013.03.003

Studer, J., Baggio, S., Mohler-Kuo, M., Dermota, P., Daeppen, J.-B., & Gmel, G. (2014). Differential association of drinking motives with alcohol use on weekdays and weekends. *Psychology of Addictive Behaviors, 28*, 651–658. https://doi.org/10.1037/a0035668

Teesson, M., Newton, N. C., Slade, T., Carragher, N., Barrett, E. L., Champion, K. E., … Conrod, P. J. (2017). Combined universal and selective prevention for adolescent alcohol use: A cluster randomized controlled trial. *Psychological Medicine, 47*, 1761–1770. https://doi.org/10.1017/S0033291717000198

Vernig, P. M., & Orsillo, S. M. (2015). Drinking motives and college alcohol problems: A prospective study. *Journal of Substance Use, 20*(5), 340–346. https://doi.org/10.3109/14659891.2014.923053

White, H. R., Anderson, K. G., Ray, A. E., & Mun, E. Y. (2016). Do drinking motives distinguish extreme drinking college students from their peers? *Addictive Behaviors, 60*, 213–218. https://doi.org/10.1016/j.addbeh.2016.04.011

Whiteside, S. P., & Lynam, D. R. (2001). The five factor model and impulsivity: Using a structural model of personality to understand impulsivity. *Personality and Individual Differences, 30*, 669–689. https://doi.org/10.1016/S0191-8869(00)00064-7

Widiger, T. A., Sellbom, M., Chmielewski, M., Clark, L. A., DeYoung, C. G., Kotov, R., … Wright, A. G. C. (2019). Personality in a hierarchical model of psychopathology. *Clinical Psychological Science, 7*, 77–92. https://doi.org/10.1177/2167702618797105

Woicik, P. A., Stewart, S. H., Pihl, R. O., & Conrod, P. J. (2009). The substance use risk profile scale: A scale measuring traits linked to reinforcement-specific substance use profiles. *Addictive Behaviors, 34*, 1042–1055. https://doi.org/10.1016/j.addbeh.2009.07.001

Young-Wolff, K. C., Kendler, K. S., & Prescott, C. A. (2012). Shared genetic contributions to early-onset drinking and drinking to cope motives. *Addictive Behaviors, 37*, 1176–1180.

Zucker, R. A. (1994). Pathways to alcohol problems and alcoholism: A developmental account of the evidence for multiple alcoholism and for contextual contributions to risk. In R. A. Zucker, J. Howard, & G. M. Boyd (Eds.), *The development of alcohol problems: Exploring the biopsychosocial matrix of risk* (NIAAA research monograph No. 26, pp. 255–289). Rockville, MD, US: Department of Health and Human Services.

Zuckerman, M. (2005). *Psychobiology of personality* (2nd ed., Revised and updated. New York, NY: Guildford Press.

Section II

Social Contextual Factors

6

The Social Contexts of Alcohol Use

Richard O. de Visser

Introduction

In many ways, drinking alcohol is like other behaviours to which health psychology models have been applied. However, in important respects, drinking is unlike other behaviours explored by health psychology. Psychology and psychologists tend to focus on individuals—they tend to look at how characteristics of individuals such as genes, personality, and attitudes influence their behaviour. In contrast, this chapter uses a biopsychosocial approach—emphasising the "-social" part of that approach. This approach is taken to provide a reminder that individual drinking and non-drinking always occur within a particular social context.

In 1977, the journal "Science" published an article by George Engel entitled "The need for a new medical model: a challenge for biomedicine". Engel (1977, p. 135) noted that:

> The dominant model of disease today is biomedical, and it leaves no room within its framework for the social, psychological, and behavioural dimensions of illness.

This paper had an impact then, and in the years since: it has been cited by over 600 publications in the PubMed database. Awareness and acceptance of the importance of psychosocial influences on health and well-being have grown, and considerable effort is put into campaigns to encourage individuals to

R. O. de Visser (✉)
Brighton and Sussex Medical School, University of Sussex, Falmer, UK
e-mail: r.o.devisser@bsms.ac.uk

R. Cooke et al. (eds.), *The Palgrave Handbook of Psychological Perspectives on Alcohol Consumption*, https://doi.org/10.1007/978-3-030-66941-6_6

engage in healthier lifestyles. Engel's (1977) biopsychosocial model argues that health and health-related behaviour are influenced by biological factors, psychological factors, and social factors. Expanding on the biomedical model—which was largely focused on diagnosis and treatment—there is a need to consider how social and psychological factors influence disease onset and disease progression and also the maintenance and enhancement of physical and psychological well-being.

The "Bio-" Part of the Biopsychosocial Model

In the context of studies of alcohol use, application of the biopsychosocial model means that we must consider biological factors such as genetic susceptibility to alcoholism and differences in metabolism. For example, the *ALDH2* and *ALD1b* genes are strongly associated with risk for alcoholism, and the distribution of *ADH1b* and *ALDH2* coding variants differs between populations, with the protective alleles most commonly found in people of East Asian origin (Edenberg, 2007; Kimura & Higuchi 2011). One review noted that data from studies of families—including studies of twins and adopted children—indicate that around half of the risk of alcoholism is due to genetic factors (Buscemi & Turchi, 2011). It also highlighted how genetic factors can influence alcohol pharmacokinetics and pharmacodynamics as well as moderating neurophysiological responses such as impulsivity, disinhibition, and sensation-seeking. Recently, epigenetic research has highlighted the importance of alcohol use (especially excessive alcohol use) on gene transcription and expression (Nieratschker, Batra, & Fallgatter, 2013).

These biomedical aspects of alcohol use are clearly important. However, the biopsychosocial model argues that in addition to biological processes such as those outlined in the previous paragraph, we must also consider psychological factors such as attitudes, beliefs, and affective states. In addition, we must consider social contextual factors. These include micro-social influences such as family environment and peer interaction and formal macro-social influences such as legislation, policy, and education, as well as informal social influences derived from the drinking culture.

The "-Psycho-" Part of the Biopsychosocial Model

The title of this collection is "Psychological perspectives of alcohol consumption", and drinking alcohol is to some extent like other behaviours to which health psychology models have been applied. This is evident in chapters in Section I of this collection, which show the important influence individuals' personality and/or beliefs have on their behaviour, and which provide evidence to support various psychological models and theories of behaviour. Not surprisingly, the "psycho" part of the biopsychosocial model is covered well in psychological research.

For example, the Theory of Planned Behaviour (TPB: Ajzen, 1991, see Chap. 2) proposes that the most important determinant of whether a person enacts a specific behaviour is their intention to do so. In turn, stronger intentions to enact a behaviour are predicted by more favourable attitudes towards the behaviour, subjective norm that are more supportive of the behaviour, and greater perceived behavioural control over the behaviour (a variable that is similar to self-efficacy). There is evidence that this model is effective in the domain of alcohol use. For example, a systematic review and meta-analysis of 40 studies indicated strong support for the TPB (Cooke, Dahdah, Norman, & French, 2016). Intentions were significantly related to attitudes, subjective norms, and perceived behavioural control, and in turn, intentions were significantly related to alcohol consumption, with an additional significant direct path from self-efficacy to alcohol consumption. One strength of the TPB is that it does include a measure of social context in the form of social norms. This social component is absent from many widely used models of health behaviour, such as the Health Belief Model (Rosenstock, 1974).

Research framed with reference to other psychological theories has also highlighted the importance of the "psycho" part of the biopsychosocial model in explanations of behaviour change. For example, the Transtheoretical Model (TTM: Prochaska & DiClemente, 1984)—often referred to as the Stages of Change model—proposes that processes of change in behaviour can be mapped onto five stages: "precontemplation"—when people have not even considered changing their behaviour; "contemplation"—when people are considering the advantages and disadvantages of changing their behaviour; "preparation"—when people who have decided to change their behaviour plan how to do so; "action"—when people have begun the process of changing their behaviour; and "maintenance"—when people have sustained their behaviour change for several months and endeavour to prevent relapse to earlier stages. The value of this model compared to the TPB is that it explores and explains processes of change, and there is evidence for its value in explaining recovery from problematic alcohol use (Heather et al., 2009).

Outside of theory-driven models, many studies have examined how well different variables assessed at the level of the individual predict or explain alcohol use. For example, in a study of university students' sensation-seeking, drinking motives in the UK, Atwell, Abraham, and Duka (2011) found that a range of variables made significant independent contributions to the explanation of variance in students' alcohol intake. Multivariate analysis highlighted the importance of age of first drink, sensation-seeking, drinking motives, self-efficacy for adhering to government guidelines and descriptive norms for student alcohol use. Such studies are important for discerning between correlates of alcohol use that are unlikely to be modifiable in interventions (e.g., personality traits such as sensation-seeking) and those that may be more amenable to change (e.g., self-efficacy). In the context of the current chapter, it is notable that descriptive norms were an independent correlate of alcohol use—that is, compared to lighter drinkers, heavier drinkers reported that peer drinking was more common and occurred in greater volumes.

To a large degree, drinking alcohol is like many other behaviours to which health psychology models have been applied. However, in important respects, drinking is unlike other behaviours to which health psychology models have been applied. For example, it is not a one-off or irregular behaviour like screening for sexually transmitted infections (STIs) (de Visser & O'Neill, 2013), and nor is it a frequent private behaviour like tooth-brushing (Anagnostopoulos, Buchanan, Frousiounioti, Niakas, & Potamianos, 2011). For most people, most of the time, drinking is something done in company and/or in public. Drinking (or non-drinking) is also part of our individual self-concept and our social identities in ways that tooth-brushing or STI screening are not. Furthermore, drinking is part of national cultures and subcultures. These social elements of the biopsychosocial model are often overlooked or under-emphasised in psychological studies of alcohol use.

The "-Social" Part of the Biopsychosocial Model

Acknowledgement of the social aspects of drinking means that psychologists must move away from a purely psychological focus—solely or predominantly focused on individual-level variables—to a psychosocial focus that also emphasises social contextual factors.

As noted with reference to the TPB, it is possible to conceptualise and operationalise the "social" in variables measured at the individual level. The

TPB does this by acknowledging that the alcohol use of an individual is influenced by her/his belief about what is appropriate (injunctive norms) as well as her/his perceptions of what other people actually do (descriptive norms). Another way to conceptualise the social at the level of the individual level is people's perceptions of drinkers and non-drinkers. In one study of university students, Conroy and de Visser (2016) found that compared to regular drinkers, prototypical non-drinkers were evaluated more negatively and were considered to be significantly less sociable by 91% of participants. Not only was this an interesting description of people's beliefs, but participants' ratings of the relative sociability of drinkers and non-drinkers also predicted their own intentions to drink to get drunk (see Chap. 3 for more on prototypes).

However, it is also possible—and indeed, necessary—to conceptualise and operationalise the social aspect of the biopsychosocial model in other ways—many of which overlap and intersect. At the national level, it is clear that there is variation in drinking cultures (see Chaps. 7 and 16). In many cultures, drinking alcohol is proscribed (as is the use of other intoxicants), whereas in other cultures, alcohol use is a normative feature of everyday life and is enmeshed in many celebrations and festivals. The World Health Organization Global status report on alcohol and health (WHO, 2018) indicates that the proportion of people aged 15 years and over who were current drinkers (i.e., had consumed alcohol in the last year) ranged from 60% of people in Europe to 3% of those in the Eastern Mediterranean Region (commonly referred to as the "Middle East"), whereas the proportion of people who had never consumed alcohol ranged from 17% in the Americas to 95% in the Eastern Mediterranean Region.

However, within the broad regions identified by the WHO—Africa, the Americas, the Eastern Mediterranean, Eastern Pacific, Europe, and South-East Asia—there is also broad variation (WHO, 2018). For example, within the Eastern Mediterranean region, the proportion of those aged 15+ years who consumed alcohol in the last year ranged from less than 2% in Jordan to 41% in Israel, which is largely a reflection of the fact that the population in Jordan is predominantly Muslim, whereas the population in Israel is predominantly Jewish (Islam proscribes alcohol use, whereas Judaism is permissive of alcohol use). In addition to variation linked to religion, there is other variation in drinking cultures. For example, within Europe there is wide variation in not only the proportions of drinkers/non-drinkers, and the volumes consumed by drinkers, but also in their patterns of drinking (WHO, 2018). One typology commonly used to explain such variation is the wet culture/dry culture distinction (Room & Mäkelä, 2000). According to this typology, "wet" cultures such as France are characterised by relatively less restrictive alcohol control structures, relatively high per-capita consumption of alcohol but lower rates of drunkenness, and relatively higher alcohol-related chronic disease and mortality. In contrast, "dry" cultures such as Sweden are characterised by relatively more restrictive legislation, less frequent but heavier drinking, and consequent higher rates of drunkenness, violence, and alcohol-related social disorder. Recently, the value of this typology has been questioned in the light of drinking cultures becoming increasingly homogenised as a result of globalisation of alcohol production and marketing (Gordon, Heim, & MacAskill, 2012; see also Chap. 7). However, the need to revise such typologies of drinking given changes at the social and global level highlights the importance of factors beyond the beliefs of the individual (see also Chap. 16).

Less important than determining whether the wet/dry distinction or another pattern is the most accurate characterisation of drinking cultures is the more fundamental need to recognise the importance of drinking cultures and drinking norms at the national level and also among sub-groups of any population. One important characteristic of a drinking culture is its norms for alcohol consumption (Room, 1975; Savic, Room, Mugavin, Pennay, & Livingston, 2016). Norms can be reported by individuals, but they belong to a culture and to interactions between people. Norms can be considered as both a reflection of people's behaviour—"descriptive norms" such as "most people in Australia drink alcohol"—and an expression of how people should behave—"injunctive norms" such as "intoxicants such as alcohol are haram, their use is forbidden in Islam" (Rivis & Sheeran, 2003). The latter conceptualisation argues that norms underlie and shape patterns of alcohol consumption. For example, Room (1975, p. 359) suggested that a norm is "a cultural rule or understanding affecting behaviour, which is to a greater or lesser degree enforced by sanctions".

It was noted above that norms belong to interactions between people. It is important to note that although norms may vary between countries, they may also vary within the same country over time, and at any one time they may also vary within cultures according to age or other demographic characteristics. Savic et al. (2016) noted that drinking cultures can be described in terms of the norms related to patterns, practices, and settings of alcohol use that operate and are enforced in a society (the macro-social level) or in a sub-group within society (the micro-social level). They noted that "drinking cultures are not homogeneous or static but are multiple and moving" (Savic et al., 2016, p. 280) and may vary according to factors such as gender, age, and social class. The sections that follow explore some of this variation.

Some quantitative research has illustrated the importance of the social context for drinking and drinking outcomes. For example, a team led by Cherpitel has explored the relative impact of drinking cultures in relation to individual characteristics and alcohol intake. Cherpitel, Korcha, Witbrodt, and Ye (2018) conducted a multi-level analysis of alcohol-related injuries that combined country-level data for ten countries and individual-level data for over 5000 people who attended hospital emergency departments. Their analyses revealed that after taking into account individual drinking, people from countries in which there was more public drinking were more likely to have experienced an alcohol-related injury in a public context than in a private context, and people from countries in which there was more private drinking were more likely to have been injured following a fall. Additional analysis of a larger data set involving over 14,000 emergency department admissions in 28 countries revealed that alcohol-related injuries are less common in countries where there are more restrictive alcohol policies (Cherpitel, Witbrodt et al., 2018). In that study, alcohol policies were measured using an index that reflects the physical availability of alcohol (e.g., legal minimum drinking age, restrictions on outlet opening times), control of transport and vehicles (e.g., legal blood alcohol limits and random testing), restrictions on advertising and marketing, and controls of drinking contexts (e.g., mandatory training of servers). Other quantitative studies have found clear evidence that alcohol-related morbidity and mortality rates are associated with socioeconomic deprivation (Erskine, Maheswaran, Pearson, & Gleeson, 2010; Jones, Bates, McCoy, & Bellis, 2015).

Quantitative analyses such as those just presented provide one perspective on social influences on alcohol use and health-related outcomes of alcohol use. However, the influence of the social context is perhaps more readily apparent in qualitative studies, because they allow an examination of not only whether social factors affect drinking behaviours and outcomes, but also how members of the population, or sub-sections of the population experience, understand and explain these associations. The sections below summarise the findings of different topics addressed in qualitative studies of social influences on drinking.

"Drinking Is Our Modern Way of Bonding"

Research with adolescents and young adults has highlighted the importance of alcohol as a key component of young people's social networks. Drinking together is a marker of belonging and provides opportunities to make shared memories. To quote to participant in one study of 13- to 25-year olds in South-East England:

> Drinking is our modern way – or the urban way at least – of bonding, of, of, you know with your comrades and your pals in the fox-holes and you've got stories to tell of what happened that night … they share those intimate moments with each other in their vulnerable states. (de Visser, Wheeler, Abraham, & Smith, 2013, p. 1466)

In that study, interviewees gave various positive reasons for using alcohol that emphasised the importance of drinking together for forming and maintaining social connections. Part of this was related to people's greater openness when they had been drinking. Another part was people making memories together and having stores to tell. Furthermore, the negative aspects of drinking served as opportunities for strengthening social bonds. Drinking together provided opportunities for close interpersonal bonding when people cared for drunk friends, were cared for by drunk friends, or when they suffered through hangovers together. These experiences of vulnerability, care, and intimacy are perceived to be unlike the kinds of interactions that may happen in other social contexts such as cinemas or cafés. Furthermore, these experiences and accounts of them were shared via social media (see also sections below):

> You'll be on Facebook and someone will be like: 'Oh I've got such a bad hangover!' and they'll post it everywhere, and then people will be, 'like it'. And people brag about it because alcohol is seen as being cool, and if you don't change how people like think about alcohol then that's not going to change. (de Visser et al., 2013, p. 1467)

Alcohol has been found to have a similar important function for forming and maintaining social connections in other studies of younger and older adults, some of which are described later in this chapter (Emslie, Hunt, & Lyons, 2013, 2015; Murphy, Hart, & Moore, 2017; Nesvåg & Duckert, 2017). For example, in a study of Norwegian workplaces, Nesvåg and Duckert (2017, p. 166) noted:

> Various efforts were also made to bring everyone together in joint conversation and drinking. But it was evident how smaller groups of employees would seek each other out for conversation and drinking. They then usually initiated the new interaction by asking if everybody had something in their glasses and then by toasting to mark how they, at least in the specific situation, formed a significant 'we'.

Such studies highlight the importance of alcohol use not as a behaviour that belongs to, and is determined by, individuals, but as something that is a fundamentally social behaviour.

"A Culture That You Can't Escape From"

The importance of the social context of drinking and its role in forming social connections is evident in studies of young people making the transition from school to university. This transition is important for many reasons: it occurs at a time when existing social networks are disrupted and new ones must be formed; it occurs at a time when many people leave the family home for the first time; it occurs at a time when young people have more individual control over how they spend their time; and it often occurs around the legal drinking age. Together, these changes mean that young people have more opportunities to drink and a need to establish new social networks. Furthermore, as indicated in the heading for this section: "It is just such a culture that you can't escape from" (Hepworth et al., 2016, p. 261). Given the centrality of alcohol in many social interactions, it is perhaps not surprising that drinking alcohol is an important part of making new interpersonal bonds at university.

Studies of university students highlight that students prepare for their arrival at university with the expectation that drinking alcohol will be a key social activity and that higher status is often conferred to those who drink excessively and are perceived to be more fun when drinking (Brown & Murphy, 2020; Davies, Law, & Hennelly, 2018). Furthermore, some studies have revealed that online social networks can be an important part of establishing social connections through alcohol-focused events (Brown & Murphy, 2020). In the accounts of students in their study, Brown and Murphy (2020) found echoes of de Visser et al.'s (2013) finding of the importance of drinking for bonding with others. For example, according to one of their interviewees:

> There is something about going out with people when they're getting drunk and having a good time that does, sort of, bring you closer together. (p.7)

Interviewees also indicated that drinking alcohol together created different and/or stronger bonds than did other social interactions such as having a cup of tea in a communal kitchen within student accommodation.

The implications of this material is that young people who do not drink, or who do not (want to) drink excessively, may need to develop tactics for avoiding excessive drinking and may find themselves excluded from activities that are important to forging new social bonds (Brown & Murphy, 2020). This is likely to be the case in both "wet" cultures (in which alcohol use is an integral part of many everyday social activities) and "dry" cultures (in which alcohol use is an important part of "time out" and celebrations). As noted above, non-drinkers and non-drinking tend to be evaluated negatively. Many young people appear to be apprehensive about "feeling like an outsider looking in" and "missing out" on a shared experience if they do not drink alcohol when socialising:

> I may feel like I've missed out on bonding with people. Sometimes when you're sober and others are drunk, nothing is as funny as you expect it to be and you can end up lagging behind in the conversations/excitement rather than getting caught up in the fun of it all when drunk. (Conroy & de Visser, 2018, p. 94)

However, other studies have found that bad or regrettable behaviour when drinking can have negative repercussions for individuals' reputations and social standing (Davies et al., 2018). The intervention-related implications of such findings are that concerns about reputations and not engaging in bad or embarrassing behaviour may be a useful focus for interventions.

"We're Doing Something Together"

Although attention is often directed towards young people's drinking—in the media and in academic research—it is important to keep in mind that alcohol use is a major (but often overlooked) cause of harm among adults in midlife. For example, in one analysis of official records for England and Wales, half of all alcohol-related deaths were found to have occurred among the 45–64 year age group, despite this group only making up one-quarter of the total population (Erskine et al., 2010).

As among younger people, alcohol use among older people is intertwined with micro-social interactions and macro-social influences. Whereas the material in the previous section focused on the role of alcohol in how young people establish new social networks, other research has highlighted the important role of alcohol for consolidating relationships and individual identities among adults in later stages of their lives. In one project, Emslie and colleagues (Emslie et al., 2013, 2015) highlighted the central role of alcohol in the social lives of Scottish men and women aged 28–52 years using data derived from single-sex and mixed-sex group interviews. In their report of men's accounts, Emslie et al. (2013) noted a close interaction between adult male friendship and drinking in pubs—especially drinking pints of beer in pubs. Participants explained that alcohol helped men to become sufficiently relaxed or disinhibited to interact in ways that allowed them to forge deeper friendships, and that men rely more on alcohol for socialising than women for because they are typically more reticent about opening up to others:

> Men don't really like to open up or chat as easily, so they need a couple of pints to try and kind of get them oiled up … Women I think are more naturally kind of gregarious and bubbly and sociable, so they don't really need to be drunk. (p. 36)

Within the context of the pub, buying rounds of drinks was an important part of the process whereby people would be included and a sense of reciprocity was developed:

> Of course the deal is, I'll buy you one back and there becomes a certain sense of comfort there. It gets round the sort of awkwardness you might have in the sort of, male-to-male relationships. (p. 37)

Although some men described experiencing negative physical and psychological effects of drinking too much—suffering hangovers or feeling regret about not having done something more productive than sitting and drinking—they also described the psychological benefits of drinking. Relaxing, laughing, and joking with friend were described as being "uplifting":

> If you go out with your mates, have a few drinks, it's great for your mental health. You don't feel lonely, you don't feel sad or depressed, it always cheers you up, you know. So I'd say that that's a huge benefit. (p. 38)

Furthermore, inviting a male friend who was having problems to the pub ensured that he was not vulnerable to loneliness and also allowed the "feminine" work of talking about emotions or vulnerability to occur in the suitably "masculine", familiar, and non-threatening context of the pub.

The parallel analyses of adult women's drinking also emphasised the importance of the social context of drinking (Emslie et al., 2015). For example, the accounts of mothers with young children indicated that alcohol use could be associated with two senses of "time out" and time that was shared with others. First, drinking at home with a partner after children had been put to bed was a symbolic marker of adult time and time out from the responsibilities of parenting alcohol use:

> it would be a kind of like, a declaration of adulthood … once they've [children] got to bed … Just trying to have a kind of bit of atmosphere with your husband … not just like sitting on the couch and staring at the telly … we're doing something together. (Emslie et al., 2015, p. 442)

Clear in this quote is the importance of the sharing of adult time with her partner. In this case, alcohol was used as a marker of adulthood, and alcohol was used to construct a relaxed atmosphere. In contrast, the second form of "time out" could also be conceived as a form of time travel to an earlier phase of the life course: a pre-family period when they were more carefree and when alcohol was used for intoxication:

> There is quite a build up to our nights out … we regress, I think! (laughter). We go back to just being teenagers, really, and we talk about what we're doing with our hair, and our shoes, we'll swap dresses … it is like going back to reliving your youth. (Emslie et al., 2015, p. 443)

Important to this account is the sharing—of alcohol, of clothes, and of the pronoun "we". Prominent in many accounts was use of the term "the girls", which indicates the continuation of long-standing friendships that have endured since childhood.

An important implication of references to femininity was the influence of gender norms on what women drank and how they drank. Even though the women interviewed used alcohol to perform many different femininities, traditional notions of appropriate feminine behaviour—including types of drinks, patterns of drinking, and physical appearance—formed the backdrop to their experiences. Emslie et al. (2015) argued that midlife women's drinking remains tied to the performance of "idealised" femininity, but at the same time represents a way of achieving "time out" from the demands of traditional feminine norms. Taken together, Emslie et al.'s (2013, 2015) papers highlight the importance of the social context of drinking: from the interpersonal (with partners), to the group, and the macro-social context of current and past gender role norms.

"I'm Trying to Develop a New Social Network"

Given the importance of alcohol to making and sustaining social connections, it is not surprising that people who stop drinking may face considerable challenges in their social lives. Evidence of such processes comes from research into people engaged with Alcoholics Anonymous (AA) as a way of managing a transition to sustained alcohol abstinence. Rodriguez-Morales' (2016, 2017) research has revealed the frustration that some people feel in not being able to control their alcohol use and the implications that this has for their social lives by distancing them from people who can drink socially and distancing them from many social interactions. This is illustrated in a quote from one study participant:

> if I'm being perfectly honest sometimes it does piss me off that some people can sit down and have a lovely meal with one or two glasses of wine and just leave it like that, that pisses me off sometimes, and it annoys me as well I don't know it annoys me, it annoys me that it annoys me that I've got this disease. (Rodriguez-Morales, 2017, p. 380)

This participant also noted that his inability to socialise in the typical adult public spaces—bars and pubs—mean that he was having to work hard to forge new social bonds in alcohol-free contexts with fellow non-drinkers:

> I avoid going to places where I think I'll be vulnerable so I avoid going in pubs and clubs … I'm trying to develop a new social network within the fellowship. (Rodriguez-Morales, 2017, p. 378)

Fortunately, this interviewee and others were able to find in their AA group not only support for managing their addiction, but also an alternative social network and social activities that did not involve drinking alcohol. These experiential accounts reflect the findings of other research (Groh, Jason, & Keys, 2008; Kaskutas, Bond, & Humphreys, 2002).

Given the social import of drinking, and the difficulty of becoming a former-drinker, it is not surprising the non-drinkers face various challenges in their social lives. As noted elsewhere in this volume (Chap. 14), they report being called on by others to explain, to justify, and to defend their non-drinking, and they must also resist pressure from others and indirect efforts to break down their resistance to drinking alcohol (Conroy & de Visser, 2014, 2015). Paradoxically, many non-drinkers found that they could only be true to themselves and not drink if they were untrue to others about their reasons for not drinking. These findings underscored the strength of the expectation that young people *should* drink when socialising unless they have a very good reason (Conroy & de Visser, 2014, 2015).

Similar findings were reported by Bartram, Eliott, Hanson-Easey, and Crabb (2017) in their study of older adults who had given up drinking or significantly reduced their alcohol intake. Respondents reported various strategies for having a fulfilling social life as a non-drinker in a (heavy) drinking culture. Strategies that involved little change to existing patterns of socialising were reported to be more acceptable to peers—for example, a former-drinker could still go to pubs or parties where others were drinking alcohol and have non-alcoholic drinks. In contrast, interviewees reported that strategies that involved more substantial changes to others' social activities—such as replacing drinking activities with other social activities—were less acceptable. Echoing the findings of studies reported in the sub-sections above, Bartram et al. (2017) highlighted that the social role and the social meaning of drinking mean that becoming a non-drinker poses challenges for individuals and their social networks.

The Importance of Drinking to Social Identity

Qualitative research has highlighted the importance of drinking for social identity—in terms of both how people are perceived because of whether, what, and how they drink, and how people use alcohol to portray a particular image or identity. Gender identity is one important aspect of overall identity that has been found to be linked to alcohol use. Women's alcohol use (particularly heavy drinking and public drunkenness) tends to be judged more harshly than men's drinking (de Visser & McDonnell, 2012; Leigh, 1995; Patterson, Emslie, Mason, Fergie, & Hilton, 2016; Plant, 2008). Whereas drinking and heavy drinking are considered acceptable for men, and even expected as part of "masculine" displays of risk taking, physical resilience, and aggression, heavy drinking is not condoned as acceptable "feminine" behaviour, because of supposed links to sexual disinhibition, and neglect of nurturing, maternal behaviour (Leigh, 1995; Plant, 2008). These beliefs have been found to persist despite the fact that there has been a convergence in men's and women's drinking over recent years (Slade et al., 2016). To use terminology introduced earlier in this chapter, there appears to be a disjuncture between descriptive norms and injunctive norms.

Not only are there different expectations of whether and how much men and women should drink, but there are gender stereotypes for appropriate drinks for men and women. Media and marketing perpetuate gendered distinctions between appropriate male and female drinks which influence people's drinking behaviour: it is considered less masculine for men to drink wine, alcopops, or champagne than to drink beer or spirits (de Visser & McDonnell, 2012; de Visser & Smith, 2007; Emslie et al., 2013; Lyons et al., 2006; Patterson et al., 2016; Towns, Parker, & Chase, 2012). The gendering of drinks has also been found to be used as a marker of sexuality among gay men and lesbian women (Emslie, Lennox, & Ireland, 2017). Many interviewees recognised a simplistic inversion of gender stereotypes such that alcopops were associated with gay men and beer with lesbians. It is notable that de Visser and McDonnell (2012) and Emslie et al. (2017) found that even when interviewees dismissed restrictive gender stereotypes around drink choice, their behaviour was still to some extent shaped by them. This again highlights that social contextual variables can sometimes have a greater influence on drinking behaviour than individual beliefs.

"It's Almost as If It's an Actual Advertisement for Drinking!"

As indicated in an earlier section, online social networks can be an important way for new university students to establishing social connections through alcohol-focused events (Brown & Murphy, 2020). Numerous studies with a broad array of population segments have indicated how online social networks are important for individual and group alcohol-related identities (see Chap. 11). They have been identified as a medium that people use to illustrate the ordinary and extraordinary aspects of alcohol use (Brown & Gregg, 2012; Hebden, Lyons, Goodwin, & McCreanor, 2015; Hendriks, van den Putte, Gebhardt, & Moreno, 2018; Jones et al., 2017; Lyons, McCreanor, Goodwin, & Barnes, 2017). Research has revealed that although some people are happy to post or be tagged in both positive and negative portrayals of social alcohol use, there is a tendency for displays of alcohol use drinking via social media to produce a positive "airbrushed" image of drinking that obscures the negative aspects (Hendriks et al., 2018; Jones et al., 2017; Niland, Lyons, Goodwin, & Hutton, 2014). However, even when negative aspects of drinking are included in posts—for example, accounts of drinking too much or suffering hangovers—their sharing on social media perhaps only serves to reinforce the point made earlier that positive *and* negative aspects of drinking can reinforce a sense of connection and belonging.

The net positive portrayal of drinking online is something of which users of social media are aware. In one study of young adults in Australia, some interviewees noted that although they were not personally influenced by such portrayals, others suggested that they and their peers could be encouraged by social media posts to engage in drinking more frequently and/or in greater volumes:

> Reading others[sic] posts about alcohol definitely persuades me to drink when I probably wouldn't be tempted otherwise. Furthermore, viewing pictures on social media of friends drinking also gets me in the mood to drink as everyone always look[sic] really happy and having a great time! Almost as if it's an actual advertisement for drinking! (Jones et al., 2017, p. 180)

The material briefly covered here indicates the importance of alcohol for identity and reputation not only in "real life", but also in the online world of social media. Earlier, it was noted that in various contexts, people often modify their drinking behaviour so that it conforms to social expectations (Conroy & de Visser, 2014, 2015; de Visser & McDonnell 2012; Emslie et al. 2017). Similar processes appear to occur online, with people tending to post material that reinforces the image of drinkers and drinking as fun and funny, with the implication that non-drinkers are missing out on this fun and can potentially detract from it. Here again we can see an interaction between macro-social influences, micro-social interactions, and individuals' behaviour.

Addressing Social Context Influences in Efforts to Change Behaviour

The material presented above highlights the importance of the social context for drinking. It would seem important, therefore, for interventions to at least acknowledge and ideally address social contextual variables. One way to do this is to address and challenge social norms to provide realistic information about other people's patterns of alcohol consumption. However, a review of social norms interventions among college/university students found that although some significant effects were found, on balance they conveyed no substantive meaningful benefits when measured at the level of individual drinking behaviours (Foxcroft, Moreira, Almeida Santimano, & Smith, 2015).

Such findings should not be taken to indicate that there is no value in addressing social norms or other social aspects of drinking. Further evidence of the effectiveness of social norms interventions may come from larger, better quality studies. It should also be noted that in many studies, the sample includes all drinkers, a large proportion of whom are not motivated to change their behaviour. Many drinkers are not concerned about their drinking (de Visser, Brown, Cooke, Cooper & Memon, 2017), and using the terminology of the TTM outlined earlier in this chapter, they would be classed as being in "precontemplation" of behaviour change (Prochaska & DiClemente, 1984).

Interventions directed towards people who are already motivated to change their behaviour often include a component of support. This could be focused on social contextual variables such as direct peer support (e.g., "buddy" schemes) and/or the creation of a community of supportive non-drinkers. Buddy schemes—in which two people seeking to change their behaviour are paired up to offer each other mutual support—have been found to increase the likelihood of successful behaviour change in contexts such as illicit drug use, smoking cessation, and physical activity (Bauld, Bell, McCullough, Richardson, & Greaves, 2009; Jepson, Harris, Platt, & Tannahill, 2010; Lüscher & Scholz, 2017; West & Stapleton, 2008). However, there is less clear evidence that such schemes are effective for changing alcohol use.

Evidence for the important of social contextual variables on alcohol use comes from studies of alcohol abstinence challenges in which people give up alcohol for one month (e.g., au.dryjuly.com, nz.dryjuly.com; www.dryjanuary.org.uk). Such campaigns are directed towards people who are in the "preparation" or "action" phases of the TTM. The remainder of this section will focus on studies of "Dry January", the UK alcohol abstinence challenge run by the charity Alcohol Change UK to encourage people to think about the way they drink and to talk about alcohol. Its popularity is growing: registrations via the website were just over 4000 in 2013, but it has been estimated that each year, over one million adults in the UK attempt a "Dry January" (de Visser, Robinson, Smith, Walmsley & Cass, 2017).

Key to the success of Dry January is the campaign's use of a range of broadcast and social media to spread the central message. It has been suggested (de Visser, Brown, et al., 2017) that awareness and acceptance of the campaign has been facilitated by processes of "social contagion"—whereby changes in the beliefs and behaviour of a sub-group of people spread through the broader population (Christakis & Fowler, 2013)—and "diffusion" of new ideas or practices between members of a social system via channels of communication including appropriate media (Rogers, 2003). The net effect of such influence is to alter social norms for alcohol and the broader drinking culture, and evidence of such change supports the arguments made earlier that rather than being homogeneous and static, drinking cultures are multiple and malleable (Room, 1975; Savic et al., 2016).

An important influence on whether individuals make a successful attempt to remain abstinent during Dry January is their engagement with the social support provided by the campaign. Dry January provides multiple forms of social support, including encouraging messages sent via email, text message, or the campaign smartphone application. It also creates and supports a community of participants via Facebook groups, a website with participant blogs, suggestions for alcohol-free drinks and alternative social activities, and live online "Q and A" sessions. These various sources of support are well received and well used by participants, and people who engage more with the support provided are more likely to make a successful attempt at Dry January (de Visser & Nicholls, 2020). These findings resonate with findings from qualitative studies that social support may help participants in alcohol abstinence challenges (Pennay, MacLean, Rankin, & O'Rourke, 2018). To repurpose the four quotes used as subheadings and the section of this chapter entitled "The "-social" part of the biopsychosocial model", social support provided via Dry January provides an alternative "modern way of bonding" so that compulsory drinking is "a culture that you *can* escape from", with the result that people are non-drinking "doing something together" with the support of "a new social network".

Conclusion

The material presented in this chapter highlights a need to give proper attention to the "social" part of the biopsychosocial model in psychological research into alcohol consumption. Much of the material presented to support the central argument came from qualitative studies, but quantitative studies of social norms interventions and campaigns such as Dry January also emphasise the importance of social context, social norms, and social support. Although much of the evidence presented came from studies of adolescents and young adults—reflecting the state of the evidence base—it is notable that among younger and older drinkers, similar findings emerged. Studies of young people, adults in midlife, non-drinkers, former-drinkers, and people seeking to reduce their alcohol use highlight the importance of social contextual influences on alcohol use. Rather than simply focusing on the beliefs and skills held by individuals, there is a need to consider the various micro-social and macro-social contexts in which individual' use (or non-use) of alcohol is situated. The social contexts of drinking range from broad drinking cultures as reflected in consumption patterns, legislation, and marketing; to sub-cultures and sub-groups including friendship groups (both real and virtual); and dyads such as drinking buddies or abstinence buddies. All of these factors need to be considered in efforts to understand unhealthy patterns of drinking and to promote healthy behaviour.

References

Ajzen, I. (1991). The theory of planned behaviour. *Organizational Behavior and Human Decision Processes, 2*, 179–211. https://doi.org/10.1016/0749-5978(91)90020-T

Anagnostopoulos, F., Buchanan, H., Frousiounioti, S., Niakas, D., & Potamianos, G. (2011). Self-efficacy and oral hygiene beliefs about toothbrushing in dental patients: A model-guided study. *Behavioral Medicine, 37*, 132–139. https://doi.org/10.1080/08964289.2011.636770

Atwell, K., Abraham, C., & Duka, T. (2011). A parsimonious, integrative model of key psychological correlates of UK university students' alcohol consumption. *Alcohol and Alcoholism, 46*, 253–260. https://doi.org/10.1093/alcalc/agr016

Bartram, A., Eliott, J., Hanson-Easey, S., & Crabb, S. (2017). How have people who have stopped or reduced their alcohol consumption incorporated this into their social rituals? *Psychology & Health, 32*, 728–744. https://doi.org/10.1080/08870446.2017.1300260

Bauld, L., Bell, K., McCullough, L., Richardson, L., & Greaves, L. (2009). The effectiveness of NHS smoking cessation services: A systematic review. *Journal of Public Health, 32*, 71–82. https://doi.org/10.1093/pubmed/fdp074

Brown, R., & Gregg, M. (2012). The pedagogy of regret: Facebook, binge drinking and young women. *Continuum, 26*, 357–369. https://doi.org/10.1080/10304312.2012.665834

Brown, R., & Murphy, S. (2020). Alcohol and social connectedness for new residential university students: Implications for alcohol harm reduction. *Journal of Further and Higher Education, 44*, 216–230. https://doi.org/10.1080/0309877X.2018.1527024

Buscemi, L., & Turchi, C. (2011). An overview of the genetic susceptibility to alcoholism. *Medicine, Science, and the Law, 51*(Suppl 1), s2–s6. https://doi.org/10.1258/msl.2010.010054

Cherpitel, C. J., Korcha, R. A., Witbrodt, J., & Ye, Y. (2018). Risk of alcohol-related injury: Does societal drinking context make a difference? *Journal of Studies on Alcohol and Drugs, 79*, 876–880. https://doi.org/10.15288/jsad.2018.79.876

Cherpitel, C. J., Witbrodt, J., Korcha, R. A., Ye, Y., Kool, B., & Monteiro, M. (2018). Multi-level analysis of alcohol-related injury, societal drinking pattern and alcohol control policy: Emergency department data from 28 countries. *Addiction, 113*, 2031–2040. https://doi.org/10.1111/add.14276

Christakis, N. A., & Fowler, J. H. (2013). Social contagion theory: Examining dynamic social networks and human behaviour. *Statistics in Medicine, 32*, 556–577. https://doi.org/10.1002/sim.5408

Conroy, D., & de Visser, R. O. (2014). Being a non-drinking student: An interpretative phenomenological analysis. *Psychology & Health, 29*, 536–551.

Conroy, D., & de Visser, R. O. (2015). The importance of authenticity for student non-drinkers: An interpretative phenomenological analysis. *Journal of Health Psychology, 20*, 1483–1493. https://doi.org/10.1177/1359105313514285

Conroy, D., & de Visser, R. O. (2016). Understanding the association between relative sociability prototypes and university students' drinking intentions. *Substance Use & Misuse, 51*, 1831–1837. https://doi.org/10.1080/10826084.2016.1197939

Conroy, D., & de Visser, R. O. (2018). Benefits and drawbacks of social non-drinking identified by British university students. *Drug and Alcohol Review, 37*(Suppl.1), s89–s97. https://doi.org/10.1111/dar.12610

Cooke, R., Dahdah, M., Norman, P., & French, D. P. (2016). How well does the theory of planned behaviour predict alcohol consumption? A systematic review and meta-analysis. *Health Psychology Review, 10*, 148–167. https://doi.org/10.1080/17437199.2014.947547

Davies, E. L., Law, C., & Hennelly, S. E. (2018). "You have to be prepared to drink": Students' views about reducing excessive alcohol consumption at university. *Health Education, 118*, 2–16. https://doi.org/10.1108/HE-04-2017-0020

de Visser, R.O. & Smith, J.A. (2007) Alcohol consumption and masculine identity among young men. *Psychology & Health, 22*, 595–614. https://doi.org/10.1080/14768320600941772

de Visser, R. O., & McDonnell, E. J. (2012). "That's OK. He's a guy": A mixed-methods study of gender double-standards for alcohol use. *Psychology & Health, 27*, 618–639. https://doi.org/10.1080/08870446.2011.617444

de Visser, R. O., & O'Neill, N. (2013). Identifying and understanding barriers to sexually transmissible infection testing among young people. *Sexual Health, 10*, 553–558. https://doi.org/10.1071/SH13034

de Visser, R. O., & Nicholls, J. (2020). Temporary abstinence during Dry January: predictors of success; impact on well-being and self-efficacy. *Psychology & Health, 35*, 1293–1305. https://doi.org/10.1080/08870446.2020.1743840

de Visser, R. O., Brown, C. E., Cooke, R., Cooper, G., & Memon, A. (2017). Using alcohol unit-marked glasses enhances capacity to monitor intake: Evidence from a mixed-method intervention trial. *Alcohol and Alcoholism, 52*, 206–212.

de Visser, R. O., Robinson, E., Smith, T., Walmsley, M., & Cass, G. (2017). The growth of "Dry January": Promoting participation and the benefits of participation. *European Journal of Public Health, 27*, 929–931.

de Visser, R. O., Wheeler, Z., Abraham, C., & Smith, J. A. (2013). "Drinking is our modern way of bonding": Young people's beliefs about interventions to encourage moderate drinking. *Psychology & Health, 28*, 1460–1480. https://doi.org/10.1080/08870446.2013.828293

Edenberg, H. J. (2007). The genetics of alcohol metabolism: Role of alcohol dehydrogenase and aldehyde dehydrogenase variants. *Alcohol Research & Health, 30*, 5–13.

Emslie, C., Hunt, K., & Lyons, A. (2013). The role of alcohol in forging and maintaining friendships amongst Scottish men in midlife. *Health Psychology, 32*, 33–41. https://doi.org/10.1037/a0029874

Emslie, C., Hunt, K., & Lyons, A. (2015). Transformation and time-out: The role of alcohol in identity construction among Scottish women in early midlife. *International Journal of Drug Policy, 26*(5), 437–445. https://doi.org/10.1016/j.drugpo.2014.12.006

Emslie, C., Lennox, J., & Ireland, L. (2017). The role of alcohol in identity construction among LGBT people: A qualitative study. *Sociology of Health & Illness, 39*, 1465–1479. https://doi.org/10.1111/1467-9566.12605

Engel, G. (1977). The need for a new medical model: The challenge for biomedicine. *Science, 196*, 129–136.

Erskine, S., Maheswaran, R., Pearson, T., & Gleeson, D. (2010). Socioeconomic deprivation, urban-rural location and alcohol-related mortality in England and Wales. *BMC Public Health, 10*, 99. https://doi.org/10.1186/1471-2458-10-99

Foxcroft, D.R., Moreira, M., Almeida Santimano, N.M.L. & Smith, L.A. (2015). Social norms information for alcohol misuse in university and college students. *Cochrane Database of Systematic Reviews, 12*. Art. No.: CD006748. doi: https://doi.org/10.1002/14651858.CD006748.pub4.

Gordon, R., Heim, D., & MacAskill, S. (2012). Rethinking drinking cultures: A review of drinking cultures and a reconstructed dimensional approach. *Public Health, 126*, 3–11. https://doi.org/10.1016/j.puhe.2011.09.014

Groh, D. R., Jason, L. A., & Keys, C. B. (2008). Social network variables in alcoholics anonymous: A literature review. *Clinical Psychology Review, 28*, 430–450. https://doi.org/10.1016/j.cpr.2007.07.014

Heather, N., Hönekopp, J., Smailes, D., & The UKATT Research Team. (2009). Progressive stage transition does mean getting better: A further test of the Transtheoretical model in recovery from alcohol problems. *Addiction, 104*, 949–958. https://doi.org/10.1111/j.1360-0443.2009.02578.x

Hebden, R., Lyons, A. C., Goodwin, I., & McCreanor, T. (2015). "When you add alcohol, it gets that much better": University students, alcohol consumption, and online drinking cultures. *Journal of Drug Issues, 45*, 214–226. https://doi.org/10.1177/0022042615575375

Hendriks, H., van den Putte, B., Gebhardt, W. A., & Moreno, M. A. (2018). Social drinking on social media: Content analysis of the social aspects of alcohol-related posts on Facebook and Instagram. *Journal of Medical Internet Research, 20*, e226. https://doi.org/10.2196/jmir.9355

Hepworth, J., McVittie, C., Schofield, T., Lindsay, J. M., Leontini, R., & Germov, J. (2016). "Just choose the easy option": Students talk about alcohol use and social influence. *Journal of Youth Studies, 19*, 251–268. https://doi.org/10.1080/13676261.2015.1059928

Jepson, R., Harris, F., Platt, S., & Tannahill, C. (2010). The effectiveness of interventions to change six health behaviours: A review of reviews. *BMC Public Health, 10*, 538. https://doi.org/10.1186/1471-2458-10-538

Jones, L., Bates, G., McCoy, E., & Bellis, M. A. (2015). Relationship between alcohol-attributable disease and socioeconomic status, and the role of alcohol consumption in this relationship: A systematic review and meta-analysis. *BMC Public Health, 15*, 400. https://doi.org/10.1186/s12889-015-1720-7

Jones, S. C., Pettigrew, S., Biagioni, N., Daube, M., Chikritzhs, T., Stafford, J., & Tran, J. (2017). Young adults, alcohol and Facebook: A synergistic relationship. *Journal of Social Marketing, 7*, 172–187. https://doi.org/10.1108/JSOCM-09-2016-0046

Kaskutas, L. A., Bond, J., & Humphreys, K. (2002). Social networks as mediators of the effect of Alcoholics Anonymous. *Addiction, 97*, 891–900. https://doi.org/10.1046/j.1360-0443.2002.00118.x

Kimura, M., & Higuchi, S. (2011). Genetics of alcohol dependence. *Psychiatry and Clinical Neurosciences, 65*, 213–225. https://doi.org/10.1111/j.1440-1819.2011.02190.x

Leigh, B. (1995). A thing so fallen, and so vile: Images of drinking and sexuality in women. *Contemporary Drug Problems, 22*, 415–434.

Lüscher, J., & Scholz, U. (2017). Does social support predict smoking abstinence in dual-smoker couples? Evidence from a dyadic approach. *Anxiety, Stress, and Coping, 30*, 273–281. https://doi.org/10.1080/10615806.2016.1270448

Lyons, A., Dalton, S., & Hoy, A. (2006). Hardcore drinking: Portrayals of alcohol consumption in women's and men's magazines. *Journal of Health Psychology, 11*, 223–232. https://doi.org/10.1177/1359105306061183

Lyons, A., McCreanor, T., Goodwin, I., & Barnes, H. M. (Eds.). (2017). *Youth drinking cultures in a digital world: Alcohol, social media and cultures of intoxication*. London, UK: Routledge.

Murphy, D. A., Hart, A., & Moore, D. (2017). Shouting and providing: Forms of exchange in the drinking accounts of young Australians. *Drug and Alcohol Review, 36*, 442–448. https://doi.org/10.1111/dar.12444

Nesvåg, S., & Duckert, F. (2017). Work-related drinking and processes of social integration and marginalization in two Norwegian workplaces. *Culture and Organization, 23*, 157–176. https://doi.org/10.1080/14759551.2015.1021800

Nieratschker, V., Batra, A., & Fallgatter, A. J. (2013). Genetics and epigenetics of alcohol dependence. *Journal of Molecular Psychiatry, 1*, 11. https://doi.org/10.1186/2049-9256-1-11

Niland, P., Lyons, A. C., Goodwin, I., & Hutton, F. (2014). "See it doesn't look pretty does it?": Young adults' airbrushed drinking practices on Facebook. *Psychology & Health, 29*, 877–895. https://doi.org/10.1080/08870446.2014.893345

Patterson, C., Emslie, C., Mason, O., Fergie, G., & Hilton, S. (2016). Content analysis of UK newspaper and online news representations of women's and men's 'binge' drinking: A challenge for communicating evidence-based messages about

single-episodic drinking? *BMJ Open, 6*, e013124. https://doi.org/10.1136/bmjopen-2016-013124
Pennay, A., MacLean, S., Rankin, G., & O'Rourke, S. (2018). Hello Sunday Morning: Strategies used to support temporary alcohol abstinence through participation in an online health promotion programme. *Health Promotion Journal of Australia, 29*, 321–327. https://doi.org/10.1002/hpja.22
Plant, M. L. (2008). The role of alcohol in women's lives. *Journal of Substance Use, 13*, 155–191.
Prochaska, J. O., & DiClemente, C. C. (1984). *The transtheoretical approach: Crossing traditional boundaries of therapy*. Homewood, IL: Dow Jones-Irwin.
Rivis, A., & Sheeran, P. (2003). Descriptive norms as an additional predictor in the theory of planned behaviour: A meta-analysis. *Current Psychology: Developmental, Learning, Personality, Social, 22*, 218–233.
Rodriguez-Morales, L. (2016). *A Hero's Journey: Becoming and Transcendence in Recovery from Addiction* (unpublished PhD dissertation). London, UK: Birkbeck College, University of London.
Rodriguez-Morales, L. (2017). In your own skin: The experience of early recovery from alcohol-use disorder in 12-step fellowships. *Alcoholism Treatment Quarterly, 35*, 372–394.
Rogers, E. (2003). *Diffusion of innovations* (5th ed.). London, UK: Free Press.
Room, R. (1975). Normative perspectives on alcohol use and problems. *Journal of Drug Issues, 5*, 358–368.
Room, R., & Mäkelä, K. (2000). Typologies of the cultural position of drinking. *Journal of Studies on Alcohol, 61*, 475–483. https://doi.org/10.15288/jsa.2000.61.475
Rosenstock, I. (1974). Historical origins of the health belief model. *Health Education & Behavior, 2*, 328–335. https://doi.org/10.1177/109019817400200403
Savic, M., Room, R., Mugavin, J., Pennay, A., & Livingston, M. (2016). Defining "drinking culture": A critical review of its meaning and connotation in social research on alcohol problems. *Drugs: Education, Prevention and Policy, 23*, 270–282. https://doi.org/10.3109/09687637.2016.1153602
Slade, T., Chapman, C., Swift, W., Keyes, K., Tonks, Z., & Teesson, M. (2016). Birth cohort trends in the global epidemiology of alcohol use and alcohol-related harms in men and women: Systematic review and metaregression. *BMJ Open, 6*, e011827. https://doi.org/10.1136/bmjopen-2016-011827
Towns, A. J., Parker, C., & Chase, P. (2012). Constructions of masculinity in alcohol advertising: Implications for the prevention of domestic violence. *Addiction Research & Theory, 20*, 389–401. https://doi.org/10.3109/16066359.2011.648973
West, R., & Stapleton, J. (2008). Clinical and public health significance of treatments to aid smoking cessation. *European Respiratory Review, 17*, 199–204. https://doi.org/10.1183/09059180.00011005
World Health Organization. (2018). *Global status report on alcohol and health, 2018*. Geneva, Switzerland: WHO.

7

Cultural Differences in Alcohol Consumption: The State of the Art and New Perspectives on Drinking Culture Research

Giovanni Aresi and Kim Bloomfield

Introduction

This chapter describes perspectives on studying cultural differences in alcohol consumption and reviews the relevant literature. After introducing the concept of culture and the main approaches used to study drinking cultures, different conceptualisations of such cultures are discussed. The chapter includes a systematic review of the recent literature on drinking cultures. It ends with a discussion of strengths and weaknesses of existing literature on drinking cultures, gaps in the field, and directions for future research.

G. Aresi (✉)
Department of Psychology, Università Cattolica del Sacro Cuore, Milan, Italy
e-mail: Giovanni.aresi@unicatt.it

K. Bloomfield
Centre for Alcohol and Drug Research, Aarhus University, Aarhus, Denmark
e-mail: Kb.crf@psy.au.dk

R. Cooke et al. (eds.), *The Palgrave Handbook of Psychological Perspectives on Alcohol Consumption*, https://doi.org/10.1007/978-3-030-66941-6_7

The Notion of Culture

From an evolutionary point of view, culture is human beings' adaptive organ, our survival mechanism to live in a social world (Ratner, 2008). Cultures are created and evolve as societies adapt to their environmental contexts. As such, culture is essentially fluid and constantly in motion to adapt to ever-changing societal and environmental conditions (Matsumoto & Yoo, 2006). Nonetheless, culture is also considered something relatively stable, accounting for durable differences across societies (Inglehart & Baker, 2000; Minkov, 2011).

There are long-standing challenges in conceptualising "culture", and most scholars agree that it remains a "social construct vaguely referring to a vastly complex set of phenomena" (Jahoda, 2012) (p. 300). Despite the variety of theoretical and methodological perspectives in the field of cultural studies (see Ratner, 2008), a classic and still relevant definition of culture is that proposed by Kroeber and Kluckhohn (1952, p. 181):

> Culture consists of patterns, explicit and implicit, of and for behaviour acquired and transmitted by symbols, constituting the distinctive achievement of human groups, including their embodiments in artefacts; the essential core of culture consists of traditional (i.e. historically derived and selected) ideas and especially their attached values; culture systems may, on the one hand, be considered as products of action, on the other as conditioning elements of further action.

What appears clear is that culture is multidimensional and a multi-layered construct that encompasses virtually all aspects of human life including food, language, morality, and, with regard to this chapter and book, whether or not, how, and under what circumstances and for what reasons we consume alcoholic beverages, that is, our drinking culture (Taras, Rowney, & Steel, 2009).

It is important to note that, far from being passive recipients of culture, individuals are involved in the processes of mutual constitution as "active agents who are socioculturally shaped shapers of themselves and their worlds" (Markus & Hamedani, 2007, p. 5). Therefore, culture shapes and is shaped by individual psychological phenomena, though this is far from being a deterministic influence. Notably, the behaviour of all individuals engaged in a particular context and cultural group (e.g., middle-class European Americans or rural tribe members in Taiwan) is by no means uniform or monolithic. This is because cultural factors (e.g., understanding of different aspects of social life) can be highly complex and diverse, are at times contradictory, and do not act uniformly on all members of the culture. Different groups of people who occupy different positions in society may be differentially exposed to various cultural factors in their individual, within-group, and between-group behaviours. There is also considerable variation in core values (e.g., autonomy) not only across cultural groups, but also within each cultural group (Fischer & Schwartz, 2011). Therefore, it should be expected that some individuals deviate from the standards of their cultural group.

Three key aspects of the sociocultural world are important for this chapter. These are meanings, practices, and products: they all contribute to determine the characteristics of a culture. Bruner (1990) used the term "meanings" and Moscovici (1998) used "representations" to refer to socially constructed entities. Others focused on "values" and "normative systems" (norms) as the core aspect of societal culture (Hofstede, 1980; Schwartz, 1999). Representations and meanings eventually go beyond individuals' contributions and become institutionalised into shared social knowledge and practices that are passed on between and within generations and learned through socialisation. Some meanings may be related to universal issues (e.g., becoming an adult), whereas others are linked to meanings of socially, historically, or context-specific significant categories such as ethnicity, regions of the world, or religion. Importantly, differences in the meanings, representations, and what is normative or of value between social groups and cultural entities imply that worlds and psyches are organised in different ways and ultimately have repercussions for social practices. These are understood as particular ways of acting and interacting in recurrent episodes of everyday life which reflect a social and moral order (Markus & Hamedani, 2007). Participation in routine activities—such as chatting with a friend, attending a meeting, parenting, or teaching—expresses in concrete form what a given context can communicate about how to be a normatively appropriate person, as well as what is regarded as "good", "right", or "real" (Miller & Goodnow, 1995). For this reason, practices are not just behaviours; they are also meaningful acts that coordinate the actions of individuals with those of others and maintain the social context.

Lastly, culture results in products (i.e., artefacts such as television commercials, newspaper articles and headlines, photographs, and social networking sites) that can be conceptualised as psychologically externalised, or as the social order objectified. Cultural products have powerful effects on action because they both reflect the ideas, images, understandings, and values of particular contexts and "re-present" and institutionalise these ideas and values as people engage with them (Markus & Hamedani, 2007).

In sum, culture as a collective product is understood as continually evolving patterns of meanings/representations, practices, and artefacts that are distributed or spread by social interaction within a social entity. Culture lends coherence to behaviour and renders actions meaningful within a given cultural context.

Drinking Cultures

The recognition of marked differences in patterns of alcohol use and the role of alcohol in daily life, beliefs and values of drinking and drinking-related behaviours has given rise to scholarly interest in drinking cultures (Heath, 1976, 1995). However, the drinking culture literature offers little in terms of explicitly defining its research object and has too often taken the concept for granted as a common-sense notion with foreseeable issues in its operationalisation (Savic, Room, Mugavin, Pennay, & Livingston, 2016). Thus, after their efforts at reviewing the literature, Savic et al. (2016, p. 12) proposed a "working definition" that states:

> Drinking cultures are generally described in terms of the norms around patterns, practices, use-values, settings and occasions in relation to alcohol and alcohol problems that operate and are enforced (to varying degrees) in a society (macro-level) or in a subgroup within society (micro-level). Drinking culture also refers to the modes of social control that are employed to enforce norms and practices [...] drinking culture is thought to influence when, where, why and how people drink, how much they drink, their expectations about the effects of different amounts of alcohol, and the behaviours they engage in before, during and after drinking.

As can be seen, this definition focuses mainly on the normative and social control aspects of culture. Norms, in particular, are thought to shape other components of culture, such as values and practices. This definition resonates with early work of Heath (1976, p. 43): "alcohol is almost universally subject to rules and regulations", and Room (1975) who argued that social problems of drinking arise because of a conflict between individual acts and social (cultural) norms. More recently, Gordon, Heim, and MacAskill (Gordon, Heim, & MacAskill, 2012) discussed how both formal (i.e., alcohol laws) and informal (social) norms play a pivotal role in regulating drinking behaviour: they are reflected in attitudes toward alcohol, identify socially permissible drinking practices, and specify the occasions when it is permissible to consume alcohol (see Chap. 4 for more on norms).

Approaches to the Study of Drinking Cultures

Two broad approaches that embrace very different perspectives on the issue of alcohol consumption have been used to study drinking cultures: the anthropological / sociological approach, and the public health approach (Wilson, 2005). Public health scholars view alcohol use and misuse as a social and public health issue. Given the traditional focus of the discipline on social determinants of health beyond the level of the individual (Berkman, Kawachi & Glymour, 2014; Marmot & Wilkinson, 2006), the notion of drinking cultures serves as a useful conceptual tool for research and intervention in this field. From the public health perspective, treating "culture" as a variable has not always been without challenges. Critiques are that the public health literature has had a tendency to oversimplify the notion of culture, either treating it as a "black box" of protective/risk factors for individual alcohol misuse and harm, or in considering it as a confounding variable to be controlled in intervention and evaluation studies (Shoveller et al., 2016).

On the other hand, anthropologists deliberately avoid a problem-oriented approach and have been more interested in the cultural and historical context of drinking (often on a smaller, context-specific scale), focusing on how alcohol fits into and makes sense in people's everyday lives (e.g., how it contributes to identity development, and individual and group identification), and its influence on cross-cultural variations in contexts, occasions and reasons for drinking (Heath, 2000; Wilson, 2005). Thus, from the anthropological and sociological perspective, drunkenness would be recognised as a socially constructed expression of culture and not only a function of pharmacological effects of alcohol on the brain (MacAndrew & Edgerton, 1969).

The Typological Tradition

Traditionally, drinking culture scholars have attempted to develop typologies of societies using various dimensions of alcohol use and related problems (Room & Mäkelä, 2000; Savic et al., 2016). A wide variety of typologies has been proposed over the last decades; however, the "wet" and "dry" cultures typology has been highly influential and is still often referred to as the basic continuum where single cultures are positioned against two ideal types (Savic et al., 2016). Wet cultures, such as France or Italy, are characterised by having alcohol as part of everyday life, of having high per capita consumption, and relatively high rates of alcohol-related chronic disease (e.g., liver cirrhosis) and mortality. Additionally, these cultures have less restrictive control policies and lower rates of drunkenness. Such a characterisation contrasts with the dry cultures of Northern Europe and English-speaking countries, such as the UK and the USA. In such countries, drinking is not part of everyday life, but is reserved for "time out", and when it does happen, drinking is more likely to lead to drunkenness (see Chap. 16). Dry drinking patterns are associated with histories of strong temperance movements in such cultures and the subsequent strict regulation (including prohibition) of alcohol consumption.

According to Room and Mäkelä (2000) reducing variations in drinking cultures to the wet/dry dichotomy is problematic both because it makes less sense as drinking patterns in Europe begin to converge in an increasingly globalised world and because of the lack of applicability to non-Western countries (e.g., Muslim countries). As a result, the authors proposed a two-dimensional framework based on prevalent consumption patterns: the regularity of drinking as an indicator of the degree to which alcohol is integrated in daily life and the cultural meanings of drunkenness ("how drunk is drunk?"). In addition, they identified other features that characterise drinking cultures, which include some of the dimensions suggested by previous typologies (e.g., alcohol use-values as nutrient or intoxicant and modes of social control of drinking).

We next describe a systematic review of the recent literature on drinking cultures. Results of this review allowed us to identify the strengths and limitations of existing literature in the field, thus offering insights for future research.

Systematic Review of the Drinking Culture Literature

Because the drinking culture literature is scattered across disciplines and fields, we have attempted to identify all relevant studies and have systematically reviewed the research to:

(a) examine the theoretical and methodological characteristics of studies of drinking cultures;
(b) contribute new information to what is already known about cross-cultural differences in alcohol use; and.
(c) provide supporting information for the future development of comprehensive theoretical frameworks.

Our review examines the literature from 1990 to 2018 on drinking cultures with the following main review questions:

1. What are the characteristics of studies on drinking cultures in terms of study design, population (e.g., age groups), and study setting (e.g., countries where the research took place)?
2. What are the theoretical approaches, if any, that studies on drinking cultures have used?
3. What are the major themes that drinking culture research has addressed?

Methods

The Preferred Reporting Items for Systematic Reviews and Meta-Analysis (PRISMA) methodology (Moher, Liberati, Tetzlaff, & Altman, 2009) was adopted as a general set of guidelines for our review.

Search Strategy

We searched ProQuest (PsycINFO and Social Science Premium Collection) and Web of Science databases. Searched fields were title and abstract. The search terms were adapted to database-specific filters. Search terms were alcohol, drinking pattern, drunk, binge drink*, and cross cultur*, drinking culture, ethnic drinking culture, cultural difference, subculture*. Boolean search operators were used (e.g., AND/OR, quotations). We restricted our searches by article type (qualitative and quantitative peer-reviewed original articles and reviews), language (English), and publication date (01 January 1990 to 31 December 2018). Date restrictions were adopted to retrieve studies of the "Contemporary Era" in drinking culture field (Castro, Barrera, Mena, & Aguirre, 2014). Opinion pieces, editorials, commentaries, letters to editors, and doctoral dissertations were excluded. Studies whose primary aim was not to examine the characteristics of one or more drinking cultures were excluded.

Screening Procedures and Data Extraction

Search results were exported to EndNote X7, which automatically removed duplicates. Review author GA assessed, by title and abstract inspection, all retrieved studies to screen out articles that did not meet basic inclusion criteria (e.g. language, publication type) or were broadly unrelated to the topic of interest. Subsequently, GA and KB independently assessed, by full-text reading, a random sample (N = 50) of the remaining studies for inclusion. The reviewers agreed 60% (N = 28) of the time. Disagreements were resolved by discussion. Subsequently, the remaining articles were screened for inclusion, and from each included study information was extracted on: bibliographic data; country in which the study was conducted; population(s) studied; study setting; study design and methods; outcomes; and predictors. Included studies were summarised descriptively and synthesised narratively. Results are structured around studies' characteristics, theoretical framework used, and major themes addressed.

Results

A total of 2729 records were retrieved. Figure 7.1 presents the study selection process. Following duplicate removal, 1462 articles were assessed for eligibility, after which another 1229 studies were excluded by title and abstract inspection. Reasons for exclusion were that alcohol use and related harm were not among the primary study outcomes (N = 654) (e.g., a study used drinking pattern variables as a covariate to predict other outcomes of interest) and the studies did not examine characteristics of one or more drinking cultures (N = 565). Other studies were excluded because they were not published in English (N = 31) or because they did not meet publication type criterion (e.g., editorials) (N = 12). Out of the 198 records screened by full-text reading 88 articles were included in the review. Of the remainder, 105 were excluded because their primary aim was not to examine the characteristics of one or more drinking cultures, and 5 were excluded because we were unable to retrieve the article full text. A summary table of each study's characteristics and themes is available from the authors on request or at: https://www.dropbox.com/s/eg21doufgolqn8n/Table%20S1.docx?dl=0

Study Characteristics

Studies could be broadly classified as theoretical (N = 5) or empirical (N = 83). Examples of theoretical articles included are those of Engs (1995), which discussed explanations for aetiology of the northern and the southern drinking cultures in antiquity, and the work of Savic et al. (2016) that, after analysing existing drinking culture definitions, proposed a new working definition of the construct.

Empirical studies are those that conducted some sort of either primary or secondary data analyses or reviewed and analysed results of other studies.

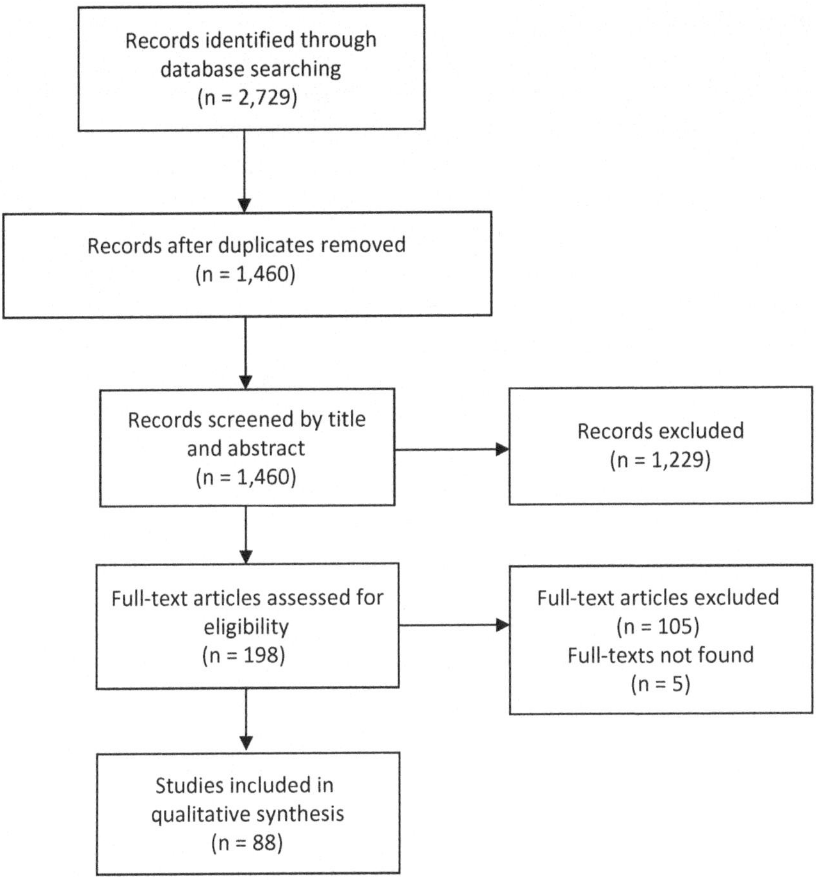

Fig. 7.1 Flowchart of study selection process

Fifty-three of these studies (60%) examined the features of a single cultural entity, generally identified with country or nation, whereas 30 (34%) used a cross-cultural approach examining differences across cultural entities. National origins of the included studies were distributed across the five continents and a total of more than 50 countries. The majority of studies were based in Europe and North America. The five most represented countries were the UK (N = 18), Finland (N = 16), Italy, the USA (N = 15 each), and Sweden (N = 11). Other countries had less representation with three or four studies each (e.g., Australia, Canada, France, India, Nigeria), and others were represented only once (e.g., Austria, Brazil, Russian Federation, Vietnam). Results of single-culture or cross-cultural studies are described separately.

Single-Culture Studies

Sixteen studies used samples drawn from the general population and 20 studies examined data from samples of subpopulations with specific socio-demographic characteristics or socio-economic status, including high-school or university students, middle-class adults, or parents (e.g., Brierley-Jones et al., 2014; Jayne, Valentine, & Gould, 2012). Thirteen studies examined a subnational cultural entity including specific ethnic groups (e.g., elderly Korean immigrants in Canada) (Kim, 2009; O'Nell & Mitchell, 1996) and four examined the drinking culture of groups with particular personal history characteristics or specific settings (e.g., marriage-based male immigrants in Taiwan, members of male sport clubs or fraternities) (Chen & Chien, 2018; Hart, 2016).

More than half (N = 31; 59%) of these single culture studies used qualitative methods (i.e., interviews or focus groups, field observations for data collection, document analysis, case studies, or a combination of these—often adopting an ethnographic approach). For example, Workman (2001) used individual interviews and participant observations to examine how high-risk drinking behaviour is constructed by the collegiate culture of fraternity members in the USA as a positive, functional activity. Fifteen studies adopted instead a quantitative design and used questionnaires to collect data. About half of these studies (N = 7) used a cross-sectional design to examine features of drinking cultures including drinking practices and problems, beverage preferences, and attitudes towards drinking (e.g., Ally, Lovatt, Meier, Brennan, & Holmes, 2016). Eight used longitudinal designs including cohort studies with data from repeated national surveys and time series analyses. For example, two studies examined changes in the Swedish and Finnish drinking cultures from the 1960s to the first decade of the new century (Bergmark, 2004; Mäkelä, Tigerstedt, & Mustonen, 2012).

Five studies were purely descriptive articles that focused on aspects of the society's drinking culture: for example, a study reflected on available data in Korea to describe the characteristics of the national drinking culture (Park, Oh, & Lee, 1998). Two were reviews of the literature on the drinking cultures of the Vietnamese (Lincoln, 2016) and the native and migrant Greek communities (Foster, Papadopoulous, Dadzie, & Jayasinghe, 2007). Only one study implemented a mixed-methods design using a survey questionnaire and individual interviews to examine the relationship between the drinking culture and gender identity among male students at a British university (Dempster, 2011).

Cross-Cultural Studies

In all cases, except two that compared two ethnic groups (Strunin, 1999), or specific areas or regions (Beccaria & Rolando, 2016), these studies compared various features of national drinking cultures. The number of cultural entities compared within these studies ranged from 2 to 30 (M = 8.1; D.S. = 8.0). Thirteen of these studies were qualitative. For example, by interviewing individuals living in wine- and non-wine-producing areas in Northern Italy, Beccaria and Rolando (2016) found differences in alcohol socialisation processes and more traditionally and family-oriented moderate alcohol use in the former (see also Chap. 16). Twelve studies implemented a quantitative approach. For example, Fjær, Pedersen, von Soest, and Gray (2016) surveyed university students in Norway and the UK to examine differences and similarities with regard to norms for the acceptability of visible drunkenness in different situations, such as with friends, with work colleagues, with family members, and situations where children are present. Four studies discussed and re-analysed existing epidemiological data, and one was a review of the alcohol literature in order to compare five European countries' drinking cultures (Gordon et al., 2012).

Definitions and Typologies of Drinking Cultures

The majority of the studies (N = 55; 63%) actually only merely mentioned the existence of drinking culture, without any attempt to define it. In nine studies (10%), the drinking culture of a particular group (often high school or university students) was negatively viewed and labelled as heavy, risky, excessive, or of intoxication (e.g., Hebden, Lyons, Goodwin, & McCreanor, 2015). Such general statements were used as a rhetorical strategy to demonstrate a need to change that particular drinking culture. For example, in one article the authors stated that an "excessive" drinking culture was dominant among university students in the UK and that in order to change this, there was a need to change norms and practices (Piacentini & Banister, 2009).

Only six studies included an explicit definition of the term drinking culture (Ander, Abrahamsson, & Bergnehr, 2017; Bloomfield, Karlsson, & Grittner 2016; Chen & Chien, 2018; Cook, Mulia, & Karriker-Jaffe, 2012; Mäkelä et al., 2012; Savic et al., 2016). All of the definitions used in these six studies mentioned shared norms for alcohol use as key to the construct. Drinking behaviour and practices were also included in most definitions, along with the functions (or use-values) of alcohol use and the idea that all of the above—that is, functions, norms, and practices—vary by social setting and context. As mentioned in the introduction, after reviewing previous definitions and the relevant literature, Savic et al. (2016) attempted to develop a new working definition that included the idea of micro- (shared by subgroups within society) and macro-level (a society as a whole) drinking cultures, including that there are informal (social) and formal (alcohol regulations) control mechanisms that "enforce" such norms and practices. The other 27 studies that did not provide an explicit definition of the drinking cultures construct mentioned some of their features—generally shared norms and habits. For example, Strunin (1999) stated that his goal was to examine aspects of US urban black adolescents' drinking culture, including norms, beliefs, and practices.

The typological tradition of studying drinking cultures seems to have had a remarkable impact on the drinking culture literature. Well over a third of the studies (N = 37; 42%) included the description of at least one typology. Different typologies were used, including some based on regional differences (e.g., Continental vs. British, Nordic/Central/Southern Europe) (e.g., Foster et al., 2007; Thurnell-Read, Brown, & Long, 2018) and dominant beverage (e.g., wine vs. spirit countries) (Pyorala, 1995), with the wet-dry distinction being referred to the most (N = 22). Generally, in such studies wet patterns are described as moderate and less risky than dry patterns. In some cases, the wet-dry types are used as a sort of independent variable whereby countries are assigned to one typology and then compared on dimensions of drinking patterns and harm. For example, Allamani, Voller, Kubicka, and Bloomfield (2000) described differences between wet and dry countries in relation to the amount of alcohol consumed, the integration of drinking in daily life, perceptions of alcohol problems, and alcohol policies.

Major Themes

The reviewed studies examined a range of issues that can be grouped into seven thematic areas: the social construction of alcohol use (N = 33), major characteristics of drinking cultures (N = 23), gender issues in relation to alcohol use (N = 10), change in national drinking cultures over time (N = 10), acculturation and ethnic drinking cultures in migrant populations (N = 5), socialisation processes (N = 4), and others (N = 3). Below we describe each thematic area and provide some examples of studies.

The Social Construction of Alcohol Use The largest group of studies consisted of those that aimed to achieve an in-depth understanding of the meanings, representations, and social constructions of drinking practices. These studies addressed several key issues of the drinking culture literature, including differences across countries in representations of what is "normal" or "pathological" alcohol use (Bennett, Jancca, Grant, & Sartorius, 1993), the construction of the meaning of drinking to intoxication among adolescents (Katainen & Rolando, 2015), and drinking practices and related representations in different settings (home vs. pub) among the middle class in the UK (Brierley-Jones et al., 2014). Other studies attempted to provide a broader perspective on the characteristics of the drinking culture in specific settings (e.g., male sports club) (Hart, 2016) or among ethnic groups. For example, Chang, Lo, and Hayter (2011) used ethnographic interviews and participant observations to identify key cultural themes concerning alcohol use (e.g., drinking to help make friends) among women from a rural tribe in Taiwan. Some studies adopted what can be considered an etic approach, studying a culture from the perspective of outsiders (e.g., non-drinkers) (Supski & Lindsay, 2017).

Major Characteristics of Drinking Cultures A large number of studies focused on variations within or between countries in the major features of drinking cultures, including drinking patterns, beverage preferences, context of drinking, and perceptions in regard to the acceptability of visible drunkenness (e.g., Bennett, Campillo, Chandrashekar, & Gureje, 1998; Fjær et al., 2016; Mäkelä et al., 2006). For example, Bergmark and Kuendig (2008) used data from the Gender, Alcohol and Culture—An International Study (GENACIS) to compare alcohol positive expectancies among a large number of countries, whereas Bräker and Soellner (2016) classified European countries into three drinking culture clusters (i.e., "mainly non-users", "mainly mild but frequent users", and "highest proportion of (heavy) episodic users") by examining dominant patterns of adolescent alcohol use.

Gender Issues in Relation to Alcohol Use Women's alcohol use and the construction of gender identities in relation to alcohol use appear as an important theme as well. Some studies were specifically interested in women's drinking patterns and related factors. For example, Ahlström (1995) used existing data to discuss cross-cultural differences in women's drinking patterns, acceptability of drinking, and public drinking. The article by Heath (1991) is instead a theoretical examination of aspects of gender differences in drinking, including cross-cultural variations, changes in drinking patterns across time, the relations between how women's drinking is portrayed in the media and the scientific literature, and the existence of gender double standards. Because aspects of women's drinking are often used as a key indicator of drinking cultures, this area partially overlaps with that of studies addressing changes in drinking culture over time (e.g., narrowing of gender gaps in alcohol use) (e.g., Stevens, Smith, Fein, Gottschalk, & Howard, 2011). Lastly, a few studies addressed issues in regard to gender identity and roles. For example, Törrönen, Rolando, and Beccaria (2017) compared how differently Finnish, Italian and Swedish men and women described their repertoire of masculinities and femininities depending on the social construction of drinking situations.

Changes in National Drinking Cultures Over Time A relatively large number of studies (ten) examined how changes occurred in the features of national drinking cultures over time. For example, Mäkelä et al. (2012) compared epidemiological data on drinking patterns and contexts of alcohol use in Finland from 1968 to 2008 and found changes in the Finnish drinking culture towards more permissiveness and a cultural shift in women's drinking. Valentine, Holloway, and Jayne (2010) used a different approach and compared attitudes towards, and consumption of, alcohol during youth experienced by three British cohort generations. Results highlighted changes in beverage preferences and how (heavy) drinking became a more widespread leisure practice in the new generations for both men and women.

Acculturation and Ethnic Drinking Cultures in Migrant Populations Another relatively recent line of research, originating from the increased interest in geographic mobility, investigated the effects of acculturation processes and ethnic drinking cultures (i.e., the culture of origin) on drinking outcomes among migrant populations. For example, Cook, Karriker-Jaffe, Bond, and Lui (2015) demonstrated that ethnic drinking cultures have enduring effects on drinking among Asian Americans.

Socialisation Processes Because socialisation is crucial to the transmission and learning of cultural norms and practices, socialisation processes represented yet another essential theme, which was examined by four of the studies included in the review. For example, Rolando, Beccaria, Tigerstedt, and Törrönen (2012) compared how alcohol socialisation experiences take place, in what kind of contexts, and what meanings and values are attributed to them in Italy and Finland (see Chap. 16 for more on this study).

Other Lastly, three studies did not fall into any of the previous groups and focused on specific aspects (i.e., the aetiology and conceptualisation of the drinking culture construct; Ames & Janes, 1992; Engs, 1995; Savic et al., 2016).

Discussion

We systematically reviewed the articles about drinking culture published between 1990 and 2018. Our findings allow us to draw some general conclusions on the state of recent drinking culture research and to remark upon the major trends as well as on theoretical and methodological gaps.

Micro- and Macro-Level Cultural Analyses

In most studies, the notion of culture was equated to country or nation, demonstrating scholars' lack of interest in sub-cultural entities such as regional or local drinking cultures (Savic et al., 2016). As Savic et al. (2016) noted, the focus on drinking cultures at the national level (i.e., the cultural entity of concern is the nation or society as a whole) reflects a macro-sociological approach and does not come without limitations. For example, in complex multicultural societies, generalisations to the whole society may not reflect the diversity and subdivisions of the society and "the drinking culture of a society may refer and 'belong' to some parts of the culture (i.e., the major ethnic group) much more than to others" (Savic et al., 2016, p. 272). To this end, important differences in how alcohol is used and understood by particular ethnic groups or other minorities may be overlooked (see, e.g., Terry-McElrath & Patrick, 2018). Alternatively, what Savic et al. (2016) label as lack of interest in research at the sub-cultural level may be due to practical hindrances with regard to access to available regionally based data. There are indeed sub-cultural or regional comparative studies of drinking practices in the literature which might not be regarded as studies of drinking cultures, such has a recent study by Bloomfield, Grittner, Kraus, and Piontek (2017). Interest in this area is growing gradually and may produce more research in the near future.

In our review, we found several examples of studies that focused attention on sex differences in alcohol use, how they vary across countries, and how they fit into the evolution of cultural and societal norms in western countries (e.g., emancipation offered women the opportunity to access drinking place and contributed to reducing gender gaps in alcohol use) (Bergmark, 2004).

This demonstrates that the research in this field has acknowledged that a gender-neutral drinking culture may be an overly simplistic description of our societies and that gender-specific analyses are almost always warranted. However, less attention has been paid to ethnic differences and other sub-societal cultural entities (Bennett, 1999).

As Savic et al. (2016) stated, studying drinking cultures at the macro- and micro-social levels should be seen as complementary. This integrated approach could provide valuable information to understand what is shared and what is distinctive of drinking (sub-)cultures across society, thus better informing intervention efforts. It would also reflect the notion that culture is a highly complex construct and that cultural factors may be diverse, can be contradictory, and need to be seen from multiple perspectives. This must be taken into account in any effort to better understand variations and discrepancies between individual behaviours and societal cultural standards, policies, and expectations of behaviour (Markus & Hamedani, 2007; Ratner, 2016).

The Qualitative – Quantitative Dichotomy

At a methodological level, only one mixed-methods study was found, demonstrating the epistemological and methodological distance between the qualitative and quantitative research traditions in the drinking culture literature. In the recent general culture literature, there has been a growing recognition that qualitative and quantitative methods can be integrated to provide more contextualised and detailed descriptions of the practices and local cultural processes that shape psychological outcomes and behaviour (Schrauf, 2017). However, we also acknowledge that mixed-methods designs are complex, require a great deal of resources and expertise, and that obtaining project financing for a type of research that funding agencies may not yet fully recognise as an established method may be particularly challenging.

Definitional Issues and New Conceptual Models

As mentioned, the reviewed studies tended to equate culture with country, but their greatest limitation perhaps lay in how they approached the construct of drinking culture. Although many articles addressed important issues for the study of drinking cultures, the actual construct was too often treated in a simplistic manner. Most studies lacked any definition of the construct, or they merely mentioned that drinking culture exists. In addition, the equation between drinking culture and heavy drinking, that is often proposed, is problematic. This is because it focuses on the negative sides of drinking cultures and overshadows the fact that drinking cultures may also promote moderation—for example, studies of the traditional Mediterranean drinking culture (Beccaria & Guidoni, 2002). For this reason, there is a need to further advance theories underlying the construct of drinking cultures and treat this notion in a neutral manner.

Among the studies we reviewed, Bloomfield et al. (2016) proposed a conceptual model to explain how a society's drinking culture changes, offering insights into what makes the construct. The model distinguished between primary (i.e., those that have a direct effect on how much alcohol is consumed or on altering the actual drinking culture) and secondary factors (which have an effect on primary factors and indirectly on the drinking culture). Primary factors include alcohol prices and taxation, and alcohol availability, alcohol advertising, societal norms and attitudes on alcohol use and misuse, and societal responses to heavy alcohol consumption and alcohol problems (e.g., educational campaigns). Secondary factors include the interaction between the population's purchasing power and alcohol prices and structural demographic changes in society. Alcohol norms and societal responses to alcohol problems are thought to have both direct and indirect effects on alcohol use in the population, for example, by changing societal attitudes towards heavy drinking. The level of alcohol-related morbidity and mortality in a society is also included in the model but is considered rather as a reflection of the drinking culture. The authors used this model to examine changes in the Danish drinking culture over the last few decades and found meaningful changes in indicators of the various components of model (e.g., shifts in drinking norms and attitudes towards a more self-critical view of Danish drinking habits). This is a working model that needs to be further refined and empirically validated in Denmark (and then in other cultures), but it may provide a general reference point to continue research in this field. A general issue in this model, however, may relate to a lack of clarity about which model components are intrinsically part of the drinking culture construct, and which influence or are influenced by it. For example, alcohol policy developments may have a circular, rather than linear, relationship with a country's drinking culture. This idea reflects early work from Christie (1965, p. 107), suggesting that:

> a drinking culture with a large degree of highly visible, non-beneficial effects of alcohol consumption leads to a strict system of control, which somewhat reduces total consumption, which again influences and most often reduces the visible problems

A further issue pointed out by the authors is that the relative weight of each one of these factors in determining shifts in the drinking culture is often unknown.

Issues in the Use of Typologies

Despite being criticised and despite more nuanced frameworks being available (Room & Mäkelä, 2000), we have found that the wet/dry typology has been, and still is, highly influential in the drinking culture field. In our review, there are examples of recently published articles that not only referred to it generally but used it to group countries and to analyse data accordingly. However, assignment of countries to each type in some studies was questionable on theoretical grounds (namely in regard to the indicator used to assign countries to each type). Furthermore, the use of this typology is intrinsically problematic in light of current trends towards cultural homogenisation, and the typology has limited applicability to non-Western countries (Room & Mäkelä, 2000). These findings suggest a need for more nuanced typologies that consider aspects other than just drinking patterns (e.g., cultural meanings of drunkenness), to be included in future research. Other more recent attempts to develop typologies (see, e.g., Gordon et al., 2012) reflect the highly debated topic regarding processes of cultural homogenisation in alcohol use towards hedonistic drinking at the expense of other use values, such as the ritualistic or convivial, taking place in Western countries and across the world. This debate parallels a similar one on the effects of globalisation on general cross-cultural research (Kitayama & Cohen, 2007). There seems to be a general understanding in the field that, over the last few decades, a reduction in cultural differences in drinking practices across countries has occurred (Kuntsche et al., 2011). General cultural and societal factors (e.g., homogenisation of lifestyles, urbanisation, globalised and integrated economies, and greater female independence) as well as alcohol-specific factors (e.g., globalisation of alcohol marketing, changes in beverage preferences, and moves towards greater homogeneity of alcohol legislation and regulation) are thought to have contributed this (Gordon et al., 2012). However, there is also a debate regarding the extent to which cultural differences still exist. For example, even though no country represented a prototypical type of drinking culture in their study (i.e., "mood-changing model" and "nutritional model"), Mäkelä et al. (2006) reported that regional differences in beverage preferences, the South-North gradient in frequency of drinking and propensity to drink in large quantities on special occasions persist. In addition, recent cross-cultural studies (Aresi et al., 2020) have highlighted remarkable differences in drinking patterns and cultural assumptions in relation to alcohol consumption among Italian and US youth.

Major Themes

We have found that many studies were interested in understanding the meanings, representations, and social constructions of drinking practices. This is not surprising given that meanings and norms are key components of drinking culture definitions (Savic et al., 2016), conceptual models (Bloomfield et al., 2016; Room & Mäkelä, 2000), and general frameworks in cultural studies (Ratner, 2008). Our reviewed studies emerged mainly from the sociological and anthropological literature, and almost all used qualitative methods and the ethnographic approach. Some of these studies attempted to provide a comprehensive picture of a micro setting-specific culture (Hart, 2016), and others were more focused on specific features of a group's drinking culture, such as the meanings of drinking to intoxication (Katainen & Rolando, 2015).

As we have seen, meanings are key to the study of drinking cultures, although another key aspect of the so-called sociocultural world, that is, practices, also has received a great deal of attention. Meanings and practices are highly interrelated. Meanings and representations shape practices that are understood as particular ways of acting and interacting in recurrent episodes of everyday life (Markus & Hamedani, 2007). Products are the third key aspect of the sociocultural world. They have apparently received comparatively little attention by drinking culture scholars. Cultural products or artefacts reflect the ideas, images, understandings, and values of particular contexts, and, as people engage with these products, they "re-present" and institutionalise these ideas and values (Markus & Hamedani, 2007). Although there is a large and growing body of research on things that, from a cultural perspective, can be considered cultural products (e.g., alcohol advertisement, posts on social media), only a few studies included in our review examined how artefacts are reflective of a particular culture. For example, McCreanor et al. (2013) examined how alcohol marketing on social network websites reflected shared understandings of drinking situations and contributed to pro-alcohol environments and promoted drinking as a result. Notably, the increasing scholarly interest in the dynamics of drinking cultures mirrors the dramatic increases in migrations of people who, for various reasons (refugees, migrants, study abroad), move to other countries and cultures (Aresi, Moore, & Marta, 2016; Zemore, 2007). We expect to see a growing body of research on this issue in the future.

Conclusions

By systematising the recent drinking culture literature and highlighting issues and gaps, this chapter offers a novel contribution to this field. We have shown that the drinking culture construct is too often poorly conceptualised and, in some cases, stereotyped into negative connotations. Conceptually, it is important to consider culture as a multidimensional and multi-layered construct. Recent attempts to develop conceptual models (e.g., Bloomfield et al., 2017) may provide the basis for future development and clarification of the construct. For example, definitions tend to highlight shared norms around alcohol use as key to the understanding of drinking cultures, although norms only partially reflect the processes of cultural production and reproduction, which include social influence and more frequent interaction with culturally similar individuals (i.e., homophily: Axelrod, 1997).

We suggest that future research should go beyond the "country/nation = culture" equation by making an effort to combine the macro- (i.e., country, region) and micro-social levels by studying sub-cultural entities and specific settings, and the relations between them. Such combinations will necessarily require integration at a methodological level between quantitative and qualitative methods. In addition, recent research using social network data suggests that in our increasingly globalised world, food habits (including drinking patterns) are more similar across cosmopolitan cities in different continents (e.g., London, New York, and Tokyo) than between these cities and other locations within single countries (Silva, de Melo, Almeida, Musolesi, & Loureiro, 2014). In this respect, social network data may be used to identify cultural boundaries. Such use of big data has implications not only for new approaches to understanding drinking cultures, but also to developing more specific targeted interventions to prevent harmful drinking and harmful drinking situations.

References

Ahlström, S. (1995). Cultural differences in women's drinking. *Contemporary Drug Problems, 22*(3), 393.

Allamani, A., Voller, F., Kubicka, L., & Bloomfield, K. (2000). Drinking cultures and the position of women in nine European countries. *Substance Abuse, 21*(4), 231–247. https://doi.org/10.1023/A:1007801223214

Ally, A. K., Lovatt, M., Meier, P. S., Brennan, A., & Holmes, J. (2016). Developing a social practice-based typology of British drinking culture in 2009–2011: Implications for alcohol policy analysis. *Addiction, 111*(9), 1568–1579. https://doi.org/10.1111/add.13397

Ames, G. M., & Janes, C. (1992). A cultural approach to conceptualizing alcohol and the workplace. *Alcohol Health and Research World, 16*(2), 112–119.

Ander, B., Abrahamsson, A., & Bergnehr, D. (2017). 'It is ok to be drunk, but not too drunk': Party socialising, drinking ideals, and learning trajectories in Swedish adolescent discourse on alcohol use. *Journal of Youth Studies, 20*(7), 841–854. https://doi.org/10.1080/13676261.2016.1273515

Aresi, G., Cleveland, M. J., Vieno, A., Beccaria, F., Turrisi, R., & Marta, E. (2020). A Mixed Methods Cross-Cultural Study to Compare Youth Drinking Cultures in Italy and the USA. *Applied Psychology: Health and Well-Being, 12*, 231–255. https://doi.org/10.1111/aphw.12181

Aresi, G., Moore, S., & Marta, E. (2016). Drinking, drug use and related consequences among university students completing study abroad experiences: A systematic review. *Substance Use and Misuse, 51*(14), 1888–1904. https://doi.org/10.1080/10826084.2016.1201116

Axelrod, R. (1997). The Dissemination of Culture: A Model with Local Convergence and Global Polarization. *Journal of Conflict Resolution, 41*(2), 203–226. https://doi.org/10.1177/0022002797041002001

Beccaria, F., & Guidoni, O. V. (2002). Young people in a wet culture: Functions and patterns of drinking. *Contemporary Drug Problems, 29*, 305–334.

Beccaria, F., & Rolando, S. (2016). The more you know, the better you drink: The new drinking culture in Italian wine production areas. *Drugs: Education, Prevention and Policy, 23*(4), 293–301. https://doi.org/10.3109/09687637.2016.1149149

Bennett, A. (1999). Subcultures or neo-tribes? rethinking the relationship between youth, style and musical taste. *Sociology, 33*(3), 599–617. https://doi.org/10.1177/s0038038599000371

Bennett, L. A., Campillo, C., Chandrashekar, C. R., & Gureje, O. (1998). Alcoholic beverage consumption in India, Mexico, and Nigeria: A cross-cultural comparison. *Alcohol Health and Research World, 22*(4), 243–252.

Bennett, L. A., Jancca, A., Grant, B. F., & Sartorius, N. (1993). Boundaries between normal and pathological drinking: A cross-cultural comparison. *Alcohol Health and Research World, 17*(3), 190–195.

Bergmark, K. H. (2004). Gender roles, family, and drinking: Women at the crossroad of drinking cultures. *Journal of Family History, 29*(3), 293–307. https://doi.org/10.1177/0363199004266906

Bergmark, K. H., & Kuendig, H. (2008). Pleasures of drinking: A cross-cultural perspective. *Journal of Ethnicity in Substance Abuse, 7*(2), 131–153. https://doi.org/10.1080/15332640802055491

Berkman, L., Kawachi, I., & Glymour, L. L. (2014). *Social Epidemiology* (2nd ed.). Oxford: Oxford University Press.

Bloomfield, K., Grittner, U., Kraus, L., & Piontek, D. (2017). Drinking patterns at the sub-national level: What do they tell us about drinking cultures in European countries? *Nordic Studies on Alcohol and Drugs, 34*(4), 342–352. https://doi.org/10.1177/1455072517712820

Bloomfield, K., Karlsson, T., & Grittner, U. (2016). How do drinking cultures change?—Or do they?: A provisional model based on evidence of transitions in Denmark. *Drugs: Education, Prevention & Policy, 23*(4), 283–292. https://doi.org/10.1080/09687637.2016.1179719

Bräker, A. B., & Soellner, R. (2016). Alcohol drinking cultures of European adolescents. *European Journal of Public Health, 26*(4), 581–586. https://doi.org/10.1093/eurpub/ckw033

Brierley-Jones, L., Ling, J., McCabe, K. E., Wilson, G. B., Crosland, A., Kaner, E. F. S., & Haighton, C. A. (2014). Habitus of home and traditional drinking: A qualitative analysis of reported middle-class alcohol use. *Sociology of Health & Illness, 36*(7), 1054–1076. https://doi.org/10.1111/1467-9566.12145

Bruner, J. S. (1990). *Acts of meaning*. Cambridge, MA: Harvard University Press.

Castro, F. G., Barrera, M., Mena, L. A., & Aguirre, K. M. (2014). Culture and alcohol use: Historical and sociocultural themes from 75 years of alcohol research. *Journal of Studies on Alcohol and Drugs. Supplement*, (s17), 36–49. https://doi.org/10.15288/jsads.2014.s17.36

Chang, L. J., Lo, S. F., & Hayter, M. (2011). Drinking behaviors: The life narratives of indigenous Bunun women in Taiwan. *Journal of Nursing Research, 19*(2), 83–92. https://doi.org/10.1097/JNR.0b013e31821cbbd0

Chen, H.-H., & Chien, L.-Y. (2018). Ethnic drinking culture, acculturation, and enculturation in relation to alcohol drinking behavior among marriage-based male immigrants in Taiwan. *American Journal of Men's Health, 12*(5), 1517–1529. https://doi.org/10.1177/1557988318772744

Christie, N. (1965). *Scandinavian experience in legislation and control.* Paper presented at the national conference on legal issues in alcoholism and alcfvohol usage, Boston, MA.

Cook, W. K., Karriker-Jaffe, K. J., Bond, J., & Lui, C. (2015). Asian American problem drinking trajectories during the transition to adulthood: Ethnic drinking cultures and neighborhood contexts. *American Journal of Public Health, 105*(5), 1020–1027. https://doi.org/10.2105/ajph.2014.302196

Cook, W. K., Mulia, N., & Karriker-Jaffe, K. (2012). Ethnic drinking cultures and alcohol use among Asian American adults: Findings from a national survey. *Alcohol and Alcoholism, 47*(3), 340–348. https://doi.org/10.1093/alcalc/ags017

Dempster, S. (2011). I drink, therefore I'm man: Gender discourses, alcohol and the construction of British undergraduate masculinities. *Gender and Education, 23*(5), 635–653. https://doi.org/10.1080/09540253.2010.527824

Engs, R. C. (1995). Do traditional western European drinking practices have origins in antiquity? *Addiction Research, 2*(3), 227–239. https://doi.org/10.3109/16066359509005208

Fischer, R., & Schwartz, S. (2011). Whence differences in value priorities?: Individual, cultural, or artifactual sources. *Journal of Cross-Cultural Psychology, 42*(7), 1127–1144. https://doi.org/10.1177/0022022110381429

Fjær, E. G., Pedersen, W., von Soest, T., & Gray, P. (2016). When is it OK to be drunk? Situational and cultural variations in the acceptability of visible intoxication in the UK and Norway. *International Journal of Drug Policy, 29*(Supplement C), 27–32. https://doi.org/10.1016/j.drugpo.2015.12.002

Foster, J., Papadopoulous, C., Dadzie, L., & Jayasinghe, N. (2007). A review of tobacco and alcohol use literature in the native and migrant Greek community. *Journal of Substance Use, 12*(5), 323–335. https://doi.org/10.1080/14659890701408766

Gordon, R., Heim, D., & MacAskill, S. (2012). Rethinking drinking cultures: A review of drinking cultures and a reconstructed dimensional approach. *Public Health, 126*(1), 3–11. https://doi.org/10.1016/j.puhe.2011.09.014

Hart, A. (2016). Good sports, drinking cultures and hegemonic masculinities in a community sporting club case study. *Drugs: Education, Prevention & Policy, 23*(4), 302–311. https://doi.org/10.3109/09687637.2015.1136267

Heath, D. B. (1976). Anthopological perspectives on alcohol: An historical review. In M. W. Everett, J. O. Waddell, & D. B. Heath (Eds.), *Cross-cultural approaches to the study of alcohol. An interdisciplinary perspective*. The Haugue, The Netherlands: Mouton Publishers.

Heath, D. B. (1991). Women and alcohol: Cross-cultural perspectives. *Journal of Substance Abuse, 3*(2), 175–185. https://doi.org/10.1016/S0899-3289(05)80035-5

Heath, D. B. (1995). *International Handbook on Alcohol and Culture*. Santa Barbara, USA: ABC-CLIO.

Heath, D. B. (2000). *Drinking occasions: Comparative perspectives on alcohol and culture*. Philadelphia, PA: Taylor and Francis.

Hebden, R., Lyons, A. C., Goodwin, I., & McCreanor, T. (2015). "When you add alcohol, it gets that much better": University students, alcohol consumption, and online drinking cultures. *Journal of Drug Issues, 45*(2), 214–226. https://doi.org/10.1177/0022042615575375

Hofstede, G. (1980). *Culture's consequences: International differences in work-related values*. Beverly Hills, CA: Sage.

Inglehart, R., & Baker, W. E. (2000). Modernization, cultural change, and the persistence of traditional values. *American Sociological Review, 65*(1), 19–51. https://doi.org/10.2307/2657288

Jahoda, G. (2012). Critical reflections on some recent definitions of "culture". *Culture & Psychology, 18*(3), 289–303. https://doi.org/10.1177/1354067X12446229

Jayne, M., Valentine, G., & Gould, M. (2012). Family life and alcohol consumption: The transmission of 'public' and 'private' drinking cultures. *Drugs: Education, Prevention & Policy, 19*(3), 192–200. https://doi.org/10.3109/09687637.2011.640720

Katainen, A., & Rolando, S. (2015). Adolescents' understandings of binge drinking in Southern and Northern European contexts – Cultural variations of 'controlled loss of control'. *Journal of Youth Studies, 18*(2), 151–166. https://doi.org/10.1080/13676261.2014.933200

Kim, W. (2009). Drinking Culture of Elderly Korean Immigrants in Canada: A Focus Group Study. *Journal of Cross-Cultural Gerontology, 24*(4), 339–353. https://doi.org/10.1007/s10823-009-9104-z

Kitayama, S., & Cohen, D. (2007). *Handbook of cultural psychology*. New York, NY: Guilford Publications.

Kroeber, A. L., & Kluckhohn, C. (1952). *Culture: A critical review of concepts and definitions*. Cambridge, MA: Peabody Museum.

Kuntsche, E., Kuntsche, S., Knibbe, R., Simons-Morton, B., Farhat, T., Hublet, A., … Demetrovics, Z. (2011). Cultural and gender convergence in adolescent drunkenness: Evidence from 23 European and North American countriesculture and gender in adolescent drunkenness. *JAMA Pediatrics, 165*(2), 152–158. https://doi.org/10.1001/archpediatrics.2010.191

Lincoln, M. (2016). Alcohol and drinking cultures in Vietnam: A review. *Drug and Alcohol Dependence, 159*, 1–8. https://doi.org/10.1016/j.drugalcdep.2015.10.030

MacAndrew, C., & Edgerton, R. B. (1969). *Drunken comportment: A social explanation*. Chicago, IL: Aldine.

Mäkelä, P., Gmel, G., Grittner, U., Kuendig, H., Kuntsche, S., Bloomfield, K., & Room, R. (2006). Drinking patterns and their gender differences in Europe. *Alcohol and Alcoholism, 41*(Suppl. 1), 8–18. https://doi.org/10.1093/alcalc/agl071

Mäkelä, P., Tigerstedt, C., & Mustonen, H. (2012). The finnish drinking culture: Change and continuity in the past 40 years. *Drug and Alcohol Review, 31*(7), 831–840. https://doi.org/10.1111/j.1465-3362.2012.00479.x

Markus, H. R., & Hamedani, M. G. (2007). Sociocultural psychology. The dynamic interdependence among self systems and social systems. In S. Kitayama & D. Cohen (Eds.), *Handbook of cultural psychology*. New York, NY: Guilford Publications.

Marmot, M., & Wilkinson, R. G. (2006). *The Social Determinants of Health* (2nd ed.). Oxford: Oxford University Press.

Matsumoto, D., & Yoo, S. H. (2006). Toward a new generation of cross-cultural research. *Perspectives on Psychological Science, 1*(3), 234–250. https://doi.org/10.1111/j.1745-6916.2006.00014.x

McCreanor, T., Lyons, A., Griffin, C., Goodwin, I., Barnes, H. M., & Hutton, F. (2013). Youth drinking cultures, social networking and alcohol marketing: Implications for public health. *Critical Public Health, 23*(1), 110–120. https://doi.org/10.1080/09581596.2012.748883

Miller, P. J., & Goodnow, J. J. (1995). Cultural practices: Toward an integration of culture and development. In J. J. Goodnow, P. J. Miller, & F. Kessel (Eds.), *Cultural practices as contexts for development* (Vol. 67, pp. 5–16). San Francisco, CA: JosseyBass.

Minkov, M. (2011). *Cultural differences in a globalizing world*. Bingley, UK: Emerald.

Moher, D., Liberati, A., Tetzlaff, J., & Altman, D. G. (2009). Preferred reporting items for systematic reviews and meta-analyses: The PRISMA statement. *PLoS Medicine, 6*(7), e1000097. https://doi.org/10.1371/journal.pmed.100009710.1371/.

Moscovici, S. (1998). The history and actuality of social representations. In U. Flick (Ed.), *The psychology of the social* (pp. 209–247). Cambridge, MA: Cambridge.

O'Nell, T. D., & Mitchell, C. M. (1996). Alcohol use among american indian adolescents: The role of culture in pathological drinking. *Social Science and Medicine, 42*(4), 565–578.

Park, S. C., Oh, S. I., & Lee, M. S. (1998). Korean status of alcoholics and alcohol-related health problems. *Alcoholism: Clinical and Experimental Research, 22*(Suppl 3), 170S–172S. https://doi.org/10.1097/00000374-199803001-00020

Piacentini, M. G., & Banister, E. N. (2009). Managing anti-consumption in an excessive drinking culture. *Journal of Business Research, 62*(2), 279–288. https://doi.org/10.1016/j.jbusres.2008.01.035

Pyorala, E. (1995). Comparing drinking cultures – Finnish and spanish drinking stories in interviews with young-adults. *Acta Sociologica, 38*(3), 217–229.

Ratner, C. (2008). *Cultural psychology, cross-cultural psychology, and indigenous psychology*. New York, NY: Nova Science Publishers.

Ratner, C. (2016). The discrepancy between macro culture and individual, lived psychology: An ethnographic example of Chinese moral behavior. *Culture & Psychology, 23*(3), 356–371. https://doi.org/10.1177/1354067X16658021

Rolando, S., Beccaria, F., Tigerstedt, C., & Törrönen, J. (2012). First drink: What does it mean? The alcohol socialization process in different drinking cultures. *Drugs: Education, Prevention, and Policy, 19*(3), 201–212. https://doi.org/10.3109/09687637.2012.658105

Room, R. (1975). Normative perspectives on alcohol use and problems. *Journal of Drug Issues, 5*(4), 358–368. https://doi.org/10.1177/002204267500500407

Room, R., & Mäkelä, K. (2000). Typologies of the cultural position of drinking. *Journal of Studies on Alcohol, 61*(3), 475–483. https://doi.org/10.15288/jsa.2000.61.475

Savic, M., Room, R., Mugavin, J., Pennay, A., & Livingston, M. (2016). Defining "drinking culture": A critical review of its meaning and connotation in social research on alcohol problems. *Drugs: Education, Prevention and Policy, 23*(4), 270–282. https://doi.org/10.3109/09687637.2016.1153602

Schrauf, R. W. (2017). Mixed methods designs for making cross-cultural comparisons. *Journal of Mixed Methods Research, 12*(4), 477–494. https://doi.org/10.1177/1558689817743109

Schwartz, S. H. (1999). Cultural value differences: Some implications for work. *Applied Psychology. An International Review, 48*, 23–47.

Shoveller, J., Viehbeck, S., Di Ruggiero, E., Greyson, D., Thomson, K., & Knight, R. (2016). A critical examination of representations of context within research on population health interventions. *Critical Public Health, 26*(5), 487–500. https://doi.org/10.1080/09581596.2015.1117577

Silva, T.H., de Melo, P.O.S.V., Almeida, J.M., Musolesi, M. & Loureiro, A.A.F. (2014). *You are what you eat (and drink): Identifying cultural boundaries by analyzing food and drink habits in foursquare.* Eighth International AAAI conference on weblogs and social media.

Stevens, B. R., Smith, T. R., Fein, K. R., Gottschalk, M., & Howard, G. J. (2011). A deadly mix? An international investigation of handgun availability, drinking culture, and homicide. *International Journal of Comparative and Applied Criminal Justice, 35*(1), 39–51.

Strunin, L. (1999). Drinking perceptions and drinking behaviors among urban Black adolescents. *Journal of Adolescent Health, 25*(4), 264–275. https://doi.org/10.1016/S1054-139X(99)00010-5

Supski, S., & Lindsay, J. (2017). 'There's something wrong with you': How young people choose abstinence in a heavy drinking culture. *Young, 25*(4), 323–338. https://doi.org/10.1177/1103308816654068

Taras, V., Rowney, J., & Steel, P. (2009). Half a century of measuring culture: Review of approaches, challenges, and limitations based on the analysis of 121 instruments for quantifying culture. *Journal of International Management, 15*. https://doi.org/10.1016/j.intman.2008.08.005

Terry-McElrath, Y. M., & Patrick, M. E. (2018). U.S. adolescent alcohol use by race/ethnicity: Consumption and perceived need to reduce/stop use. *Journal of Ethnicity in Substance Abuse*, 1–25. doi:https://doi.org/10.1080/15332640.2018.1433094

Thurnell-Read, T., Brown, L., & Long, P. (2018). International students' perceptions and experiences of british drinking cultures. *Sociological Research Online, 23*(3), 572–588. https://doi.org/10.1177/1360780418761207

Törrönen, J., Rolando, S., & Beccaria, F. (2017). Masculinities and femininities of drinking in Finland, Italy and Sweden: Doing, modifying and unlinking gender in relation to different drinking places. *Geoforum, 82*, 131–140. https://doi.org/10.1016/j.geoforum.2017.04.005

Valentine, G., Holloway, S. L., & Jayne, M. (2010). Generational patterns of alcohol consumption: Continuity and change. *Health & Place, 16*(5), 916–925. https://doi.org/10.1016/j.healthplace.2010.05.003

Wilson, T. M. (2005). *Drinking culture.* Oxford, UK: Berg.

Workman, T. A. (2001). Finding the meanings of college drinking: An analysis of fraternity drinking stories. *Health Communication, 13*(4), 427–447. https://doi.org/10.1207/s15327027hc1304_05

Zemore, S. E. (2007). Acculturation and alcohol among Latino adults in the United States: A comprehensive review. *Alcoholism, Clinical and Experimental Research, 31*(12), 1968–1990. https://doi.org/10.1111/j.1530-0277.2007.00532.x

8

Alcohol Use and Problems at the Event Level: Theory, Methods, and Intervention

John D. Clapp and Danielle R. Madden

Introduction

Alcohol consumption is a complex behaviour involving the interplay of physiological, psychological, social, and environmental factors. Alcohol science, however, seldom examines these interrelated domains simultaneously. Likewise, preventive and harm reduction approaches to alcohol-related problems often focus on a single domain (e.g. interventions designed to change misperceptions of normative behaviour). Naturally occurring drinking events present a unique opportunity to understand the social ecology of drinking behaviour. From an intervention standpoint, drinking events are temporally proximal to drinking outcomes both good and bad. In theory, understanding drinking events has great potential for preventing and minimizing harm related to acute alcohol problems (e.g. fights, injuries, drunk driving, sexual assaults, etc.). This chapter focuses on the theory, methods, and interventions common to alcohol event research.

J. D. Clapp (✉) • D. R. Madden
Suzanne Dworak-Peck School of Social Work, University of Southern California, Los Angeles, CA, USA
e-mail: john.clapp@usc.edu; dmadden@usc.edu

R. Cooke et al. (eds.), *The Palgrave Handbook of Psychological Perspectives on Alcohol Consumption*, https://doi.org/10.1007/978-3-030-66941-6_8

Theoretical and Conceptual Approaches to Understanding Drinking at the Event Level

Historically, research concerning the aetiology of alcohol use and alcohol-related problems has focused on one or two conceptual domains independently or as they relate to one another (e.g. drinking expectancies, social influence, etc.). Historical methodological approaches to studying alcohol consumption have included ethnographic observations (Cavan, 1966), retrospective surveys (Wechsler, Davenport, Dowdall, Moeykens, & Castillo, 1994), and field studies using breathalyzers and interviews (Clapp et al., 2009; Clapp, Min, Shillington, Reed, & Croff, 2008).

Given the focus of research into drinking events noted above, interventions to limit heavy event-level drinking often fail to focus on individual behaviour or are mistimed (i.e., not during risk behaviour). Currently, there are few attempts to intervene during critical moments such as when individuals make decisions to drink more, drive a car when intoxicated, or engage in risky sexual behaviour (discussed below). More work that addresses drinking at the event level and avenues to intervene is sorely needed.

What Is a Drinking Event?

Operationally, drinking events can be difficult to define. While a drinking event starts with the first sip of alcohol, operationalizing the end of a drinking event can be tricky. For instance, the bulk of research on "pre-gaming"—that is, drinking at home before going out to licensed venues (see Chap. 13)—tends to focus on the earliest part of a drinking event as a predictor of either estimated peak blood alcohol concentration (BAC) or harmful outcomes (Barry, Stellefson, Piazza-Gardner, Chaney, & Dodd, 2013). In our early work, we defined drinking events as beginning with the first sip of alcohol and ending with the last sip, over the course of several hours (Clapp et al., 2018). This definition is limited in that BAC decays long after the last sip. One may argue that drinking events begin with the first sip of alcohol on a given occasion, and end when BAC reaches zero. However, this definition is also problematic for two reasons. First, for people meeting criteria for an alcohol use disorder, BAC may never reach zero. Second, for people who do not have an alcohol use disorder an event (e.g. a party or wedding) might include a few drinks over the course of several hours where BAC hits "zero" more than once. Thus, it is important to consider drinking events as an ecological system where environmental, individual, and social factors are considered in the operational definition. For instance, "a drinking event begins when one takes the first sip of alcohol, drinks over a period of at least one hour, for personal (e.g., to enhance a meal, reduce stress, have fun, etc.) or social reasons (e.g., to celebrate with friends, etc.) in one or more environments where alcohol is available. The drinking event ends when the drinker's BAC reaches zero after all drinking for the event has ended."

Drinking events are direct antecedents to numerous acute alcohol-related problems including burns, crashes, crime injuries, falls, and sexual and other violence (National Institute of Health, 2000). Acute problems have a huge global impact (Rehm et al., 2009); for instance, approximately 25% of all unintentional, and 10% of intentional injuries in the world can be attributed to drinking events. When alcohol-related disease and death are considered, 5% of all deaths in the world and 5% of disability adjusted life years lost are alcohol related (World Health Organization, 2018). In aggregate, drinking events represent patterns of consumption that drive alcohol-related disease and premature death (Holder, 2006).

Over the past five decades, a subfield of alcohol research has emerged with the goal of better understanding the ecology of drinking behaviour as it naturally occurs. Reflecting the inherent multidisciplinary nature of alcohol research, such studies vary in conceptual foci, methods, and operational definitions. Independently, studies on "drinking contexts," "drinking situations," and "drinking environments" (see also Chap. 9) offer related but unique insights into drinking behaviour in situ. Recent work has focused on drinking at the event level (Clapp, Reed, & Ruderman, 2014; Thrul & Kuntsche, 2015; Verster, Benjaminsen, van Lanen, van Stavel, & Olivier, 2015; Wells et al., 2015) as a way of examining drinking as it occurs. For example, Wells et al. (2015) found that drinkers who pre-drank in a bar district, had a higher breath estimates of blood alcohol concentration (BAC) than those drinking in other settings. The study controlled for typical drinking pattern and also found a drinker-by-group interaction in which individual pre-drinkers influenced group-level BAC. In a study of over 1700 partygoers nested in 226 parties, Clapp et al. (2014) found that playing drinking games resulted in a higher likelihood of continued drinking, and that the presence of drinking games at a party predicted intent to drive after drinking—regardless of whether the drinker engaged in them.

Riley et al. (2011, p. 54) noted the importance of developing "health behaviour models that have dynamic, regulatory system components to guide rapid intervention adaptation based on the individual's current and past behaviour and situational context" (p. 54). However, until recently, understanding the aetiology of alcohol related problems at the event level has been rudimentary. Although conceptual models and theory have long guided alcohol studies (Denzin, 1987; Gusfield, 1996), models for drinking events rarely build on previous work or transcend levels of abstraction in ways that integrate theoretical streams or acknowledge dynamics and complexity (e.g. non-linearity, feedback loops—see Sect. 1 of this volume for a description of commonly used alcohol models). Although there is a small body of system dynamics alcohol studies at the community level (Holder, 2006; Scribner et al., 2009), and some recent notable exceptions employing agent-based modelling (Fitzpatrick & Martinez, 2011; Gorman, Mezic, Mezic, & Gruenewald, 2006) at the population and event levels, dynamic modelling in alcohol research is still largely underdeveloped.

The conceptualization of drinking events began over 40 years ago when the US National Institute on Alcoholism and Alcohol Abuse published a monograph titled *Social Drinking Contexts* (Harford & Gaines, 1979). In the introduction to that collection of conference papers, the authors noted, "While context, or frame of reference, may hold the key to understanding drinking behaviour, no single idiom describes context" (p. 1). The authors went on to say that the multidisciplinary nature of alcohol studies related to context reflect a spectrum of terms and units of analysis. The nomenclature and taxonomies used today to frame drinking events still reflect such diversity (see Chap. 9).

In that same monograph, drawing from the basic social psychology theory of Lewin (1951), Harford and Gaines (1979) offered a simple linear multilevel representation (person × environment leads to drinking behaviour).This path model explicitly defined "context" as "environment," and the authors went on to conceptualize environment into five elements: (1) physiogeographical (e.g. geospatial), (2) group level (e.g. demographics, size, gender ratio), (3) social or situational (e.g. a party), (4) theoretical (e.g. alcohol availability, social control, norms), and (5) how it is perceived by the individuals embedded in it (see Chap. 9). They also noted two important considerations. First, "(the environment) persists in being a concept of disturbing *complexity*" (p. 230). And second, "the *dynamics* of situations give rise to changes in situations and behaviour over time … an obvious source of such change is … alcohol ingestion … and its disinhibition effects" (p. 231; emphasis added).

Since the publication of *Social Drinking Contexts* (Harford & Gaines, 1979), there have been numerous publications examining drinking events which have varied in the conceptualization, measurement, and analysis of drinking events. In a mapping review of the existing literature on drinking events, 278 papers published between 2010 and 2019 were identified (Stevely, Holmes, & Meier, 2020). Most studies looked at a very limited set of contextual variables (e.g. affect, timing, number or type of people, venue), were US based, and focused on college students.

The implicit notion of a drinking event is often embedded in another conceptual focus. For instance, a number of studies have examined behaviours conceptually couched in drinking events such as "pre-partying" (Reed et al., 2011) or "drinking games" (Zamboanga et al., 2014). Others have correlated typical drinking settings with drinking behaviours or problem outcomes (Saltz, Paschall, McGaffigan, & Nygaard, 2010). Alcohol epidemiology—quantity, frequency, variability measures (e.g. heavy episodic drinking) (Wechsler et al., 1994)—is also a simple form of enumerating drinking events.

Although segmenting drinking events into time-specific (e.g. pre-gaming), social (e.g. drinking games), or geospatial (e.g. bars) elements allows one to study behaviour more easily, such segmentation obscures an understanding of the systemic and complex nature of events (Miller & Page, 2009), and potentially results in ineffective policy solutions to alcohol-related problems (Wells, Graham, & Purcell, 2009). For instance, over the course of an individual's drinking event, pre-gaming can occur in a small private setting (e.g. a few friends), followed by drinking games in a larger party setting, and culminating in a public setting like a bar. Each activity and setting comes with its own dynamics (Clapp et al., 2008, 2009; Fitzpatrick & Martinez, 2011), resulting in complexity (i.e. multilevel) and transitory risk (and protection) across an entire event (Ally, Lovatt, Meier, Brennan, & Holmes, 2016). The segmentation approach to studying drinking events, however, may soon be changing. For instance, Ally et al. (2016) conducted latent class analyses of over 180,000 drinking events across over 60,000 drinkers to develop a typology of British drinking culture. The study was able to identify risk events, including multi-location events, across population demographics, offering a richer understanding of drinking contexts as they relate to other key factors.

Conceptually, the social ecology of drinking events is complex and dynamic (Clapp et al., 2018; Giraldo, Passino, & Clapp, 2017 ; Giraldo, Passino, Clapp, & Ruderman, 2017). Systems dynamics models (Giraldo, Passino, & Clapp, 2017; Giraldo, Passino, Clapp, & Ruderman, 2017) based on field data have illustrated how biological factors (e.g. gender, body weight, etc.), motives, peer influence and the environment interact in complex feedback systems that influence intoxication (both peak blood alcohol content [BAC] and rate of BAC change). Although such models are useful to guide theory and pre-test potential interventions (Hawe, Shiell, & Riley, 2009), validation and tuning of computational models with empirical data is critical.

Understanding drinking event dynamics and complexity associated with individuals, groups, social context, the built environment, and shifting BAC remains a vexing problem, but recent studies have advanced this literature. Clapp et al. (2018) presented a dynamical model of drinking events including "micro," "mezzo," and "macro" elements that we have provided in Fig. 1. In the model, "environmental wetness" (i.e. the mean level of intoxication in the environment coupled with alcohol availability) was influenced by, and influenced, "group wetness" (i.e. the average level of intoxication in a social group drinking together). In turn, "group wetness" influenced drinkers' desired states of intoxication and drinking. A drinker's level of intoxication was influenced by the rate and amount of drinking (metabolic and elimination factors). In a series of computational systems dynamics studies grounded in empirical field data, the same research team modelled the various aspects of the conceptual drinking event system (Fig. 8.1).

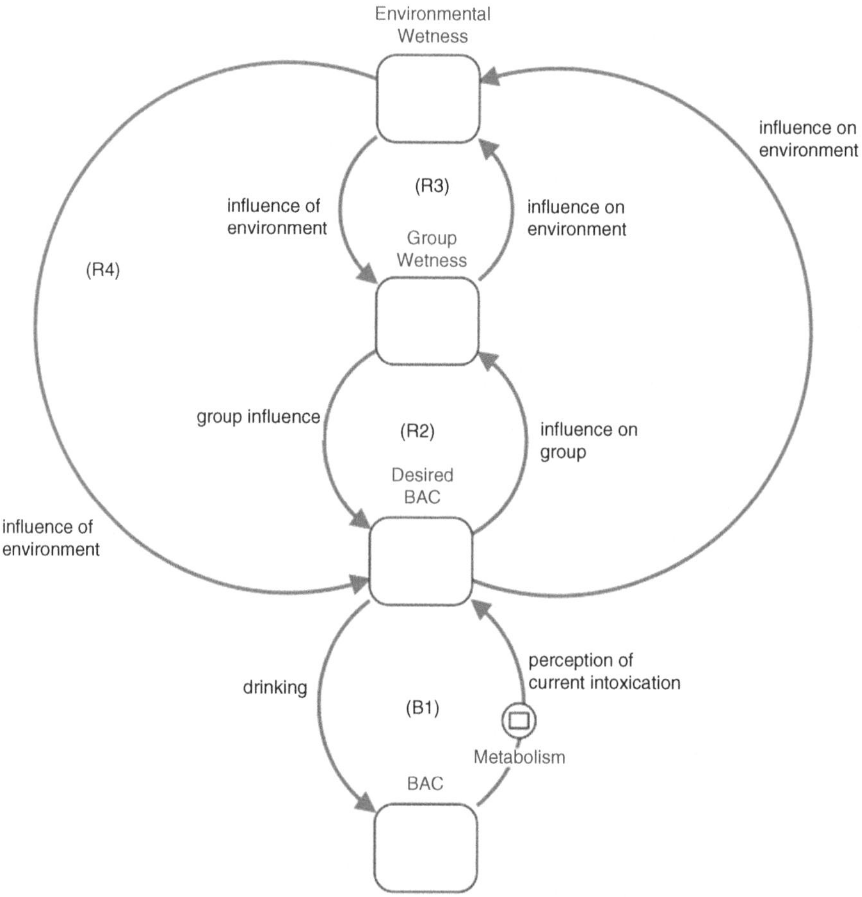

Fig. 8.1 Dynamic model of drinking events ('B' indicates balancing influences, 'R' indicates reinforcing influences)

Giraldo, Passino, and Clapp (2017) illustrated how decision-making concerning drinking influences and is influenced by the rate of alcohol intake, where intoxication accelerates as decision making becomes impaired. Similarly, a second study (Giraldo, Passino, Clapp, & Ruderman, 2017) illustrated the social influence a single heavy drinker at drinking events, where that heavier drinker could pull their lighter drinking peers into heavy drinking at the event level. Wetter environments were also influenced, and were influenced by, social groups.

Methodological Approaches to Studying and Intervening During Drinking Events

Capturing the complexity of drinking events is methodologically challenging. Historically, research into drinking behaviour in situ has relied on retrospective survey methods, observation, or field interviews (Patrick & Lee, 2010; Quinn & Fromme, 2011). Beyond self-reports, many field studies of drinking have used breathalyzers to estimate BAC. Although breathalyzers provide biological estimates of drinking that are arguably better than self-reports, the logistics of collecting breath tests in the field are difficult (Clapp et al., 2007). Logistically, collecting quality breath samples requires calibrated law enforcement grade breathalyzers, respondents who have not consumed alcohol in the past 20 minutes (some argue 10 minutes is adequate) to avoid mouth alcohol contamination, and trained staff. Further, with few exceptions (Clapp et al., 2009; Wells et al., 2015) most studies using breathalyzers collect one sample per participant making them cross-sectional.

Although point-estimates of BAC have utility (as do estimates of peak BAC), they are limited in providing useful data related to blood alcohol curves or how drinking shifts over the course of an event. Computational simulations of the dynamics of drinking events and the pharmacokinetics of BAC (Giraldo, Passino, & Clapp, 2017) strongly suggest that repeated measures of drinking during an event are needed to understand BAC curves and the ecology of drinking events. Understanding the overall dynamics of drinking events and how BAC "behaves over time" is critical to identifying leverage points for intervention (Stokols, 2000) and to avoid interventions based on simplistic models grounded in potentially spurious findings (Miller & Page, 2009). Regarding spurious findings, Miller and Page (Miller & Page, 2009) note that theory based on assumptions of mathematical normality, and cross-sectional studies that make inferences to guide such theory, can result in inaccurate inferences regarding complex phenomena. For example, a cross-sectional study of BAC at a drinking event (i.e. a single breath sample) predicting peak BAC cannot account for variations in the blood alcohol curve over the course of event. For some study participants peak BAC may have already occurred. For others, there may be multiple peaks.

There is a rapidly growing body of research that leverages the widespread use of mobile phones to survey individuals in natural environments ideally as risk behaviour is occurring. Ecological momentary assessments (EMA) are repeated, short, often smartphone-based surveys that allow researchers to sample important temporal features of risk behaviour as it occurs in natural environments (Smyth & Stone, 2003). These studies minimize recall error, maximize ecological validity (Stone & Shiffman, 1994), and help capture complex and dynamic behavioural data. The use of EMA methods seems particularly applicable to the study of event-level risky behaviour as well as event-level social interactions because both are dynamic and difficult to recall (Wray, Merrill, & Monti, 2014). For example, Thrul and Kuntsche (Thrul & Kuntsche, 2015) utilized EMA methods to survey young adult drinkers on weekend evenings to determine if consumption was affected by the number of friends present and interactions with either same-sex or other-sex peers. In this study, men tended to drink at a faster pace than women initially, but group dynamics negated gender differences later in the evening. Larger group size also predicted heavier drinking. The use of EMA allowed these researchers to view drinking as it was occurring over the course of multiple weekends.

EMA studies, however, do have several potential limitations. On the technical side, internet and cellular coverage can cause delays in subjects getting EMA notifications as well as in participants responding. Coupled with participants selectively responding (e.g. response fatigue, etc.), technical issues can result in missing data which can compromise the overall quality of findings. Although there are numerous imputation approaches to handle missing data in EMA studies, drinking event studies benefit from triangulation of data collection approaches (Shiffman, 2009). For instance, drinking event studies might include a retrospective and geo-grounded follow up interview to fill missing values (i.e. "last night at 11:00 pm you were at Bill's Bar, at 9:00 pm you reported having had three rounds of beer, do you recall what you drank between 9:00 and 11:00). Other potential methods include using the subject's recent drinking events or group member data from the same event (if available) to help impute missing values.

Transdermal alcohol monitors represent a potential alternative to breathalyzers, observation or self-reported drinking during drinking events (Marques & McKnight, 2009). Whereas breathalyzers provide BAC, transdermal alcohol monitors provide estimates based on alcohol perspired through the skin (transdermal alcohol content: TAC). One major potential advantage of using transdermal monitors over other methods is their capacity to take repeated TAC samples from the same subject over time. This feature has potential for enhancing event-level research, treatment outcome studies, and the like. In a recent study of a college bar crawl, Clapp et al., (Clapp, Madden, Mooney, & Dahlquist, 2017) tracked a group of college drinkers over the course of an organized drinking event. Using EMA data, transdermal monitors, and observation, the study was able to plot TAC curves for each participant relative to geographic location, perceived intoxication, and motivations related to drinking. Transdermal biosensors can be an improvement over self-report measures, but there are still some caveats. There is not yet a standard approach to reliably convert TAC to comparable BAC values (Luczak et al., 2018). In addition, there is a time lag between alcohol consumption and skin detection that may have subject-to-subject variability or within-person variability at higher doses of alcohol. Although the current reliability of TAC measures is still in development, when coupled with other measures of drinking at the event level, TAC data augments the overall ecological validity of event-level studies. The proliferation of Global Positioning System (GPS) and Bluetooth-equipped smartphones, smart "apps" and newer generations of smaller (wristwatch size) wearable alcohol or "tattoo" like monitors will likely improve our ability to study and intervene in alcohol events in real time.

To date, however, there are only a few notable examples of empirical research that has utilized transdermal monitors to observe everyday drinking contexts (Clapp et al., 2017; Fairbairn, Rosen, Luczak, & Venerable, 2018; Leffingwell et al., 2013). Thus far, research with ethanol biochemical sensors has mostly focused on either estimating BAC based on transdermal data (Luczak et al., 2018) or exploring contingency management interventions that promote abstinence (Barnett et al., 2017; Barnett, Tidey, Murphy, Swift, & Colby, 2011; Dougherty et al., 2014). The devices are more typically utilized as an intervention in a criminal justice setting to decrease the propensity of reoccurring harm such as drink-driving (McKnight, Fell, & Auld-Owens, 2012). Otherwise, event-level studies still fail to include more continuous objective measures of alcohol consumption. Although recent advances in data collection technologies (Leffingwell et al., 2013; Riley et al., 2011) have the potential to advance our understanding of event-level drinking behaviour, Riley et al. (Riley et al., 2011) noted that our ability to collect individualized, context-specific data and to intervene in situ has surpassed our current theories. The authors noted that "health behaviour models that have dynamic, regulatory system components to guide rapid intervention adaptation based on the individual's current and past behaviour and situational context" (p. 54) are greatly needed.

Intervention

Intervening during an event to prevent extreme intoxication makes good sense, because individual decision making can be markedly impaired leading to problems such as interpersonal conflicts, unprepared sexual activity, drunk driving, or violence (Abernathy, Chandler, & Woodward, 2010). In addition, drinking behaviour is contextually bound to one's current situation (Monk, Heim, Qureshi, & Price, 2015). In order to intervene during risk behaviour, recent studies have begun to embrace mobile technology such as smartphones, geolocators, or wearable biosensors (e.g. accelerometers). Internet-connected mobile devices are near ubiquitous and provide feasible instruments for both data collection and intervention delivery (Beckjord & Shiffman, 2014). New "smart" technologies have the potential to complement universal prevention efforts by targeting "leverage points" in events (Stokols, 2000).

Interventions delivered on mobile devices in real-world settings are often referred to as ecological momentary interventions (EMI) or mobile health (mHealth) interventions (Morgenstern, Kuerbis, & Muench, 2014). EMI are based on the notion of consumer self-control or individuals can change their own behaviour when prompted. Mobile-based interventions can be cost-effective options to more traditional in-person methods and have the potential to reach individuals during risk behaviour (Yu, Wu, Yu, & Xiao, 2006). Mobile-based interventions have become increasingly used in related behaviour change efforts (Riley et al., 2011), such as management of depressive symptoms (Agyapong, McLoughlin, & Farren, 2013). Furthermore, smartphone applications are now being utilized to implement interventions for at-risk individuals with drug use issues or other addictions such as gambling (Zhang & Ho, 2016). These types of interventions are also becoming more common for alcohol use particularly in US college student populations (Kauer, Reid, Sanci, & Patton, 2009), though interventions have been conducted with both young and older adults and deployed in educational, clinical, or community-based settings (Song, Qian, & Yu, 2019). In a recently published systematic review, mobile-based interventions have resulted in significant behavioural change such as decreased number of self-reported drinks consumed during an event (Song et al., 2019), fewer self-reported heavy drinking days during the past month (Alessi & Petry, 2013; Gustafson et al.,

2014; Hasin, Aharonovich, & Greenstein, 2014), lower prevalence of alcohol-related injury (Suffoletto et al., 2014, 2015), or increased number of days abstinent post-treatment (Agyapong et al., 2013).

mHhealth interventions are generally delivered either by short message service (i.e. text messaging), apps, or interactive voice response (IVR). Text-based interventions primarily remind individuals of protective strategies and risk-based knowledge via repeated messages (Bock et al., 2016; Muench et al., 2017) while app-based and IVR interventions tend to monitor current use, provide personalized visual feedback (Gonzalez & Dulin, 2015; Gustafson et al., 2014), or even generate answers to consumer questions (Hasin et al., 2014). The content of mHealth interventions is typically based on two main theoretical constructs: behavioural change (e.g. planned behaviour, health belief model, cognitive-behavioural therapy, or social learning theory) and psychological motivation (e.g. self-determination, contingency management) (Song et al., 2019). Content is both informational (e.g. general or personalized information about risks of alcohol) and motivational (e.g. encouragement messages, committing to drinking goals) (Heron & Smyth, 2010). Interventions can be delivered at fixed times, on-demand by participants, randomly, or in response to contextual data such as geospatial coordinates (Song et al., 2019). For example, EMIs can be implemented throughout the course of an intervention period (e.g. three months post-treatment), during pre-identified high-risk times (i.e. weekends or holidays), or when an individual enters an area of risk (i.e. geographically close to alcohol outlets (Dulin & Gonzalez, 2017; Gustafson et al., 2014)).

While reviews have generally pointed to the effectiveness of mobile-based substance use interventions (Song et al., 2019), continuous monitoring of risk behaviour as a means of understanding triggers for either relapse or dangerous intoxication is still underdeveloped. We do not yet have a solid theoretical understanding of the underlying relationship between indicators and triggers (Kennedy et al., 2015). In randomized control trials, mHealth interventions for alcohol use tend to be more effective if the intervention period is longer, there are more frequent delivery of prompts or messages, and there are tangible incentives (Fowler, Holt, & Joshi, 2016; Mason, Ola, Zaharakis, & Zhang, 2015; Song et al., 2019). Alarmingly, very few commercially available mHealth apps incorporate empirically based strategies (Cohn, Hunter-Reel, Hagman, & Mitchell, 2011). Furthermore, most mHealth interventions fail to intervene during an event with content that is tailored both to the person and the current context (Fjeldsoe, Marshall, & Miller, 2009).

Ideally, mobile health interventions would be adaptable to individual circumstances in the moment. Just-in-time adaptive interventions (JITAI) hypothetically utilize the power of mobile phone technology, geospatial trackers, and wearables to intervene at *just* the right time to alter the trajectory of an individual's behaviour (Nahum-Shani et al., 2018). JITAI are deployed based on decision rules that are affected by an individual's demographics, past behaviour and their current context (Lagoa, Bekiroglu, Lanza, & Murphy, 2014). Not all mHealth interventions are adaptive however, even though mobile devices provide intensive context-specific longitudinal data. Furthermore, there are few examples of JITAI that have incorporated objective measures of intoxication (Barnett et al., 2011; Dougherty et al., 2014).

The combined use of both transdermal monitors and sensors embedded in smartphones is a promising avenue for preventive applications. Almost all mHealth applications rely on self-reported data from participants, but self-assessed drinking behaviour can be biased or inaccurate (Beckjord & Shiffman, 2014). Inferring drunkenness at any point in time is precluded by the dynamic process of metabolizing ethanol (Clapp et al., 2018). In a small field-based pilot study of drinking behaviour during a bar crawl, subjectively inferring one's intoxication was less reliable when consumption increased (Clapp et al., 2017). A sensor-based application could feasibly detect a dangerous drinking episode before even the drinker is capable of realizing they have consumed too much alcohol or too quickly.

Passively collected smartphone data have been connected to drinking behaviour (Bae, Chung, Ferreira, Dey, & Suffoletto, 2018) but not yet employed in an intervention. Transdermal monitors have been utilized as additions to contingency management interventions to promote overall abstinence (Barnett et al., 2011), but have not yet been included in attempts to intervene during drinking events to decrease event-level intoxication. Commercial-based transdermal companies are already in the process of developing monitors that can be worn on a wrist and can communicate with app-based software (Langley, 2017). Unfortunately, consumer-oriented technology is being crafted and sold to the public before our health-related theories have detailed how factors interact during an event. We were able to find only one example of an mHealth intervention that utilizes biosensor data. The Mind the Moment (MtM) intervention relies on continuous readings from a wrist-worn electrodermal activity (EDA) sensor to intervene at moments when individuals are experiencing heightened emotional arousal (i.e. stress or anxiety) (Leonard et al., 2017) which has been linked to alcohol use disorders (Nees, Diener, Smolka, & Flor, 2012). When EDA rose to a certain threshold, participants were provided with Cognitive Behavioural Therapy (CBT) informed strategies and protective behavioural strategies for drinking (Leonard et al., 2017). Initial findings were promising but it is not yet clear if these types of interventions can mitigate event-level issues such as violence, sexual risk taking, or acute alcohol poisoning.

Despite limited research to date, the real-time delivery of interventions aimed at reducing alcohol consumption shows great promise (Free et al., 2010). In the least, the practice of self-monitoring and the use of real-time assessment during drinking events may result in positive behavioural change (Kazemi et al., 2017). Furthermore, tying geographically explicit information to momentary responses (McQuoid, Thrul, & Ling, 2018) may provide the opportunity to physically map areas of risk in an entertainment district (i.e. "hotspots"). In the future, it will be important to continue to blend engineering principles with intervention design to identify optimal points to intervene and at what frequency (Gonzalez Villasanti, Passino, Clapp, & Madden, 2018; Lagoa et al., 2014). Tools often employed in control engineering could allow researchers to test interventions at various time points with existing data. In this case, interventions are designed based on an algorithm that utilizes an individual's current status and a prediction of the individual's future status and the intervention can be adjusted when individuals deviate (Lagoa et al., 2014). System dynamics frameworks can provide guidelines for behavioural interventions at the individual, group, and environmental levels and how we may be able to complement population-level or environmental interventions (i.e. RBS, increased prices) with personalized individual strategies. Technologies like global positioning systems (GPS), Bluetooth networking, SMS-based ecological momentary assessments, and transdermal alcohol sensors may greatly increase both our understanding of drinking events and our ability to intervene in real time and in a tailored manner (Riley et al., 2011).

In order to design real-time interventions with emergent technologies and engineering principles, it is critical to better understand the conceptualization of drinking events. When considering the field in its current state, several areas of inquiry are needed. First, conceptual work to help understand and frame the complexity of drinking events must continue. Our understanding of interplay between drinking rate, motives, social influence and environment as part of an ecological system is still rudimentary. As noted earlier, such work is critical for identifying leverage points for just-in-time interventions. Second, further development of methods to capture drinking behaviour at the event level is needed. Methods to augment and triangulate EMA and other self-report data might include artificial intelligence approaches using GPS, accelerometer and or other smart-phone data (Bae et al., 2018). Third, as noted earlier, transdermal alcohol monitors have not yet been fully developed, though researchers in the field are moving this important innovation forward (Leffingwell et al., 2013). Finally, as a field, alcohol science would benefit of better understanding drinking at the event level to inform epidemiology (i.e. context to drinking trends), the trajectories of alcohol use disorders, and the development of environmental alcohol prevention policies and programs. To this end, papers, special issue journals, books and conferences that help alcohol researchers and prevention professionals better understand alcohol use across the spectrum of levels of abstraction (i.e. de-segmentation) is greatly needed.

Conclusion

Understanding alcohol use as it naturally occurs remains a relatively understudied but potentially very important area of alcohol science given the prevalence of acute alcohol-related problems. Advances in real-time data collection methods, the transdermal estimation of blood alcohol concentrations, and complex multi-level modelling increase both our understanding of the complex ecology of alcohol use and our potential to strategically intervene to influence drinking in real time. This chapter begins to layout the framework for future work in this area.

References

Abernathy, K., Chandler, L. J., & Woodward, J. J. (2010). Alcohol and the prefrontal cortex. *International Review of Neurobiology, 91*, 289–320. https://doi.org/10.1016/S0074-7742(10)91009-X

Agyapong, V. I. O., McLoughlin, D. M., & Farren, C. K. (2013). Six-months outcomes of a randomised trial of supportive text messaging for depression and comorbid alcohol use disorder. *Journal of Affective Disorders, 151*(1), 100–104. https://doi.org/10.1016/j.jad.2013.05.058

Alessi, S. M., & Petry, N. M. (2013). A randomized study of cellphone technology to reinforce alcohol abstinence in the natural environment: Portable CM for alcohol abstinence. *Addiction, 108*(5), 900–909. https://doi.org/10.1111/add.12093

Ally, A. K., Lovatt, M., Meier, P. S., Brennan, A., & Holmes, J. (2016). Developing a social practice-based typology of British drinking culture in 2009–2011: Implications for alcohol policy analysis. *Addiction (Abingdon, England), 111*(9), 1568–1579. https://doi.org/10.1111/add.13397

Bae, S., Chung, T., Ferreira, D., Dey, A. K., & Suffoletto, B. (2018). Mobile phone sensors and supervised machine learning to identify alcohol use events in young adults: Implications for just-in-time adaptive interventions. *Addictive Behaviours, 83*, 42–47. https://doi.org/10.1016/j.addbeh.2017.11.039

Barnett, N. P., Celio, M. A., Tidey, J. W., Murphy, J. G., Colby, S. M., & Swift, R. M. (2017). A preliminary randomized controlled trial of contingency management for alcohol use reduction using a transdermal alcohol sensor: Contingency management for alcohol use reduction. *Addiction, 112*(6), 1025–1035. https://doi.org/10.1111/add.13767

Barnett, N. P., Tidey, J., Murphy, J. G., Swift, R., & Colby, S. M. (2011). Contingency management for alcohol use reduction: A pilot study using a transdermal alcohol sensor. *Drug and Alcohol Dependence, 118*(2–3), 391–399. https://doi.org/10.1016/j.drugalcdep.2011.04.023

Barry, A. E., Stellefson, M. L., Piazza-Gardner, A. K., Chaney, B. H., & Dodd, V. (2013). The impact of pregaming on subsequent blood alcohol concentrations: An event-level analysis. *Addictive Behaviours, 38*(8), 2374–2377. https://doi.org/10.1016/j.addbeh.2013.03.014

Beckjord, E., & Shiffman, S. (2014). Background for real-time monitoring and intervention related to alcohol use. *Alcohol Research: Current Reviews, 36*(1), 9–18.

Bock, B. C., Barnett, N. P., Thind, H., Rosen, R., Walaska, K., Traficante, R., ... Scott-Sheldon, L. A. J. (2016). A text message intervention for alcohol risk reduction among community college students: TMAP. *Addictive Behaviours, 63*, 107–113. https://doi.org/10.1016/j.addbeh.2016.07.012

Cavan, S. (1966). *Liquor license: An ethnography of bar behaviour*. Chicago, IL: Aldine Transaction.

Clapp, J. D., Holmes, M. R., Reed, M. B., Shillington, A. M., Freisthler, B., & Lange, J. E. (2007). Measuring college students' alcohol consumption in natural drinking environments: Field methodologies for bars and parties. *Evaluation Review, 31*(5), 469–489. https://doi.org/10.1177/0193841X07303582

Clapp, J. D., Madden, D. R., Gonzalez Villasanti, H., Giraldo, L. F., Passino, K. M., Reed, M. B., & Fernandez Puentes, I. (2018). A system dynamic model of drinking events: Multi-level ecological approach: A system dynamic model of drinking events. *Systems Research and Behavioural Science, 35*(3), 265–281. https://doi.org/10.1002/sres.2478

Clapp, J. D., Madden, D. R., Mooney, D. D., & Dahlquist, K. E. (2017). Examining the social ecology of a bar-crawl: An exploratory pilot study. *PLoS One, 12*(9), e0185238. https://doi.org/10.1371/journal.pone.0185238

Clapp, J. D., Min, J. W., Shillington, A. M., Reed, M. B., & Croff, J. K. (2008). Person and environment predictors of blood alcohol concentrations: A multi-level study of college parties. *Alcoholism: Clinical and Experimental Research, 32*(1), 100–107. https://doi.org/10.1111/j.1530-0277.2007.00547.x

Clapp, J. D., Reed, M. B., Min, J. W., Shillington, A. M., Croff, J. M., Holmes, M. R., & Trim, R. S. (2009). Blood alcohol concentrations among bar patrons: A multi-level study of drinking behaviour. *Drug and Alcohol Dependence, 102*(1–3), 41–48. https://doi.org/10.1016/j.drugalcdep.2008.12.015

Clapp, J. D., Reed, M. B., & Ruderman, D. E. (2014). The relationship between drinking games and intentions to continue drinking, intentions to drive after drinking, and adverse consequences: Results of a field study. *The American Journal of Drug and Alcohol Abuse, 40*(5), 374–379. https://doi.org/10.3109/00952990.2014.933838

Cohn, A. M., Hunter-Reel, D., Hagman, B. T., & Mitchell, J. (2011). Promoting behaviour change from alcohol use through Mobile technology: The future of ecological momentary assessment. *Alcoholism: Clinical and Experimental Research, 35*(12), 2209–2215. https://doi.org/10.1111/j.1530-0277.2011.01571.x

Denzin, N. K. (1987). *The alcoholic self.* London, England: Sage.

Dougherty, D. M., Hill-Kapturczak, N., Liang, Y., Karns, T. E., Cates, S. E., Lake, S. L., … Roache, J. D. (2014). Use of continuous transdermal alcohol monitoring during a contingency management procedure to reduce excessive alcohol use. *Drug and Alcohol Dependence, 142*, 301–306. https://doi.org/10.1016/j.drugalcdep.2014.06.039

Dulin, P. L., & Gonzalez, V. M. (2017). Smartphone-based, momentary intervention for alcohol cravings amongst individuals with an alcohol use disorder. *Psychology of Addictive Behaviours, 31*(5), 601–607. https://doi.org/10.1037/adb0000292

Fairbairn, C. E., Rosen, I. G., Luczak, S. E., & Venerable, W. J. (2018). Estimating the quantity and time course of alcohol consumption from transdermal alcohol sensor data: A combined laboratory-ambulatory study. *Alcohol, 81*, 111. https://doi.org/10.1016/j.alcohol.2018.08.015

Fitzpatrick, B., & Martinez, J. (2011). Agent-based modeling of ecological niche theory and assortative drinking. *Journal of Artificial Societies and Social Simulation, 15*(2), 4.

Fjeldsoe, B. S., Marshall, A. L., & Miller, Y. D. (2009). Behaviour change interventions delivered by mobile telephone short-message service. *American Journal of Preventive Medicine, 36*(2), 165–173. https://doi.org/10.1016/j.amepre.2008.09.040

Fowler, L. A., Holt, S. L., & Joshi, D. (2016). Mobile technology-based interventions for adult users of alcohol: A systematic review of the literature. *Addictive Behaviours, 62*, 25–34. https://doi.org/10.1016/j.addbeh.2016.06.008

Free, C., Phillips, G., Felix, L., Galli, L., Patel, V., & Edwards, P. (2010). The effectiveness of M-health technologies for improving health and health services: A systematic review protocol. *BMC Research Notes, 3*, 250. https://doi.org/10.1186/1756-0500-3-250

Giraldo, L. F., Passino, K. M., & Clapp, J. D. (2017). Modeling and analysis of group dynamics in alcohol-consumption environments. *IEEE Transactions on Cybernetics, 47*(1), 165–176. https://doi.org/10.1109/TCYB.2015.2509444

Giraldo, L. F., Passino, K. M., Clapp, J. D., & Ruderman, D. (2017). Dynamics of metabolism and decision making during alcohol consumption: Modeling and analysis. *IEEE Transactions on Cybernetics, 47*(11), 3955–3966. https://doi.org/10.1109/TCYB.2016.2593009

Gonzalez, V. M., & Dulin, P. L. (2015). Comparison of a smartphone app for alcohol use disorders with an internet-based intervention plus bibliotherapy: A pilot study.

Journal of Consulting and Clinical Psychology, 83(2), 335–345. https://doi.org/10.1037/a0038620

Gonzalez Villasanti, H., Passino, K. M., Clapp, J. D., & Madden, D. R. (2018). A control-theoretic assessment of interventions during drinking events. *IEEE Transactions on Cybernetics, 49*, 1–12. https://doi.org/10.1109/TCYB.2017.2782010

Gorman, D. M., Mezic, J., Mezic, I., & Gruenewald, P. J. (2006). Agent-based Modeling of drinking behaviour: A preliminary model and potential applications to theory and practice. *American Journal of Public Health, 96*(11), 2055–2060. https://doi.org/10.2105/AJPH.2005.063289

Gusfield, J. R. (1996). *Contested meanings: The construction of alcohol problems.* Madison, WI: University of Wisconsin Press.

Gustafson, D. H., McTavish, F. M., Chih, M. Y., Atwood, A. K., Johnson, R. A., Boyle, M. G., ... Shah, D. (2014). A smartphone application to support recovery from alcoholism: A randomized clinical trial. *JAMA Psychiatry, 71*(5), 566–572. https://doi.org/10.1001/jamapsychiatry.2013.4642

Harford, T. C., & Gaines, L. S. (1979). Social drinking contexts. In *Proceedings of a Workshop* (DHHS-ADM-81-1097). National Institute of Alcohol Abuse and Alcoholism. https://files.eric.ed.gov/fulltext/ED227373.pdf

Hasin, D. S., Aharonovich, E., & Greenstein, E. (2014). HealthCall for the smartphone: Technology enhancement of brief intervention in HIV alcohol dependent patients. *Addiction Science & Clinical Practice, 9*. https://doi.org/10.1186/1940-0640-9-5

Hawe, P., Shiell, A., & Riley, T. (2009). Theorising interventions as events in systems. *American Journal of Community Psychology, 43*(3–4), 267–276. https://doi.org/10.1007/s10464-009-9229-9

Heron, K. E., & Smyth, J. M. (2010). Ecological momentary interventions: Incorporating mobile technology into psychosocial and health behaviour treatments. *British Journal of Health Psychology, 15*(1), 1–39. https://doi.org/10.1348/135910709X466063

Holder, H. D. (2006). *Alcohol and the community: A systems approach to prevention.* Cambridge, England: Cambridge University Press.

Kauer, S. D., Reid, S. C., Sanci, L., & Patton, G. C. (2009). Investigating the utility of mobile phones for collecting data about adolescent alcohol use and related mood, stress and coping behaviours: Lessons and recommendations. *Drug and Alcohol Review, 28*(1), 25–30. https://doi.org/10.1111/j.1465-3362.2008.00002.x

Kazemi, D. M., Borsari, B., Levine, M. J., Li, S., Lamberson, K. A., & Matta, L. A. (2017). A systematic review of the mHealth interventions to prevent alcohol and substance abuse. *Journal of Health Communication, 22*(5), 413–432. https://doi.org/10.1080/10810730.2017.1303556

Kennedy, A. P., Epstein, D. H., Jobes, M. L., Agage, D., Tyburski, M., Phillips, K. A., ... Preston, K. L. (2015). Continuous in-the-field measurement of heart rate: Correlates of drug use, craving, stress, and mood in polydrug users. *Drug and*

Alcohol Dependence, 151, 159–166. https://doi.org/10.1016/j.drugalcdep.2015.03.024

Lagoa, C. M., Bekiroglu, K., Lanza, S. T., & Murphy, S. A. (2014). Designing adaptive intensive interventions using methods from engineering. *Journal of Consulting and Clinical Psychology, 82*(5), 868–878. https://doi.org/10.1037/a0037736

Langley, H. (2017). *Bactrack's wearable will tell you how drunk you are*. Wareable. https://www.wareable.com/health-and-wellbeing/bactrack-sync-wearable-alcohol-monitor-release-date-price-3735

Leffingwell, T. R., Cooney, N. J., Murphy, J. G., Luczak, S., Rosen, G., Dougherty, D. M., & Barnett, N. P. (2013). Continuous objective monitoring of alcohol use: Twenty-first century measurement using transdermal sensors. *Alcoholism: Clinical and Experimental Research, 37*(1), 16–22. https://doi.org/10.1111/j.1530-0277.2012.01869.x

Leonard, N. R., Silverman, M., Sherpa, D. P., Naegle, M. A., Kim, H., Coffman, D. L., & Ferdschneider, M. (2017). Mobile health technology using a wearable sensorband for female college students with problem drinking: An acceptability and feasibility study. *JMIR mHealth and uHealth, 5*(7), e90. https://doi.org/10.2196/mHealth.7399

Lewin, K. (1951). *Field theory in social science: Selected theoretical papers* (Ed. D. Cartwright). Harpers.

Luczak, S. E., Hawkins, A. L., Dai, Z., Wichmann, R., Wang, C., & Rosen, I. G. (2018). Obtaining continuous BAC/BAC estimates in the field: A hybrid system integrating transdermal alcohol biosensor, Intellidrink smartphone app, and BAC estimator software tools. *Addictive Behaviours, 83*, 48–55. https://doi.org/10.1016/j.addbeh.2017.11.038

Marques, P. R., & McKnight, A. S. (2009). Field and laboratory alcohol detection with 2 types of transdermal devices. *Alcoholism: Clinical and Experimental Research, 33*(4), 703–711. https://doi.org/10.1111/j.1530-0277.2008.00887.x

Mason, M., Ola, B., Zaharakis, N., & Zhang, J. (2015). Text messaging interventions for adolescent and young adult substance use: A meta-analysis. *Prevention Science: The Official Journal of the Society for Prevention Research, 16*(2), 181–188. https://doi.org/10.1007/s11121-014-0498-7

McKnight, A. S., Fell, J. C., & Auld-Owens, A. (2012). *Transdermal alcohol monitoring: Case studies*. Washington, DC: National Highway Traffic Safety Administration.

McQuoid, J., Thrul, J., & Ling, P. (2018). A geographically explicit ecological momentary assessment (GEMA) mixed method for understanding substance use. *Social Science & Medicine, 202*, 89–98. https://doi.org/10.1016/j.socscimed.2018.02.014

Miller, J. H., & Page, S. E. (2009). *Complex adaptive systems: An introduction to computational models of social life*. Princeton, NJ: Princeton University Press.

Monk, R. L., Heim, D., Qureshi, A., & Price, A. (2015). "I have no clue what I drunk last night" using smartphone technology to compare in-vivo and retrospective self-reports of alcohol consumption. *PLoS One, 10*(5). https://doi.org/10.1371/journal.pone.0126209

Morgenstern, J., Kuerbis, A., & Muench, F. (2014). Ecological momentary assessment and alcohol use disorder treatment. *Alcohol Research: Current Reviews, 36*(1), 101–110.

Muench, F., van Stolk-Cooke, K., Kuerbis, A., Stadler, G., Baumel, A., Shao, S., McKay, J. R., & Morgenstern, J. (2017). A randomized controlled pilot trial of different mobile messaging interventions for problem drinking compared to weekly drink tracking. PLoS One, 12(2), e0167900. https://doi.org/10.1371/journal.pone.0167900.

Nahum-Shani, I., Smith, S. N., Spring, B. J., Collins, L. M., Witkiewitz, K., Tewari, A., & Murphy, S. A. (2018). Just-in-time adaptive interventions (JITAIs) in Mobile Health: Key components and design principles for ongoing health behaviour support. *Annals of Behavioural Medicine: A Publication of the Society of Behavioural Medicine, 52*(6), 446–462. https://doi.org/10.1007/s12160-016-9830-8

National Institute of Health. (2000). *10th special report to the U.S. Congress on Alcohol and Health*. Bethesda, MD: U.S. Department of Health and Human Services.

Nees, F., Diener, C., Smolka, M. N., & Flor, H. (2012). The role of context in the processing of alcohol-relevant cues. *Addiction Biology, 17*(2), 441–451. https://doi.org/10.1111/j.1369-1600.2011.00347.x

Patrick, M. E., & Lee, C. M. (2010). Comparing numbers of drinks: College students' reports from retrospective summary, followback, and prospective daily diary measures. *Journal of Studies on Alcohol and Drugs, 71*(4), 554–561.

Quinn, P. D., & Fromme, K. (2011). Predictors and outcomes of variability in subjective alcohol intoxication among college students: An event-level analysis across 4 years. *Alcoholism: Clinical and Experimental Research, 35*(3), 484–495. https://doi.org/10.1111/j.1530-0277.2010.01365.x

Reed, M. B., Clapp, J. D., Weber, M., Trim, R., Lange, J., & Shillington, A. M. (2011). Predictors of partying prior to bar attendance and subsequent BAC. *Addictive Behaviours, 36*(12), 1341–1343. https://doi.org/10.1016/j.addbeh.2011.07.029

Rehm, J., Mathers, C., Popova, S., Thavorncharoensap, M., Teerawattananon, Y., & Patra, J. (2009). Global burden of disease and injury and economic cost attributable to alcohol use and alcohol-use disorders. *Lancet, 373*(9682), 2223–2233.

Riley, W. T., Rivera, D. E., Atienza, A. A., Nilsen, W., Allison, S. M., & Mermelstein, R. (2011). Health behaviour models in the age of mobile interventions: Are our theories up to the task? *Translational Behavioural Medicine, 1*(1), 53–71. https://doi.org/10.1007/s13142-011-0021-7

Saltz, R. F., Paschall, M. J., McGaffigan, R. P., & Nygaard, P. M. O. (2010). Alcohol risk management in college settings: The safer California universities randomized trial. *American Journal of Preventive Medicine, 39*(6), 491–499. https://doi.org/10.1016/j.amepre.2010.08.020

Scribner, R., Ackleh, A. S., Fitzpatrick, B. G., Jacquez, G., Thibodeaux, J. J., Rommel, R., & Simonsen, N. (2009). A systems approach to college drinking: Development of a deterministic model for testing alcohol control policies. *Journal of Studies on Alcohol and Drugs, 70*(5), 805–821.

Shiffman, S. (2009). Ecological momentary assessment (EMA) in studies of substance use. *Psychological Assessment, 21*(4), 486–497. https://doi.org/10.1037/a0017074

Smyth, J. M., & Stone, A. A. (2003). Ecological momentary assessment research in behavioural medicine. *Journal of Happiness Studies; Dordrecht, 4*(1), 35–52. http://dx.doi.org.libproxy1.usc.edu/10.1023/A:1023657221954

Song, T., Qian, S., & Yu, P. (2019). Mobile health interventions for self-control of unhealthy alcohol use: Systematic review. *JMIR mHealth and uHealth, 7*(1). https://doi.org/10.2196/10899

Stevely, A. K., Holmes, J., & Meier, P. S. (2020). Contextual characteristics of adults' drinking occasions and their association with levels of alcohol consumption and acute alcohol-related harm: A mapping review. *Addiction, 115*(2), 218–229. https://doi.org/10.1111/add.14839

Stokols, D. (2000). Social ecology and behavioural medicine: Implications for training, practice, and policy. *Behavioural Medicine (Washington, D.C.), 26*(3), 129–138. https://doi.org/10.1080/08964280009595760

Stone, A. A., & Shiffman, S. (1994). Ecological momentary assessment (Ema) in behavioural medicine. *Annals of Behavioural Medicine, 16*(3), 199–202. https://doi.org/10.1093/abm/16.3.199

Suffoletto, B., Kristan, J., Callaway, C., Kim, K. H., Chung, T., Monti, P. M., & Clark, D. B. (2014). A text message alcohol intervention for young adult emergency department patients: A randomized clinical trial. *Annals of Emergency Medicine, 64*(6), 664–672.e4. https://doi.org/10.1016/j.annemergmed.2014.06.010

Suffoletto, B., Kristan, J., Chung, T., Jeong, K., Fabio, A., Monti, P., & Clark, D. B. (2015). An interactive text message intervention to reduce binge drinking in young adults: A randomized controlled trial with 9-month outcomes. *PLoS One, 10*(11), e0142877. https://doi.org/10.1371/journal.pone.0142877

Thrul, J., & Kuntsche, E. (2015). The impact of friends on young adults' drinking over the course of the evening-an event-level analysis: Impact of friends on young adults' drinking. *Addiction, 110*(4), 619–626. https://doi.org/10.1111/add.12862

Verster, J. C., Benjaminsen, J. M. E., van Lanen, J. H. M., van Stavel, N. M. D., & Olivier, B. (2015). Effects of mixing alcohol with energy drink on objective and subjective intoxication: Results from a Dutch on-premise study. *Psychopharmacology, 232*(5), 835–842. https://doi.org/10.1007/s00213-014-3715-y

Wechsler, H., Davenport, A., Dowdall, G., Moeykens, B., & Castillo, S. (1994). Health and behavioural consequences of binge drinking in college: A National Survey of students at 140 campuses. *JAMA, 272*(21), 1672–1677. https://doi.org/10.1001/jama.1994.03520210056032

Wells, S., Dumas, T. M., Bernards, S., Kuntsche, E., Labhart, F., & Graham, K. (2015). Predrinking, alcohol use, and breath alcohol concentration: A study of young adult bargoers. *Psychology of Addictive Behaviours, 29*(3), 683–689. https://doi.org/10.1037/adb0000065

Wells, S., Graham, K., & Purcell, J. (2009). Policy implications of the widespread practice of "pre-drinking" or "pre-gaming" before going to public drinking establishments: Are current prevention strategies backfiring? *Addiction (Abingdon, England), 104*(1), 4–9. https://doi.org/10.1111/j.1360-0443.2008.02393.x

World Health Organization. (2018). *Global status report on alcohol and health 2018*. Geneva, Switzerland: World Health Organization.

Wray, T. B., Merrill, J. E., & Monti, P. M. (2014). Using ecological momentary assessment (EMA) to assess situation-level predictors of alcohol use and alcohol-related consequences. *Alcohol Research: Current Reviews, 36*(1), 19–27.

Yu, P., Wu, M. X., Yu, H., & Xiao, G. Q. (2006). The challenges for the adoption of M-health. In *2006 IEEE International Conference on Service Operations and Logistics, and Informatics* (pp. 181–186). https://doi.org/10.1109/SOLI.2006.329059

Zamboanga, B. L., Kenney, S. R., Van Tyne, K., Olthuis, J. V., Correia, C. J., Ham, L. S., & Borsari, B. (2014). Not just fun and games: A review of college drinking games research from 2004 to 2013. Psychology of Addictive Behaviours: Journal of the Society of Psychologists in Addictive Behaviours, 28(3), 682–695. https://doi.org/10.1037/a0036639.

Zhang, M. W. B., & Ho, R. C. M. (2016). Tapping onto the potential of smartphone applications for psycho-education and early intervention in addictions. *Frontiers in Psychiatry, 7*. https://doi.org/10.3389/fpsyt.2016.00040

9

The Contextual Milieu of Alcohol Consumption

Rebecca Monk and Derek Heim

Introduction

This chapter provides a critical overview of current understanding about how contextual factors influence alcohol consumption and related cognitions. The chapter begins by outlining current knowledge regarding the role of external contextual factors—environmental location and social interaction—in shaping people's alcohol consumption and affecting their cognitions. Next, we argue that when exploring alcohol consumption in drinking contexts, it is more useful to focus on the gender composition of the group, as opposed to the individual's own gender, because one's social group potentially acts as a prompt-level factor (i.e. something that may change from one point to the next as opposed to a static variable) which can mediate consumption. The chapter will then highlight internal factors such as mood and intoxication, which we argue may change the context of consumption and are also important considerations. We highlight how technological advances afford researchers the capacity to better track dynamic changes in such influences. Finally, the chapter explores how to deepen our limited understanding of how factors interact within the *contextual milieux* of consumption to drive or inhibit drinking. We conclude that alcohol consumption can be best understood as an interactive culmination of a complex interplay of contextually varying

R. Monk (✉) • D. Heim
Department of Psychology, Edge Hill University, Ormskirk, UK
e-mail: monkre@edgehill.ac.uk; heimd@edgehill.ac.uk

R. Cooke et al. (eds.), *The Palgrave Handbook of Psychological Perspectives on Alcohol Consumption*, https://doi.org/10.1007/978-3-030-66941-6_9

predictors. We believe that continued work in this area will improve our understanding of alcohol consumption and, with it, our ability to develop effective interventions.

What Do We Mean by Context?

Context refers to the setting in which an event takes place. In the case of consumption, our research has sought to examine the influence of the broadest contextual categories in which consumption takes place, such as the physical environment (e.g. bars, homes, restaurants) and social setting (e.g. friends, colleagues). We have also sought to examine how potentially more subtle factors such as sights, sounds and smells within an environment may also be important contextual considerations, in that they have the capacity to affect drinking, as well as associated beliefs and cognitive processes. We also suggest that factors such as gender are part of the context of much consumption. For example, although a person's gender is a static, individual-level factor, the gender composition of one's drinking group can vary between different drinking occasion, as well as within the same consumption occasion. When viewed through the lens of ecological momentary assessment, which assesses behaviour by collecting data at multiple time points over an extended period of time, contextual factors such as environmental and social context, and group gender composition can be viewed as prompt-level variables—variables that can change from one data collection point to another. By way of example, it is possible that at 8 pm a person may be drinking alone in their flat, by 10 pm, they have joined a group of all-male friends in a bar, and by 1 am, some female friends may have joined the group. This exemplar highlights important elements of the social and environmental context which change dynamically with differential potential impacts on alcohol-related beliefs and behaviours. By capturing and modelling such prompt-level variables, it is possible to demonstrate this statistically, providing a more nuanced understanding of the influence of drinking contexts.

This way of viewing an individual's drinking as the product of complex interactions between internal and exogenous factors (i.e. social or environmental influences) is summarised nicely by conceptual models produced by Clapp et al. (2018). As such, we define drinking contexts in their most inclusive sense, examining the wide ecological system where individual, social and environmental factors interact to drive consumption (see Chap. 8). In this chapter, we outline the growing literature in this regard and argue that is incumbent on researchers to continue to explore this research area in order to better inform alcohol-related interventions.

The Role of External Contexts in Shaping Alcohol-Related Cognitions and Consumption

Alcohol-related cognitions are widely recognised psychological influences on alcohol consumption (see Sect. 1). Belief variables include drinking motives, that is, the reasons why people decide to drink (e.g. Cooper, 1994), drinking refusal self-efficacy, that is, the ability to refuse the offer of an alcoholic drink, outcome expectancies, that is, the positive and negative anticipated outcomes of consumption (Oei & Baldwin, 1994) and perceived social norms (i.e. what is viewed as typical or standard in the group: Beck & Treiman, 1996). There is also a sizeable literature applying health psychology theories, such as Ajzen's (1991) Theory of Planned Behaviour or Gibbons and Gerrard's (1995) Prototype Willingness Model, to the prediction of alcohol consumption (see Sect. 1 for more on the application of these theories to the prediction of alcohol consumption). Alcohol-related cognitions typically explain a greater proportion of the variance in alcohol consumption than do background and demographic variables. Furthermore, because beliefs are modifiable, interventions can be designed to tackle excessive alcohol consumption by altering these cognitions (e.g. Lau-Barraco & Dunn, 2009; Wood, Capone, Laforge, Erickson, & Brand, 2007).

However, research studies testing the effects of alcohol-related cognitions as predictors of alcohol consumption have typically used research methods that downplay the extent to which both consumption and associated cognitions can be affected by the external social and environmental contexts in which people consume alcohol. For example, our own research has shown that beliefs about the likely positive consequences of consumption are higher when participants are exposed to alcohol-related (as opposed to neutral) visual cues in the laboratory (Monk & Heim, 2013a) and when assessed in a bar (as opposed to lecture) environment (Monk & Heim, 2013b). Likewise, participants' attitudes, intentions and perceived behavioural control were found to be significantly more positive when they were elicited from people in a university bar, as opposed to a university library (Cooke & French, 2011). Context matters when measuring alcohol-related cognitions.

In light of such concerns, research has begun to assess alcohol-related cognitions in more realistic testing environments. Real-time observations in semi naturalistic bar environments, for instance, indicate that positive outcome expectancies are associated with greater alcohol consumption (Larsen, Engels, Wiers, Granic, & Spijkerman, 2012). Similarly, norms governing consumption have also been highlighted as potential influences on consumption in pseudo naturalist drinking environments (e.g. Fugitt & Ham, 2018; Kuendig & Kuntsche, 2012). For example, at a staged wine tasting event (Kuendig & Kuntsche, 2012), consumption was lower in the solitary condition than in the subsequent group tasting condition and the authors posited that this may be due to the prevailing belief that it would not be appropriate, or normative, to drink large quantities in this isolated setting in comparison to a group context. Indeed, the assertion that normative beliefs are at play is supported further by the observation that when the order of testing was reversed, consumption was higher when participants were alone than when they consumed alcohol as part of a group. For these participants, their first experience of this environment involved interacting and drinking as part of a group; Kuendig and Kuntsche (2012) suggest that this group interaction may have shaped individual norms such that during subsequent, solitary testing, a more permissive behavioural norm had been established, potentially overwriting the previously more restrictive injunctive norm. Although it should be noted that normative beliefs were not directly measured in that study—making such assertions tentative and in need of further exploration—such ecologically aware semi-naturalistic testing environments have contributed important insights concerning the nature of contextually varying alcohol-related beliefs, and how these can shape consumption.

Such approaches go some way to mitigating concerns about the extent to which environments where alcohol research is conducted mirror real world contexts. Recently, smartphone technology has also been used to move alcohol research into the real world. Cumulatively, this more contextually aware body of work has indicated that different social contexts and environments can be associated with changes in positive expectancies (e.g. Monk & Heim, 2014) and motives (Kuntsche & Labhart, 2013; Labhart, Kuntsche, Wicki, & Gmel, 2017). For example, Monk and Heim (2014) found that participants' accounts from smartphone-enabled ecological momentary assessment suggest that positive outcome expectancies are heightened in a pub, bar or club and in a social group of friends, in contrast to reports from within more socially isolated contexts. Such research is supported by latent class analyses of weekly drinking accounts that identified eight typologies of drinking in a sample of over 60,000 UK adults (Ally et al., 2016). In that typology, drinking practices were characterised by variability in quantities (e.g. light, heavy), social company (e.g. with friends, with a partner) and location (e.g. at someone's house, at home with a partner). Research using Smartphone technology therefore suggests that alcohol-related cognitions are contextually constructed to a degree. These studies highlight that where, and with whom, people are can play important roles influencing alcohol-related cognitions.

External Factors That Affect Consumption

Studies investigating prediction of people's alcohol consumption have been criticised for being overly reliant on the use of retrospective reports (Monk & Heim, 2014; Monk, Heim, Qureshi, & Price, 2015) which can be problematic for several reasons. First, providing ex post facto accounts of alcohol-related consumption is cognitively demanding and may be fallible as such accounts are reliant on retrospective sense-making of the behaviours in question rather than on recollections of "facts" stored unchanged in memory. This problem may be further exacerbated by the alcohol consumption in question, which can inhibit recall (see Walker & Hunter, 1978). Second, if assessment takes place in a non-alcohol-related environment (e.g. a laboratory) this necessitates recall in the absence of any associated environmental stimuli to aid memory (Godden & Baddeley, 1975), and one's ability to recall drinking behaviours after the fact has also been found to be shaped by drinking contexts (e.g. Monk et al., 2015). For example, comparisons between records provided in vivo, using a smartphone application, and daily and weekly retrospective reports suggest that there is a substantial underestimation of the amounts of alcohol consumed when relying on memory, although being with two or more friends (as opposed to being alone) decreased the discrepancy between real-time and retrospective reports (Monk et al., 2015). Finally, self-report explanations of substance use can be shaped by the motives and contexts in which these are elicited, as well as by the perceived demands of the interviewer (Davies, 1997; Davies, McConnochie, Ross, Heim, & Wallace, 2004).

Environmental Factors and Consumption: Where Does Consumption Take Place?

Acknowledging these limitations, an emerging body of work has begun to yield insights into how alcohol consumption is shaped by the environmental in which alcohol consumption takes place. The environment comprises both the location drinking takes place in (i.e. home drinking, drinking in licensed premises) and the cues present in the environment. Regarding the influence of drinking location, it has become apparent that actual alcohol preference (see Mueller, Charters, Agnoli, Begalli, & Capitello, 2011) and quantities of consumption can vary as a function of the drinking location. For example, drinking in bars and clubs (Monk et al., 2015) and at special events (Callinan,

Livingston, Room, & Dietze, 2016) has been associated with heightened alcohol intake. Furthermore, irrespective of location, consumption that takes place within a social group tends to be heavier than solitary drinking (e.g. Kuendig & Kuntsche, 2012). Real-time research further suggests that throughout the course of an evening, increasing quantities of alcoholic drinks are often consumed per hour (Kuntsche & Labhart, 2012; Kuntsche, Otten, & Labhart, 2015; Thrul & Kuntsche, 2015).

Beyond the macro-environment where drinking takes place, a range of micro-environmental cues present within drinking locations have been shown to influence alcohol consumption (see Chap. 8). For example, one cue to alcohol consumption is the music played before or during consumption; Engels, Rutger, Poelen, Spijkerman and ter Bogt (2012) found that prior exposure to classical music increased people's alcohol consumption. Similarly, Jacob (2006) found that playing popular music commonly played in bars increased the time and money customers spent in a bar. Musical cues may trigger alcohol consumption through conditioning processes which result from the pairing of stimuli and behaviours/cognitions. Further research efforts are required to unpick these effects.

Time of the Week and Consumption: When Does Consumption Take Place?

Time of week is another external factor that can affect consumption. For many people drinking levels tend to be higher at weekends than during the week, where the majority of people are likely to have work commitments (Kuntsche & Gmel, 2013; Kuntsche & Labhart, 2012). However, not all research has produced consistent findings. For example, recent real-time observations revealed consistent drinking practices on Thursday (a common night for student consumption) in addition to weekend drinking on Friday and Saturday evenings (Groefsema & Kuntsche, 2019). Specifically, acceleration in drinking pace throughout the course of an evening was apparent on all these days.

Such inconsistent findings may, to a degree, undermine the notion that there are consistent (and therefore predictable) drivers of consumption. Support for this idea comes from research which has shown that participants who were asked to report their cognitions about drinking tonight reported significantly less positive cognitions compared to participants asked to report their cognitions about the next week (Cooke & French, 2011). However, when comparing research findings, it is important to consider the specific demographics of the populations studied. For example, a university student might consider Thursday to be a "popular drinking night" (Groefsema & Kuntsche, 2019) whereas someone in full-time employment may not. A potential limitation of research in this area is an over-reliance on student and adolescent samples, who tend to have different work/life commitments—around which alcohol consumption must be negotiated—when compared to the wider population from which they are drawn. This limitation is likely to have shaped current understanding of how contextual factors influence consumption.

Social Factors and Consumption: Who Is Present When Consumption Takes Place?

As argued in this book, alcohol consumption is usually an inherently social behaviour (see Chap. 6). Following this proposal, we would expect social interactions before and during drinking may affect alcohol consumption. Work in this area documents, for example, that interpersonal exchanges such as being shouted at (negative) or being complimented (positive) can mediate the extent to which being in a group of friends is associated with increased alcohol consumption; people who reported having positive interpersonal experiences during a day were more likely to report drinking with others, although those who reported experiencing negative interpersonal interactions were more likely to report drinking alone (Mohr et al., 2001; Mohr, Arpin, & McCabe, 2015). Alcohol consumption has also been observed to increase to match the perceived pace of others' drinking (e.g. Borsari & Carey, 2001; Quigley & Collins, 1999). Beverage choice also seems to be affected by the selections made by others (e.g. Larsen et al., 2012), and the gender composition of the group present in the drinking context.

The gender composition of one's drinking group has been shown to shape alcohol behaviours. However, this effect varies across different drinking contexts. For example, pre-drinking (where people consume alcohol with the goal of achieving intoxication prior to going out socialising, see Chap. 13) among women in mixed-gender groups appears to be greater than that observed in all-female groups (e.g. Paves, Pedersen, Hummer, & LaBrie, 2012).

Recently, Thrul, Labhart and Kuntsche (2017) found that in contrast to drinking as part of a female-only group, women drank less when they were the only woman in an otherwise all-male group). Similarly, men consumed more when drinking in all-male groups compared to when drinking within an otherwise all-female group. Whereas men's drinking as part of an evenly mixed or majority male group was higher than when in all-male groups, the number of drinks that women consumed was higher in mixed-gender groups (of any composition) than within all-females groups. Such findings may, in part, be the product of an equilibrium effect, with men observing that women drink slower and imitating their rate of consumption, although women may notice that men drink faster than them and imitate their rate of consumption. Indeed, gender differences in drinking rates over the course of an evening have been observed, such that men appear to increase their drinking rate more quickly than women (Kuntsche et al., 2015; Kuntsche & Labhart, 2012). However, gender-based differences in pace of consumption are not replicated consistently; for example, research found that both female and male adolescents drink faster as the evening progresses (Groefsema & Kuntsche, 2019). Continued exploration in this domain is therefore warranted.

Nevertheless, Thrul et al.'s (2017) work marks an important step towards understanding how the gender composition of a group can shape alcohol consumption; gender composition of groups can be viewed as a prompt-level variable (i.e. that can change from one data collection point to another) in the same way as one's current situational (e.g. with friends) or environmental context (e.g. a bar), with potential consequences for consumption levels (Heim & Monk, 2017). Thrul et al.'s (2017) work therefore differs from more traditional approaches which treat gender, along with other sociodemographic characteristics, as a static (individual-level) factor. Rather, it highlights that the gender composition of a social group may be an influential variable, and one which is dynamic, with the potential to change throughout a drinking episode, as people leave/join a group. Work in this vein alerts us to the importance of examining the influence of demographic variables as part of the wider social contexts in which consumption occurs. Those designing interventions should acknowledge how temporally immediate factors may be targeted as a more effective way of bringing about immediate behaviour change, in contrast to targeting predictors such as deprivation which, probably require longer-term, multidimensional interventions. We have summarised briefly here how varying contextual factors may be important influences on the decision to drink or exercise restraint and the development of interventions could arguably benefit from being more sensitive to these variable influences.

Overall, although there is an increasing awareness of the myriad of environmental factors that may shape consumption, there remains a need for further research to unpick the role of contextual forces on alcohol consumption. It is particularly important to conduct research that seeks to disentangle the effects of environment, time and social factors like gender composition of group, to more fully understand alcohol consumption patterns.

Within-Person Variability in Mood and Intoxication Can Also Affect Consumption

In addition to examining how external factors like the environment (i.e. where we are), the time of day (i.e. when we are drinking) and social context (i.e. who we are with) shape alcohol consumption, research has also shown that some internal factors can influence consumption. Such factors include "inhibitory control"—that is, the ability to regulate prepotent (dominant) attentional and behavioural responses (see Chap. 22), and "attentional control/bias"—that is. where attention is focussed (e.g. Qureshi, Monk, Pennington, Wilcockson, & Heim, 2019). These factors can be changed by alcohol-related sights (e.g. Christiansen, Cole, Goudie, & Field, 2012), sounds (Spence & Shankar, 2010) and smells (Monk, Sunley, Qureshi, & Heim, 2016). In addition to these executive function factors, emotional (mood) and pharmacological (intoxication) factors vary within-people and can also have an impact. It is therefore possible to conceptualise these as variable and contextually shaped influences on alcohol consumption.

Mood: Laboratory mood-induction and priming studies have found that participants who are manipulated to experience negative moods show an increase in the perceived incentive value of alcohol (e.g. Amlung & MacKillop, 2014), as well as heightened alcohol-related attentional biases (e.g. Field & Quigley, 2009; Hepworth, Mogg, Brignell, & Bradley, 2010) and approach tendencies (e.g. Cousijn, Luijten, & Wiers, 2014). Likewise, those primed with negative words have been found to drink more alcohol than those exposed to neutral or positive priming conditions (Zack, Poulos, Fragopoulos, Woodford, & MacLeod, 2006).

In addition, retrospective self-reports of daily/weekly mood indicate that variability in mood can predict the quantity (Rankin & Maggs, 2006) and frequency of alcohol consumption (Gottfredson & Hussong, 2013) and that changes in enhancement motives—that is, drinking motivated by the belief that alcohol will make people feel better about themselves may mediate the relationship between mood and consumption (see Chap. 4). Experiential sampling data also indicate that alcohol consumption is generally associated with lower reported levels of nervousness (Swendsen et al., 2000), and with increasing or sustained positive mood (Kuntsche & Bruno, 2015).

Nevertheless, such retrospective self-reports may not always be sufficiently sensitive to capture the rapid fluctuations that can characterise changes in mood, particularly as people react to daily events (Swendsen et al., 2000). In addition, laboratory-based research may lack ecological validity and may therefore underplay the importance of changes in mood over time. Fortunately, technological advances now afford researchers better opportunities to assess phenomena in real time. Indeed, technology has been used to capture variability in individuals' mood (e.g. Ebner-Priemer & Trull, 2009) and to record how real-time events may affect it (Swendsen et al., 2000). For example, research suggests that real-time mood is higher whilst people are drinking (Peacock, Cash, Bruno, & Ferguson, 2015). There is also growing evidence for the self-medication/affect dampening hypothesis—that is, the notion that people may use alcohol as part of coping with negative affect (e.g. Gottfredson & Hussong, 2013). Specifically, negative mood (Jones, Tiplady, Houben, Nederkoorn, & Field, 2018), nervousness (Swendsen et al., 2000), higher day-to-day positive affect (Peacock et al., 2015) and greater variability in negative affect (Mohr et al., 2015) have all been found to be associated with real-time increases in beverage alcohol consumption.

Technological advances afford researchers improved means of accurately measuring the interplay between mood, context and alcohol consumption by assessing participants in real time, rather than relying on retrospective self-reports. For example, in one study, people reporting better quality friendships were found to be less vulnerable to the negative effect of mood on real-time recorded consumption (Shadur, Hussong, & Haroon, 2015). However, the study did not examine social support at the time of testing, meaning this was a static variable assessed using a one-off self-report measure. So, assertions about the in vivo effect of friendship quality alongside context and mood may be limited (Monk et al., 2020). In a similar vein, Mohr et al. (2015) found that positive and negative mood variability affected respondents' solitary and social alcohol consumption. However, in this study mood was treated as an individual-level variable (i.e. mood was assessed only at the start of testing, rather than being assessed regularly at the prompt level, see above), which undermines our ability to ascertain how mood may vary alongside, and in response to, real-time changes in social context. Also, as consumption was measured three times a day (e.g. a 10:00–11:30 a.m. prompt would ask participants to report their drinking since the previous prompt at 8:30–10:00 p.m.), there was heightened reliance on retrospective memory which, to an extent, may limit the insights that can be drawn from this work. Although research in this domain has been important in developing and enhancing our understanding, there therefore remains a need to explore in more depth how real-time mood and current context interact to shape in vivo consumption.

Alcohol priming: "The alcohol priming effect" (de Wit, 1996) describes the finding that initial doses of alcohol can elevate subsequent consumption. For example, participants primed with alcohol (as opposed to a placebo) have been shown to prefer alcohol over monetary rewards (Fillmore & Rush, 2001). In this way, varying levels of intoxication (and indeed people's sensitivity to the pharmacological effect of alcohol) can be viewed as another within-person factor, variability in which can contribute to prediction of alcohol consumption behaviours. Alcohol priming effects on subsequent consumption may from this perspective be, at least partly, explained by alcohol-related impairments in inhibitory control (Field, Wiers, Christiansen, Fillmore, & Verster, 2010). Anticipation of reward, for instance, has been associated with heightened activations in areas of the brain associated with inhibitory control, including the dorsolateral prefrontal cortex (Luijten, Schellekens, Kühn, Machielse, & Sescousse, 2017) and impairing this area using Transcranial Magnetic Stimulation has been shown to impair inhibitory control and to be associated with increases in consumption, relative to sham stimulation (McNeill, Monk, Qureshi, Makris, & Heim, 2018). However, this effect of alcohol priming seems to be apparent even when intoxication is insufficient to result in global impairments (Field et al., 2010). Therefore, models of consumption postulate that even low doses of alcohol may result in changes in alcohol-related cognitions, such as motivations (e.g. Rose et al., 2010), craving (e.g. Schoenmakers, Wiers, & Field, 2008) and attentional bias (e.g. Schoenmakers et al., 2008) and that it is therefore possible that alcohol priming interacts with other factors, such as inhibitory control (Field et al., 2010), to influence alcohol seeking behaviours. Finally, it is also noteworthy that previous research has tended to examine effects of alcohol on inhibition control in participants tested individually and in isolation (e.g. Stautz & Cooper, 2013). There remains, therefore, a need to explore more fully whether such findings hold true in the social contexts in which people commonly drink.

Using Technology: Limitations and Possibilities

So far, this chapter has highlighted the importance of considering contextual influences on alcohol consumption. We have also noted how technology can be harnessed to examine the impact of these influences. As we near the end of this chapter it is important to briefly consider some of the limitations of methods currently used in this area, as well as outlining how technological advances can be harnessed in future studies.

Smartphone technologies have several limitations. First, there is variation among researchers in how data are classed as being collected in *real time*. Although some researchers limit the amount of time that can elapse between a request for information and a participant response, to provide increased assurances that responses represent data that is “in the moment” rather than retrospective (e.g. Monk & Heim, 2014), this is not universal. Many researchers use prompts that ask participants to reflect back and record their consumption in the period since last responding, with a lag of up to five hours (e.g. Mohr et al., 2015). In such cases, there is an increased reliance on participants' memory which may limit response reliability (Kuntsche & Labhart, 2012). Furthermore, reports about behaviour obtained within hours of the event in question are likely to be considerably more accurate than reports about behaviour performed, say, a week or a month ago. Nevertheless, such temporal variability should be borne in mind by researchers as they continue to explore the contextually varying nature of consumption and related cognitions (see Cooke & French, 2011; Monk, Qureshi and Heim, in press).

As touched on earlier, real-time reports may also be prone to demand characteristics, such as socially desirable responses, despite assurances of participant anonymity (Monk et al., 2015). Prompts may be ignored, or responses may be impaired by the amount of alcohol that has been consumed which may restrict or alter the type of information participants can be expected to provide (e.g. Altman, Schreiber Compo, McQuiston, Hagsand, & Cervera, 2018; Schreiber Compo et al., 2011). Furthermore, participants might have difficulties in monitoring which drinks they had previously recorded—a telescoping effect. This alerts us to the possibility that some “double counting” of drinks can occur when using these methods. Finally, it should be noted that although data may be recorded in real time, this does not preclude the possibility that participants forget to record every single drink (Monk et al., 2015). Similarly, participants may have consumed alcohol on days when they did not use the data-collection application, meaning that these data are effectively missed. Technological advances may therefore be needed to help overcome such limitations (Labhart et al., 2019).

Turning to emerging methods in the field, Secure Continuous Remote Alcohol Monitoring (SCRAM) is one technology which may represent a solution to the some of the challenges faced when seeking to track alcohol consumption more accurately (Leffingwell et al., 2013). Such devices, securely fitted around the ankle, measure levels of alcohol in perspiration approximately every 30 minutes throughout a 24-hour period, recording and sending these data remotely. These devices have been shown to offer some promise as intervention tools (Leffingwell et al., 2013) and for the monitoring of consumption in those who are, for example, released on licence with the condition of sobriety (Flango & Cheesman, 2009). Furthermore, scientists are increasingly highlighting SCRAM's potential to be used to develop our understanding of real-world consumption (see Caluzzi et al., 2019), and possibly even as a tool that may promote reductions in drinking—also by offering wearers an "excuse" from drinking in situations where they may perceive social pressure to do so (e.g. Neville, Williams, Goodall, Murer, & Donnell, 2013). Furthermore, there is growing interest in examining the utility of such instruments in research projects which seek to identify more objective means of measuring consumption, away for self-reports (e.g. Caluzzi et al., 2019). Despite some enthusiasm for this approach, however, they are rather expensive, limiting their application for large-scale research, and there are notable concerns about their comfort, appearance and susceptibility to tampering (Barnett et al., 2017; Caluzzi et al., 2019). It has also been suggested that transdermal alcohol levels can lag breath alcohol levels (Leffingwell et al., 2013) and, although they may reliably detect two drinks or more (Sakai, Mikulich-Gilbertson, Long, & Crowley, 2006), they may be less accurate at detecting lower levels of consumption (Roache et al., 2015). See Chap. 8 for more on transdermal measures of alcohol consumption.

In theory, SCRAM may also lead to the development of more acceptable devices to monitor consumption, such as smartwatches designed to track intoxication using similar transdermal technology (Gutierrez et al., 2015). However, at the time of writing, there are no established criteria of what might represent a SCRAM-measured "true" drinking episode, which limits their interpretable use for researchers, particularly for real-world testing where the onset of a drinking occasion or event cannot be established independently by the researcher when using these methods (see Chap. 8 for more on defining the onset and end of a drinking event). There also remains a need to refine methods for converting transdermal alcohol to blood alcohol concentration (Wang, Fridberg, Leeman, Cook, & Porges, 2019). Finally, these new biosensors require further validation, examining potential individual differences (e.g. skin thickness, gender differences) and environmental factors (e.g. humidity, temperature) that may contribute to variations in transdermal alcohol readings (Wang et al., 2019). Researchers may need to expand the tools they employ as part of their methodological arsenal. One such approach may be the use of various alcohol-related biomarkers (e.g. 5-hydroxytrptophol, ethyl glucuronide and fatty acid ethyl esters, see Piano, Mazzuco, Kang, &

Phillips, 2017 for review) though research in this area is in its relative infancy, and their use outside of clinical and forensic settings appears to rare at this moment in time (see Ghosh, Jain, Jhanjee, Rao, & Mishra, 2019). Nevertheless, as the use of these biomarkers develops, it may be feasible for researchers to harness these tests as a "gold standard" alcohol consumption measurement, to compare and calibrate against self-report.

Similarly, technology may offer us greater insights into the internal contextual states that influence consumption. Previous examinations of mood and consumption, for example, have been largely dependent on self-reported mood (Kuntsche & Bruno, 2015). However, such self-reports rely on a participants' ability to accurately self-introspect and reliably report their current affective state, which cannot be guaranteed (Paulhus & Vazire, 2007). It is also possible that responses are an artefact of having posed the question—asking a question about mood may elicit a process of reflection that influences mood (Ruby, Smallwood, Engen, & Singer, 2013) or causes a response that is merely a demand characteristic (e.g. Allen & Smith, 2012. Objective measures of mood such as cortisol levels (e.g. Schlotz, 2011) or implicit measures which may ameliorate demand characteristics (Ito, Matsuzaki, & Kawahara, 2018) may therefore also warrant future consideration. In short, as researchers continue to explore the interplay of contextual factors that appear to influence consumption and related cognitions, they are likely to harness the increasingly sophisticated technologies available to overcome existing methodological limitations and increase our understanding of contextual influences on alcohol consumption.

Conclusion

Research has considered how external factors such as environmental locations (e.g. bars, wine tasting) and the gender composition of one's social group (e.g. how many men and women are present during a drinking event) can affect: (1) the way that people think about alcohol; (2) the frequency of alcohol consumption; (3) the amounts and pace at which drinking happens; and (4) the beverages selected. Furthermore, internal factors such as variability in mood and intoxication levels appear to be important in shaping patterns of alcohol use. It will be exciting to see how our understanding of alcohol consumption will be refined by future research that considers how these variables interact. There is still much more to be learn about how external contextual factors interact (or not) with internal factors to drive/inhibit the alcohol consumption. It is incumbent on researchers to continue work in this area to improve our understanding of consumption and to refine our methodological approaches to aid this endeavour. In so doing, we will expand our ability to develop more effective interventions that can more effectively shape the complex and contextually varying alcoholic beverage drinking practices.

References

Ajzen, I. (1991). The theory of planned behavior. *Organizational Behavior and Human Decision Processes, 50*, 179–211.

Allen A. P., & Smith, A. P. (2012). Demand characteristics, pre-test attitudes and time-on-task trends in the effects of chewing gum on attention and reported mood in healthy volunteers. *Appetite, 59*, 349–356.

Ally, A. K., Lovatt, M., Meier, P. S., Brennan, A., & Holmes, J. (2016). Developing a social practice-based typology of British drinking culture in 2009–2011. *Implications for alcohol policy analysis. Addiction, 111*(9), 1568–1579.

Altman, C. M., Schreiber Compo, N., McQuiston, D., Hagsand, A. V., & Cervera, J. (2018). Witnesses' memory for events and faces under elevated levels of intoxication. *Memory, 26*, 946–959.

Amlung, M., & MacKillop, J. (2014). Understanding the effects of stress and alcohol cues on motivation for alcohol via behavioral economics. *Alcoholism, Clinical and Experimental Research, 38*, 1780–1789. https://doi.org/10.1111/acer.12423

Barnett, N. P., Celio, M. A., Tidey, J. W., Murphy, J. G., Colby, S. M., & Swift, R. M. (2017). A preliminary randomized controlled trial of contingency management for alcohol use reduction using a transdermal alcohol sensor. *Addiction, 112*, 1025–1035.

Beck, K. H., & Treiman, K. A. (1996). The relationship of social context of drinking, perceived social norms, and parental influence to various drinking patterns of adolescents. *Addictive Behaviors, 21*, 633–644.

Borsari, B., & Carey, K. B. (2001). Peer influences on college drinking: A review of the research. *Journal of Substance Abuse, 13*, 391–424.

Callinan, S., Livingston, M., Room, R., & Dietze, P. (2016). Drinking contexts and alcohol consumption: How much alcohol is consumed in different Australian locations? *Journal of Studies on Alcohol and Drugs, 77*, 612–619.

Caluzzi, G., Pennay, A., Cook, M., Wright, C., Norman, T., & Kuntsche, E. (2019). Transdermal monitors to assess alcohol consumption in real-time and real-life–a qualitative study on user-experience. *Addiction Research & Theory, 27*, 354–361.

Christiansen, P., Cole, J. C., Goudie, A. J., & Field, M. (2012). Components of behavioural impulsivity and automatic cue approach predict unique variance in hazardous drinking. *Psychopharmacology, 219*, 501–510.

Clapp, J. D., Madden, D. R., Gonzalez Villasanti, H., Giraldo, L. F., Passino, K. M., Reed, M. B., & Fernandez Puentes, I. (2018). A system dynamic model of drinking events: Multi-level ecological approach. *Systems Research and Behavioral Science, 35*, 265–281.

Cooke, R., & French, D. P. (2011). The role of context and timeframe in moderating relationships within the theory of planned behaviour. *Psychology & Health, 26*, 1225–1240. https://doi.org/10.1080/08870446.2011.572260

Cooper, M. L. (1994). Motivations for alcohol use among adolescents: Development and validation of a four-factor model. *Psychological assessment, 6*(2), 117–128.

Cousijn, J., Luijten, M., & Wiers, R. W. (2014). Mechanisms underlying alcohol-approach action tendencies: The role of emotional primes and drinking motives. *Frontiers in Psychiatry, 5*, 44. https://doi.org/10.3389/fpsyt.2014.00044

Davies, J. B. (1997). *The myth of addiction* (2nd ed.). Amsterdam, The Netherlands: Harwood Academic Publishers.

Davies, J. B., McConnochie, F., Ross, A. J., Heim, D., & Wallace, B. (2004). Evidence for social learning in the self-presentation of alcohol problems. *Alcohol & Alcoholism, 39*, 346–350.

de Wit, H. (1996). Priming effects with drugs and other reinforcers. *Experimental and Clinical Psychopharmacology, 4*, 5–10. https://doi.org/10.1037/1064-1297.4.1.5

Ebner-Priemer, U. W., & Trull, T. J. (2009). Ecological momentary assessment of mood disorders and mood dysregulation. *Psychological Assessment, 21*, 463–475. https://doi.org/10.1037/a0017075

Engels, R. C. M. E., Poelen, E. A. P., Spijkerman, R., & ter Bogt, T. (2012). The effects of music genre on young people's alcohol consumption: An experimental observational study. *Substance Use & Misuse, 47*, 180–188. https://doi.org/10.3109/10826084.2012.637461

Field, M., & Quigley, M. (2009). Mild stress increases attentional bias in social drinkers who drink to cope: A replication and extension. *Experimental and Clinical Psychopharmacology, 17*, 312–319. https://doi.org/10.1037/a0017090

Field, M., Wiers, R. W., Christiansen, P., Fillmore, M. T., & Verster, J. C. (2010). Acute alcohol effects on inhibitory control and implicit cognition: Implications for loss of control over drinking. *Alcoholism: Clinical and Experimental Research, 34*, 1346–1352. https://doi.org/10.1111/j.1530-0277.2010.01218.x

Fillmore, M. I., & Rush, C. R. (2001). Alcohol effects on inhibitory and activational response strategies in the acquisition of alcohol and other reinforcers: Priming the motivation to drink. *Journal of Studies on Alcohol, 62*, 646–656. https://doi.org/10.15288/jsa.2001.62.646

Flango, V. E., & Cheesman, F. L. (2009). Effectiveness of the SCRAM alcohol monitoring device: A preliminary test. *Drug Court Review, 6*, 109–134. Available from: http://www.ndci.org/sites/default/files/ndci/DCRVolume6_Issue2.pdf#page=119

Fugitt, J. L., & Ham, L. S. (2018). Beer for "brohood": A laboratory simulation of masculinity confirmation through alcohol use behaviors in men. *Psychology of Addictive Behaviors, 32*, 358.

Ghosh, S., Jain, R., Jhanjee, S., Rao, R., & Mishra, A. K. (2019). Alcohol biomarkers and their relevance in detection of alcohol consumption in clinical settings. *International Archives of Substance Abuse and Rehabilitation, 1*, 1–8.

Gibbons, F. X., & Gerrard, M. (1995). Predicting young adults' health risk behavior. *Journal of personality and social psychology, 69*(3), 505–517.

Godden, D. R., & Baddeley, A. D. (1975). Context-dependent memory in two natural environments: On land and underwater. *British Journal of Psychology, 66*, 325–331. https://doi.org/10.1111/j.2044-8295.1975.tb01468.x

Gottfredson, N. C., & Hussong, A. M. (2013). Drinking to dampen affect variability: Findings from a college student sample. *Journal of Studies on Alcohol and Drugs, 74*, 576–583. https://doi.org/10.15288/jsad.2013.74.576

Groefsema, M., & Kuntsche, E. (2019). Acceleration of drinking pace throughout the evening among frequently drinking young adults in the Netherlands. *Addiction, 114*, 1295–1302. https://doi.org/10.1111/add.14588

Gutierrez, M. A., Fast M. L., Ngu A. H., & Gao B. J. (2016). Real-time prediction of blood alcohol content using smartwatch sensor data In X. Zheng, D. Zeng, H. Chen, & S. Leischow (Eds.), *Smart Health. ICSH 2015* (Lecture Notes in Computer Science, Vol. 9545). Cham, Switzerland: Springer.

Heim, D., & Monk, R. (2017). Commentary on Thrul et al. (2017): A welcome step towards a more context-aware addiction science. *Addiction, 112*, 440–441. https://doi.org/10.1080/14746689.2017.1294803

Hepworth, R., Mogg, K., Brignell, C., & Bradley, B. P. (2010). Negative mood increases selective attention to food cues and subjective appetite. *Appetite, 54*, 134–142. https://doi.org/10.1016/j.appet.2009.09.019

Ito, M., Matsuzaki, N., & Kawahara, J. (2018). Measurement of mood states following light alcohol consumption: Evidence from the implicit association test. *Behavioral Sciences, 8*, 79.

Jacob, C. (2006). Styles of background music and consumption in a bar: An empirical evaluation. *International Journal of Hospitality Management, 25*, 716–720. https://doi.org/10.1016/j.ijhm.2006.01.002

Jones, A., Tiplady, B., Houben, K., Nederkoorn, C., & Field, M. (2018). Do daily fluctuations in inhibitory control predict alcohol consumption? An ecological momentary assessment study. *Psychopharmacology, 235*, 1487–1496. https://doi.org/10.1007/s00213-018-4860-5

Kuendig, H., & Kuntsche, E. (2012). Solitary versus social drinking: An experimental study on effects of social exposures on in situ alcohol consumption. *Alcoholism: Clinical and Experimental Research, 36*, 732–738. https://doi.org/10.1111/j.1530-0277.2011.01663.x

Kuntsche, E., & Bruno, R. (2015). Moody booze: Introducing the special section on affect regulation and substance use. *Drug and Alcohol Review, 34*, 569–570. https://doi.org/10.1111/dar.12349

Kuntsche, E., & Gmel, G. (2013). Alcohol consumption in late adolescence and early adulthood – Where is the problem? *Swiss Medical Weekly, 143*, w13826. https://doi.org/10.4414/smw.2013.13826

Kuntsche, E., & Labhart, F. (2012). Investigating the drinking patterns of young people over the course of the evening at weekends. *Drug and Alcohol Dependence, 124*, 319–324. https://doi.org/10.1016/j.drugalcdep.2012.02.001

Kuntsche, E., & Labhart, F. (2013). Drinking motives moderate the impact of pre-drinking on heavy drinking on a given evening and related adverse consequences–an event-level study. *Addiction, 108*, 1747–1755. https://doi.org/10.1111/add.12253

Kuntsche, E., Otten, R., & Labhart, F. (2015). Identifying risky drinking patterns over the course of saturday evenings: An event-level study. *Psychology of Addictive Behaviors, 29*, 744–752. https://doi.org/10.1037/adb0000057

Labhart, F., Kuntsche, E., Wicki, M., & Gmel, G. (2017). Reciprocal influences of drinking motives on alcohol use and related consequences: A full cross-lagged panel study among young adult men. *Behavioral Medicine, 43*, 277–284. https://doi.org/10.1080/08964289.2016.1157057

Labhart, F., Tarsetti, F., Bornet, O., Santani, D., Truong, J., Landolt, S., … Kuntsche, E. (2019). Capturing drinking and nightlife behaviours and their social and physical context with a smartphone application–investigation of users' experience and reactivity. *Addiction Research & Theory*, 1–14.

Larsen, H., Engels, R. C. M. E., Wiers, R. W., Granic, I., & Spijkerman, R. (2012). Implicit and explicit alcohol cognitions and observed alcohol consumption: Three studies in (semi)naturalistic drinking settings. *Addiction, 107*, 1420–1428. https://doi.org/10.1111/j.1360-0443.2012.03805.x

Lau-Barraco, C. & Dunn, M.E. (2009). Environmental context effects on alcohol cognitions and immediate alcohol consumption. *Addiction Research & Theory, 17*, 306–314.

Leffingwell, T. R., Cooney, N. J., Murphy, J. G., Luczak, S., Rosen, G., Dougherty, D. M., & Barnett, N. P. (2013). Continuous objective monitoring of alcohol use: Twenty-first century measurement using transdermal sensors. *Alcoholism: Clinical and Experimental Research, 37*, 16–22.

Luijten, M., Schellekens, A. F., Kühn, S., Machielse, M. W., & Sescousse, G. (2017). Disruption of reward processing in addiction: An image-based meta-analysis of functional magnetic resonance imaging studies. *JAMA Psychiatry, 74*, 387–398. https://doi.org/10.1001/jamapsychiatry.2016.3084

McNeill, A., Monk, R. L., Qureshi, A. W., Makris, S., & Heim, D. (2018). Continuous theta burst transcranial magnetic stimulation of the right dorsolateral prefrontal cortex impairs inhibitory control and increases alcohol consumption. *Cognitive, Affective, & Behavioral Neuroscience, 18*, 1198–1206. https://doi.org/10.3758/s13415-018-0631-3

Mohr, C. D., Armeli, S., Tennen, H., Carney, M. A., Affleck, G., & Hromi, A. (2001). Daily interpersonal experiences, context, and alcohol consumption: Crying in your beer and toasting good times. *Journal of Personality and Social Psychology, 80*(3), 489–500. https://doi.org/10.1037/0022-3514.80.3.489

Mohr, C. D., Arpin, S., & McCabe, C. T. (2015). Daily affect variability and context-specific alcohol consumption. *Drug and Alcohol Review, 34*, 581–587. https://doi.org/10.1111/dar.12253

Monk, R. L., & Heim, D. (2013a). Panoramic projection: Affording a wider view on contextual influences on alcohol-related cognitions. *Experimental and Clinical Psychopharmacology, 21*, 1.

Monk, R. L., & Heim, D. (2013b). Environmental context effects on alcohol-related outcome expectancies, efficacy, and norms: A field study. *Psychology of Addictive Behaviors, 27*, 814–818. https://doi.org/10.1037/a0033948

Monk, R. L., & Heim, D. (2014). A real-time examination of context effects on alcohol cognitions. *Alcoholism: Clinical and Experimental Research, 38*, 2454–2459. https://doi.org/10.1111/acer.12504

Monk, R. L., Heim, D., Qureshi, A., & Price, A. (2015). "I have no clue what I drunk last night" using smartphone technology to compare in-vivo and retrospective self-reports of alcohol consumption. *PLoS One, 10*(5), e0126209. https://doi.org/10.1371/journal.pone.0126209

Monk, R.L., Qureshi, A.W., & Heim, D (2020). An examination of the extent to which mood and context are associated with real-time alcohol consumption. *Drug & Alcohol Dependence, 208*, 107880.

Monk, R. L., Sunley, J., Qureshi, A. W., & Heim, D. (2016). Smells like inhibition: The effects of olfactory and visual alcohol cues on inhibitory control. *Psychopharmacology, 233*, 1331–1337. https://doi.org/10.1007/s00213-016-4221-1

Mueller, S., Charters, S., Agnoli, L., Begalli, D., & Capitello, R. (2011). Generation Y's perception of wine and consumption situations in a traditional wine-producing region. *International Journal of Wine Business Research, 23*(2), 176–192.

Neville, F., Williams, D. J., Goodall, C. A., Murer, J. S., & Donnell, P. D. (2013). An experimental trial exploring the impact of continuous transdermal alcohol monitoring upon alcohol consumption in a cohort of male students. *PLoS One, 8*(6), e67386. https://doi.org/10.1371/journal.pone.0067386

Oei, T. P. S., & Baldwin, A. R. (1994). Expectancy theory: A two-process model of alcohol use and abuse. *Journal of Studies on Alcohol, 55*, 525–534.

Paulhus, D. L., & Vazire, S. (2007). The self report method. In R. W. Robins, R. C. Fraley, & R. F. Krueger (Eds.), *Handbook of research methods in personality psychology* (pp. 224–239). New York, NY: Guilford.

Paves, A. P., Pedersen, E. R., Hummer, J. F., & LaBrie, J. W. (2012). Prevalence, social contexts, and risks for prepartying among ethnically diverse college students. *Addictive Behaviors, 37*, 803–810.

Peacock, A., Cash, C., Bruno, R., & Ferguson, S. G. (2015). Day-by-day variation in affect, arousal and alcohol consumption in young adults. *Drug and Alcohol Review, 34*, 588–594. https://doi.org/10.1111/dar.12238

Piano, M. R., Mazzuco, A., Kang, M., & Phillips, S. A. (2017). Binge drinking episodes in young adults: How should we measure them in a research setting? *Journal of Studies on Alcohol and Drugs, 78*(4), 502–511.

Quigley, B. M., & Collins, R. L. (1999). The modelling of alcohol consumption: A meta-analytic review. *Journal of Studies on Alcohol, 60*(1), 90–98.

Qureshi, A., Monk, R. L., Pennington, C. R., Wilcockson, T. D. W., & Heim, D. (2019). Alcohol-related attentional bias in a gaze contingency task: Comparing appetitive and non-appetitive cues. *Addictive Behaviors, 90*, 312–317. https://doi.org/10.1016/j.addbeh.2018.11.034

Rankin, L. A., & Maggs, J. L. (2006). First-year college student affect and alcohol use: Paradoxical within- and between-person associations. *Journal of Youth and Adolescence, 35*, 925–937. https://doi.org/10.1007/s10964-006-9073-2

Roache, J. D., Karns, T. E., Hill-Kapturczak, N., Mullen, J., Liang, Y., Lamb, R. J., & Dougherty, D. M. (2015). Using transdermal alcohol monitoring to detect low-level drinking. *Alcoholism: Clinical and Experimental Research, 39*, 1120–1127.

Rose, A. K., Hobbs, M., Klipp, L., Bell, S., Edwards, K., O'hara, P., & Drummond, C. (2010). Monitoring drinking behaviour and motivation to drink over successive doses of alcohol. *Behavioural Pharmacology, 21*, 710–718. https://doi.org/10.1097/FBP.0b013e32833fa72b

Ruby, F. J., Smallwood, J., Engen, H., & Singer, T. (2013). How self-generated thought shapes mood – The relation between mind-wandering and mood depends on the socio-temporal content of thoughts. *PLoS One, 8*(10), e77554.

Sakai, J. T., Mikulich-Gilbertson, S. K., Long, R. J., & Crowley, T. J. (2006). Validity of transdermal alcohol monitoring: Fixed and self-regulated dosing. *Alcoholism: Clinical and Experimental Research, 30*, 26–33.

Schlotz, W. (2011). Ambulatory psychoneuroendocrinology: Assessing salivary cortisol and other hormones in daily life. In M. R. Mehl & T. S. Conner (Eds.), *Handbook of research methods for studying daily life*. New York, NY: Guilford Press.

Schoenmakers, T., Wiers, R. W., & Field, M. (2008). Effects of a low dose of alcohol on cognitive biases and craving in heavy drinkers. *Psychopharmacology, 1*, 169–178. https://doi.org/10.1007/s00213-007-1023-5

Schreiber Compo, N., Evans, J. R., Carol, R. N., Kemp, D., Villalba, D., Ham, L. S., & Rose, S. (2011). Alcohol intoxication and memory for events: A snapshot of alcohol myopia in a real-world drinking scenario. *Memory, 19*, 202–210.

Shadur, J. M., Hussong, A. M., & Haroon, M. (2015). Negative affect variability and adolescent self-medication: The role of the peer context. *Drug and Alcohol Review, 34*, 571–580. https://doi.org/10.1111/dar.12260

Spence, C., & Shankar, M. U. (2010). The influence of auditory cues on the perception of, and responses to, food and drink. *Journal of Sensory Studies, 25*, 406–430. https://doi.org/10.1111/j.1745-459X.2009.00267.x

Stautz, K., & Cooper, A. (2013). Impulsivity-related personality traits and adolescent alcohol use: A meta-analytic review. *Clinical Psychology Review, 33*, 574–592.

Swendsen, J. D., Tennen, H., Carney, M. A., Affleck, G., Willard, A., & Hromi, A. (2000). Mood and alcohol consumption: An experience sampling test of the self-medication hypothesis. *Journal of Abnormal Psychology, 109*, 198–204. https://doi.org/10.1037/0021-843X.109.2.198

Thrul, J., & Kuntsche, E. (2015). The impact of friends on young adults' drinking over the course of the evening--an event-level analysis. *Addiction, 110*, 619–626. https://doi.org/10.1111/add.12862

Thrul, J., Labhart, F., & Kuntsche, E. (2017). Drinking with mixed-gender groups is associated with heavy weekend drinking among young adults. *Addiction, 112*, 432–439. https://doi.org/10.1111/add.13633

Walker, D. W., & Hunter, B. E. (1978). Short-term memory impairment following chronic alcohol consumption in rats. *Neuropsychologia, 16*, 545–553. https://doi.org/10.1016/0028-3932(78)90082-9

Wang, Y., Fridberg, D. J., Leeman, R. F., Cook, R. L., & Porges, E. C. (2019). Wrist-worn alcohol biosensors: Strengths, limitations, and future directions. *Alcohol, 81*, 83–92.

Wood, M. D., Capone, C., Laforge, R., Erickson, D. J., & Brand, N. H. (2007). Brief motivational intervention and alcohol expectancy challenge with heavy drinking college students: A randomized factorial study. *Addictive Behaviors, 32*, 2509–2528.

Zack, M., Poulos, C. X., Fragopoulos, F., Woodford, T. M., & MacLeod, C. M. (2006). Negative affect words prime beer consumption in young drinkers. *Addictive Behaviors, 31*, 169–173. https://doi.org/10.1016/j.addbeh.2005.04.016

10

Altering Choice Architecture to Alter Drinking Behaviour: Evidence from Research on Lower Strength Alcohol Labelling and Glass Design

Milica Vasiljevic and Rachel Pechey

Introduction

The harms of alcohol consumption are well-known—alcohol consumption is the seventh leading risk factor for burden of disease worldwide (World Health Organization, 2018), with 5% of deaths and 5% of disability-adjusted life years attributable to alcohol use. Drink-related harm costs the UK Government £21 billion (approx. USD25.5 billion) per year (Home Office et al., 2014). Any increase in alcohol consumption exacerbates harm—even at low levels of consumption—adding to calls to take a population level approach to

Milica Vasiljevic and Rachel Pechey contributed equally to the writing of this chapter.

M. Vasiljevic (✉)
Behaviour and Health Research Unit, Institute of Public Health, University of Cambridge, Cambridge, UK

Department of Psychology, Durham University, Durham, UK
e-mail: milica.vasiljevic@durham.ac.uk; milica.vasiljevic@medschl.cam.ac.uk

R. Pechey
Behaviour and Health Research Unit, Institute of Public Health, University of Cambridge, Cambridge, UK

Nuffied Department of Primary Care Health Sciences, University of Oxford, Oxford, UK
e-mail: rachel.pechey@phc.ox.ac.uk

R. Cooke et al. (eds.), *The Palgrave Handbook of Psychological Perspectives on Alcohol Consumption*, https://doi.org/10.1007/978-3-030-66941-6_10

reducing consumption (Griswold et al., 2018). In this chapter, we present the current evidence for the efficacy of two types of choice architecture interventions on modifying perceptions of alcoholic drinks, willingness to purchase and alcohol consumption itself. The first intervention we evaluate concerns the use of labels indicating lower alcohol strength. In the second part of this chapter, we then examine the evidence for changing the size and/or shape of wine and beer glasses in order to reduce alcohol purchasing and consumption.

What Is Choice Architecture?

Recently there has been growing interest in interventions targeting changes in small-scale physical environments ("the physical micro-environment")—for example, within shops, bars or restaurants (Hollands, Marteau, & Fletcher, 2016; Thaler & Sunstein, 2008). Such interventions are often referred to as choice architecture or nudge interventions. This approach emphasises the automatic or habitual side to human behaviour that has been relatively neglected in models of human behaviour (Gawronski & Bodenhausen, 2006; Hofmann, Friese, & Wiers, 2008; Strack & Deutsch, 2004). As choice architecture interventions involve altering physical or social environments to cue particular behaviours, they are hypothesised to act principally via the engagement of automatic cognitive processes.

Choice architecture interventions can alter the properties of drinks within the physical microenvironment in myriad ways—categorised in a recent typology (TIPPME: Hollands et al., 2017). This includes changing their availability (e.g. fewer alcoholic drinks on sale), position (e.g. removing alcohol from end-of-aisle displays), functionality (e.g. making it harder to open a bottle or can), presentation (e.g. removing branding), size (e.g. changing the size of wine glasses) or the information provided on the products (e.g. labels on alcoholic drinks). A 2013 review found few choice architecture interventions targeting alcohol-related behaviours (Hollands et al., 2013), but evidence has gradually accumulated since this time. We begin by evaluating the use of labels indicating lower alcohol strength on consumption.

Choice Architecture Interventions That Use Labels to Indicate "Lower" Alcohol Strength

Lower strength alcohol labels carry verbal descriptors such as "low," "lighter," or "super low" to denote reduced strength alcohol content in alcoholic beverages (i.e. products containing lower-than-average percentage alcohol by volume [% ABV]). Current European Union (EU) legislation limits the number of verbal descriptors that can be used and further restricts the use of such terms to drinks of ≤1.2% ABV (The European Parliament and the Council of the European Union, 2011). Globally, similar legislation restricts the use of lower strength alcohol verbal descriptors to beverages of below ≤1.15% ABV (e.g. Food Standards Australia & New Zealand, 2014). See Chap. 19 for more on alcohol labelling legislation.

It has been suggested that wider availability and marketing—through the use of explicit labelling of lower strength alcoholic beverages—have the potential to reduce alcohol consumption at the population level if they attract more consumers towards these products. Even though sales of regular or average strength alcoholic beverages still dominate the market (ONS, 2017), there is a growing trend—especially in high income countries such as the UK, the US, Canada and Germany—for consumers to opt for lower strength alcohol and alcohol-free products (Nielsen, 2018).

Interest in revisions to this legislation to expand lower strength alcohol labelling to cover a wider range of lower alcohol strengths was captured in the 2012 UK government's Alcohol Strategy—for example, including an industry pledge through the Responsibility Deal to take one billion units of alcohol out of the market by 2015, primarily through increasing consumer selection of lower strength alcoholic beverages (Department of Health, 2012). Studies have however disputed whether this pledge has been met (Holmes, Angus, & Meier, 2015). UK regulations covering the use of terms to describe lower strength alcohol products were repealed at the end of December 2014, with January 2019 set as the date for the enactment of new legislation in this area.

In the next section we discuss the potential impact of extending the use of lower strength alcohol terms to promote products with alcohol content higher than the currently legislated threshold of 1.2% ABV, but lower than the current average on the market (which in the UK is 12.9% for wine and 4.2% for beer; see Department of Health, 2014).

Does Lower Strength Content Labelling Alter Perceptions and Consumption of Products That Are Harmful to Health?

Increasing the availability and marketing of lower strength alcohol products could reduce the number of alcohol units consumed, but only if certain assumptions are met. There are two key risks to realising the potential of lower strength alcohol labelling to reduce alcohol harm at the population level. First, lower strength alcohol products could increase total alcohol consumption if these products increase the number of occasions perceived to be appropriate for consuming alcohol (see also Anderson & Rehm, 2016; Rehm, Lachenmeier, Llopis, Imtiaz, & Anderson, 2016). Second, these drinks could result in a paradoxical self-licensing effect (whereby individuals give themselves permission to act indulgently following a virtuous choice; see Khan & Dhar, 2006). If alcohol-drinking occasions increase and/or self-licensing occurs such that individuals over-consume lower strength alcohol products to the extent that they consume more units than would have been consumed from higher strength products, overall alcohol consumption at the population level would increase.

Studies examining the impact of warning labels and labels showing alcohol units may provide indirect evidence regarding the possible impact of lower alcohol strength labels. These studies show that warning labels displaying recommended alcohol consumption levels and possible harms increase awareness of these labels and recommendations, but no studies report effects of these types of labels on alcohol consumption (Agostinelli & Grube, 2002; Stockwell, 2006; Wilkinson & Room, 2009). Similarly, although consumers support labelling in several forms—for example, alcohol units, recommended intake and standard drinks (Coomber, Jones, Martino, & Miller, 2017)—actual knowledge of alcohol strength arising from such labels seems to be limited, raising questions as to the potential utility of lower alcohol strength labelling. Furthermore, labels displaying alcohol units can be used paradoxically as a reference cue to identify and purchase stronger or cheapest-for-strength alcohol products, highlighting a possible negative effect of more prominent labelling of the alcohol content of drinks (Bui, Burton, Howlett, & Kozup, 2008; Jones & Gregory, 2009).

Labels indicating low or light versions of products harmful to health (high fat foods and tobacco) also suggest the potential for unintended paradoxical effects, including greater appeal and energy (kcal) consumption when foods are labelled "low fat," and perceived lower harm from cigarettes labelled as "light" (e.g. Borland et al., 2004; McCann et al., 2013). A recent systematic review including studies of food (k = 19) and tobacco (k = 6) labelling that identified options with low contents (low-calorie food; low-tar tobacco) showed that such labels can alter people's perceptions concerning the content of products. Moreover, with respect to food, these labels also altered what consumers' judged to be an appropriate serving, with the potential to license greater consumption of the labelled product (Shemilt, Hendry, & Marteau, 2017). The same review identified no studies regarding lower alcohol content labelling.

Since that review, one set of studies has explored whether lower strength alcohol labelling may successfully decrease alcohol consumption and associated harms at the population level—looking at whether lower strength alcohol labelling alters both alcohol-related perceptions and consumption. The following section provides an overview of these studies and showcases current knowledge relating to how lower strength alcohol labelling alters consumers' perceptions and consumption.

Does Lower Strength Alcohol Labelling Affect Perceptions and Consumption of Alcoholic Drinks?

There remains a paucity of empirical evidence pertaining to this question. To provide the first evidence to address the above question, we studied the content of marketing messages on producers' and retailers' websites for lower and regular strength wines and beers sold online by the four main UK supermarkets (Vasiljevic, Coulter, Petticrew, & Marteau, 2018). Our analyses showed that lower strength drinks were significantly more likely than regular strength drinks to be marketed as suitable for everyday consumption. Consumption during lunch-times, outdoor events and sports/fitness occasions were also significantly more likely to appear in the marketing messages for the lower strength products (e.g. "Perfect for all occasions from a lunchtime barbeque to an evening celebration"). Lower strength alcoholic drinks were also significantly more likely to be marketed with health-related claims (e.g. "You don't have to give up on the Pinot Grigio when you're cutting back on calories"; "Who said dieting couldn't be fun?"). These analyses were the first to demonstrate that lower strength alcoholic drinks are marketed not as substitutes for higher strength products but as ones that can be consumed on additional occasions, whilst also implying the purported healthiness of the lower strength products.

In a related experimental study, we found that weekly drinkers in the UK perceived that alcohol-free and lower alcohol strength drinks were targeting pregnant women, dieters, drivers, sportspeople and underage drinkers (Vasiljevic, Couturier, & Marteau, 2019). Furthermore, lower strength and alcohol-free drinks were perceived as targeting consumption during weekday lunchtimes. On the other hand, weekend lunches were considered as the target occasions for both lower and higher strength wines and beers. Taken together, these findings suggest that the general population of weekly drinkers may perceive lower strength alcoholic drinks as an extension to regular strength alcoholic drinks, rather than solely as a substitute product.

Alongside the potential for lower strength alcoholic drinks to reduce actual alcohol consumption, lower strength alcohol labelling may change the self-reported perceptions and knowledge of such drinks. We conducted an online survey of a nationally representative sample of 3390 UK adults to assess the impact of labelling wine and beer with different verbal descriptors—denoting lower alcohol strength, with and without % ABV—on product appeal and participants' understanding of the alcohol strength of a given product (e.g. units contained in the drink; whether consumption falls within the drink-drive limit) (Vasiljevic, Couturier, & Marteau, 2018). Weekly wine and beer drinkers were randomised to one of 18 experimental groups. We found that lower alcohol strength products had lower appeal than regular strength products (with appeal decreasing as % ABV decreased). Understanding of strength was generally high across the different drinks, with the majority of participants correctly identifying or erring on the side of caution when estimating: the units and calories in a given drink, appropriateness for consumption by children and drinking within the driving limit. Interestingly, understanding of strength was better amongst those randomised to the lower strength verbal/numerical labels, when compared to those randomised to see the regular strength labels.

However, this better understanding of alcohol strength when drinks have lower alcohol content may not necessarily translate into decreased (less harmful) consumption levels. To this end, we examined wine and beer consumption in a bar laboratory amongst a sample of weekly wine and beer drinkers sampled from an existing representative panel of the general population of England (Vasiljevic, Couturier, Frings, Moss, Albery, & Marteau, 2018). We found that participants drank approximately 20% more wine and beer (measured in ml) when it was labelled as lower in alcohol strength, suggesting that lower strength alcoholic drinks may engender paradoxical effects. Overconsumption of wines and beers was observed despite the better understanding of alcohol strength displayed by those participants randomised to drink products labelled as lower in alcohol strength compared to those randomised to drink products labelled as regular strength. In the next section we consider policy implications arising from these recent studies.

Does Current Evidence Support Changes to Existing Policies on Lower Strength Alcohol Labelling?

Industry representatives have expressed real interest in policy changes regarding lower strength alcohol labelling, suggesting that such changes in policy have the potential to reduce total alcohol consumption and associated harms at the population level (Department of Health, 2012). For lower strength alcoholic drinks to achieve their full potential for reduced consumption at the population level, two conditions need to be met: (1) the occasions during which alcohol is consumed must not increase (potentially extending the total time during which alcohol is consumed); and (2) consumers must not compensate for the lower strength of these drinks by consuming more (thereby resulting in higher overall alcohol consumption).

Our studies found that marketing materials used by both producers and retailers in the UK suggested extending the occasions suitable for alcohol consumption. Weekly consumers of wine and beer sampled from the UK population mirrored such claims, by reporting that they perceived lower strength alcoholic drinks to be suitable for consumption on more occasions and by more varied consumer groups when compared to regular strength drinks. Furthermore, although weekly drinkers' understanding of the alcohol content of lower strength alcoholic drinks was better when compared to knowledge of content of regular strength alcoholic drinks, this better understanding did not translate into less harmful consumption. In fact, participants consumed 20% more wine or beer when it was labelled as lower in strength. Combined, these findings suggest that—contrary to recent suggestions made by industry—extending the use of lower strength alcohol labels to alcoholic drinks of higher % ABV than currently legislated is likely to have limited potential for reducing alcohol-related harms at the population level.

The limited evidence base suggests any changes to existing policies will need to account for the possibility of paradoxical increases in alcohol purchasing during extended drinking occasions. Careful monitoring of future sales data will be needed to ascertain if the marketing messages and consumers' perceptions analysed in our studies will translate into actual increases in overall alcohol consumption.

Furthermore, the dissociation we found between self-reported understanding of alcohol content and actual consumption of the drinks suggests that labelling of lower strength alcoholic drinks may affect consumers' behaviours largely via implicit processes without conscious awareness, leading to self-licensing mechanisms as described above (see Strack & Deutsch, 2004). This indicates that policy options other than explicit labelling of lower strength alcoholic drinks may be more effective at encouraging consumers to switch to lower content alternatives. These include preferential tax treatment for lower content alcoholic drinks (Burton et al., 2016), resulting in reduced price per container whilst at the same time not highlighting the lower alcohol content of the products (see Geller, Kalsher, & Clarke, 1991).

We next turn our attention to another choice architecture intervention which has been proposed as a viable tool to decrease alcohol consumption; alterations in shape or size of drinking glasses used to serve alcoholic drinks.

Choice Architecture Interventions That Manipulate the Size/Shape of Drinking Glasses

Glasses for serving alcohol are available in a myriad of different sizes and shapes, features that may change drinking behaviour—indeed, a whole industry exists around the impact of the glass on taste, for wine in particular: see Spence and Wan (2015) and Spence and van Doorn (2017) for reviews of the impact of glass design on taste and enjoyment. Glass shape and size may help to drive sales, with their design featuring in industry marketing (Stead, Angus, Macdonald, & Bauld, 2014). Notably, wine glass size underwent a marked increase in the 1990s (Zupan, Evans, Couturier, & Marteau, 2017), which may have played a part in the almost doubling of wine consumption between 1980 and 2004 in the UK (see Nicholls, 2010; Smith & Foxcroft, 2009). Yet the extent to which glass design affects alcohol purchasing and consumption, key to public health concerns, is uncertain. A Cochrane review, showing that tableware size influences consumption for food and non-alcoholic drinks, found an absence of evidence relating to alcoholic drinks (Hollands et al., 2015). This gap in the literature has now begun to be filled, providing initial evidence on the roles of glass size and glass shape with regard to drinking behaviour.

Does Changing Glass Size Influence Drinking Behaviour?

A series of studies conducted in Cambridge in the UK has examined the impact of changing wine glass size (without changing the portion sizes served) on purchasing (Clarke et al., 2019; Pechey et al., 2016; Pechey et al., 2017). The first of these studies, conducted in a single establishment in 2015, suggested that daily wine sales increased by 9% when the establishment served wine in larger (370 ml) glasses compared to their standard (300 ml) glasses (a 23% increase in glass size; Pechey et al., 2016). This was followed up with a replication study in two further bars in 2016 (Pechey et al., 2017). This replication study found that in one of the participating bars, daily wine volume purchased was 11% higher when sold in 510 ml compared to 370 ml glasses (a 38% increase in glass size), but findings were inconclusive when comparing 370 ml to 300 ml glasses as used in the first study (see Fig. 10.1). Moreover, no significant differences in sales were seen in the second bar—comparing serving wine in 300 ml vs. 510 ml glasses (a 70% increase in glass size). This mixed pattern of results could reflect a moderating influence (e.g. the effect was dependent on the portion sizes that tend to be purchased or the type of establishment in the studies). It could also be that these results reflected random fluctuations rather than true effects.

To try to clarify possible effects, the study design was repeated in two bars and one restaurant. One of these bars had already participated in the replication study, while the other was its sister bar, offering the same drinks menu. The restaurant participated twice, once in 2017 and then repeating the study in 2018, to compare results across these time periods. As before, however, results were mixed (Clarke et al., 2019). Daily wine volume sold was 21% higher when served with 450 ml vs. 350 ml glasses (a 29% increase in glass size) in the bar from the replication study, but this effect was not observed in their sister bar. Nor were any meaningful differences observed when comparing between other glass sizes in bars. In the restaurant, daily wine volume sold was 13% higher when served with 350 ml vs. 290 ml glasses (a 21% increase in glass size) in 2017, but although a similar direction of effect (6% higher) was seen in 2018, this was not statistically significant. Figure 10.1 shows the results across all studies and establishments.

Across these studies, the only statistically significant differences in purchasing suggest that larger glasses increased purchasing, across a wide range of glass sizes. Yet Fig. 10.1 clearly shows that for the majority of glass comparisons, no conclusive findings were observed. It also highlights that effects of glass size may differ between bars and restaurants. There are some obvious differences in these settings—they may attract different clientele, drinking while dining could be a substantially different experience to drinking wine in a bar—but beyond this, key distinctions to be drawn between these types of establishment relate to the mechanisms that could explain any impact of glass size.

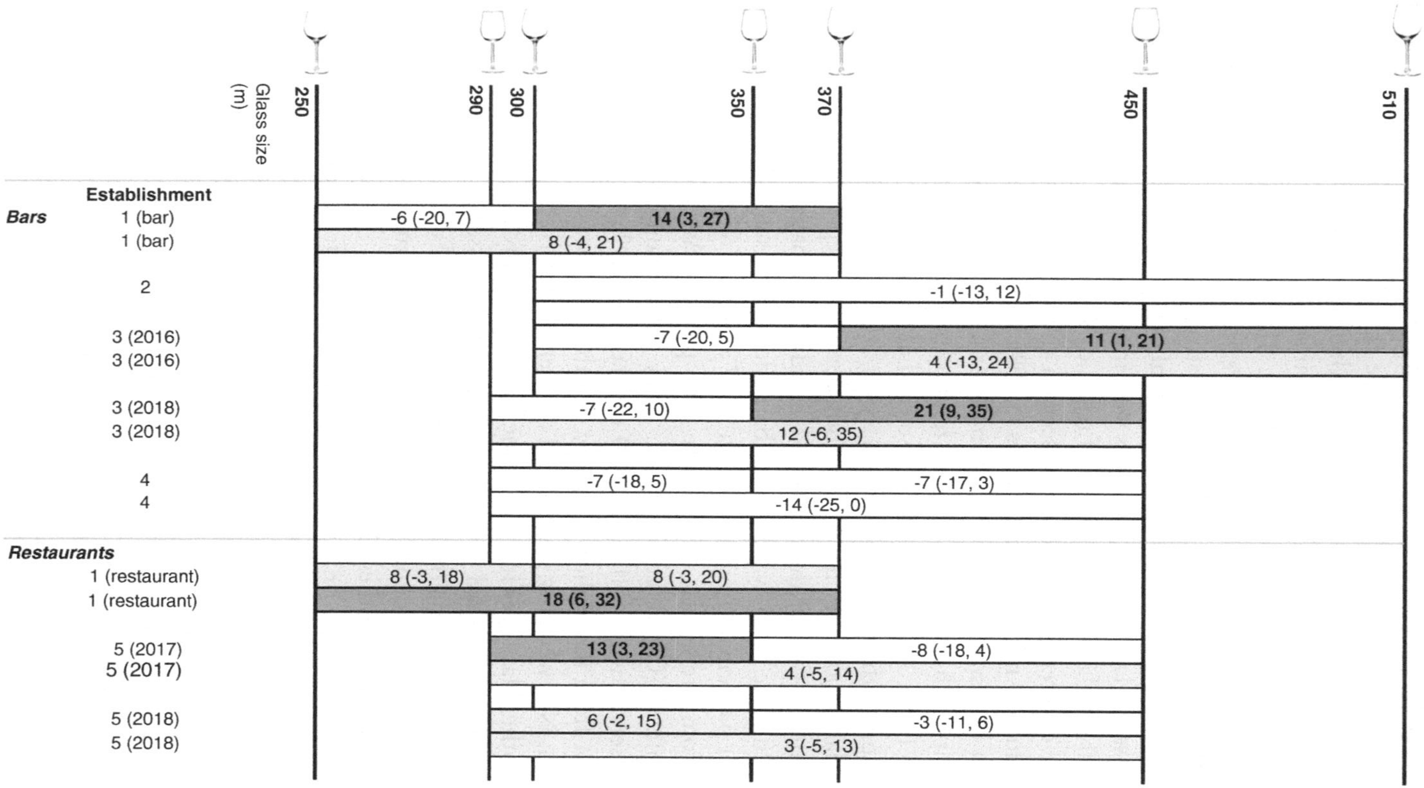

Fig. 10.1 Percentage change (95% CI) in wine sales when wine is served in glasses varying in capacity (larger compared to smaller glasses). (Notes. Comparisons that suggest a significant increase in sales with larger glasses are shaded dark grey, comparisons suggesting a non-significant increase are shaded light grey, and comparisons suggesting a non-significant decrease in sales with larger glasses are not shaded. Statistically significant results ($p < 0.05$) are in bold. Studies are described elsewhere (Clarke et al., 2019; Pechey et al., 2016; Pechey et al., 2017); Additional comparisons reported in Pilling et al., 2020)

First, a greater proportion of wine was purchased by the glass in the bars (around 90% of sales, compared to around two-thirds of sales in restaurants). The impact of glass size may vary depending on whether the drink is poured freely into the glass from a bottle or purchased as a fixed portion (e.g. wine purchased by the glass). When a drink is freely poured into the glass, this may result in different portions being poured into larger vs. smaller glasses. Indeed, portion size poured (and thus alcohol content) has been shown to be influenced by the glass size used (Kerr, Patterson, Koenen, & Greenfield, 2009; White, Kraus, McCracken, & Swartzwelder, 2003), with larger glasses promoting larger portions.

Second, none of the restaurants in this set of studies offered a 250 ml portion of wine (in the UK, establishments standardly offer portions of 125 ml, 175 ml and/or 250 ml when serving wine by the glass). In contrast, all but one of the bars offered this larger serving size, meaning the mean portion size for purchases of glasses of wine was larger in the bars than in the restaurants. When purchasing wine by the glass, customers purchase a fixed portion, so any influence of glass size may be due to perceptual differences. For example, individuals may perceive a 175 ml portion of wine in a smaller glass as a larger portion than the same 175 ml portion in a larger glass. Moreover, any perceptual differences might vary depending on the portion size purchased. An online study where participants filled wine glasses to match a portion shown in a reference glass suggested some perceptual differences by glass size and shape, whereby participants underfilled a wider glass and overfilled a larger glass (Pechey et al., 2015). These results also suggested some variation in these effects depending on the portion size they were trying to match (Pechey et al., 2015). For a review of perceptual differences and mechanisms that might underlie an effect of glass size or shape on drinking behaviour, see Langfield et al. (2020).

A mega-analysis—that is, combining the raw daily sales data from each venue in each of the above field studies into one regression analysis—was conducted for all the data from bars, and a second for the data from restaurants (Pilling, Clarke, Pechey, Hollands, & Marteau, 2020). A literature search identified no other studies to include in the analysis; the studies by Kersbergen et al. (2018) were not included as the focus of these studies was on altering portion size, with glass size being simultaneously altered to hold relative fullness constant. As such, it was not possible to isolate the effect of glass size in these studies. For bars, no statistically significant effects of glass size on wine sales were evident. For restaurants, however, using 350 ml or 370 ml glasses increased sales by 7.3% over using 290 ml or 300 ml glasses (95% CI 1.5% to 13.5%). Using 250 ml glasses suggested decreased sales compared to

290 ml or 300 ml glasses, although confidence intervals crossed zero (-9.6%, 95% CI -19.0 to 7.2). There was no evidence that 450 ml glasses increased sales over 290 ml or 300 ml glasses (0.9%, 95% CI -5.5 to 7.7). This suggests that the relationship between glass size and purchasing in restaurants may not be linear. Glasses sized between 300 ml and 370 ml may be seen as "typical" sizes—for example, glass sizes of between 300 ml and 350 ml were commonly used in the study establishments before their participation, so drinkers may not have noticed the size of these glasses. In contrast, larger—450 ml and 510 ml—glasses may be noticeably larger than "typical" glasses, leading individuals to change their behaviour to avoid consuming more than intended—for example, pacing their drinking from these glasses or being more aware of the volume poured into them.

This could reflect the unit bias heuristic, which postulates that people consume in "units" (e.g. one plate or one glass), perceiving it as an appropriate amount to consume, albeit perhaps only if it is above a certain "minimum" amount (Geier, Rozin, & Doros, 2006). In this context, portions served in "typical size" wine glasses (including the range between 250 ml and 370 ml) may be perceived as "a typical glass of wine"—even if more wine is poured into the glasses as they increase in size. As such, within the boundaries of what is considered a "typical size" wine glass, increasing glass size might increase purchases and consumption. Beyond this size threshold, however, if larger glasses (e.g. 450 ml and 510 ml) are regarded as holding more than a typical glass of wine, then individuals may adapt their behaviour when drinking from these glasses. If so, there may be a threshold past which the relationship between glass size and purchasing is altered, so that increasing glass size no longer increases purchasing or consumption. In the next section we review current evidence on the impact of glass shape on drinking behaviour.

Does Changing Glass Shape Influence Drinking Behaviour?

Fewer studies have been conducted altering the shape of glasses. Four studies are identified here, of which three examined speed of drinking as the outcome of interest. First, Cliceri, Petit, Garrel, Monteleone and Giboreau (2018) compared consumption of an alcoholic cocktail between two straight-sided glasses (tall and narrow vs. short and wide), with results suggesting 7% slower consumption from the tall and narrow glass, although the confidence intervals for this difference crossed zero. This could tie in with the "elongation effect," whereby shorter cylinders are perceived to have smaller volumes than taller (or longer, depending on which is the most salient dimension) cylinders of equal volume (Pearson, 1964; Raghubir & Krishna, 1999). The elongation effect relates to the classic experiments which indicated that young children based their judgements of the volume of a liquid on the height of its container, suggesting that the volume of liquid in the glass decreased after they saw the contents being poured from a tall narrow container to a short wide one (Piaget & Inhelder, 1969). Although older children and adults correctly identify that the volume of liquid remains constant in this experiment, our judgements of volume may still be subject to similar biases when observing tall or short glasses without direct comparison between these.

The influence of this effect may vary with the size of glasses, diminishing with increasing volume (Frayman & Dawson, 1981). Moreover, given beverage glasses are often not filled to capacity (pints of beer being a notable exception), it is possible individuals' judgements of volume in glasses might be influenced by the height of the glasses and/or by the height of the volumes of liquid contained within. Indeed, if both these factors have an impact, the percentage of a glass that has been filled (i.e. relative fullness) may also affect perceptions of volume. Judgements of proportions may therefore also come into play in this context, with evidence from studies of simple geometric shapes suggesting proportions less than 0.5 are overestimated whereas proportions over 0.5 are underestimated (Hollands & Dyre, 2000; Varey, Mellers, & Birnbaum, 1990). Perceptual effects might therefore vary with portion size (and moreover, with relative fullness, that is, a glass size x portion size interaction effect—see, e.g, Pechey et al., 2015). One study of pouring behaviour suggested drawing attention to the empty space remaining (rather than the volume of liquid filling a glass) could reverse an elongation effect (perhaps as the perceptual effects now acted similarly on the empty space) (Caljouw & van Wijck, 2014). As such, if pouring into a glass that was close to capacity, perceptual effects may reverse compared to pouring into a glass with considerable capacity remaining. This might offer an explanation for the results of one study looking at speed of consumption, which found a 175 ml portion of wine was consumed more slowly from a larger (370 ml) compared to a smaller (250 ml) glass (contrary to the expected effect) (Zupan, Pechey, Couturier, Hollands, & Marteau, 2017). Combining the potential influences of each of these factors suggests the resulting effects on perception may not be straightforward to predict with increasing glass size or glass shape.

Two studies focused on differences in speed of consumption between curved/sloped and straight-sided glasses. Attwood, Scott-Samuel, Stothart, and Munafò (2012) found 60% slower beer consumption from straight, compared with outward-curved, beer glasses, but found no differences in speed of consumption for a soft drink or when using smaller half-portions. Langfield, Pechey, Pilling and Marteau (2018) similarly found drinking was around 20% faster when using outward-sloped rather than straight-sided tumblers, although this study used a soft drink (one possible explanation for the difference between this and Attwood et al.'s (2012) study is that the soft drink in this study had similar colouring to beer, compared to the clear soft drink used by Attwood and colleagues).

Finally, the only field study investigating the impact of glass shape—a feasibility study conducted in three bars over two weekends—demonstrated that sales of beer were 24% lower when served using straight-sided compared with outward-curved glasses, although again confidence intervals crossed zero (Troy, Maynard, Hickman, Attwood, & Munafò, 2015). Further field studies are currently underway, attempting to replicate this finding in a larger sample, but as yet, the evidence for changing glass shape to alter purchasing or consumption of alcoholic drinks remains limited.

These studies highlight the idea that a "midpoint bias" might underlie the impact of some glass designs on drinking behaviour. This proposes that people's rate of drinking is guided by perceptual judgements of when approximately half a beverage has been consumed (Attwood et al., 2012). These misjudgements of the midpoint may also relate to the elongation effect, if misjudgements are resulting from individuals using the height of the glass to estimate the volume within. In these studies, people were more likely to underestimate the midpoint when glasses have outwardly sloped walls (compared to straight parallel walls), using both beer glasses and tumblers (Attwood et al., 2012; Langfield et al., 2018; Troy et al., 2018). Such a bias would suggest that individuals might be more likely to drink more from outwardly sloped glasses. However, findings have as yet been inconclusive as to whether there is any relationship between greater misjudgements of the midpoint and drinking behaviour.

In summary, there is some evidence that glass size might impact on purchasing, at least in restaurants. Studies also indicate the potential for glass shape to influence drinking behaviour, but evidence to date is insufficient to draw any robust conclusions. Given these findings, it is worth considering the implications for policies to reduce alcohol purchasing and consumption.

Does Current Evidence Support Advocating Changes with Regard to Glass Size and/or Shape?

Twice as much alcohol is purchased for consumption at home than is drunk in pubs or restaurants in the UK (Institute of Alcohol Studies, 2019), reflecting a greater volume of alcohol being sold off-trade than on-trade across Western Europe and North America (Euromonitor, 2010). In terms of glass size, it is likely that pouring behaviour would be the key factor at play when people drink at home (for example, de Beukelaar, Janse, Sierksma, Feskens, & de Vries, 2019, though it is not possible to distinguish between glass size and shape in this study). Given that the predictions relating to this mechanism are relatively clear-cut: larger glasses afford larger amounts of wine to be poured (and perceptual biases may make people unaware of increased quantities poured), it may be that reducing the size of wine glasses in the home could lead to a substantial reduction in alcohol consumed. However, no studies to date have been conducted looking at the influence of glass design on in-home alcohol consumption. This gap in our evidence base needs addressing. In addition, if further evidence suggests that outwardly sloped glasses lead to increased beer consumption, consideration could also be given to advocating straight-sided beer glasses for in-home consumption.

That said, to focus on advocating changes within the home (i.e. to place the onus on individuals) runs the risk of only reaching those populations who are actively interested in healthy behaviour change, and so may exacerbate existing inequalities in the burden of ill-health due to alcohol consumption (Probst, Roerecke, Behrendt, & Rehm, 2014). Instead, it may be fruitful to consider capping wine glass to a maximum size outside the home (and if evidence accumulates with regard to glass shape, mandating the use of straight-sided beer glasses), via local licensing regulations. Population-level interventions have the means to reach individuals across all socioeconomic groupings and levels of alcohol consumption. Given that this involves a relatively minor change to the choice architecture in consumers' environments (there is considerable variety in glass design across establishments), it would be expected that such a change would have little impact other than potentially to consumption. Moreover, if the use of smaller glasses became widespread, this might then affect social norms for appropriate glass size. Such social norms may then in turn encourage the use of smaller glasses in other contexts (Higgs, 2015; Perkins, 2002), such as the home.

One disadvantage of such an approach is that at present it is by no means certain that there is an optimum glass size (or cap threshold) that could be advocated across establishments, given that the relationship between glass size and consumption may be non-linear. Although there has been no statistical evidence to suggest smaller sizes lead to increased consumption in bars and restaurants, the presence of multiple inconclusive results, alongside the mega-analysis results finding no evidence for an effect in bars, might lead some to question the utility of a cap on glass size. Further exploration of the underlying mechanisms and the contexts in which these effects seem to occur could help strengthen the basis for targeting glass design as a strategy to reduce alcohol consumption. In what follows we provide some avenues for future research that would give further insights into the impact of the two choice architecture interventions discussed in this chapter.

Future Research Directions

The limited evidence base indicates that we need to be cautious about any changes to regulations pertaining to lower strength alcohol labelling or introducing any regulations with regard to wine glass size or shape. There is a need for further studies to explore underlying mechanisms, in order to understand how and why lower strength alcohol labelling and changes in glass size/shape may change behaviour. For example, regarding the potential impact of altering glass size, it would be beneficial to establish (a) whether the effects of glass size are largely limited to occasions when drinks are freely poured, alongside (b) whether there is a minimum and maximum glass size beyond which a linear relationship between glass size and portion poured breaks down, or indeed whether there is a linear relationship or some other pattern. Exploring the extent to which the unit bias heuristic may play a role in the effects of glass size may help to shed light onto these questions. Similarly, examining contexts in which self-licensing effects could be ameliorated would advance our understanding of the impact of lower strength alcohol labelling. As such, elucidating underlying mechanisms may help identify boundary conditions and contexts in which the proposed interventions may be effective, ineffective or even counterproductive.

Future studies should also explore the extent to which effects persist over time. For example, glass size may affect pouring via non-conscious processes, which in turn might influence consumption in a relatively consistent manner over time. Perceptual effects may be more vulnerable to change, however. For example, immediately following the introduction of different-sized glasses, people may perceive portions served in these new glasses as more or less than a typical glass of wine. Over time, however, they may adjust so that portions in these glasses start to be perceived as a typical glass of wine. Such effects—whereby the norm of what is "standard" changes over time—may also be apparent with expansion in lower strength alcohol labelling: the norm of what is lower in strength may shift if drinks higher than 1.2% ABV start to be labelled as lower strength. Therefore, establishing the likely persistence of any positive behaviour change resulting from changing glass design, or expanding the use of lower strength alcohol labels, is key if we wish to optimise policies to reduce alcohol consumption.

Alongside the exploration of mechanisms and the persistence of effects, there is a need for rigorous studies testing the robustness of obtained effects. For example, it is clear from the series of wine glass size studies that multiple studies need to be conducted in different settings (given that bars and restaurants often cater for a particular clientele) using variants of each choice architecture intervention (i.e. different glass and portion size combinations). Such work should then be subjected to evidence synthesis to establish whether interventions work as expected across different contexts. Although there is clearly a role for controlled laboratory studies—particularly in the exploration of mechanisms—these should be supported by field studies to help contextualise drinking behaviour—for example, the social context of drinking with others, or the cumulative effects of an intervention as an individual consumes a series of drinks over a drinking occasion (see Chap. 9). Moreover, although studies to date have focused on quantifying any perceptual effects arising from the manipulation of glass size/shape and lower strength labelling, our understanding of such effects would be greatly enriched by extending protocols to incorporate qualitative and mixed method explorations of how people interpret and respond to these type of interventions.

Future studies should also examine potential moderators of the effects arising from altered glass size/shape or lower strength alcohol labelling. For example, laboratory studies for both interventions discussed in this chapter sampled regular (weekly) drinkers. Whether these effects would be replicated among individuals who do not regularly consume alcohol deserves further exploration. Furthermore, testing the impact of the interventions on different types of alcoholic drinks would better elucidate the impact of the two interventions. For example, the impact of glass size has only been tested in relation to wine glass size, whereas the impact of lower strength alcohol labelling has only been applied to wine and beer thus far. Future studies should examine whether the effects obtained to date would translate to other types of alcoholic drinks, such as cider, alcopops, mixed drinks and spirits. Finally, testing the impact of altered glass size/shape or lower strength alcohol labelling across time within the same individuals would enable us to better understand the long-term impacts of these interventions. Triangulating findings using different methodologies, including qualitative studies, would help advance our understanding of how and why lower strength alcohol labelling and glass size/shape affect drinking-related behaviours.

Conclusion

This chapter has outlined two possible choice architecture modes of intervention suggested to affect drinking-related behaviours. We have also outlined the potential mechanisms underlying these intervention modes. The existing evidence base is small and equivocal, and the current chapter highlights the need for further research. Overall, these serve to illustrate that robust exploration of intervention efficacy is needed. Future studies designed to examine choice architecture interventions should evaluate not only how people respond to these labels and glass design variants, but also, by taking a whole systems approach (Petticrew et al., 2017), how the alcohol industry and retailers respond through branding and marketing.

References

Agostinelli, G., & Grube, J. (2002). Alcohol counter-advertising and the media. *Alcohol Research & Health, 26*(1), 15–21.

Anderson, P., & Rehm, J. (2016). Evaluating alcohol industry action to reduce the harmful use of alcohol. *Alcohol and Alcoholism, 51*(4), 383–387. https://doi.org/10.1093/alcalc/agv139

Attwood, A. S., Scott-Samuel, N. E., Stothart, G., & Munafò, M. R. (2012). Glass shape influences consumption rate for alcoholic beverages. *PLoS One, 7*(8), e43007. https://doi.org/10.1371/journal.pone.0043007

Borland, R., Yong, H. H., King, B., Cummings, K. M., Fong, G. T., Elton-Marshall, T., … McNeill, A. (2004). Use of and beliefs about light cigarettes in four countries: Findings from the International Tobacco Control Policy Evaluation Survey. *Nicotine & Tobacco Research, 6*(Suppl 3), S311–S321. https://doi.org/10.1080/14622200412331320716

Bui, M., Burton, S., Howlett, E., & Kozup, J. (2008). What am I drinking? The effects of serving facts information on alcohol beverage containers. *Journal of Consumer Affairs, 42*(1), 81–99. https://doi.org/10.1111/j.1745-6606.2007.00095.x

Burton, R., Henn, C., Lavoie, D., O'Connor, R., Perkins, C., Sweeney, K., … Musto, V. (2016). A rapid evidence review of the effectiveness and cost-effectiveness of alcohol control policies: An English perspective. *The Lancet, 389*(10078), 1558–1580. https://doi.org/10.1016/S0140-6736(16)32420-5

Caljouw, S. R., & van Wijck, R. (2014). Is the glass half full or half empty? How to reverse the effect of glass elongation on the volume poured. *PLoS One, 9*(10), e109374. https://doi.org/10.1371/journal.pone.0109374

Clarke, N., Pechey, R., Pilling, M., Hollands, G. J., Mantzari, E., & Marteau, T. M. (2019). Wine glass size and wine sales: Four replication studies in one restaurant and two bars. *BMC Research Notes, 12*(1), 426. https://doi.org/10.1186/s13104-019-4477-8

Cliceri, D., Petit, E., Garrel, C., Monteleone, E., & Giboreau, A. (2018). Effect of glass shape on subjective and behavioral consumer responses in a real-life context of drinking consumption. *Food Quality and Preference, 64*, 187–191. https://doi.org/10.1016/j.foodqual.2017.09.008

Coomber, K., Jones, S. C., Martino, F., & Miller, P. G. (2017). Predictors of awareness of standard drink labelling and drinking guidelines to reduce negative health effects among Australian drinkers. *Drug and Alcohol Review, 36*(2), 200–209. https://doi.org/10.1111/dar.12383

de Beukelaar, M. F. A., Janse, M. L., Sierksma, A., Feskens, E. J. M., & de Vries, J. H. M. (2019). How full is your glass? Portion sizes of wine, fortified wine and straight spirits at home in the Netherlands. *Public Health Nutrition, 22*(10), 1727–1734. https://doi.org/10.1017/S1368980019000442

Department of Health. (2012). *Public health responsibility deal – A8(a) Alcohol Unit reduction.* Retrieved from: https://responsibilitydeal.dh.gov.uk/pledges/pledge/?pl=22 on 11th October 2016.

Department of Health. (2014). *Responsibility Deal Alcohol Network – Pledge to remove 1 billion units of alcohol from the market by end 2015 – First interim monitoring report.* Retrieved from: https://www.gov.uk/government/uploads/system/uploads/attachment_data/file/389573/RDAN_-_Unit_Reduction_Pledge_-_1st_interim_monitoring_report.pdf on 22nd June 2017.

Euromonitor. (2010). *Best performing channel in alcoholic drinks in 2010: On-trade vs. Off-trade volume.* Retrieved from: https://blog.euromonitor.com/best-performing-channel-in-alcoholic-drinks-in-2010-on-trade-vs-off-trade-volume/on 6th July 2020.

Food Standards Australia & New Zealand. (2014). *Labelling of alcoholic beverages: User guide.* Retrieved from: https://www.foodstandards.gov.au/code/userguide/pages/labellingofalcoholic4967.aspx on 5th February 2021.

Frayman, B., & Dawson, W. (1981). The effect of object shape and mode of presentation on judgments of apparent volume. *Perception & Psychophysics, 29*(1), 56–62. https://doi.org/10.3758/BF03198840

Gawronski, B., & Bodenhausen, G. V. (2006). Associative and propositional processes in evaluation: An integrative review of implicit and explicit attitude change. *Psychological Bulletin, 132*(5), 692–731. https://doi.org/10.1037/0033-2909.132.5.692

Geier, A. B., Rozin, P., & Doros, G. (2006). Unit bias: A new heuristic that helps explain the effect of portion size on food intake. *Psychological Science, 17*(6), 521–525. https://doi.org/10.1111/j.1467-9280.2006.01738.x

Geller, E. S., Kalsher, M. J., & Clarke, S. W. (1991). Beer versus mixed-drink consumption at fraternity parties: A time and place for low-alcohol alternatives. *Journal of Studies on Alcohol, 52*(3), 197–204. https://doi.org/10.15288/jsa.1991.52.197

Griswold, M. G., Fullman, N., Hawley, C., Arian, N., Zimsen, S. R. M., Tymeson, H. D., … Gakidou, E. (2018). Alcohol use and burden for 195 countries and territories, 1990–2016: A systematic analysis for the global burden of disease study 2016. *The Lancet, 392*(10152), 1015–1035. https://doi.org/10.1016/S0140-6736(18)31310-2

Higgs, S. (2015). Social norms and their influence on eating behaviours. *Appetite, 86*, 38–44. https://doi.org/10.1016/j.appet.2014.10.021

Hofmann, W., Friese, M., & Wiers, R. W. (2008). Impulsive versus reflective influences on health behavior: A theoretical framework and empirical review. *Health Psychology Review, 2*(2), 111–137. https://doi.org/10.1080/17437190802617668

Hollands, G. J., Bignardi, G., Johnston, M., Kelly, M. P., Ogilvie, D., Petticrew, M., … Marteau, T. M. (2017). The TIPPME intervention typology for changing environments to change behaviour. *Nature Human Behaviour, 1*, 0140. https://doi.org/10.1038/s41562-017-0140. https://www.nature.com/articles/s41562-017-0140#supplementary-information

Hollands, G. J., Marteau, T. M., & Fletcher, P. C. (2016). Non-conscious processes in changing health-related behaviour: A conceptual analysis and framework. *Health Psychology Review, 10*(4), 381–394. https://doi.org/10.1080/17437199.2015.1138093

Hollands, G. J., Shemilt, I., Marteau, T. M., Jebb, S. A., Kelly, M. P., Nakamura, R., … Ogilvie, D. (2013). Altering micro-environments to change population health behaviour: Towards an evidence base for choice architecture interventions. *BMC Public Health, 13*(1), 1218. https://doi.org/10.1186/1471-2458-13-1218

Hollands, G. J., Shemilt, I., Marteau, T. M., Jebb, S. A., Lewis, H. B., Wei, Y., … Ogilvie, D. (2015). Portion, package or tableware size for changing selection and consumption of food, alcohol and tobacco. *Cochrane Database of Systematic Reviews, 9*, CD011045. https://doi.org/10.1002/14651858.CD011045.pub2

Hollands, J., & Dyre, B. P. (2000). Bias in proportion judgments: The cyclical power model. *Psychological Review, 107*(3), 500-524. https://doi.org/10.1037/0033-295X.107.3.500

Holmes, J., Angus, C., & Meier, P. S. (2015). UK alcohol industry's "billion units pledge": Interim evaluation flawed. *BMJ, 350*(h), 1301. https://doi.org/10.1136/bmj.h1301

Home Office, Department of Health, Baker, N., Ellison, J., Hunt, J., & May, T. (2014). Alcohol industry takes action to tackle irresponsible drinking. Retrieved from https://www.gov.uk/government/news/alcohol-industry-takes-action-to-tackle-irresponsible-drinking

Institute of Alcohol Studies. (2019). *Consumption of alcohol: Factsheets*. Retrieved from: http://www.ias.org.uk/uploads/images/Consumption/Slide15.png

Jones, S. C., & Gregory, P. (2009). The impact of more visible standard drink labelling on youth alcohol consumption: Helping young people drink (ir) responsibly? *Drug and Alcohol Review, 28*(3), 230–234. https://doi.org/10.1111/j.1465-3362.2008.00020.x

Kerr, W. C., Patterson, D., Koenen, M. A., & Greenfield, T. K. (2009). Large drinks are no mistake: Glass size, not shape, affects alcoholic beverage drink pours. *Drug and Alcohol Review, 28*(4), 360–365. https://doi.org/10.1111/j.1465-3362.2009.00056.x

Kersbergen, I., Oldham, M., Jones, A., Field, M., Angus, C., & Robinson, E. (2018). Reducing the standard serving size of alcoholic beverages prompts reductions in alcohol consumption. *Addiction, 113*, 1598–1608. https://doi.org/10.1111/add.14228

Khan, U., & Dhar, R. (2006). Licensing effects in consumer choice. *Journal of Marketing Research, 43*(2), 259–266. https://doi.org/10.1509/jmkr.43.2.259

Langfield, T., Pechey, R., Pilling, M., & Marteau, T. M. (2018). Impact of glass shape on time taken to drink a soft drink: A laboratory-based experiment. *PLoS One, 13*(8), e0202793. https://doi.org/10.1371/journal.pone.0202793

Langfield, T., Pechey, R., Pilling, M. A., & Marteau, T. M. (2020). Glassware design and drinking behaviours: a review of impact and mechanisms using a new typology of drinking behaviours. *Health Psychology Review,* 1–23. https://doi.org/10.1080/17437199.2020.1842230

McCann, M. T., Wallace, J. M., Robson, P. J., Rennie, K. L., McCaffrey, T. A., Welch, R. W., & Livingstone, M. B. E. (2013). Influence of nutrition labelling on food portion size consumption. *Appetite, 65*, 153–158. https://doi.org/10.1016/j.appet.2013.02.013

Nicholls, J. (2010). *Drinking cultures and consumption in England: Historical trends and policy implications*. Retrieved from https://www.publications.parliament.uk/pa/cm200910/cmselect/cmhealth/151/151we21.htm#note 66.

Nielsen. (2018). *The rise of no and low alcohol*. Retrieved from: https://www.nielsen.com/uk/en/insights/article/2018/rise-of-no-and-low-alcohol/ on 14th August 2019.

ONS. (2017). *Adult drinking habits in Great Britain: 2005 to 2016*. Newport, England: Office for National Statistics.

Pearson, R. G. (1964). Judgment of volume from photographs of complex shapes. *Perceptual and Motor Skills, 18*(3), 889–900. https://doi.org/10.2466/pms.1964.18.3.889

Pechey, R., Attwood, A. S., Couturier, D.-L., Munafò, M. R., Scott-Samuel, N. E., Woods, A., & Marteau, T. M. (2015). Does glass size and shape influence judgements of the volume of wine? *PLoS One, 10*(12), e0144536. https://doi.org/10.1371/journal.pone.0144536

Pechey, R., Couturier, D.-L., Hollands, G. J., Mantzari, E., Munafò, M. R., & Marteau, T. M. (2016). Does wine glass size influence sales for on-site consumption? A multiple treatment reversal design. *BMC Public Health, 16*(1), 390. https://doi.org/10.1186/s12889-016-3068-z

Pechey, R., Couturier, D.-L., Hollands, G. J., Mantzari, E., Zupan, Z., & Marteau, T. M. (2017). Wine glass size and wine sales: A replication study in two bars. *BMC Research Notes, 10*(1), 287. https://doi.org/10.1186/s13104-017-2610-0

Perkins, H. W. (2002). Social norms and the prevention of alcohol misuse in collegiate contexts. *Journal of Studies on Alcohol, Supplement*, (s14), 164–172. https://doi.org/10.15288/jsas.2002.s14.164

Petticrew, M., Shemilt, I., Lorenc, T., Marteau, T. M., Melendez-Torres, G. J., O'Mara-Eves, A., … Thomas, J. (2017). Alcohol advertising and public health: Systems perspectives versus narrow perspectives. *Journal of Epidemiology and Community Health, 71*(3), 308–312. http://dx.doi.org/10.1136/jech-2016-207644

Piaget, J., & Inhelder, B. (1969). *The child's conception of space*. New York, NY: Basic Books.

Pilling, M., Clarke, N., Pechey, R., Hollands, G. J., & Marteau, T. M. (2020). Wine glass size and sales: A mega-analysis of studies in bars and restaurants. *Addiction, 115*, 1660–1667. https://doi.org/10.1111/add.14998

Probst, C., Roerecke, M., Behrendt, S., & Rehm, J. (2014). Socioeconomic differences in alcohol-attributable mortality compared with all-cause mortality: A systematic review and meta-analysis. *International Journal of Epidemiology, 43*(4), 1314–1327. https://doi.org/10.1093/ije/dyu043

Raghubir, P., & Krishna, A. (1999). Vital dimensions in volume perception: Can the eye fool the stomach? *Journal of Marketing Research, 36*(3), 313–326. https://doi.org/10.1177/002224379903600302

Rehm, J., Lachenmeier, D. W., Llopis, E. J., Imtiaz, S., & Anderson, P. (2016). Evidence of reducing ethanol content in beverages to reduce harmful use of alcohol. *The Lancet Gastroenterology & Hepatology, 1*, 78–83. https://doi.org/10.1016/S2468-1253(16)30013-9

Shemilt, I., Hendry, V. L., & Marteau, T. M. (2017). What do we know about the effects of exposure to 'low alcohol' and equivalent product labelling on the amounts of alcohol, food and tobacco people select and consume? A systematic review. *BMC Public Health, 17*, 29. https://doi.org/10.1186/s12889-016-3956-2

Smith, L., & Foxcroft, D. (2009). *Drinking in the UK: An exploration of trends*. York: Joseph Rowntree Foundation. Retrieved from https://www.jrf.org.uk/sites/default/files/jrf/migrated/files/UK-alcohol-trends-FULL.pdf

Spence, C., & Van Doorn, G. (2017). Does the shape of the drinking receptacle influence taste/flavour perception? A review. *Beverages, 3*(3), 33. https://doi.org/10.3390/beverages3030033

Spence, C., & Wan, X. (2015). Beverage perception and consumption: The influence of the container on the perception of the contents. *Food Quality and Preference, 39*, 131–140. https://doi.org/10.1016/j.foodqual.2014.07.007

Stead, M., Angus, K., Macdonald, L., & Bauld, L. (2014). Looking into the glass: Glassware as an alcohol marketing tool, and the implications for policy. *Alcohol and Alcoholism, 49*(3), 317–320. https://doi.org/10.1093/alcalc/agt178

Stockwell, T. (2006). *A review of research into the impacts of alcohol warning labels on attitudes and behaviours*. Victoria, Canada: Centre for Addictions Research of BC. Retrieved from: https://dspace.library.uvic.ca/bitstream/handle/1828/4785/Alcohol%20Warning%20Labels%202006.pdf?s

Strack, F., & Deutsch, R. (2004). Reflective and impulsive determinants of social behavior. *Personality and Social Psychology Review, 8*(3), 220–247. https://doi.org/10.1207/s15327957pspr0803_1

Thaler, R. H., & Sunstein, C. R. (2008). *Nudge: Improving decisions about health, wealth and happiness* (2nd ed.). London, England: Penguin.

The European Parliament and the Council of the European Union. (2011). Regulation (EU) No 1169/2011 of the European Parliament and the Council of the European Union of 25 October 2011 on the provision of food information to consumers. Retrieved from: http://eur-lex.europa.eu/legal-content/EN/ALL/?uri=CELEX:32011R1169 on 8th August 2017.

Troy, D. M., Attwood, A. S., Maynard, O. M., Scott-Samuel, N. E., Hickman, M., Woods, A., & Munafò, M. R. (2018). Effect of glass shape on the pouring accuracy of liquid volume. *PLoS One, 13*(10), e0204562. https://doi.org/10.1371/journal.pone.0204562

Troy, D. M., Maynard, O. M., Hickman, M., Attwood, A. S., & Munafò, M. R. (2015). The effect of glass shape on alcohol consumption in a naturalistic setting: A feasibility study. *Pilot and Feasibility Studies, 1*(1), 27. https://doi.org/10.1186/s40814-015-0022-2

Varey, C. A., Mellers, B. A., & Birnbaum, M. H. (1990). Judgments of proportions. *Journal of Experimental Psychology: Human Perception and Performance, 16*(3), 613–625. https://doi.org/10.1037/0096-1523.16.3.613

Vasiljevic, M., Coulter, L., Petticrew, M., & Marteau, T. M. (2018). Marketing messages accompanying online selling of low/er and regular strength wine and beer products in the UK: A content analysis. *BMC Public Health, 18*, 147. https://doi.org/10.1186/s12889-018-5040-6

Vasiljevic, M., Couturier, D. L., Frings, D., Moss, A. C., Albery, I. P., & Marteau, T. M. (2018). Impact of lower strength alcohol labeling on consumption: A randomized controlled trial. *Health Psychology, 37*(7), 658–667. https://doi.org/10.1037/hea0000622

Vasiljevic, M., Couturier, D. L., & Marteau, T. M. (2018). Impact on product appeal of labeling wine and beer with (a) lower strength alcohol verbal descriptors and (b) percent alcohol by volume (% ABV): An experimental study. *Psychology of Addictive Behaviors, 32*(7), 779–791. https://doi.org/10.1037/adb0000376

Vasiljevic, M., Couturier, D. L., & Marteau, T. M. (2019). What are the perceived target groups and occasions for wines and beers labelled with verbal and numerical descriptors of lower alcohol strength? An experimental study. *BMJ Open, 9*(6), e024412. http://dx.doi.org/10.1136/bmjopen-2018-024412

White, A. M., Kraus, C. L., McCracken, L. A., & Swartzwelder, H. S. (2003). Do College students drink more than they think? Use of a free-pour paradigm to determine how college students define standard drinks. *Alcoholism: Clinical and Experimental Research, 27*(11), 1750–1756. https://doi.org/10.1097/01.ALC.0000095866.17973.AF

Wilkinson, C., & Room, R. (2009). Warnings on alcohol containers and advertisements: International experience and evidence on effects. *Drug and Alcohol Review, 28*, 426–435. https://doi.org/10.1111/j.1465-3362.2009.00055.x

World Health Organization. (2018). Global, regional, and national comparative risk assessment of 84 behavioural, environmental and occupational, and metabolic risks or clusters of risks for 195 countries and territories, 1990–2017: A systematic analysis for the Global Burden of Disease Study 2017. *The Lancet, 392*(10159), 1923–1994. https://doi.org/10.1016/S0140-6736(18)32225-6

Zupan, Z., Evans, A., Couturier, D.-L., & Marteau, T. M. (2017). Wine glass size in England from 1700 to 2017: A measure of our time. *BMJ, 359*, j5623. https://doi.org/10.1136/bmj.j5623

Zupan, Z., Pechey, R., Couturier, D. L., Hollands, G. J., & Marteau, T. M. (2017). Micro-drinking behaviours and consumption of wine in different wine glass sizes: A laboratory study. *BMC Psychology, 5*(1), 17. https://doi.org/10.1186/s40359-017-0183-2

Section III

Drinking Identities

11

Young Adults and Online Drinking Identities

Antonia Lyons and Ian Goodwin

Introduction

The meanings and functions of alcohol consumption depend upon the social and cultural environments in which it takes place (see Sect. 2). Factors such as age, ethnicity, gender, sexuality and socio-economic status also work together to impact the meanings, functions and experiences of drinking alcohol (Day, 2012; Hunt & Antin, 2019; Lyons, McCreanor, Goodwin, & Moewaka Barnes, 2017). Alcohol has long been linked to creating and performing specific identities, particularly among youth and young adults. This chapter provides an overview of some of the research on young adults, alcohol consumption and identities, before turning our attention to the rapidly changing digital environment and social media. Social media are essential to consider in any work exploring young people's lives and identities, given that they are now the fundamental infrastructure for young people's social worlds in Western societies (Dobson, Robards, & Carah, 2018). The chapter also explores how social media have changed drinking practices and cultures, and the implications of this for young people's identities, focusing on gender identities primarily.

A. Lyons (✉)
School of Health, Victoria University of Wellington, Wellington, New Zealand
e-mail: antonia.lyons@vuw.ac.nz

I. Goodwin
School of English and Media Studies, Massey University, Wellington, New Zealand
e-mail: i.goodwin@massey.ac.nz

R. Cooke et al. (eds.), *The Palgrave Handbook of Psychological Perspectives on Alcohol Consumption*, https://doi.org/10.1007/978-3-030-66941-6_11

Finally, the chapter considers social media platforms in terms of their recent mobility on smartphones, their diversity and their commercialised nature, drawing on recent research to show how they may open up new opportunities for youth to develop their identities around drinking.

Youth and young adults drink more alcohol, and drink more frequently, than other population groups (e.g. World Health Organisation, 2018). Recent surveys conducted in Western societies show that overall alcohol consumption is declining in teenagers (Livingston & Vashishtha, 2019), although this decline is apparent in younger teenagers rather than older teenagers or adults, suggesting there is a delay in starting to drink (Twenge & Park, 2019). Furthermore, even in younger teenagers there are some groups whose consumption levels have stayed the same or increased, including ethnic minorities and those with poor mental health (Fat, Shelton, & Cable, 2018). Subgroups of heavier younger drinkers have also not displayed decreased consumption levels, perhaps due to homogenous drinking groups where (heavy) drinking is normative (Caluzzi, 2019).

There has also been a global convergence of young people's drinking cultures. Gordon, Heim and MacAskill (2012) have argued that the dichotomy between 'wet' and 'dry' drinking cultures that has been such a feature of European drinking cultures in the past is no longer relevant (Chap. 7). This is due to a shift in many societies towards more liberalised alcohol policies, as well as multinational alcohol corporations and a globalised culture of social media. Many young people drink heavily, actively seeking intoxication and drunkenness, because it is fun, pleasurable and social (see Chap. 1). Researchers have conceptualised such drinking patterns using notions of 'determined drunkenness' and 'calculated hedonism' where young people actively aim to drink until intoxicated as a form of pleasure, excitement and self-expression (Measham, 2006, 2011; Measham & Brain, 2005; Szmigin et al., 2008). Research highlights a number of reasons why young people engage in drinking to intoxication with groups of friends. These include providing ways to challenge or escape (albeit temporarily) social roles and societal expectations (Bannister & Paicentini, 2008; Haydock, 2016), as well as to build friendships and collective forms of belonging (Niland, Lyons, Goodwin, & Hutton, 2013; Szmigin et al., 2008). They also use alcohol to explore, create and perform their identities (Lennox, Emslie, Sweeting, & Lyons, 2018).

Young Adults, Alcohol Consumption and Identities

Much of the research in the field of alcohol and identities has focused on gender, and particularly masculinities and femininities. Traditionally, consuming alcohol in public, and drinking beer, was a male past-time linked to masculine identities (Lemle & Mishkind, 1989). Research has shown that drinking to intoxication has been a way for young men to demonstrate hegemonic masculinity in Western societies (Campbell, 2000; Hunt & Antin, 2019; Peralta, 2007; Willott & Lyons, 2012). With changes in drinking contexts, such as an increase in women's drinking, greater diversity in places to drink and a greater choice of alcoholic products, there are alternative masculine identities available in relation to alcohol consumption and drinking practices (Emslie, Hunt, & Lyons, 2013; Mullen, Watson, Swift, & Black, 2007; Thurnell-Read, 2011). Some young men also use alcohol to engage in alternative masculine identities, such as portraying particular class identities through specific products (e.g. drinking 'craft' beer vs. lager; Lyons, 2009; Lyons & Gough, 2017; Mullen et al., 2007). Furthermore, alcohol has been found to provide a way for men to transgress notions of dominant (heterosexual) masculinity by allowing behaviour that is not associated with masculinity, such as sharing and displaying emotion to other men (Emslie et al., 2013; Peralta, 2008) and engaging in homosexual behaviour (Peralta, 2008).

Historically, women's drinking was considered non-respectable and unfeminine (Ettore, 2004), associated with lower- or working-class women (Lindsay & Supski, 2017). This has changed in recent years with women's increased economic and social freedoms (Lyons & Willott, 2008). Most women engage in particular forms of drinking, drinking particular products, and drinking in particular ways, to produce idealised notions of femininities. However, while a drinking femininity is acceptable, a 'drunken femininity' is not (Hutton, Griffin, Lyons, Niland, & McCreanor, 2016). The 'ladette' culture of the 1990s and 2000s in the UK saw young women challenging gender stereotypes around alcohol by engaging in patterns of drinking and behaviour traditionally associated with young men ('lads'). This included drinking beer and drinking excessively in public, behaving boisterously, assertively, drunkenly and outrageously. Such behaviour drew severe criticism of young—particularly working-class—women in the UK press, where ladettes became the 'figurehead of the British tabloid newspaper portrayal of the so-called binge drinking epidemic' (Watts, Linke, Murray, & Barker, 2015, p.220). Media accounts portrayed these young women as lacking self-control and self-esteem, thus transgressing social norms and expectations around femininity. This led to moral panic about women's drinking (Day, Gough, & McFadden, 2004), highlighting ongoing gendered double standards around alcohol consumption and drinking patterns.

Young women's drinking has also been linked to broader theorisations of neoliberal imperatives that individuals should be actively engaged in continual self-transformation and improvement, performing authentic feminine identities in the night time economy (Goodwin, Griffin, Lyons, McCreanor, & Moewaka Barnes, 2016; Griffin, Szmigin, Bengry-Howell, Hackley, & Mistral, 2013). By engaging in cultures of intoxication, young women have been drinking in more traditional masculine ways, transgressing ideal femininity, although many—particularly middle-class women—are also feminising these practices (Lyons & Willott, 2008). They are drinking heavily, but drinking more 'feminine' drinks, such as sparkling wine, drinking in glamorous places, such as clubs and bars, and feminising their appearance through make-up and clothing. In whatever ways they engage in cultures of intoxication, women face contradictions in creating their identities as they are expected drink heavily but at the same time maintain a hypersexual and attractive appearance (Griffin et al., 2013; Lindsay & Supski, 2017).

More recent research has explored the role of social practices around alcohol consumption for both sexual and gender identities (Hunt, Antin, Sanders, & Sisneros, 2019). This work highlights the importance of safe and comfortable spaces where hegemonic masculinity and heteronormativity are absent or less dominant for lesbian, gay, bisexual, transgender, queer and intersex people to socialise and engage in identity performances involving alcohol consumption (Hunt et al., 2019). Other work also demonstrates that people consume particular drinks to convey or express specific sexual identities and to challenge dominant preconceptions about gender (Emslie, Lennox, & Ireland, 2017). Gender also intersects with class in creating particular identities (e.g. Bailey, Griffin, & Shankar, 2015). Thus research suggests there are many ways in which alcohol consumption is linked to creating identities in young people. In recent years this has shifted, as it has extended into new digital environments with the proliferation of new technologies and social media platforms.

Alcohol Consumption, Social Media and Creating Identities

Young people have enthusiastically embraced emerging digital technologies, particularly social media platforms. Social media are digital technologies that allow people to interact, share and consume online content. They have become increasingly diverse and include social networking sites that tend to have profiles, feeds, comments and can be public, such as Facebook, Instagram, YouTube, WeChat and Twitter, as well as social media platforms that allow communication and sharing of digital content with others—both individuals and groups—such as WhatsApp, Snapchat and Viber. The latter were developed primarily for use on mobile devices; some social networking sites have their own mobile messaging platforms, such as Facebook Messenger and WeChat Messenger. Social media platforms are central to young people's processes of identity construction (Zhao, Grasmuck, & Martin, 2008), allowing them to express, explore and experiment with their identities (Gündüz, 2017). They can be viewed as 'identity-making toolboxes' for young people (Doster, 2013, p. 267). These platforms now play a key part in many young people's drinking practices, and in their associated identity practices and displays (Lyons et al., 2017).

Contemporary online drinking cultures include a diverse range of content and activities, such as posting and sharing photos and videos of drinking occasions, organising social events, socialising online while preloading (see Chap. 13) in different locations, meeting up, hooking up, commenting and tagging on alcohol-related content, hashtagging and communicating about alcohol-sponsored events, taking up promotions and engaging in competitions (e.g. see Moreno & Whitehill, 2016; Ridout, 2016; Westgate & Holliday, 2016 for overviews). Research has explored the ways in which young adults use social media in their drinking practices and their drinking cultures more generally to perform and forge their identities (e.g. Goodwin & Griffin, 2017; Lindsay & Supski, 2017). This work highlights how identity is created through both offline socialising and online sociality, which is the crux of social media platforms. Drinking-related activities on social media function to reinforce and maintain young adults' friendships and social relationships (e.g. Niland, Lyons, Goodwin, & Hutton, 2015), solidifying bonds between people and creating identities linked to friendship groups and friendship practices. Young people share images and posts on social media of themselves and their friends engaging in drinking practices, representations that have become integral to drinking as a locus of identity for young adults. This online material gains a lot of attention, and often gets circulated around networks as humorous and fun content within and beyond peer networks (Carah & Dobson, 2016; Lyons, Goodwin, Griffin, McCreanor, & Moewaka Barnes, 2016).

These practices take place within an online environment in which alcohol-related content is pervasive, and contributes to the normalisation of drinking and alcohol within young people's everyday lives (Cavazos-Rehg, Krauss, Sowles, & Bierut, 2015; Nicholls, 2012). According to Westgate and Holliday (2016), posting and engaging with alcohol-related online content affects perceived social norms and the creation of individual and group identities. Research demonstrates that the sheer amount of alcohol content on social networking sites affects alcohol consumption through influencing social norms (Ridout, 2016; Westgate & Holliday, 2016). Yet young people also exercise considerable agency in curating online individual and collective identities through alcohol consumption practices, sharing content, communicating, uploading photos and performing particular kinds of online drinking identities. Importantly, young people are encouraged, in both online and offline spaces, to perform a 'calculated hedonism' where conspicuous (and over-) consumption of alcohol are celebrated, although simultaneously bodily control and deportment are expected (Szmigin et al., 2008).

While these virtual spaces and practices provide important ways through which young adults craft and actively create their own identities, how this plays out—and the work involved—varies across social dimensions such as gender, class and ethnicity, and the intersectionality of these dimensions. Factors such as gender influence how young adults take part in and engage with online drinking cultures (e.g. Atkinson & Sumnall, 2016; Hutton et al., 2016; Moewaka Barnes, Niland, Samu, Sciasia, & McCreanor, 2017). As noted previously (Goodwin & Lyons, 2019), drinking and its online display is a way for young adults to exercise considerable agency as they narrate their own identities, but these practices can also reproduce broader power relations that limit, constrain or shape young adults' lives. This will be outlined more fully in the next section.

Masculinities and Femininities in Online Drinking Cultures

Within online drinking cultures, research suggests that societal expectations of appropriate and inappropriate masculinities and femininities are negotiated as young people display, share and comment on drinking photos on social media (Brown & Gregg, 2012; Dobson, 2014). Social media platforms, and social networking sites particularly, have always been used as a way for users to construct and perform gendered identities (Cook & Hasmath, 2014). Generally, such performances reflect traditional notions of masculinity and femininity (e.g. Haferkamp, Eimler, Papadakis, & Kruck, 2012; Kapidzic & Herring, 2014). In an early study in this field, Mendelson and Papacharissi (2010) explored the photos on US college students' personal Facebook photo galleries, and found that women had more casual photos and photos that involved sexy and flirtatious posing. Men tended to have more formal photos that emphasised friendships and 'drinking buddies'. The researchers concluded that posting and sharing drinking photos enabled users to perform gendered identities (Mendelson & Papacharissi, 2010).

The practices involved in sharing drinking-related content on social media platforms are themselves gendered, highlight how these issues go beyond online representations of gender. Taking and uploading photos, checking, tagging and untagging during a night out drinking with friends have been found to be practices engaged in more frequently, and more intensely, by young women (Goodwin et al., 2016; Lyons et al., 2016). Women also engage in much greater self-surveillance during drinking practices than men, orienting to cameras and ensuring their appearance is appropriate, as well as checking, deleting and untagging photos on Facebook (Atkinson & Sumnall, 2016; Hutton et al., 2016; Lyons et al., 2016). Drinking photos appear to be highly valued by both men and women, although the acceptability of the 'drunken' photo was much greater for men than women (Hutton et al., 2016). Unruly, unrestrained and carnivalesque-type behaviours are expected and also highly valued among young men during events that involve excessive drinking (e.g. Hubbard, 2013; Thurnell-Read, 2011); indeed, the loss of bodily control during these situations is 'condoned and encouraged within the strictures of hegemonic masculinity' (Thurnell-Read, 2011, p. 978).

In the UK, research has examined the Facebook photographs of white, heterosexual male university students and found over half of these photos involved alcohol, drinking and partying (Scoats, 2015). Many of the drinking-related photos involved displays of homosocial behaviours (e.g. men touching, kissing and dancing together), reinforcing previous findings that alcohol enables transgression of heteronormative boundaries (de Visser & Smith, 2007; Peralta, 2008). With the advent of social media, these transgressions can be captured and posted online. Although they may suggest there is a broadening of acceptable masculinities in certain circumstances, often gender transgressions are posted ironically by (privileged) young men in their identity performances, while dominant forms of masculinity are reinforced (Manago,

2013; Nagel & Mora, 2010). Such transgressions, therefore, can effectively function to reinforce heteronormativity by positioning them as a 'spectacle', enabled through (apparent) excessive drinking, and thus highlighting that they are not normally acceptable within the group.

While much of the research exploring identities within online drinking cultures has focused on gendered identities, some has examined how gender intersects with other aspects of identity, such as class and ethnicity. Little research work has explored sexuality, or forms of non-binary gender identities. Initial research has found that in the UK, class intersects heavily with depictions—and judgements—of women's drinking online (Bailey & Griffin, 2017). Here the concern for achieving respectable femininities while drinking on a night out, and ensuring online displays represent such respectability, is important for many young women. Working-class women drinkers are 'othered' and positioned in derogatory ways due to not meeting the standards of 'respectable' femininities (Bailey & Griffin, 2017; Lennox et al., 2018). The performances of femininities in online drinking cultures reflect the contradictory pressures young women experience in public drinking spaces (Lindsay & Supski, 2017).

Ethnicity is also important in processes of online identity creation, although again there has been little research in this field. Moewaka-Barnes and colleagues (Moewaka Barnes et al., 2017) explored young Māori, Pasifika and Pākehā New Zealanders' drinking practices and the role of social networking sites in their drinking cultures. They highlighted that cultural factors influenced social media use and representations of drinking online, while societal power relations meant that some groups were much more reluctant to engage in portrayals of drinking online. It is important for future research to consider intersectional identities, drinking practices and online drinking cultures, as these highlight social power relations that are often left unseen. The changing nature of the digital environment is also highly relevant to young people's identities within online drinking cultures.

The Shifting Social Media Environment: Multiple and Mobile Platforms

Although much of the previous research on young adults, online identities, drinking practices and cultures focused on Facebook (Boyle, Earle, LaBrie, & Ballou, 2017), the recent proliferation of social media has meant that young people now use multiple platforms that are more image-based (e.g. Instagram) with content that is not as permanent (e.g. Snapchat) (Anderson & Jiang,

2018). As young people manage multiple social media platforms, social norms and practices are evolving around what is acceptable and desirable to post on different platforms (and what is not; Boczkowski, Matassi, & Mitchelstein, 2018). These have implications for alcohol use and identity performances.

Previous research into drinking cultures highlights how drinking photos have been a key part of young adults' Facebook content (Goodwin et al., 2016), and central to drinking cultures and identity performances across Facebook, Instagram, Snapchat, Twitter and WhatsApp (see Atkinson & Sumnall, 2016 for more detail). People have different expectations around the kinds of drinking photos and content that should appear on different social media sites, thereby potentially creating a range of identities—simultaneously—often for different audiences (Zhao, Lampe, & Ellison, 2016). In a study employing hypothetical, photographic vignettes of alcohol consumption, Boyle et al. (2017) found that young adults viewed Instagram as where they would likely see attractive and glamorous photos, and Snapchat as where they would likely see photos depicting the negative consequences of drinking. Other work has found that alcohol was positively and socially framed on both Facebook and Instagram, promoting young adults' drinking (Hendriks, den Putte, Winifed, & Moreno, 2018). Glamorous depictions of alcohol use 'fit' with Instagram, a space that is tailored to stylised self-presentations, while more negative depictions 'fit' with the temporary and more playful nature of Snapchat (Boczkowski et al., 2018; Boyle et al., 2017).

Evidence suggests that drinking cultures are 'airbrushed' on social media sites where content is more permanent (such as Facebook) to present positive, fun and enjoyable images and content about drinking with friends (Niland, Lyons, Goodwin, & Hutton, 2014), and desirable identity performances (Hutton et al., 2016; Lyons et al., 2016). By excluding explicit images or content about the negative outcomes of drinking events and practices, drinking cultures reinforce and normalise the view that drinking alcohol is always pleasurable without negative consequences, and always involves positive and desirable gender and identity displays. In contrast, as a platform in which content disappears after a few seconds, Snapchat is perceived to be appropriate to share more negative content around drinking (Boyle et al., 2017). This sharing may be important given that young adults often share and re-work their 'negative' drinking events into 'good drinking stories' that function to reinforce friendships and have a laugh (Griffin, Bengry-Howell, Hackley, Mistral, & Szmigin, 2009). Such sharing may also make it possible for young people to portray less conventionally desirable identity displays, and engage in a broader range of identity performances with friends. The temporary nature of Snapchat posts and Instagram stories may be particularly valuable for drinkers who feel they could be marginalised for their drinking, so this provides a way to share with friends without the potential of disapproval from others within their broader networks with whom they do not want to share drinking photos.

The widespread availability and use of smartphones has also led to an intensification of social media use. Smartphones have become increasingly embedded within everyday life (Mackey, 2016), providing young people with access to ubiquitous virtual environments that are increasingly where social life is playing out (Anderson & Jiang, 2018; Twenge, 2017). This allows for continuous access to 'mobile' social media platforms, providing an environment in which physical and virtual worlds are enmeshed. Mobile social media allow young people to micro-coordinate their social and drinking events (Bertel & Ling, 2016) and share their 'fun' drinking photos with friends in the moment, enhancing the pleasure they get from drinking with friends (e.g. Lyons & Willott, 2008; Niland et al., 2013). Furthermore, while getting ready to go out drinking with friends and/or while preloading (Chap. 13) prior to a night out, young adults can be, and are often expected to be, in continual contact with friends who are getting ready and preloading in other places (McCreanor et al., 2016). This intensification of social media use in drinking practices and cultures—used routinely and regularly on smartphones, and in different ways on different platforms—enables users more flexibility to construct their individual and collective identities through alcohol consumption. However, this intensification is occurring on platforms owned by corporations that have profit as their main goal.

The Commercial Nature of Social Media

Social media are commercialised platforms that operate through selling user-data to third parties. Alcohol companies and other commercial alcohol interests have been quick to use young adults' enthusiasm for sharing alcohol-related content on social media sites (Nicholls, 2012; Niland, McCreanor, Lyons, & Griffin, 2017). They use a range of sophisticated marketing techniques to promote drinking among young people, linking alcohol products to processes of identity creation (Lyons et al., 2017; McCreanor et al., 2013). The branded messages of corporate marketers are increasingly subtle, pervasive and tailored in real time to fit seamlessly with young people's identities and social practices (Carah & Angus, 2018; Niland et al., 2017). This makes it difficult to distinguish between user generated and commercial content on social media (Lyons et al., 2017).

The new marketing practices of alcohol corporations are more covert than 'offline' practices, mimicking user cultures, drawing on users' everyday identity-making processes and sociality and recruiting users to do free work for their brands. Young people's social activities while drinking reinforce individualised, branded identifications with drinks, venues and practices. Instagram influencers are sponsored to create user-generated branded content and post images with alcohol brand hashtags linked to specific highly valued cultural events (Carah, 2017). Such forms of digital alcohol marketing encourage both consumption-based identities and alcohol-driven socialising (McCreanor et al., 2013; Niland et al., 2017). Additionally, mobile social media platforms have locational affordances that allow commercial establishments to target and interact with young people as they engage in nights out drinking with their peers (Carah, 2014b). Social media marketing techniques based on virtual tracking allow commercial establishments to encourage young people to visit and attend specific nightlife locations and events (Carah & Dobson, 2016; Niland et al., 2017). Alcohol companies also encourage drinking and promote particular drinking identities by using augmented reality and immersive, interactive apps (e.g. Zaitsev, 2017).

Overall, marketing and branding activities used by alcohol companies within the evolving social media environment are highly effective and generate lucrative income from and for mobile social media platforms (Carah, 2014a; Carah & Angus, 2018). These changes have enhanced novel forms of (often real-time) alcohol marketing in ways that stimulate young people's drinking, socialising and identity work. A systematic review of 47 studies in this field concluded that young adults find alcohol-related branded marketing messages highly appealing, and also that exposure to digital alcohol marketing is linked with higher levels of drinking (Jernigan, Noel, Landon, Thornton, & Lobstein, 2017; Lobstein, Landon, Thornton, & Jernigan, 2017). This has led to public concerns about the difficulties of regulating the marketing of unhealthy commodities—including alcohol—on social media (Mart, 2017).

Conclusion

Diverse, mobile, 'always-on' social media open up a range of new opportunities for young people to develop their identities around alcohol consumption and drinking practices. They provide a way for young people to engage in processes of individual and collective forms of identity creation, but within an environment that is heavily laden with alcohol marketing. Social media are primarily visual, providing novel, immediate and fun ways for young people to create their identities linked to drinking and socialising, although this is more easily achieved by some groups than others (Atkinson, Ross-Houle, Begley, & Sumnall, 2017; Lyons et al., 2017). Although they are commercialised platforms, social media also provide spaces of belonging where young people can engage with collective identities around alcohol consumption. Researchers need to expand their focus to the multiple forms of mobile social media platforms that diverse groups of young people are now using in their drinking cultures (Goodwin & Lyons, 2019), and consider what this means for their processes of identity construction across different social groups and in different geographical locations.

References

Anderson, M., & Jiang, J. (2018). *Teens, social media and technology 2018*. Washington, DC: Pew Research Center.

Atkinson, A. M., Ross-Houle, K. M., Begley, E., & Sumnall, H. (2017). An exploration of alcohol advertising on social networking sites: An analysis of content, interactions and young people's perspectives. *Addiction Research & Theory, 25*, 91–102.

Atkinson, A. M., & Sumnall, H. R. (2016). 'If I don't look good, it just doesn't go up': A qualitative study of young women's drinking cultures and practices on social network sites. *International Journal of Drug Policy, 38*, 50–62.

Bailey, L., & Griffin, C. (2017). Social locations: Class, gender and young people's alcohol consumption in a digital world. In *Youth Drinking Cultures in a Digital World* (pp. 31–48). Abingdon, England: Routledge.

Bailey, L., Griffin, C., & Shankar, A. (2015). 'Not a good look': Impossible dilemmas for young women negotiating the culture of intoxication in the United Kingdom. *Substance Use and Misuse, 50*, 747–758.

Bannister, E., & Paicentini, M. (2008). Drunk and (dis)orderly: The role of alcohol in supporting liminality. *NA – Advances in Consumer Research, 35*, 311–318.

Bertel, T., & Ling, R. (2016). "It's just not that exciting anymore": The changing centrality of SMS in the everyday lives of young Danes. *New Media and Society, 18*, 1293–1309.

Boczkowski, P., Matassi, M., & Mitchelstein, E. (2018). How young users deal with multiple platforms: The role of meaning-making in social media repertoires. *Journal of Computer Mediated Communication, 23*, 245–259.

Boyle, S., Earle, A., LaBrie, J., & Ballou, K. (2017). Facebook dethroned: Revealing the more likely social media destinations for college students' depiction of underage drinking. *Addictive Behaviours, 65*, 63–67.

Brown, R., & Gregg, M. (2012). The pedagogy of regret: Facebook, binge drinking and young women. *Continuum, 26*, 357–369.

Caluzzi, G. (2019). Changing but resistant: The importance of integrating heavier young drinkers within a declining drinking culture. *Drugs: Education, Prevention and Policy, 26*, 517–521.

Campbell, H. (2000). The glass phallus: Pub(lic) masculinity and drinking in rural New Zealand. *Rural Society, 65*, 562–581.

Carah, N. (2014a). Brand value: How affective labour helps create brands. *Consumption, Markets and Culture, 17*, 346–366.

Carah, N. (2014b). Watching nightlife: Affective labor, social media, and surveillance. *Television & New Media, 15*, 250–265.

Carah, N. (2017). Alcohol corporations and marketing in social media. In A. C. Lyons, T. McCreanor, I. Goodwin, & H. Moewaka Barnes (Eds.), *Youth drinking cultures in a digital world: Alcohol, social media and cultures of intoxication* (pp. 115–131). Abingdon, England: Routledge.

Carah, N., & Angus, D. (2018). Algorithmic brand culture: Participatory labour, machine learning and branding on social media. *Media, Culture and Society, 40*, 178–194.

Carah, N., & Dobson, A. (2016). Algorithmic hotness: Young women's 'promotion' and 'reconnaissance' work via social media body images. *Social Media + Society, 2*. https://doi.org/10.1177/2056305116672885

Cavazos-Rehg, P., Krauss, M., Sowles, S., & Bierut, L. (2015). "Hey everyone, I'm drunk." An evaluation of drinking-related Twitter chatter. *Journal of Studies on Alcohol and Drugs, 76*, 635–643.

Cook, J., & Hasmath, R. (2014). The discursive construction and performance of gendered identity on social media. *Current Sociology, 62*, 975–993.

Day, K. (2012). Social class, socioeconomic status and 'health-risk' behaviours: A critical analysis. In C. Horrocks & S. Johnson (Eds.), *Advances in health psychology: Critical approaches* (pp. 61–73). New York, NY: Palgrave Macmillan.

Day, K., Gough, B., & McFadden, M. (2004). "Warning! Alcohol can seriously damage your feminine health": A discourse analysis of recent British newspaper coverage of women and drinking. *Feminist Media Studies, 4*, 165–183.

de Visser, R. O., & Smith, J. A. (2007). Alcohol consumption and masculine identity among young men. *Psychology and Health, 22*, 595–614.

Dobson, A. S. (2014). Laddishness online: The possible significations and significance of 'performative shamelessness' for young women in the postfeminist context. *Cultural Studies, 28*, 142–164.

Dobson, A. S., Robards, B., & Carah, N. (Eds.). (2018). *Digital intimate publics and social media*. Cham, Switzerland: Palgrave Macmillan.

Doster, L. (2013). Millennial teens design and redesign themselves in online social networks. *Journal of Consumer Behaviour, 12*, 267–279.

Emslie, C., Hunt, K., & Lyons, A. C. (2013). The role of alcohol in forging and maintaining friendships amongst Scottish men in midlife. *Health Psychology, 32*, 33–41.

Emslie, C., Lennox, J., & Ireland, L. (2017). The role of alcohol in identity construction among LGBT people: A qualitative study. *Sociology of Health & Illness, 39*, 1465–1479.

Ettore, E. M. (2004). Revisioning women and drug use: Gender sensitivity, gendered bodies and reducing harm. *International Journal of Drug Policy, 15*, 327–335.

Fat, L. N., Shelton, N., & Cable, N. (2018). Investigating the growing trend of non-drinking among young people; analysis of repeated cross-sectional surveys in England 2005–2015. *BMC Public Health, 18*, 1090.

Goodwin, I., & Griffin, C. (2017). Neoliberalism, alcohol, and identity. In A. C. Lyons, T. McCreanor, I. Goodwin, & H. Moewaka Barnes (Eds.), *Youth drinking cultures in a digital world* (pp. 15–30). London, England: Routledge.

Goodwin, I., Griffin, C., Lyons, A. C., McCreanor, T., & Moewaka Barnes, H. (2016). Precarious popularity: Facebook drinking photos, the attention economy, and the regime of the branded self. *Social Media + Society, 2*, 1–13.

Goodwin, I., & Lyons, A. (2019). Social media and young adults' drinking cultures: Orienting research towards multiplicity and mobility. In D. Conroy & F. Meashem (Eds.), *Young adult drinking styles: Current perspectives on research, policy and practice* (pp. 133–152). London, England: Palgrave Macmillan.

Gordon, R., Heim, D., & MacAskill, S. (2012). Rethinking drinking cultures: A review of drinking cultures and a reconstructed dimensional approach. *Public Health, 126*, 3–11.

Griffin, C., Bengry-Howell, A., Hackley, C., Mistral, W., & Szmigin, I. (2009). Every time I do it I absolutely annihilate myself': Loss of (self-) consciousness and loss of memory in young people's drinking narratives. *Sociology, 43*, 457–476.

Griffin, C., Szmigin, I., Bengry-Howell, A., Hackley, C., & Mistral, W. (2013). Inhabiting the contradictions: Hypersexual femininity and the culture of intoxication among young women in the UK. *Feminism and Psychology, 23*, 184–206.

Gündüz, U. (2017). The effect of social media on identity construction. *Mediterranean Journal of Social Sciences, 8*, 85–92.

Haferkamp, N., Eimler, S. C., Papadakis, A. M., & Kruck, J. V. (2012). Men are from Mars, women are from Venus? Examining gender differences in self-presentation on social networking sites. *Cyberpsychology, Behavior and Social Networking, 15*, 91–98.

Haydock, W. (2016). The consumption, production and regulation of alcohol in the UK: The relevance of the ambivalence of the carnivalesque. *Sociology, 50*, 1056–1071.

Hendriks, H., den Putte, B., Winifed, A., & Moreno, M. (2018). Social drinking on social media: Content analysis of the social aspects of alcohol-related posts on Facebook and Instagram. *Journal of Medical Internet Research, 20*, 1–12.

Hubbard, P. (2013). Carnage! Coming to a town near you? Nightlife, uncivilised behaviour and the carnivalesque body. *Leisure Studies, 32*, 265–282.

Hunt, G., & Antin, T. (2019). Gender and intoxication: From masculinity to intersectionality. *Drugs: Education, Prevention & Policy, 26*, 70–78.

Hunt, G., Antin, T., Sanders, E., & Sisneros, M. (2019). Queer youth, intoxication and queer drinking spaces. *Journal of Youth Studies, 22*, 380–400.

Hutton, F., Griffin, C., Lyons, A. C., Niland, T., & McCreanor, T. (2016). "Tragic girls" and "crack whores": Alcohol, femininity and Facebook. *Feminism and Psychology, 26*, 73–93.

Jernigan, D., Noel, J., Landon, J., Thornton, N., & Lobstein, T. (2017). Alcohol marketing and youth alcohol consumption: A systematic review of longitudinal studies published since 2008. *Addiction, 112*(Suppl 1), 7–20.

Kapidzic, S., & Herring, S. C. (2014). Race, gender, and self-presentation in teen profile photographs. *New Media & Society, 17*, 958–976.

Lemle, R., & Mishkind, M. E. (1989). Alcohol and masculinity. *Journal of Substance Abuse Treatment, 6*, 213–222.

Lennox, J., Emslie, C., Sweeting, H., & Lyons, A. (2018). The role of alcohol in constructing gender and class identities among young women in the age of social media. *International Journal of Drug Policy, 58*, 13–21.

Lindsay, J., & Supski, S. (2017). Curating identity: Drinking, young women, femininities and social media practices. In A. C. Lyons, T. McCreanor, I. Goodwin, & H. Moewaka Barnes (Eds.), *Youth drinking cultures in a digital world: Alcohol, social media and cultures of intoxication*. Abingdon, England: Routledge.

Livingston, M., & Vashishtha, R. (2019). Have recent declines in adolescent drinking continued into young adulthood? In D. Conroy & F. Meashem (Eds.), *Young adult drinking styles: Current perspectives on research, policy and practice* (pp. 21–46). London, England: Palgrave Macmillan.

Lobstein, T., Landon, J., Thornton, N., & Jernigan, D. (2017). The commercial use of digital media to market alcohol products: A narrative review. *Addiction, 112*, 21–27.

Lyons, A., & Willott, S. (2008). Alcohol consumption, gender identities and women's changing social positions. *Sex Roles, 59*, 694–715.

Lyons, A. C. (2009). Masculinities, femininities, behaviour and health. *Social and Personality Psychology Compass, 3-4*, 394–412.

Lyons, A. C., Goodwin, I., Griffin, C., McCreanor, T., & Moewaka Barnes, H. (2016). Facebook and the fun of drinking photos: Reproducing gendered regimes of power. *Social Media and Society, 2*, 1–13. https://doi.org/10.1177/2056305116672888

Lyons, A. C., & Gough, B. (2017). Youth drinking cultures in a digital world. In A. C. Lyons, T. McCreanor, I. Goodwin, & H. M. Barnes (Eds.), *Alcohol, social media and cultures of intoxication* (pp. 66–79). Abingdon Routledge.

Lyons, A. C., McCreanor, T., Goodwin, I., & Moewaka Barnes, H. (Eds.). (2017). *Youth drinking cultures in a digital world: Alcohol, social media and cultures of intoxication*. Abingdon, England: Routledge.

Mackey, A. (2016). Sticky e/motional connections: Young people, social media, and the re-orientation of affect. *Safundi, 17*, 156–173.

Manago, A. M. (2013). Negotiating a sexy masculinity on social networking sites. *Feminism & Psychology, 23*, 478–497.

Mart, S. (2017). New marketing, new policy? Emerging debates over regulating alcohol campaigns on social media. In A. C. Lyons, T. McCreanor, I. Goodwin, & H. Moewaka Barnes (Eds.), *Youth drinking cultures in a digital world* (pp. 218–219). London, England: Routledge.

McCreanor, T., Lyons, A. C., Griffin, C., Goodwin, I., Moewaka Barnes, H., & Hutton, F. (2013). Youth drinking cultures, social networking and alcohol marketing: Implications for public health. *Critical Public Health, 23*, 110–120. https://doi.org/10.1080/09581596.2012.748883

McCreanor, T., Lyons, A. C., Moewaka Barnes, H., Hutton, F., Goodwin, I., & Griffin, C. (2016). 'Drink a 12 box before you go': Pre-loading among young people in Aotearoa New Zealand. *Kotuitui: New Zealand Journal of Social Sciences, 11*, 36–46. https://doi.org/10.1080/1177083X.2015.1037314

Measham, F. (2006). The new policy mix: Alcohol, harm minimisation, and determined drunkenness in contemporary society. *International Journal of Drug Policy, 17*, 258–268. https://doi.org/10.1016/j.drugpo.2006.02.013

Measham, F. (2011). Drunkeness – A historical and contemporary cross-cultural perspective: "A voluntary madness". In A. Fox & M. MacAvoy (Eds.), *Expressions of drunkenness: (Four hundred rabbits)* (pp. 121–153). New York, NY: Routledge.

Measham, F., & Brain, K. (2005). 'Binge' drinking, British alcohol policy and the new culture of intoxication. *Crime, Media, Culture, 1*, 262–283. https://doi.org/10.1177/1741659005057641

Mendelson, A., & Papacharissi, Z. (2010). Look at us: Collective narcissism in college student Facebook photo galleries. In Z. Papacharissi (Ed.), *The networked self: Identity, community and culture on social network sites*. New York, NY: Routledge.

Moewaka Barnes, H., Niland, P., Samu, L., Sciasia, A. D., & McCreanor, T. (2017). Ethnicity/culture, alcohol and social media. In A. C. Lyons, T. McCreanor, I. Goodwin, & H. Moewaka Barnes (Eds.), *Youth drinking cultures in a digital world* (pp. 80–98). London, England: Routledge.

Moreno, M. A., & Whitehill, J. M. (2016). # Wasted: The intersection of substance use behaviors and social media in adolescents and young adults. *Current Opinion in Psychology, 9*, 72–76.

Mullen, K., Watson, J., Swift, J., & Black, D. (2007). Young men, masculinity and alcohol. *Drugs: Education, Prevention and Policy, 14*, 151–165.

Nagel, E. G., & Mora, R. (2010). Book reviews: Inclusive masculinity: The changing nature of masculinities. *The Journal of Men's Studies, 18*, 109–112.

Nicholls, J. (2012). Everyday, everywhere: Alcohol marketing and social media – Current trends. *Alcohol and Alcoholism, 47*, 486–493.

Niland, P., Lyons, A. C., Goodwin, I., & Hutton, F. (2013). "Everyone can loosen up and get a bit of a buzz on": Young adults, alcohol and friendship practices. *International Journal of Drug Policy, 24*, 530–537.

Niland, P., Lyons, A. C., Goodwin, I., & Hutton, F. (2014). "See it doesn't look pretty does it?": Young adults' airbrushed drinking practices on Facebook. *Psychology and Health, 29*, 877–895.
Niland, P., Lyons, A. C., Goodwin, I., & Hutton, F. (2015). Friendship work on Facebook: Young adults' understandings and practices of friendship. *Journal of Community and Applied Social Psychology, 25*, 123–137. https://doi.org/10.1002/casp.2201
Niland, P., McCreanor, T., Lyons, A. C., & Griffin, C. (2017). Alcohol marketing on social media: Young adults engage with marketing moments on Facebook. *Addiction: Research and Theory, 25*, 273–284. https://doi.org/10.1080/16066359.2016.1245293
Peralta, R. L. (2007). College alcohol use and the embodiment of hegemonic masculinity among European American men. *Sex Roles, 56*, 741–756.
Peralta, R. L. (2008). "Alcohol allows you to not be yourself": Toward a structured understanding of alcohol use and gender difference among gay, lesbian, and heterosexual youth. *Journal of Drug Issues, 38*, 373–399.
Ridout, B. (2016). Facebook, social media and its application to problem drinking among college students. *Current Opinion in Psychology, 9*, 83–87.
Scoats, R. (2015). Inclusive masculinity and Facebook photographs among early emerging adults at a British university. *Journal of Adolescent Research*, 0743558415607059.
Szmigin, I., Griffin, C., Mistral, W., Bengry-Howell, A., Weale, L., & Hackley, C. (2008). Re-framing 'binge drinking' as calculated hedonism: Empirical evidence from the UK. *International Journal of Drug Policy, 19*, 359–366.
Thurnell-Read, T. (2011). Off the leash and out of control: Masculinities and embodiment in Eastern European stag tourism. *Sociology, 45*, 977–991.
Twenge, J. M. (2017). *iGen: Why today's super-connected kids are growing up less rebellious, more tolerant, less happy*. New York, NY: Atria Books.
Twenge, J. M., & Park, H. (2019). The decline in adult activities among US adolescents, 1976–2016. *Child Development, 90*, 638–654.
Watts, R., Linke, S., Murray, E., & Barker, C. (2015). Calling the shots: Young professional women's relationship with alcohol. *Feminism & Psychology, 25*, 219–234.
Westgate, E. C., & Holliday, J. (2016). Identity, influence, and intervention: The roles of social media in alcohol use. *Current Opinion in Psychology, 9*, 27–32.
Willott, S., & Lyons, A. C. (2012). Consuming male identities: Masculinities, gender relations and alcohol consumption in Aotearoa New Zealand. *Journal of Community and Applied Social Psychology, 22*, 330–345.
World Health Organization. (2018). *Global status report on alcohol and health 2018.* Retrieved from https://www.who.int/substance_abuse/publications/global_alcohol_report/en/. Accessed 18 Sep 2019.

Zaitsev, D. (2017). *It's not just the booze talking: How augmented reality brought wine and spirits to life*. Retrieved from https://blog.theroar.io/its-not-just-the-booze-talking-how-augmented-reality-brought-wine-and-spirits-to-life-dc256905ac7f. Accessed 17 June 2018.

Zhao, S., Grasmuck, S., & Martin, J. (2008). Identity construction on Facebook: Digital empowerment in anchored relationships. *Computers in Human Behavior, 24*, 1816–1836.

Zhao, X., Lampe, C., & Ellison, N. B. (2016). The social media ecology: User perceptions, strategies and challenges. In *Proceedings of the 2016 CHI Conference on Human Factors in Computing Systems* (pp. 89–100). New York, NY: Association for Computing Machinery.

12

Deconstructing the Alcohol-Sport Paradox: Why Do Student Athletes Misuse Alcohol and How Can We Change Behaviour?

Sarah Partington and Elizabeth Partington

Introduction

This chapter provides an overview of current research into university and college student athlete alcohol consumption. In so doing, the chapter will attempt to shed light on why student athletes consume more alcohol and drink alcohol more frequently than their non-athlete counterparts and will also discuss approaches that hold promise for moderating drinking behaviours reported by student athletes. The chapter begins by defining the alcohol-sport paradox—the finding that athletic participation has been shown to increase heavy episodic drinking. The chapter then goes on to outline the relationship between alcohol consumption and student sport participation. Following this, the chapter discusses potential risk factors for student athlete drinking. Then, current interventions targeted at student athletes will be reviewed, and potential future alcohol interventions consider. The chapter closes with suggested avenues for further research.

S. Partington (✉) • E. Partington
Department of Sport, Exercise, and Rehabilitation, Northumbria University, Newcastle upon Tyne, UK
e-mail: sarah.partington@northumbria.ac.uk; elizabeth.partington@northumbria.ac.uk

R. Cooke et al. (eds.), *The Palgrave Handbook of Psychological Perspectives on Alcohol Consumption*, https://doi.org/10.1007/978-3-030-66941-6_12

The Alcohol-Sport Paradox

Participation in university and college sports has been found to be a protective factor against performing health behaviours which carry risks to physical health such as, cigarette consumption and illicit recreational drug use (Lisha & Sussman, 2010). Despite this, student athletes have also been identified as a subgroup within the wider student population who are particularly at risk for heavy episodic drinking (HED; see Chap. 1 for a definition). In studies conducted across different countries, student athletes have been found to consume greater quantities of alcohol, to be drunk more often, to engage in HED more frequently and to experience more alcohol-related harms than students who do not participate in sport (Martens, Dams-O'Connor, & Beck, 2006; Partington et al., 2013; Zhou & Heim, 2014).

Such findings regarding student athletes' alcohol consumption can be understood as something of a paradox, with sports participation operating as a site for both health-promoting behaviours (e.g. healthy eating, regular physical activity) and health compromising behaviours (e.g. HED). This paradox has been recognised by alcohol researchers (e.g. Lisha & Sussman, 2010; Zhou, Heim, & O'Brien, 2015), as well as by professionals involved in the management, organisation and delivery of student sport. However, to date the paradox has yet to be resolved.

The Alcohol-Sport Relationship in University and College Sport

Heavy episodic drinking in athletes seems counterintuitive. As well as being subject to the same risks as other young people who engage in this pattern of behaviour (e.g. poor academic performance, contact with the police, unplanned sexual activity, sexual assault and physical injury—see O'Neill, Martin, Birch, Oldam, & Newbury-Birch, 2015), high levels of alcohol consumption result in physical and cognitive deficits that can negatively impact on an athlete's performance (Grossbard, Hummer, LaBrie, Pederson, & Neighbors, 2009) and cause injuries that pose a serious risk to both current and future sport performance (Howell, Barry, & Pitney, 2015). In addition, scholarship athletes who engage in HED also risk the loss of their scholarship funding through either poor performance or sanctions related to problematic behaviours associated with inebriation (Williams Jr et al., 2006).

Despite the substantial risks outlined above, a positive relationship between alcohol consumption and sport participation has been found in both high school and college students (Lisha & Sussman, 2010; Partington et al., 2013), and this relationship exists for both men and women and across ethnic groups (Green, Nelson, & Hartmann, 2014; O'Brien, Blackie, & Hunter, 2005). Of particular concern is the finding that when student athletes drink alcohol, they are most likely to engage in HED (Nelson & Wechsler, 2001) or similar behaviours such as pre-drinking (see Chap. 13). Participation in college and university sport, has been found to be associated with a higher percentage of HED than a comparable group who has not participated in sport, irrespective of gender or ethnicity (Green et al., 2014).

Whilst it is clear that there is a relationship between sport participation and alcohol consumption, capturing the nuances of that relationship has proved challenging. For example, whilst starting athletic involvement has been shown to be associated with HED and ceasing athletic involvement with reductions in drinking (Cadigan, Littlefield, Martens, & Sher, 2013), there is also evidence to suggest that for some athletes, the alcohol-sport relationship extends beyond their time of active engagement in sport. Ex-athletes have been found to be 15% more likely to engage in HED than those who have never played sport at all, a statistic that is analogous to continuation of sporting involvement (e.g. Green et al., 2014). Such findings suggest there may be a contextual and temporal element to sports participation and alcohol consumption that has not been considered previously.

Conflicting findings have also been reported in relation to competitive level and drinking behaviour. Some studies have found that university students that participate in provincial- or regional-level, national- or international-level competition, have higher rates of HED than recreational sports participants and non-participants (e.g. O'Brien et al., 2005), whereas other research has failed to find any significant differences in the drinking behaviours of athletes participating at different competitive levels (e.g. Partington et al., 2013). Differences in the sporting culture between New Zealand (O'Brien et al., 2005) and the UK (Partington et al., 2013), and the small number of athletes in the Partington et al. (2013) study who were involved at national and international levels may partially explain these contradictory findings, but still the relationship between competitive level and drinking behaviour remains unclear.

There is more consensus in terms of establishing the relationship between type of sport and alcohol consumption. Students involved in team sports, for example, rugby, football, hockey, have largely been found to drink significantly more, to engage in more frequent HED, and to be at greater risk for alcohol-related harm than athletes whose sporting activities are not team-based, for example, swimmers, track and field athletes (e.g. Martha, Grelot, & Peretti-Watel, 2009; Partington et al., 2013). However, Martens, Watson and Beck (2006), found that within their sample, individual sports athletes exhibited both the lowest levels of consumption (track and field) and the highest (swimming and diving). These inconsistent findings suggest that the relationship between alcohol consumption and sport type is more complex than the team-individual dichotomy. The different drinking behaviours observed between athletes across sports may be more reflective of the specific culture of the particular team or club to which the athlete is affiliated, and that team/club's attitude towards substance use than to the characteristics of the sport per se (Smith et al., 2010).

Whilst these findings do not give a definitive picture of the nature and extent of student athlete drinking, they offer a starting point for recognising and seeking to further understand the relationship between alcohol and sport in student populations. The next section turns to identify the alcohol risk factors associated with being a student athlete.

Cognitive and Motivational Risk Factors

As student athletes are students as well as athletes, literature pertaining to alcohol consumption in the wider student population provides a useful starting point for understanding risk factors for student athlete drinking (Weaver et al., 2013). Common risk factors that have been identified in student drinking include being a white male (Wechsler, Lee, Nelson, & Kuo, 2002), being involved with a Fraternity/Sorority (Cashin, Presley, & Meilman, 1998), having high levels of impulsivity (Littlefield, Sher, & Steinley, 2010), holding positive alcohol expectancies (Zamboanga, Schwartz, Ham, Borsari, & Van Tyne, 2010), possessing strong drinking motives (Martens, Pedersen, Smith, Stewart, & O'Brien, 2011) and experiencing perceived heavy drinking norms (Borsari & Carey, 2003; Dams-O'Connor, Martin, & Martens, 2007; Grossbard et al., 2009). In terms of student athlete drinking, researchers have focused in particular on both dispositional and identity-related risk factors and three cognitive or motivational risk factors: Alcohol expectancies, drinking motives and perceived norms (see Chap. 4 for a review of the evidence that these factors predict university student consumption). The focus will first be on dispositional and identity-related risk factors before going on to cover research on expectancies, motives and norms.

Dispositional and Identity-Related Risk Factors

Certain personality traits found to be associated with participation in sport such as sensation seeking and the drive to achieve, are also associated with higher levels of alcohol use (Weaver et al., 2013; Yusko, Buckman, White, & Pandina, 2008; Chap. 5). It has been speculated that high levels of competitiveness among athletes may translate from the practice and playing arenas into competitive alcohol related behaviours such as attempting to out-drink peers (Martens, 2012; Martens, Dams-O'Connor, & Beck, 2006). However, findings by Weaver et al. (2013) suggest that this relationship is more complex than originally thought. In Weaver et al.'s study, specific sport-related achievement motivations were associated with alcohol use, but most of these relationships were moderated by other variables. Higher levels of competitiveness were only associated with greater alcohol consumption among male student athletes and this relationship was strongest when the student athletes were in their competitive season. In contrast, competitiveness was associated with less alcohol use in female student athletes both in season and during the off season. Further research is necessary to more fully understand the role of competitiveness in student athlete drinking behaviours.

Student sports teams and clubs are social groups that encourage and facilitate alcohol consumption (Martens, 2011, see Chaps. 6 and 8). They have been described as more intense and with more highly defined social structures and behaviours than other drinking groups on campus (Christmas & Seymour, 2014). Sparkes, Partington and Brown (2007) provide some potential insights into student athlete drinking culture from their three-year ethnographic study of one university setting in which a 'jock culture' dominated the campus. They identified 'the 12 commandments' of this jock culture—practices for student athletes that governed behaviour if one was to become and remain a 'successful' jock. Significantly, 4 of the 12 commandments identified were guidelines for student athlete drinking behaviour: *commandment 4*, be committed to the social life; *commandment 5*, excessive alcohol consumption and associated behaviours are obligatory; *commandment 9*, attend socials regularly; and *commandment 10*, attend post-match drinking sessions, combined to provide a road map for student athletes in terms of their relationship with alcohol within this specific culture.

Such 'road maps' not only guide behaviours but play a role in the development of cultural identities (see also Chaps. 7 and 16) and, in the case of student athletes, athletic identities (see Ronkainen, Kavoura, & Ryba, 2016). Athletic identity can be defined as the extent to which an individual identifies with the athlete role (Brewer, Van Raalte, & Linder, 1993). An individual with a strong athletic identity places great importance on their involvement in sport and will appraise an event in terms of its potential impact on their athletic participation. Although a strong sense of athletic identity has been found to be associated with a range of positive outcomes in student athlete populations (e.g. strong sense of self-identity, more social interactions, high level of self-confidence), negative outcomes have also been found (Heird & Steinfeldt, 2013). Individuals presenting with a strong and exclusive athletic identity can be vulnerable to increased risk for depression, anxiety, disordered eating and substance-abuse as well as exhibiting lower levels of well-being (Carter, 2009).

In relation to alcohol consumption, previous research has highlighted the importance of social and athletic identity in determining the alcohol consumption of student athletes (Zhou & Heim, 2016; Zhou, Heim, & Levy, 2015; Zhou, Heim, & O'Brien, 2015). Zhou, Heim and Levy (2015) reported that among a sample of UK student athletes, social identity was positively associated with alcohol consumption, whereas athletic identity was associated with lower levels of alcohol use. However, several researchers (e.g. K. E. Miller, Melnick, Barnes, Sabo, & Farrell, 2007), have recognised that engagement with sport is a multidimensional experience and that this should be reflected in the way in which athletic identity is measured. For example, researchers have differentiated between objective athletic activity (e.g. team membership, frequency of athletic activity) and subjective identity (how the individual perceives themselves/is perceived by others).

In a series of studies directly contrasting objective (behavioural) and subjective (identity) measures of athletic involvement, K. E. Miller and colleagues identified two distinct trends. A beneficial effect of athletic participation (objective) but an exacerbating effect of athletic identity (subjective) on a wide range of health compromising behaviours including; problem drinking (K. E. Miller et al., 2003), sexual risk-taking (K. E. Miller, Farrell, Barnes, & Melnick, 2005), interpersonal violence (K. E. Miller, Melnick, Farrell, Sabo, & Barnes, 2006) and delinquency (K. E. Miller et al., 2007). However, K. E. Miller (2009) reflected that the limited measures used in the studies meant that it was impossible to know whether these findings indicated a dichotomy between sport-related activity and sport-related identity or between different types of sport-related identities.

K. E. Miller (2009) went on to suggest 'athlete' and 'jock' as two distinct sport-related identities that have different implications for health risk behaviours, including drinking. According to K. E. Miller (2009), the 'jock' identity is developed via participation in high status, physically violent sports that focus on individual achievement, external measures of success and conformity to conventional masculine norms. In contrast, the 'athlete' identity is associated with a task orientation (mastery of skills, development of personal excellence). K. E. Miller suggests that female athletes are more likely to adopt an 'athlete' identity, whereas male athletes could develop either identity. However, women who adopt a 'jock' identity will exhibit the same characteristics and behaviours found in male 'jocks.' Although the two sport-related identities are distinct, it is possible to hold both identities. In K. E. Miller's (2009) study, participants were more likely to have an athlete identity, and whilst most self-identified jocks also had a strong athlete identity, those with a strong 'athlete' identity did not always score highly on 'jock' identity.

Based upon this line of research, K. E. Miller put forward the 'toxic jock theory', characterising the specific sport-related identity of 'jock' as one that makes the individual more prone to health compromising behaviour including hazardous and harmful alcohol consumption. In contrast, the 'athlete' identity should act as a protective factor against such behaviours. However, K. E. Miller recommends caution when interpreting and applying the results of her study. The toxic jock theory has not been tested outside of the specific demographic of undergraduates at one US public university. In addition, the data is cross-sectional in nature, meaning that it is not possible to draw firm conclusions regarding the causality of the relationships (see Chap. 2). Further work testing the theory across different cultures and populations of athletes is needed.

Sparkes et al. (2007) in their exploration of sport culture on a university campus in the south of England encountered a 'jock' identity that was very similar to that described by K. E. Miller (2009). Although not explicitly discussing the 'athlete' identity, Sparkes et al. did identify a group that they termed 'sport-scholars', who were elite-level athletes on university-based scholarships. These sport scholars did exhibit the characteristics of K. E. Miller's 'athlete' identity. Interestingly, Sparkes et al. (2007) also described several other sport-related identities operating on the campus. The 'also rans', a group of students who desired the 'jock' identity but were precluded from it because of a lack of physical proficiency. The 'wanna-bees', individuals who had assimilated the values of the 'jock' identity but were not viewed by others as 'jocks' because they were studying a non-sport-related degree course. The 'broken jocks', those who formerly embodied the 'jock' identity but were no longer able to participate at university level due to a career-ending injury. Finally, the 'anti-jocks', those who embraced the 'athlete' identity, to use K. E. Miller's term, but were also openly critical towards and actively rejecting of the 'jock' identity. These individuals defined themselves specifically in opposition to the 'jock' identity. Further research exploring the range of different sport-related identities held by student athletes and their differential association with drinking behaviour could prove insightful. For example, certain sports may have cultures that facilitate the rejection of the 'jock' identity, whereas other may encourage 'jock' ideals.

Alcohol Expectancies

Alcohol expectancies represent perceived expectations of the effects of alcohol use (Jones, Corbin, & Fromme, 2001). Expectancies can be either positive or negative. Positive alcohol expectancies include the view that alcohol enhances social bonding, increases sexual attractiveness, improves mood and heightens social status (Hallett, McManus, Maycock, Smith, & Howat, 2014). Negative alcohol expectancies include views that alcohol increases aggression and depression, and causes cognitive motor impairment (Lewis & O'Neill, 2000; Pilatti, Cupani, & Pautassi, 2015; see Chap. 4).

Positive alcohol expectancies have been associated with high levels of alcohol consumption in student athletes (Zamboanga, Horton, Leitkowski, & Wang, 2006). There is some indication that this relationship may be gendered, as for example, Lewis, Milroy, Wyrik, Hebard and Lamberson (2017) found that whilst positive outcome expectancies were related to drinking status for female student athletes this relationship did not exist for the male student athletes in their sample. Based on current research, it is difficult to explain how and why positive alcohol expectancies may operate differently for male and female athletes, if indeed they do. Lewis et al. have suggested that college women may have differing expectations of behaviour than college men. However, the findings of this study need to be replicated in further student athlete samples in order to further establish the role of gender differences in the relationship between outcome expectancies and drinking behaviours in student athletes.

Research regarding negative alcohol expectancies in student athletes has produced inconclusive results (Ham, Stewart, Norton, & Hope, 2005). For example, Lewis et al. (2017) found that negative alcohol expectancies decreased the odds of being a binge drinker (i.e. someone who engages in HED; see Chap. 1). In contrast, Zamboanga et al. (2006) found no impact of negative alcohol expectancies on drinking among student athletes. It has been suggested that these contrasting findings may be because expectancy outcomes that researchers assume are 'negative' could actually be viewed by some participants as 'positive'. Zamboanga and Ham (2008) addressed this issue by examining both researcher definitions and participant valuations of expectancies. They found that more favourable student athlete valuations of researcher-defined 'negative expectancies' were associated with higher frequencies of heavy alcohol use in student athletes.

Drinking Motives

Cooper (1994), utilising Cox and Klinger's (1988) incentive motivation model of alcohol use, suggested four types of drinking motives. Two are categorised as internally driven motives: coping (drinking to decrease negative emotional states) and enhancement (drinking to increase positive emotional states). Two are classified as externally driven motives: conformity (drinking to fit in) and social (drinking to be sociable). Chapter 2 provides further detail about this model, while Chap. 4 reviews the evidence that drinking motives predict alcohol use in students. Studies on student athletes have shown that social and enhancement motives are primary reasons for drinking, suggesting that student athletes drink to increase positive mood states and social enjoyment (Doumas & Midgett, 2015).

Based on the premise that being a student athlete creates a different kind of student experience, Martens, Watson, Royland and Beck (2005) suggested that student athlete drinking motives are likely formed from a combination of the general drinking motives described by Cooper (1994) and also sport-related drinking motives specific to the athletic environment. Examples of sport-related motives include, positive reinforcement (e.g. "I work hard at my sport, so I should be able to drink to have a good time"), team/group (e.g. "I feel pressure from my teammates to drink") and sport-related coping (e.g. "I drink to help me deal with poor performances").

Of the sport-related motives, Martens, Watson, et al. (2005) found that positive reinforcement accounted for the most variance in both alcohol consumption and alcohol-related problems, after accounting for general drinking motives and demographic variables. Sport-related coping was only shown to be positively associated with alcohol-related problems. Team/group motives did not seem to be related to alcohol consumption or alcohol-related problems. This result is somewhat surprising given the general findings around higher levels of alcohol consumption amongst team sport athletes. Interestingly, further exploration of the influence of sport type on drinking motives has produced more results that appear counterintuitive. For example, although Taylor, Ward and Hardin (2017) found no differences in sport-related drinking motives for team versus individual sport athletes, when scored on general drinking motives those athletes involved in individual sports had higher enhancement and conformity motives than team sport athletes did. Taylor et al. (2017) suggest that it might not be the team structure of team sports that is important in terms of motives, but rather the specific culture created by the student athletes and coaches.

In relation to competitive level, findings are inconclusive. Some studies have found that National Collegiate Athletic Association Division III athletes are more likely to drink for social and conformity reasons than are those in Division I and Division II (e.g. Milroy et al., 2014). Note that the Divisions differ in terms of their athletic budget, with Division I schools having the largest budget and Division III the smallest. Others found no differences in drinking motives, alcohol consumption, or alcohol-related negative consequences between athletes competing at different divisional levels (e.g. Taylor et al., 2017). Commenting on previous contradictory findings, Pitts, Chow and Donohue (2018) have argued that the relationship between drinking motives, alcohol use and alcohol-related consequences in student athletes has not been examined with appropriate analyses nor have studies statistically controlled for effects of gender, sport type, or competitive season status. In a study specifically designed to address these limitations, they found that student athletes who drink for individual reasons (e.g. positive reinforcement and enhancement) demonstrate higher levels of consumption than those who drink for social reasons. It is worth noting here that this association between positively reinforcing motives and heavy drinking has also been found in the general student population (Cadigan, Martens, & Herman, 2015). It could therefore be that those student athletes who are drinking for enhancement motives would be classed as heavy drinkers irrespective of their involvement in sport. In contrast, those student athletes drinking for social motives maybe drinking more heavily in order to fit in with their teammates. Those drinking because of perceived pressure to conform experience more negative alcohol-related consequences. Results also highlight the use of alcohol by student athletes as a reward both for hard work and/or for good athletic performance (Doumas & Midgett, 2015; Martens & Martin, 2010; Pitts et al., 2018).

In summary, sport-related drinking motives have proved to be somewhat helpful in predicting alcohol consumption and alcohol-related problems in student athletes after accounting for demographic variables and general drinking motives (Martens, Watson, et al., 2005). However, the diverse methods used to study these effects, methodological and statistical limitations in the studies, and the inconclusive findings preclude definitive conclusions on the relationship between sport-related drinking motives and alcohol outcomes among student athletes.

Social Norms

Social norms theory (Perkins & Berkowitz, 1986) is a general theory that describes situations in which individuals misperceive the attitudes or behaviours of others. The theory has been applied to explain student alcohol consumption across multiple studies (Borsari & Carey, 2003), and predicts that a student will increase their alcohol consumption to match the misperceived norm in order to fit in. Accordingly, HED is predicted to occur when students overestimate the amount of drinking that is taking place by their peers/ in their social community compared to what is actually happening in reality (see Chaps. 6 and 8). Correcting such misperceptions is central to web-based personalised feedback interventions discussed in Chap. 20.

Researchers have identified two specific types of social norms: descriptive and injunctive (Berkowitz, 2004; Borsari & Carey, 2003; McAlaney, Bewick, & Hughes, 2011). Descriptive social norms are based on perceptions of how much or how often others drink on a 'typical occasion' (Borsari & Carey, 2003). Injunctive social norms relate to perceptions of whether or not the drinking behaviour is approved of (Borsari & Carey, 2003). In essence, descriptive norms are based on actual drinking behaviour, whereas injunctive norms are based on ideas about and attitudes towards drinking behaviour (see Chaps. 4, 11 and 13).

Strong support has been found for the influence of descriptive norms on quantity and frequency of alcohol consumption in student athletes. The biggest impact has been shown to come from perceptions of close friends, particularly same-sex teammates (Lewis, 2008; Lewis et al., 2017; Lewis & Paladino, 2008). Support for the role of injunctive norms in influencing student athlete drinking behaviour is less convincing. In a study specifically exploring injunctive norms and student athlete drinking, teammates were perceived to have higher levels of approval of drinking alcohol than coaches had, and perceived approval from both teammates and coaches were independently associated with student athletes' drinking behaviours (Seitz, Wyrick, Rulison, Strack, & Fearnow-Kenney, 2014). In contrast, Lewis et al. (2017) found that whilst descriptive norms were significant predictors of HED in student athletes, injunctive norms were not. Such findings are consistent with theoretical discussions of how norms influence behaviour or behavioural antecedents like intentions (see Chap. 2).

When comparing the impact of descriptive versus injunctive norms, as well as other variables such as sociodemographic factors and drinking motives, on student athlete drinking, Hummer, LaBrie and Lac (2009) found that both norm types were strong predictors. However, descriptive norms had the biggest influence on student athlete drinking behaviour compared to all other variables. Additional research is needed to clarify the mechanisms underpinning the influence of specific social norms (injunctive versus descriptive) within the student athlete culture. In the meantime, existing research evidence suggests that prevention and intervention efforts for student athletes that are norm-based, should focus more on the use of descriptive norms. In the next section we will turn from psychological factors as explanations for student athlete drinking to risk factors associated with the broader socio-cultural context in which these activities take place.

Socio-cultural Risk Factors

Student athletes exist within a different social environment at university to their non-athlete peers (Sparkes et al., 2007; Tewksbury, Higgins, & Mustaine, 2008; Wicki, Kuntsche, & Gmel, 2010; Zhou & Heim, 2014). For example, student athletes have a greater number of friends, are more socially connected (Nelson & Wechsler, 2001) and have higher social status due to their athletic achievements (Martens, Dams-O'Connor, & Beck, 2006). This elevated social status provides student athletes with more opportunities to attend social events, particularly those that involve alcohol consumption (Martens, 2011). Heavy alcohol consumption, drinking games and associated forfeits are activities typical of social events following sports matches at university (Sparkes et al., 2007). Hazing and initiation ceremonies, characterised by excessive alcohol consumption, are also commonplace (Clayton, 2013; Clayton & Harris, 2008; Groves, Griggs, & Leflay, 2012; Chap. 13). It has therefore been suggested that there is value in taking a socio-cultural approach (see Chap. 6) to exploring risk factors for student athlete drinking (Zhou & Heim, 2014).

Within this cultural and social context, a number of 'sport-related' factors have been highlighted as potentially influential in shaping the drinking behaviours of student athletes. The longstanding and implicit cultural link between alcohol and sport is reinforced in student sport via repeated experiences of alcohol consumption when watching sport and by the alcohol sponsorship of college sporting teams and sporting events (Groves et al., 2012; O'Brien & Kypri, 2008; Vamplew, 2013). The use of alcohol to cope with sport-related pressures and to manage associated anxiety or stress, has also been suggested as a potential explanation for student athlete drinking (Smith et al., 2010; Vamplew, 2013).

However, findings around sport-related coping as a drinking motive have been inconsistent.

Alcohol consumption has been found to be associated with team bonding among student athletes (Clayton & Harris, 2008; Taylor et al., 2017; Zhou, O'Brien, & Heim, 2014). In a study involving UK student athletes, Clayton and Harris (2008) found that football provided a basis for male student athletes' friendships, whilst alcohol consumption was the method by which those friendships were created and reinforced. It has also been suggested that student athletes may harbour the belief that athletic training regimes and resultant high levels of physical fitness provide immunity to the negative effects of alcohol (Vamplew, 2013). In the next section we move from risk factor to consider interventions for high risk alcohol consumption among student athletes.

Interventions Designed to Reduce Harmful Drinking Among Student Athletes

At present, the development, implementation and evaluation of interventions specifically targeted at managing the harmful effects of HED in student athletes is lacking (Cimini et al., 2015). In this section we will discuss what is currently known about alcohol interventions for student athletes and will suggest potential future interventions that are worthy of consideration for use with student athletes.

Interventions Using the Social Norms Approach

The majority of alcohol interventions developed for student athletes have adopted a social norms approach (Perkins & Berkowitz, 1986). Most often these interventions utilise descriptive norms (quantity and/or frequency of drinking, e.g. McAlaney et al., 2011). This approach has been somewhat successful in terms of tackling college student drinking (Alfonso, Hall, & Dunn, 2013; Cronce & Larimer, 2011), and it is therefore not surprising that social norms have been the 'go to' intervention, for student athletes.

General social norms-based interventions have proven successful in correcting student athletes' normative misperceptions but have failed to have any impact on their alcohol consumption (Nelson & Wechsler, 2001; Thombs & Hamilton, 2002). A potential explanation for the lack of success is that the interventions were not 'athlete specific' (Cimini et al., 2015; Lewis et al., 2017). According to Lewis et al. (2017), information on 'typical student' drinking behaviours would most likely be ignored by most student athletes, because the reference group is one with which they do not 'connect'. More successful social norms based interventions have sought to appeal to student athletes by modifying the information given. For example, providing student athlete drinking norms (Cimini et al., 2015) and summarising athlete specific consequences of drinking (e.g. being hung-over at a game or practice and the impact of heavy alcohol use on athletic performance) (Cimini et al., 2015; Martens, Kilmer, Beck, & Zamboanga, 2010).

These athlete-focused interventions have achieved some success. Although Martens et al. (2010) found no group differences in alcohol outcomes between control and experimental conditions, the student athlete focused condition did lead to significantly lower peak drinking when heavy drinkers were examined. Similarly, Cimini et al. (2015) found that their athlete-focused intervention—that combined personalised feedback on drinking (see Chap. 20) with motivational interviewing (W. R. Miller & Rollnick, 2002)—was effective in reducing reports of alcohol use, frequency, quantity and alcohol-related negative consequences three months post intervention. Those who participated in the athlete-focused intervention reported an increase in scores on the protective behaviours strategies manner of drinking sub-scale (meaning they reported drinking more slowly; Martens et al., 2005), demonstrated statistically significant corrections in their norm misperceptions and also demonstrated greater corrections of norm misperceptions and greater use of protective behavioural strategies than did a comparison group of student athletes not participating in the intervention.

Although there are limitations to both of the studies described above, the findings highlight the potential relevance of examining the type of normative information that may be meaningful to student athletes. Identifying 'credible sources' for alcohol messaging for student athletes, a behaviour change technique identified in the Behaviour Change Technique Taxonomy (Michie et al., 2013) may also help. Given that student athletes perceive their coaches as having more lenient attitudes towards drinking behaviour (Lewis, 2008), involving the coach in normative feedback messaging may be beneficial. Parents too, have been shown to have some influence on reducing student athlete drinking (Turrisi et al., 2009; see Chap. 17 for more on how parents can influence consumption). Inviting athletes to self-select a significant other (e.g. coach, teammate, friend, parent) to engage in the alcohol-intervention programme with them has shown promise (Donohue et al., 2016), but larger scale studies of this type are needed.

Current thinking on alcohol-interventions for student athletes recommends moving beyond a 'single focus' approach to incorporate more than one mediator, that is, descriptive norms, alcohol expectancies, of alcohol behaviour change (Fearnow-Kenney et al., 2016). Drawing on existing literature on risk factors Fearnow-Kenney et al. (2016) targeted not only normative misperceptions, but also student athletes' negative alcohol expectancies and intentions to use alcohol-related harm prevention strategies. They created a 'myPlaybook' programme comprised of a series of learning activities focused on perceived social norms of student athlete alcohol use, student athletes' expectations about the effects of alcohol use and also strategies to prevent or reduce the negative consequences of alcohol use. The intervention had a significant effect on social norms perceptions and intentions to use harm prevention strategies. The treatment group did not actually increase intentions to prevent harm, but a buffering effect was observed. Student athletes who received the intervention maintained their intentions to prevent harm during their 'Freshman' year when risk of substance use usually increases. The effect on alcohol expectancies was not significant. The authors claimed that positive alcohol expectancies in student athletes may be strongly established and therefore more difficult to impact than other variables. Unfortunately, a limitation of the study was that there were no behavioural measures included, so it is not possible to determine whether or not the intervention had any influence on actual behaviour.

In line with Fearnow-Kenney et al.'s findings, Lewis et al. (2017) reported that the student athletes in their sample did not hold strong negative expectancies related to drinking, suggesting that student athletes may not be consciously aware of the negative outcomes of heavy alcohol use or it may be that potential negative outcomes are in fact viewed by student athletes in a positive light. These findings suggest that working with athletes to develop clear discrepancies between drinking behaviours and their athletic goals and values, as well as other motivational interviewing-based techniques may be more effective methods to help student athletes to accurately assess the pros and cons of their heavy-drinking behaviour.

More Recent Interventional Approaches

As heavy alcohol use has been found to be an element of certain student athlete sport-related identities (K. E. Miller, 2009), it is perhaps not surprising that current thinking around interventions focuses on exploring how social identity can be used to reduce alcohol-related harm (Zhou, Heim, & Levy,

2015). One potential approach for exploring and addressing identity is narrative therapy. Based on the idea that identities are created within and through the stories individuals tell about their experiences, narrative therapy focuses on exposing dominant 'or problem' stories that are shaping people's lives and identities in a negative way (Gardner & Poole, 2009). Narrative therapists help clients to understand the dominant narratives that are shaping their identities and behaviours, and work with clients to help them to retell their stories in alternative ways that will enable them to create more positive identities (Gardner & Poole, 2009). Gardner and Poole (2009) developed a three-stage model of narrative therapy, starting with deconstructing the problem-saturated dominant story, then re-authoring a new story/stories and finally making the new story/stories real and salient. By changing the story/stories, the participant is able to create new, more productive identities, resulting in new, more productive behaviours.

Narrative therapy has been used successfully in a psychoeducational context to promote the development of positive body image in elite young female athletes (Leahy & Harrigan, 2006) and as an effective discussion tool for athletes with serious mental illness (Carless & Sparkes, 2008). There are currently no studies on the use of narrative as an intervention for either student or student athlete drinking. However, narrative therapy has been found to be effective in the treatment of alcohol addiction in adults (Szabo, Toth, & Pakai, 2014).

Future Directions

In terms of understanding and explaining student athlete drinking behaviour and developing effective interventions for combating student athlete drinking, success is associated with consideration of both general student factors and more specific athlete-related factors. Taking this a step further, there are grounds for exploring subgroups within the wider student athlete group in more detail. In particular, future research should explore further the role of sport, team and club culture as well as the different sport-related identities held by student athletes, to ascertain how these different cultural values and identities might shape drinking motives, expectancies, norms and engagement with alcohol interventions.

A related area ripe for investigation is student athletes who choose not to drink. Understanding student athletes' motives for abstinence would provide useful information in terms of prevention and intervention design. To date, only four studies have assessed student athletes' motives for not drinking

(Evans, Weinberg, & Jackson, 1992; Green, Uryasz, Petr, & Bray, 2001; Martin, 1998; Nelson & Wechsler, 2001). Unfortunately, these studies are dated, and more recent studies of student athlete drinking have not included athletes who choose not to drink (e.g. Fetherman & Grossman, 2018). Beyond the sport domain, Conroy and de Visser (2018) outlined benefits and drawbacks perceived in social non-drinking (i.e. not drinking during social occasions when friends/peers may be drinking themselves) among UK-based university students (see also Chap. 14). Their findings indicated that promoting moderate drinking by highlighting the benefits of, or challenging the perceived drawbacks of, social non-drinking may be of merit, particularly among female students. There may be value in replicating this study in a student athlete group. Likewise, whilst there are studies on drink refusal self-efficacy in student populations (e.g. Oei, Hasking, & Young, 2005), none of these studies have as yet, been carried out on student athletes. Further investigation of these alternative areas of research may be of benefit.

Conclusion

There is clear evidence that student athletes are at risk of engaging in HED. Whilst this initially appears to be a paradox, in that athletic pursuits promote health yet may also increase the likelihood of engaging in health risk behaviours like harmful alcohol consumption levels, the culture of student sport offers potential explanations. Whilst student athletes share some similarities with their non-athlete peers, in terms of their disposition and cognitive or motivational factors it is clear that there are additional identity and socio-cultural factors associated with being a student athlete that are different to the general student experience. Existing interventions targeting a reduction in alcohol consumption have been relatively unsuccessful at changing drinking behaviour so there is a need for further research to identify the best way to bring about changes.

References

Alfonso, J., Hall, T. V., & Dunn, M. (2013). Feedback-based alcohol interventions for mandated students: An effectiveness study of three modalities. *Clinical Psychology & Psychotherapy, 20*(5), 411–423. https://doi.org/10.1002/cpp.1786

Berkowitz, A. D. (2004). *The social norms approach: Theory, research, and annotated bibliography*. Trumansburg, NY: Independent Consultant.

Borsari, B., & Carey, K. B. (2003). Descriptive and injunctive norms in college drinking: A meta-analytic integration. *Journal of Studies on Alcohol, 64*, 331–341. https://doi.org/10.15288/jsa2003.64.331

Brewer, B. W., Van Raalte, J. L., & Linder, D. E. (1993). Athletic identity: Hercules' muscles or Achilles' heel? *International Journal of Sport Psychology, 24*, 237–254.

Cadigan, J. M., Littlefield, A. K., Martens, M. P., & Sher, K. J. (2013). Transitions into and out of intercollegiate athletic involvement and risky drinking. *Journal of Studies on Alcohol and Drugs, 74*(1), 21–29. https://doi.org/10.15288/jsad.2013.74.21

Cadigan, J. M., Martens, M. P., & Herman, K. C. (2015). A latent profile analysis of drinking motives among heavy drinking college students. *Addictive Behaviors, 51*(Dec), 100–105. https://doi.org/10.1016/j.addbeh.2015.07.029

Carless, D., & Sparkes, A. C. (2008). The physical activity experiences of men with serious mental illness: Three short stories. *Psychology of Sport and Exercise, 9*(2), 191–210. https://doi.org/10.1016/j.psychsport.2007.03.008

Carter, J. E. (2009). Disordered eating in college student-athletes. In E. F. Etzel, A. P. Ferrante, & J. W. Pinkney (Eds.), *Counselling college student-athletes: Issues and interventions* (2nd ed., pp. 303–322). Morgantown, WV: Fitness Information Technology.

Cashin, J. R., Presley, C. A., & Meilman, P. W. (1998). Alcohol use in the Greek system: Follow the leader? *Journal of Studies on Alcohol and Drugs, 59*, 63–70. https://doi.org/10.15288/jsa.1998.59.63

Christmas, S., & Seymour, F. (2014). *Drunken nights out: Motivations, norms and rituals in the night-time economy*. https://www.drinkaware.co.uk/media/1567/drinkaware_drunken-nights-out-report_full-report_vfinal-pdf-version-without-page-breaks-_dec-2014-amend.pdf

Cimini, M. D., Monserrat, J. M., Sokolowski, K. L., Dewitt-Parker, J. Y., Rivero, E. M., & McElroy, L. A. (2015). Reducing high-risk drinking among student-athletes: The effects of a targeted athlete-specific brief intervention. *Journal of American College Health, 63*, 343–352. https://doi.org/10.1080/07448481.2015.1031236

Clayton, B. (2013). Initiate: Constructing the 'reality' of male team sport initiation rituals. *International Review for the Sociology of Sport, 48*(2), 204–219. https://doi.org/10.1177/10126902.11432659

Clayton, B., & Harris, J. (2008). Our friend Jack: Alcohol, friendship and masculinity in university football. *Annals of Leisure Research, 11*(3–4), 311–330. https://doi.org/10.1080/11745398.2008.9686800

Conroy, D., & De Visser, E. O. (2018). Benefits and drawbacks of social non-drinking identified by British university students. *Drug and Alcohol Review, 37*(Suppl. 1), S89–S97. https://doi.org/10.1111/dar.12610

Cooper, M. L. (1994). Motivations for alcohol use among adolescents: Development and validation of a four-factor model. *Psychological Assessment, 6*(2), 117–128. https://doi.org/10.1037/1040-3590.6.2.117

Cox, W. M., & Klinger, E. (1988). A motivational model of alcohol use. *Journal of Abnormal Psychology, 97*(2), 168–180. https://doi.org/10.1037/0021-843x.97.2.168

Cronce, J. M., & Larimer, M. E. (2011). Individual-focused approaches to the prevention of college student drinking. *Alcohol Research & Health, 34*(2), 210.

Dams-O'Connor, K., Martin, J. L., & Martens, M. P. (2007). Social norms and alcohol consumption among intercollegiate athletes: The role of athlete and non-athlete reference groups. *Addictive Behaviors, 32*(11), 2657–2666. https://doi.org/10.1016/j.addbeh.2007.04.030

Donohue, B., Dowd, A., Philips, C., Plant, C. P., Loughran, T., & Gavrilova, Y. (2016). Controlled evaluation of a method to assist recruitment of participants into treatment outcome research and engage student-athletes into substance abuse intervention. *Journal of Clinical Sport Psychology, 10*, 272–288. https://doi.org/10.1123/jcsp.2015-0022

Doumas, D. M., & Midgett, A. (2015). Ethnic differences in drinking motives and alcohol use among college athletes. *Journal of College Counselling, 18*, 116–128. https://doi.org/10.1002/jocc.12009

Evans, M., Weinberg, R., & Jackson, A. (1992). Psychological factors related to drug use in college athletes. *The Sport Psychologist, 6*, 24–41. https://doi.org/10.1123/tsp.6.1.24

Fearnow-Kenney, M., Wyrick, D. L., Milroy, J. J., Reifsteck, E. J., Day, T., & Kelly, S. E. (2016). The effects of a web-based alcohol prevention program on social norms, expectancies, and intentions to prevent harm among college student-athletes. *The Sport Psychologist, 30*, 113–122. https://doi.org/10.1123/tsp.2015-0016

Fetherman, D. L., & Grossman, J. C. (2018). Exploring the experiences of Division III athletes drinking alcohol with their teams: A qualitative study. *Journal of Intercollegiate Sport, 11*, 129–148. https://doi.org/10.1123/jis.2017-0044

Gardner, P. J., & Poole, J. M. (2009). One story at a time: Narrative therapy, older adults, and addictions. *Journal of Applied Gerontology, 28*(5), 600–920. https://doi.org/10.1177/0733464808330822

Green, G. A., Uryasz, F. D., Petr, T. A., & Bray, C. D. (2001). NCAA study of substance use and abuse habits of college student-athletes. *Clinical Journal of Sports Medicine, 11*(1), 51–56. https://doi.org/10.1177/1012690213509257

Green, K., Nelson, T. F., & Hartmann, D. (2014). Binge drinking and sports participation in college: Patterns among athletes and former athletes. *International Review for the Sociology of Sport, 49*(3–4), 417–434. https://doi.org/10.1177/1012690213509257

Grossbard, J. R., Hummer, J. F., LaBrie, J. W., Pederson, E., & Neighbors, C. (2009). Is substance use a team sport? Attraction to team, perceived norms, and alcohol and marijuana use among males and female intercollegiate athletes. *Journal of Applied Sport Psychology, 21*, 247–261. https://doi.org/10.1080/10413200903019145

Groves, M., Griggs, G., & Leflay, K. (2012). Hazing and initiation ceremonies in university sport: Setting the scene for further research in the United Kingdom. *Sport in Society, 15*(1), 117–131. https://doi.org/10.1080/03031853.2011.625287

Hallett, J., McManus, A., Maycock, B. R., Smith, J., & Howat, P. M. (2014). "Excessive drinking: An inescapable part of university life?" A focus group study of Australian undergraduates. *Open Journal of Preventive Medicine, 04*(07), 616–629. https://doi.org/10.4236/ojpm.2014.47071

Ham, L. S., Stewart, S. H., Norton, P. J., & Hope, D. A. (2005). Psychometric assessment of the comprehensive effects of alcohol questionnaire: Comparing a brief version to the original full scale. *Journal of Psychopathology and Behavioural Assessment, 27*, 141–158. https://doi.org/10.1007/s10862-005-0631-9

Heird, E. B., & Steinfeldt, J. A. (2013). An interpersonal psychotherapy approach to counselling student athletes: Clinical implications of athletic identity. *Journal of College Counselling, 16*, 143–157. https://doi.org/10.1002/j.2161-1882.2013.00033.x

Howell, S. M., Barry, A. E., & Pitney, W. A. (2015). Exploring the athletic trainers role in assisting student-athletes presenting with alcohol-related unintentional injuries. *Journal of Athletic Training, 50*(9), 977–980. https://doi.org/10.4085/1062-6050-50.5.09

Hummer, J. F., LaBrie, J. W., & Lac, A. (2009). The prognostic power of normative influences among NCAA student-athletes. *Addictive Behaviors, 34*, 573–580. https://doi.org/10.1016/j.addbeh.2009.03.021

Jones, B. T., Corbin, W., & Fromme, K. (2001). A review of expectancy theory and alcohol consumption. *Addiction, 96*(1), 57–72. https://doi.org/10.1080/09652140020016969

Leahy, T., & Harrigan, R. (2006). Using narrative therapy in sport psychology practice: Application to a psychoeducational body image program. *The Sport Psychologist, 20*(4), 480–494. https://doi.org/10.1123/tsp.20.4.480

Lewis, B. A., & O'Neill, H. K. (2000). Alcohol expectancies and social deficits relating to problem drinking among college students. *Addictive Behaviors, 25*(2), 295–299. https://doi.org/10.1016/S0306-4603(99)00063-5

Lewis, T. F. (2008). An explanatory model of student-athlete drinking: The role of team leadership, social norms, perceptions of risk, and coaches' attitudes toward alcohol consumption. *College Student Journal, 42*, 818–831.

Lewis, T. F., Milroy, J., Wyrik, D., Hebard, S. P., & Lamberson, K. A. (2017). Binge-drinking and non-binge-drinking student-athletes: The role of proximal norms, negative expectancies, and selected sociodemographic variables. *Journal of Child & Adolescent Substance Abuse, 26*(2), 141–151. https://doi.org/10.1080/1067828x.2016.1222978

Lewis, T. F., & Paladino, D. (2008). Proximal norms, selected socio-demographics, and drinking behaviour among university student-athletes. *Journal of*

Addictions and Offender Counselling, 29, 7–21. https://doi.org/10.1002/j.2161-1874.2008.tb00040.x

Lisha, N. E., & Sussman, S. (2010). Relationship of high school and college sports participation with alcohol, tobacco, and illicit drug use: A review. *Addictive Behaviors, 35*, 399–407. https://doi.org/10.1016/j.addbeh.2009.12.032

Littlefield, A. K., Sher, K. J., & Steinley, D. (2010). Developmental trajectories of impulsivity and their association with alcohol use and related outcomes during emerging and young adulthood I. *Alcoholism, Clinical and Experimental Research, 34*, 1409–1416. https://doi.org/10.1111/j.1530-0277.2010.01224.x

Martens, M. P. (2011). Alcohol interventions for college student-athletes. In H. R. White & D. L. Rabiner (Eds.), *College drinking and drug use*. New York, NY: Guilford Press.

Martens, M. P. (2012). Alcohol interventions for college student athletes. In H. R. White & D. L. Rabiner (Eds.), *College drinking and drug use* (pp. 203–220). New York, NY: The Guilford Press.

Martens, M. P., Dams-O'Connor, K., & Beck, N. C. (2006). A systematic review of college student-athlete drinking: Prevalence rates, sport-related factors, and interventions. *Journal of Substance Abuse Treatment, 31*(3), 305–316. https://doi.org/10.1016/j.jsat.2006.05.004

Martens, M. P., Ferrier, A. G., Sheehy, M. J., Corbett, K., Anderson, D. A., & Simmons, A. (2005). Development of the protective behavioral strategies survey. *Journal of Studies on Alcohol and Drugs, 66*, 698–705.

Martens, M. P., Kilmer, J. R., Beck, N. C., & Zamboanga, B. L. (2010). The efficacy of a targeted personalized drinking feedback intervention among intercollegiate athletes: A randomized controlled trial. *Psychology of Addictive Behaviours, 24*(4), 660–669.

Martens, M. P., & Martin, J. L. (2010). College athletes' drinking motives and competitive seasonal status: Additional assessment of the athlete drinking scale. *Addiction Research & Theory, 18*(1), 23–32. https://doi.org/10.3109/16066350902867882

Martens, M. P., Pedersen, E. R., Smith, A. E., Stewart, S. H., & O'Brien, K. (2011). Predictors of alcohol-related outcomes in college athletes: The roles of trait urgency and drinking motives. *Addictive Behaviours, 36*, 456–464. https://doi.org/10.1016/j.addbeh.2010.12.025

Martens, M. P., Watson, J. C., & Beck, N. C. (2006). Sport-type differences in alcohol use among intercollegiate athletes. *Journal of Applied Sport Psychology, 18*(2), 136–150. https://doi.org/10.1080/10413200600653758

Martens, M. P., Watson, J. C., Royland, E. M., & Beck, N. C. (2005). Development of the athlete drinking scale. *Psychology of Addictive Behaviours, 19*(2), 158–164. https://doi.org/10.1037/0893-164x.19.2.158

Martha, C., Grelot, L., & Peretti-Watel, P. (2009). Participants' sports characteristics related to heavy episodic drinking among French students. *International Journal of Drug Policy, 20*(2), 152–160. https://doi.org/10.1016/j.drugpo.2007.11.023

Martin, M. (1998). The use of alcohol among NCAA Division I female college basketball, softball, and volleyball athletes. *Journal of Athletic Training, 33*(2), 163–167.

McAlaney, J., Bewick, B., & Hughes, C. (2011). The international development of the "social norms" approach to drug education and prevention. *Drugs: Education, Prevention, and Policy, 18*(2), 81–89. https://doi.org/10.3109/09687631003610977

Michie, S., Richardson, M., Johnston, M., Abraham, C., Francis, J., Hardeman, W., … Wood, C. E. (2013). The behaviour change technique taxonomy (vi) of 93 hierarchically clustered techniques: Building an international consensus for the reporting of behaviour change interventions. *Annals of Behavioral Medicine, 46*, 81–95.

Miller, K. E. (2009). Sport-related identities and the 'toxic jock. *Journal of Sport Behavior, 32*, 69–91.

Miller, K. E., Farrell, M. P., Barnes, G. M., Melnick, M. J., & Sabo. (2005). Gender/racial differences in jock identity, dating, and adolescent sexual risk. *Journal of Youth and Adolescence, 34*, 123–136.

Miller, K. E., Hoffman, J. E., Barnes, G. M., Farrell, M. P., Sabo, D., & Melnick, M. J. (2003). Jocks, gender, race, and adolescent problem drinking. *Journal of Drug Education, 33*, 445–462.

Miller, K. E., Melnick, M. J., Barnes, G. M., Sabo, D., & Farrell, M. P. (2007). Athletic involvement and adolescent delinquency. *Journal of Youth and Adolescence, 36*, 711–723. https://doi.org/10.1007/s10964-006-9123-9

Miller, K. E., Melnick, M. J., Farrell, M. P., Sabo, D. F., & Barnes, G. M. (2006). Jocks, gender, binge drinking and adolescent violence. *Journal of Interpersonal Violence, 21*, 105–120. https://doi.org/10.1177/0886260505281662

Miller, W. R., & Rollnick, S. (2002). *Motivational interviewing: Preparing people for change* (2nd ed.). New York, NY: Guildford Press.

Milroy, J. J., Orsini, M., Wyrick, D. L., Fearnow-Kenney, M., Kelly, S. E., & Burley, J. (2014). A National study of the reasons for use and non-use of alcohol among college student-athletes by sex, race, and NCAA division. *Journal of Alcohol and Drug Education, 58*(3), 67–87.

Nelson, T. F., & Wechsler, H. (2001). Alcohol and college athletes. *Medicine & Science in Sports & Exercise, 33*(1), 43–47.

O'Brien, K. S., Blackie, J. M., & Hunter, J. A. (2005). Hazardous drinking in elite New Zealand sportspeople. *Alcohol and Alcoholism, 40*(3), 239–241. https://doi.org/10.1093/alcalc/agh145

O'Brien, K. S., & Kypri, K. (2008). Alcohol industry sponsorship and hazardous drinking among sportspeople. *Addiction, 103*, 1961–1966. https://doi.org/10.1111/j.1360-0443.2008.0237

O'Neill, G., Martin, N., Birch, J., Oldam, A., & Newbury-Birch, D. (2015). The drinkers degree: Risk taking behaviours amongst undergraduate student drinkers. *Journal of Addiction*, 965438. https://doi.org/10.1155/2015/965438

Oei, T. P. S., Hasking, P. A., & Young, R. M. D. (2005). Drinking refusal self-efficacy questionnaire-revised (DRSEQ-R): A new factor structure with confirmatory factor analysis. *Drug and Alcohol Dependence, 78*(3), 297–307. https://doi.org/10.1016/j.drugalcdep.2004.11.010

Partington, S., Partington, E., Heather, N., Longstaff, F., Allsop, S., Jankowski, M., … Gibson, A. S. C. (2013). The relationship between membership of a university sports group and drinking behaviour among students at English Universities. *Addiction Research & Theory, 21*(4), 339–347. https://doi.org/10.3109/16066359.2012.727508

Perkins, H. W., & Berkowitz, A. D. (1986). Perceiving the community norms of alcohol use among students: Some research implications for campus alcohol education programming. *International Journal of the Addictions, 21*, 971–976. https://doi.org/10.3109/10826088609077249

Pilatti, A., Cupani, M., & Pautassi, R. M. (2015). Personality and alcohol expectancies discriminate alcohol consumption patterns in female college students. *Alcohol and Alcoholism, 50*(4), 385–392. https://doi.org/10.1093/alcalc/agvo25

Pitts, M., Chow, G. M., & Donohue, B. (2018). Relationship between general and sport-related drinking motives and athlete alcohol use and problems. *Substance Use & Misuse*, 146–155. https://doi.org/10.1080/10826084.2018.1512624

Ronkainen, N. J., Kavoura, A., & Ryba, T. V. (2016). Narrative and discursive perspectives on athletic identity: Past, present, and future. *Psychology of Sport and Exercise, 27*, 128–137. https://doi.org/10.1016/j.psychsport.2016.08.010

Seitz, C. M., Wyrick, D. L., Rulison, K. L., Strack, R. W., & Fearnow-Kenney, M. (2014). The association between coach and teammate injunctive norm reference groups and college student-athlete substance use. *Journal of Alcohol and Drug Education, 58*, 7–26.

Smith, A. C. T., Stewart, B., Oliver-Bennetts, S., McDonald, S., Ingerson, L., Anderson, A., … Graetz, F. (2010). Contextual influences and athlete attitudes to drugs in sport. *Sport Management Review, 13*(3), 181–197. https://doi.org/10.1016/j.smr.2010.01.008

Sparkes, A. C., Partington, E., & Brown, D. H. K. (2007). Bodies as bearers of value: The transmission of jock culture via the 'twelve commandments'. *Sport, Education and Society, 12*(3), 295–316. https://doi.org/10.1080/13573320701464150

Szabo, J., Toth, S., & Pakai, A. K. (2014). Narrative therapy for alcohol dependent patients. *International Journal of Mental Health and Addiction, 12*(4), 470–476. https://doi.org/10.1007/s11469-014-9478-1

Taylor, E. A., Ward, R. M., & Hardin, R. (2017). Examination of drinking habits and motives of collegiate student-athletes. *Journal of Applied Sport Management, 9*(1). https://doi.org/10.18666/jasm-2017-v9-i1-7470

Tewksbury, R., Higgins, G. E., & Mustaine, E. E. (2008). Binge drinking among college athletes and non-athletes. *Deviant Behavior, 29*(3), 275–293. https://doi.org/10.1080/01639620701588040

Thombs, D. L., & Hamilton, M. (2002). Effects of a social norm feedback campaign on the drinking norms and behaviour of Division I student-athletes. *Journal of Drug Education, 3*, 227–244. https://doi.org/10.2190/2UYU-6X9M-RJ65-3YYH

Turrisi, R., Larimer, M. E., Mallet, K. A., Kilmer, J. R., Ray, A. E., Mastroleo, N. R., … Montoya, H. (2009). A randomized clinical trial evaluating a combined alcohol intervention for high-risk college students. *Journal of Studies on Alcohol and Drugs, 70*, 555–567. https://doi.org/10.15288/jsad.2009.70.555

Vamplew, W. (2013). Alcohol and the sportsperson: An anomalous alliance. In P. Dimeo (Ed.), *Drugs, alcohol and sport: A critical history*. London, England: Routledge.

Weaver, C. C., Martens, M. P., Cadigan, J. M., Takamatsu, S. K., Treloar, H. R., & Pedersen, E. R. (2013). Sport-related achievement motivation and alcohol outcomes: An athlete-specific risk factor among intercollegiate athletes. *Addictive Behaviours, 38*(12), 2930–2936. https://doi.org/10.1016/j.addbeh.2013.08.021

Wechsler, H., Lee, J. E., Nelson, T. F., & Kuo, M. (2002). Underage college students' drinking behaviour, access to alcohol, and the influence of deterrence policies: Findings from the Harvard School of Public Health College Alcohol Study. *Journal of American College Health, 50*, 223–236. https://doi.org/10.1080/07448480209595714

Wicki, M., Kuntsche, E., & Gmel, G. (2010). Drinking at European universities? A review of students' alcohol use. *Addictive Behaviors, 35*(11), 913–924. https://doi.org/10.1016/j.addbeh.2010.06.015

Williams, R. D., Jr., Perko, M., Belcher, D., Leaver-Dunn, D. D., Usdan, S. L., & Leeper, J. D. (2006). Use of social ecology model to address alcohol use among college athletes. *American Journal of Health Studies, 21*(4), 228–237.

Yusko, D. A., Buckman, J. F., White, H. R., & Pandina, R. J. (2008). Risk for excessive alcohol use and drinking-related problems in college student athletes. *Addictive Behaviors, 33*(12), 1546–1556. https://doi.org/10.1016/j.addbeh.2008.07.010

Zamboanga, B. L., & Ham, L. S. (2008). Alcohol expectancies and context-specific drinking behaviours among female college athletes. *Behaviour Therapy, 39*(2), 162–170. https://doi.org/10.1016/j.beth.2007.06.002

Zamboanga, B. L., Horton, N. J., Leitkowski, L. K., & Wang, S. C. (2006). Do good things come to those who drink? A longitudinal investigation of drinking expectancies and hazardous alcohol use in female college athletes. *Journal of Adolescent Health, 39*, 229–236. https://doi.org/10.1016/j.jadohealth.2005.11.019

Zamboanga, B. L., Schwartz, S. J., Ham, L. S., Borsari, B., & Van Tyne, K. (2010). Alcohol expectancies, pregaming, drinking games, and hazardous alcohol use in a multiethnic sample of college students. *Cognitive Therapy and Research, 34*(2), 124–133. https://doi.org/10.1007/s10608-009-9234-1

Zhou, J., & Heim, D. (2014). Sports and spirits: A systematic qualitative review of emergent theories for student-athlete drinking. *Alcohol and Alcoholism, 49*(6), 604–617. https://doi.org/10.1093/alcalc/agu061

Zhou, J., & Heim, D. (2016). A qualitative exploration of alcohol use among student sportspeople: A social identity perspective. *European Journal of Social Psychology, 46*(5), 581–594. https://doi.org/10.1002/ejsp.2195

Zhou, J., Heim, D., & Levy, A. (2015). Sports participation and alcohol use: Associations with sports-related identities and well-being. *Journal of Studies on Alcohol and Drugs, 77*(1), 170–179. https://doi.org/10.15288/jsad.2016.77170

Zhou, J., Heim, D., & O'Brien, K. S. (2015). Alcohol consumption, athlete identity, and happiness among student sportspeople as a function of sport type. *Alcohol and Alcoholism, 50*(5), 617–623. https://doi.org/10.1093/alcalc/agv030

Zhou, J., O'Brien, K. S., & Heim, D. (2014). Alcohol consumption in sportspeople: The role of social cohesion, identity and happiness. *International Review for the Sociology of Sport, 49*(3–4), 278–293. https://doi.org/10.1177/1012690213493105

13

Determinants and Effects of Pre-drinking

Kim M. Caudwell and Martin S. Hagger

Introduction

A considerable amount of research has investigated hazardous patterns of alcohol consumption and their relation to the experience of alcohol-related harm. One hazardous pattern is "binge" drinking, a pattern of drinking characterised by excessive alcohol consumption over a discrete period. Such drinking patterns place individuals at increased risk of alcohol-related harm and are associated with substantial costs in terms of health care and workplace absenteeism. More recently, other patterns of excessive or problematic alcohol consumption have been considered, which are characterised by specific temporal and contextual components (see O'Rourke, Ferris, & Devaney, 2015). Such research has primarily considered *pre-drinking*—the practice of consuming

K. M. Caudwell (✉)
School of Health, Medical and Applied Sciences, CQUniversity, Rockhampton, QLD, Australia

School of Psychology, Curtin University, Perth, WA, Australia
e-mail: k.caudwell@cqu.edu.au

M. S. Hagger
Department of Psychological Sciences, University of California, Merced, Merced, CA, USA

Faculty of Sport and Health Sciences, University of Jyväskylä, Jyväskylä, Finland
e-mail: mhagger@merced.edu

R. Cooke et al. (eds.), *The Palgrave Handbook of Psychological Perspectives on Alcohol Consumption*, https://doi.org/10.1007/978-3-030-66941-6_13

alcohol prior to a social event. The present chapter aims to review the nascent literature on pre-drinking, providing definitions and theoretical explanations, and reviewing the evidence for psychological interventions aimed at reducing pre-drinking.

What Is Pre-drinking?

"Binge" drinking (Wechsler & Isaac, 1992, Chap. 1) is a pattern of drinking characterised by excessive alcohol consumption over a discrete period (also known as Heavy Episodic Drinking; HED; see Chap. 1) that has received considerable interest from psychological and health behaviour theorists and researchers (Cooke, Dahdah, Norman, & French, 2016; Hagger et al., 2012; see Chaps. 2 and 3). Such drinking patterns place individuals at increased risk of alcohol-related harm and are associated with substantial costs in terms of health care and workplace absenteeism (Doran, Hall, Shakeshaft, Vos, & Cobiac, 2010; Chap. 1).

More recently, other patterns of excessive or problematic alcohol consumption have been considered, that are characterised by specific temporal and contextual components (see O'Rourke et al., 2015). Such research has primarily considered *pre-drinking*—the practice of consuming alcohol prior to a social event. This pattern of drinking is known by many other terms, including *pre-loading*, *pre-funking*, *prepartying*, *pregaming*[1], and, in Argentina, *previa* (Borsari et al., 2007; J. H. Foster & Ferguson, 2013; LaBrie, Hummer, Kenney, Lac, & Pedersen, 2011; LaBrie & Pedersen, 2008; Pilatti & Read, 2018). For the present chapter, the term pre-drinking will be used to refer to this general pattern of alcohol consumption, however other terms used in pre-drinking measures will be retained.

Wells, Graham, and Purcell (2009) suggest that pre-drinking may have emerged in part due to the increased level of policy focus directed at reducing excessive alcohol consumption in licensed premises, such as bars and clubs. For example, mandatory "lockout" laws and regulations regarding the service of alcohol have been implemented to reduce excessive consumption in such premises (Chikritzhs et al., 2009; Miller et al., 2012). Subsequent research in the form of multi-site in situ studies have investigated pre-drinking at the population level in Australia (e.g. Miller et al., 2012), finding that 65% of

[1] Note that the term pre-gaming appears to overlap with drinking games—skill- or chance-based games that facilitate alcohol consumption and socialisation, which can, but do not always occur during pre-drinking sessions (Read et al., 2010; Zamboanga, Schwartz, Ham, Borsari, & Van Tyne, 2010).

participants reported pre-drinking on the occasion they were approached by researchers. Pre-drinking has also been observed in college or university settings and in associated populations, who tend to consume more alcohol than their non-student peers (Slutske et al., 2004), and for whom alcohol consumption is inherent to the university experience (Hallett, McManus, Maycock, Smith, & Howat, 2014). University students also appear to be highly aware of the perceived strategic benefits of pre-drinking (i.e. to become sufficiently intoxicated at low cost)—for example, researchers seeking to measure the breath alcohol concentration of university students prior to their entering a university concert were unable to collect data from over 40% of those intercepted as the students had consumed alcohol within the previous ten minutes (Riordan et al., 2018). Pre-drinking also appears to be more popular among younger undergraduate students, and less frequent in postgraduate students (Rutledge, Bestrashniy, & Nelson, 2016).

An early review of research on pre-drinking found the practice was related to increased alcohol consumption, intoxication, and the experience of alcohol-related harm (Foster & Ferguson, 2013). Initially, there had been debate over the utility of pursuing pre-drinking as a distinct alcohol consumption behaviour (Room & Livingston, 2009; Wells et al., 2009), however conceptualising pre-drinking as a form of off-premise alcohol consumption that occurs prior to subsequent alcohol consumption elsewhere (e.g. on-premise), appears an important distinction. Research has since confirmed that the pre-drinking environment (see Chaps. 8 and 9) plays a considerable role in determining the nature of alcohol consumption, and by extension, places pre-drinkers at unique risk for the experience of alcohol-related harm. Various event-level designs have been used to quantify the contribution of pre-drinking to total alcohol consumption, appearing to conclude that pre-drinking can be considered a specific case of HED (e.g. Labhart, Graham, Wells, & Kuntsche, 2013). Research evidence shows high rates of intoxication among pre-drinkers who are approached by researchers prior to attending their destination social event (Cameron, Roskruge, Droste, & Miller, 2018). The social dynamics conferred by the pre-drinking environment appears to have a contextual effect on alcohol consumption behaviour. For instance, individuals consume alcohol faster when pre-drinking (e.g. Kuntsche, Otten, & Labhart, 2015), which may be influenced by the size and composition of pre-drinking groups (Wells et al., 2015).

Given the substantive health and economic costs associated with all types of HED, and the problems caused by pre-drinking in particular, researchers have aimed to identify what factors make pre-drinking more or less likely. Such an endeavour may inform the development of strategies to reduce the frequency of pre-drinking and duration of pre-drinking sessions, which may subsequently reduce overall alcohol consumption during drinking occasions. Identification of the determinants of pre-drinking that may be targeted for intervention is, therefore, important. Knowledge of some determinants, such as alcohol availability and the density of retail outlets selling alcohol in the neighbourhood or pre-drinkers, may signal the importance of legislation to reduce the effects of the "drinking environment" on pre-drinking, such determinants may not be readily changeable. However, identifying highly modifiable determinants, such as psychological factors derived from theories of motivation may inform the content of behavioural interventions targeting change in these factors (see Chap. 21, for further justification). Much of the psychological theory-based research on pre-drinking draws from a variety of motivational and social cognition approaches, and the current chapter is organised according to the theoretical approaches and measures used. The following sections provide (1) a narrative overview of existing research on pre-drinking motives, (2) a summary of research applying motivational and social cognition approaches to the study of pre-drinking motives and behaviour, (3) discussion of interventions designed to target pre-drinking reduction and (4) limitations and extensions of pre-drinking research.

Measuring Pre-drinking

Motive-Based Measures

Cox and Klinger's (1988) incentive motivation model of alcohol use (see Chap. 2) suggests that decisions to approach or avoid alcohol are dependent on the likelihood that positive affect will be enhanced (hope), or reduced (disappointment), or that negative affect will be reduced (relief) or intensified (fear), by alcohol consumption. The balance of these anticipated affective responses influences an individual's decision regarding whether or not they will consume alcohol. Based on this framework, Cooper (1994) developed a four-factor questionnaire of drinking motives: The Drinking Motives Questionnaire-Revised (DMQ-R), that outlines four distinct motive dimensions that reflect those of Cox and Klinger's model: *enhancement*, *social*, *coping*, and *conformity*. Specifically, *enhancement* and *social* motives pertain to consuming alcohol to attain positive affective states (i.e. positive reinforcement), while *coping* and *conformity* relate to consuming alcohol to alleviate negative affective states (i.e. negative reinforcement). See Chap. 4 for more on prediction of consumption by drinking motives.

Early theory-based research on pre-drinking used the DMQ-R to investigate relationships between the four motives, self-reported pre-drinking frequency and alcohol consumption. Pedersen and LaBrie (2007) found statistically significant correlations between pre-drinking frequency and all four DMQ-R subscales in men, but pre-drinking frequency in women only significantly correlated with the *social* and *enhancement* motives (i.e. the positive subscales). In their regression analyses, *social* motives were the only significant predictor of pre-drinking frequency in men and women. None of the DMQ-R subscales correlated with nor were predictive of pre-drinking alcohol consumption. Read, Merrill, and Bytschkow (2010) generated a range of statements with dichotomous response scales based on reasons for pre-drinking from existing literature, and experience in researching alcohol consumption among college students. These reasons pertained to enhancement, socialisation, tension reduction, and financial and practical considerations, including becoming intoxicated prior to going out. The most commonly endorsed reason for pre-drinking was to save money. Correlation and regression analyses were conducted on the DMQ-R subscales, and pre-drinking frequency and alcohol consumption. Of the DMQ-R subscales, the authors noted marginally significant correlations and standardised regression coefficients between *enhancement* motives and pre-drinking frequency, suggesting that pre-drinkers are likely motivated to drink as they expect positive affective effects of alcohol consumption. Researchers have since sought to develop measures of motives that pertain to pre-drinking specifically, with some attempting to reconcile these within the broader DMQ-R, rooted in Cox and Klinger's incentive motivation model. These measures are described in the following section.

The Prepartying Motives Inventory Study findings discussed above led LaBrie, Hummer, Pedersen, Lac, and Chithambo (2012) to determine the whether or not pre-drinking motives differed from "general" drinking motives as captured by the DMQ-R (Cooper, 1994). LaBrie et al. (2012) recruited a random sample of students from two universities (stratified by class year) in the US and asked them to respond to an open-ended question regarding their reasons for pre-drinking (i.e. "for what reasons do you typically preparty?"). These reasons were then grouped according to similarity, with the 27 most frequently reported reasons administered to a second sample the following year. Factor analysis of responses revealed a four-factor structure of the Prepartying Motives Inventory (PMI), comprised of *interpersonal enhancement* (i.e. pre-drinking to facilitate or improve social interactions); *situational control* (i.e. pre-drinking for reasons related to alcohol supply and consumption); *barriers to consumption* (i.e. pre-drinking to compensate for a lack of access to alcohol at the intended destination), and; *intimate pursuit* (i.e. pre-drinking to facilitate romantic or sexual interactions with individuals). Higher scores on all four subscales were statistically significantly and positively correlated with pre-drinking behaviour with correlations ranging from 0.13 to 0.35, reflecting small to small- to medium-sized effects.

Interestingly, a cost item (i.e. pertaining to pre-drinking for reasons related to the relative cheaper cost of alcohol) was included in the PMI. However, this item failed to load on any dimension within the factor structure. Based on research evidence that suggested the alcohol consumption behaviours of undergraduate students may be sensitive to cost of alcohol (Miller & Droste, 2013), Caudwell and Hagger (2014) administered an online survey to a sample of university students in Australia comprising the PMI that omitted an item related to being under the legal age to purchase alcohol (as participants were of legal drinking age), but also included the single cost item (i.e. "I pre-drink because it is cheaper than purchasing drinks at the destination"), as well as measures of pre-drinking alcohol consumption, and alcohol-related harm as measured using the Brief Young Adult Alcohol Consequences Questionnaire (Kahler, Strong, & Read, 2005). In their path analysis, the single-item indicator of cost positively predicted both measures, indicating its importance in determining pre-drinking behaviour. *Interpersonal enhancement* and *barriers to consumption* also predicted higher alcohol consumption and alcohol-related harm; whereas *situational control* predicted lower scores on these measures.

Subsequent research by O'Neil, Lafreniere, and Jackson (2016) tested the factor structure of the PMI in a Canadian sample. The authors used a mixed-method approach, including questions about participants' experiences and reasons for pre-drinking. Their confirmatory factor analysis replicated the factor structure of the PMI adequately, observing improved fit following the removal of a *barriers to consumption* item. In terms of their correlational findings, all factors except *situational control* were significantly correlated with some aspect of pre-drinking behaviour, with small- to medium-sized effects (i.e. 0.14–0.43). The qualitative analysis of participant experiences revealed limited endorsement for *barriers to consumption*, and *situational control*, and no endorsement for *intimate pursuit*. The most commonly occurring themes were *monetary concern* (54%), *socialisation* (31%), *inebriation* (22%), *peer influence* (11%), and *boredom relief* (10%). These findings suggest that the PMI factor structure is replicable in a different national context, however the qualitative findings indicate that it may not encompass all factors that likely explain why individuals engage in pre-drinking behaviour.

A study of UK college students aged 16–18 years and university students aged 18 and over investigated relations between PMI subscales and pre-drinking (Howard, Albery, Frings, Spada, & Moss, 2019). The authors predicted that different motives determined the pre-drinking behaviour of participants in these age groups. In the college student sample, *interpersonal enhancement* was positively correlated with pre-drinking frequency, and *barriers to consumption* negatively correlated with pre-drinking alcohol consumption. Regression analyses revealed that participant AUDIT-C (Bush, Kivlahan, McDonell, Fihn, & Bradley, 1998) scores—a brief measure of hazardous alcohol use—were the only predictor of pre-drinking frequency; gender, AUDIT-C scores, and *barriers to consumption* were predictors of pre-drinking alcohol consumption (with the effect of *barriers to consumption* being negative). In the university student sample, *interpersonal enhancement* was correlated with pre-drinking frequency, and *interpersonal enhancement* and *intimate pursuit* correlated with pre-drinking alcohol consumption. Regression analysis revealed that AUDIT-C scores and *interpersonal enhancement* predicted pre-drinking frequency, and AUDIT-C scores alone significantly predicted alcohol consumption. The authors note the limited relevance of the situational control motives in both samples. While both younger and older samples of UK students endorsed *interpersonal enhancement* motives, the influence of *barriers to consumption* was largely confined to the younger sample, whereas *intimate pursuit* motives were more salient in the older sample. The negative correlations observed between *barriers to consumption* and pre-drinking behaviour suggests that UK participants may pre-drink for reasons related to alcohol access but moderate their alcohol consumption when pre-drinking.

The Pregaming Motives Measure Similar to LaBrie et al. (2012), Bachrach, Merrill, Bytschkow, and Read (2012) suspected that general drinking motives captured in the DMQ-R, may not adequately capture motives for engaging in "unique types of alcohol use" (p. 3). Specifically, they argue that pre-drinking may be primarily driven by positive affect. Accordingly, Bachrach et al. (2012) developed the Pregaming Motives Measure (PGMM). Based on initial focus group data and motives identified in the literature, a factor analysis of an initial PGMM item pool identified three factors. These were: *inebriation/fun* (positive affect), *instrumentality* (practicality, generally related to alcohol availability), and *social ease* (social relaxation, or to "loosen up").

In contrast to the findings of LaBrie et al. (2012), Bachrach et al. found PGMM factors were correlated with the *social*, *coping*, *enhancement*, and *conformity* dimensions from the DMQ-R, with effect sizes ranging from small to large (i.e. 0.12–0.71). Regression analysis showed that the DMQ-R motive *enhancement* predicted pre-drinking quantity/frequency, however this became non-significant when the PGMM subscales were included in the analysis, suggesting some redundancy across the scales. The only predictors of pregaming quantity/frequency in the analysis were the PGMM factors *inebriation/fun*, and *instrumentality*, after controlling for gender. Bachrach et al. noted that while *social ease* did not predict pre-drinking behaviour, it was positively correlated with it, suggesting that "social reasons may explain *why* one would engage in this behaviour, but do not necessarily predict *how much* or *how often*" (p. 11). This suggests that there may be some relationship between general drinking motives and pre-drinking-specific motives; however, the contribution of *instrumentality* appears a relevant finding, given that it is not represented in the DMQ-R.

Like O'Neil et al. (2016), Bachrach et al. (2012) suggested that their data indicated that pre-drinking may be highly context-specific—for example, in a scenario where students are under the legal drinking age, they may more strongly endorse reasons related to alcohol access (e.g. *instrumental*, *barriers to consumption* motives). Given that the average age of participants in LaBrie et al. (2012) was under 21, a large proportion of the sample may not have been legally allowed to procure alcohol. Bachrach et al. also sought to establish whether the relationship between pre-drinking motives and alcohol-related consequences was mediated by pre-drinking quantity/frequency. The authors found evidence for an indirect effect via both the *inebriation/fun* and *instrumental* variables, respectively, suggesting that effects of motives determined outcomes via behaviour. These findings indicate the process by which motives lead to outcomes, which presents a potentially viable avenue for intervention development.

The Pre-drinking Motives Questionnaire In response to the development and validation of the PGMM and PMI, Labhart and Kuntsche (2017) developed a Pre-drinking Motives Questionnaire (PMQ), using the same or similar items to those in the PGMM and PMI, as well as those elicited from focus group interviews. Data were collected from participants in French- and German-speaking Switzerland. Factor analysis of the initial item pool revealed a three-factor structure comprising *fun/intoxication* (i.e. to maximise drunkenness at minimal cost), *conviviality* (i.e. pre-drinking to socialise in an appropriate environment), and *facilitation* (i.e. to overcome difficulty with social interactions). Regression analyses indicated associations between the *fun/intoxication*, and *social* and *enhancement* subscales of the PMQ, and the *facilitation*, and *social* and *conformity* dimensions of the DMQ-R. In terms of participant group differences, those in the French-speaking region scored higher on the conviviality subscale than those in the German-speaking region, suggesting some regional variation in pre-drinking motives. Males scored higher than females on the fun/intoxication and facilitation subscales. There were no statistically significant age group, nor student status differences in subscale scores, which may suggest some degree of universality in pre-drinking motives measured by the PMQ. The authors stated that a key contribution of the PMQ was that *conviviality* was not associated with any of the DMQ-R subscales.

The Pregaming Motives Questionnaire (PMQ-Arg) Pilatti and Read (2018) considered the factor structure of pre-drinking/pre-gaming motives in Argentinean pre-drinkers, based on research that suggesting that underlying pre-drinking motives may vary between countries. The authors first identified frequently endorsed motives, rated for correspondence, quality, and adequacy, generating a pool of 28 items, before subjecting these to factor analysis in a different sample. Their analysis yielded four factors: *intoxication and fun*; *gathering and social enhancement*; *going with the flow*; and *beverage preference*—comprising the Pregaming Motives Questionnaire (PMQ-Arg). These motives significantly correlated with pre-drinking frequency, and all but *going with the flow* were significantly correlated with pre-drinking alcohol consumption. The authors also included the DMQ-R and PGMM in their analysis and found that *enhancement* motives from the DMQ-R significantly correlated with pre-drinking frequency. In contrast to LaBrie et al.'s (2012) study, all PMI subscales were significantly correlated with the DMQ-R subscales with the exception of the correlation between *situational control* and *conformity*. Results revealed that none of the PMQ-Arg dimensions accounted for significant variance in pre-drinking frequency beyond total alcohol consumed in the previous year. The *intoxication and fun*, and *beverage preference* accounted for significant variance in pre-drinking alcohol consumption, beyond that of gender, and total alcohol consumption.

Original work on establishing pre-drinking motives is grounded in Cox and Klinger's incentive motivation model (Cox & Klinger, 1988, see Chap. 2), and indeed many of the constructs that form the basis of pre-drinking questionnaires and inventories are broadly consistent with these dimensions.

Specifically, most motives regarding pre-drinking relate to the positive expected affective responses relating to alcohol consumption, represented by the *social* and *enhancement* motives (e.g. *interpersonal enhancement, inebriation/fun*). However, there appear some deviations from the dimensional framework in relation to the expected effects of alcohol consumption, pertaining to positive and negative affect. For example, some motives (e.g. *interpersonal enhancement, conviviality*) are perhaps tangentially related to the negative expected effects of alcohol consumption, such as *conformity* and *coping*. However, correlational research on pre-drinking motives has not provided conclusive evidence for consistent relationships with drinking motives measured using the DMQ-R, nor provide support for the universality of pre-drinking motives (see Table 13.1 for a summary). A number of motives emerging from research on pre-drinking motives relate to barriers, facilitation, and control-related factors (e.g. situational *control, barriers to consumption, instrumental*), and appear less concerned with anticipated affect. It is possible that motives measures developed in one country do not adequately capture the relevant contextual factors that underpin pre-drinking motives in other countries (Labhart & Kuntsche, 2017). A study by Ferris, Puljević, Labhart, Winstock, and Kuntsche (2019) supports this proposition; considerable heterogeneity was observed in an analysis of 27 countries' pre-drinking behaviours, indicating an individual country focus may be best for identifying relevant motives, and therefore developing effective pre-drinking interventions that target these motives, at both individual and policy levels.

Motivational and Social Cognition Research

Recent attempts to integrate psychological models and theories to better explain the reasons why individuals engage in a range of health behaviours, have led to new insights (Hagger & Chatzisarantis, 2009). Two such perspectives include self-determination theory, and the theory of planned behaviour, which have been applied to the broader alcohol consumption research domain (e.g. Hagger et al., 2012). In relation to pre-drinking, Caudwell and Hagger (2015) used an integrated theoretical model that comprised elements of self-determination theory (Deci & Ryan, 1985) and the theory of planned behaviour (Ajzen, 1991, see Chap. 2) to explore pre-drinking among undergraduates, based on the premise that motivational orientations from self-determination theory lead to the development of belief-based evaluations in the theory of planned behaviour, which will subsequently influence behaviour (Hagger & Chatzisarantis, 2009). In their prospective-correlational study, Caudwell and

Table 13.1 Pre-drinking motive measures, their factors, and associations with DMQ-R subscales

Measure (*n* factors)	Dimension (*n* items)	Highest-loading item (reported loading)	Associations with DMQ-R[a]			
			Social	Coping	Enh.	Conf.
PMI (4)	Interpersonal enhancement (6)	"To relax or loosen up before I go out" (0.85)	<0.01	−0.05	−0.04	−0.07
	Situational control (4)	"So I don't have to worry about whether someone has tampered with the drinks at a party" (0.82)	−0.03	−0.06	−0.05	−0.08
	Barriers to consumption (3)	"To avoid getting caught with alcohol on the way to, or at, the final destination" (0.85)	0.04	−0.01	0.04	−0.03
	Intimate pursuit (3)	"To increase the likelihood of hooking up" (0.85)	0.09	<0.01	0.01	0.04
PGMM (3)	Inebriation/fun (5)	"To have fun." (0.84)	0.71**	0.34**	0.64**	0.26**
	Instrumentality (5)	"Because there will not be enough alcohol at the event" (0.82)	0.17**	0.35**	0.21**	0.44**
	Social ease (5)	"To become more social before going to the event" (0.94)	0.49**	0.60**	0.43**	0.42**
PMQ (3)	Fun/ intoxication (6)	"To get in a party mood" (0.84)	0.41***	0.09	0.28***	0.00
	Conviviality (5)	"Because we can listen to the music we like" (0.75)	0.13	0.00	−0.01	0.06
	Facilitation (4)	"Because it helps for hitting on someone, flirting or being charming ""(0.90)	0.44***	0.00	−0.04	0.31***

(*continued*)

Table 13.1 (continued)

Measure (*n* factors)	Dimension (*n* items)	Highest-loading item (reported loading)	Associations with DMQ-R[a]			
			Social	Coping	Enh.	Conf.
PMQ-Arg (4)	Intoxication and fun (8)	"To get uninhibited at the event" (0.84)	0.70**	0.33**	0.59**	0.30**
	Gathering and social enhancement (5)	"To go out in group" (0.79)	0.24**	0.08	0.24**	0.12
	Going with the flow (6)	"Because this is what my friends do" (0.74)	0.35**	0.16	0.18**	0.37**
	Beverage control (4)	"To drink better quality alcoholic beverages than the ones at the event" (0.78)	0.30**	0.22**	0.31**	0.04

Note: DMQ-R = drinking motives questionnaire revised (Cooper, 1994); PMI = prepartying motives inventory (LaBrie et al., 2012); PGMM = pregaming motives measure (Bachrach et al., 2012); PMQ = pre-drinking motives questionnaire (Labhart & Kuntsche, 2017); PMQ-Arg = pregaming motives questionnaire (Pilatti & Read, 2018); Enh = enhancement; Conf. = conformity. Loadings and correlations have been rounded to two decimal places for interpretability

[a]The PMI and PGMM were correlated with the subscales of the 20-item DMQ-R (Cooper, 1994), whereas the PMQ was regressed on the subscales of the 12-item DMQ-R short form (DMQ-R-SF; Kuntsche & Kuntsche, 2009), and the PMQ-Arg correlated with the subscales of the Spanish version of the DMQ-R-SF (Mezquita et al., 2016)

*$p < 0.05$ ** $p < 0.01$ *** $p < 0.001$ (reported)

Hagger (2015) found that autonomous motivation from self-determination theory was associated with Australian students' intentions to pre-drink, and this pathway was partially mediated by attitudes and subjective norms pertaining to pre-drinking. These results suggest that undergraduates consider pre-drinking as serving some internalised goal (e.g. becoming intoxicated), or being inherently enjoyable. This appears to echo the dimensions identified in pre-drinking motive research (Bachrach et al., 2012; Labhart & Kuntsche, 2017; LaBrie et al., 2012; Pilatti & Read, 2018).

Caudwell and Hagger (2015) also found modest relationships between pre-drinking frequency and both intentions and perceived behavioural control (i.e. higher scores in perceived behavioural control were associated with less frequent pre-drinking), which are somewhat different to what has been found in other studies (see Chap. 4).

The authors suggested that dual systems theories could overcome limitations in the prediction of behaviour by reflective processes, by incorporating measures of impulsive processes (Hofmann, Friese, & Wiers, 2008), such as implicit alcohol identity—the degree to which an individual exhibits a non-conscious bias towards alcohol and identity-related stimuli (Lindgren, Foster, Westgate, & Neighbors, 2013). Caudwell and Hagger (2014) tested this proposition by including a measure of implicit drinking identity alongside the Prepartying Motives Inventory in a cross-sectional study on pre-drinking in undergraduate students. Implicit drinking identity was correlated with alcohol consumption frequency, predicted alcohol-related harm, and was a marginally significant predictor of pre-drinking alcohol consumption. However, because a cross-sectional design was used in this study caution must be taken when applying results to studies using prospective designs (see Chap. 2 for more on this issue).

Expanding on this line of research, Caudwell, Keech, Hamilton, Mullan, and Hagger (2019) incorporated a measure of implicit alcohol identity alongside measures from self-determination theory and the theory of planned behaviour in a prospective-correlational design, measuring intentions to reduce alcohol consumption during pre-drinking sessions, and subsequent behaviour. Results showed that implicit alcohol identity and perceived behavioural control (i.e. regarding reducing alcohol consumption during pre-drinking sessions) both significantly predicted alcohol consumption at follow-up. This suggests that both implicit and reflective factors can influence individuals' alcohol consumption during pre-drinking sessions, consistent with O'Neil et al. (2016), who suspect that peer influence to engage in pre-drinking may incorporate explicit and implicit factors.

Interventions Designed to Target Pre-drinking

In light of the converging evidence on the risks of pre-drinking, and the psychological factors that influence pre-drinkers, the next step has been to develop interventions to reduce alcohol consumption and alcohol-related harm among pre-drinkers (Pedersen, 2016). Caudwell, Mullan, and Hagger (2016) developed an intervention aimed at changing pre-drinking determinants identified in theory-based and formative research applied to pre-drinking. The intervention was based on the model of action-phases, comprising elements to target the motivational and volitional phases of behavioural engagement (Heckhausen, 1991). The motivational phase required participants to provide responses to autonomy-supportive text prompts, in order to facilitate autonomous motivation to change behaviour (Ng et al., 2012). The volitional phase asked participants to select or form their own implementation intentions—a planning technique that facilitates linking an environmental cue with a goal-intended behaviour (Gollwitzer, 1999; Gollwitzer & Sheeran, 2006, Chap. 21). Research has identified that the provision of autonomy support, coupled with such a planning technique, is likely more efficacious in changing behaviour than either approach alone (Caudwell et al., 2016; Koestner et al., 2006). The intervention adopted a randomised controlled design with pre-screened pre-drinking undergraduates randomly assigned to receive either the autonomy support or the implementation intention component of the intervention, both, and a control group (neither). The intervention was delivered online, with participants completing initial pre-intervention measures of alcohol consumption behaviour, and theory-based motivational and volitional constructs, before viewing national guidelines pertaining to reducing health risks associated with alcohol consumption. Participants then received motivational and/or volitional intervention components, or neither, depending on the condition to which they were allocated. All participants were sent a summary email reminder and weekly SMS messages consistent with their allocated intervention condition (the control group received brief restatements of the national guidelines).

Results revealed alcohol consumption and experience of alcohol-related harm decreased for all groups following the intervention, with no main effects for the motivational and volitional components of the intervention on pre-drinking alcohol consumption at four-week follow-up (Caudwell, Mullan, & Hagger, 2018). However, Caudwell et al. (2018) speculated that the combination of providing the national guidelines, baseline measurement of alcohol consumption, and provision of a summary email and related SMS messages, likely conferred a substantial treatment effect that led to reductions in the outcome measures. This is consistent with the findings of Livingston (2012) who concluded that Australian drinkers were generally unaware of the national guidelines pertaining to alcohol consumption and health, meaning that some participants may have been unaware of them prior to commencing the intervention, and changed their behaviour accordingly. Similarly, the "mere measurement" effect (i.e. the effect of measuring alcohol consumption behaviour at baseline on subsequent pre-drinking behaviour) may have contributed to behaviour change across conditions (see Kypri, Langley, Saunders, & Cashell-Smith, 2007), obscuring the effect of the motivation and planning elements. Ultimately, these findings suggest that the provision of basic information on the risks of alcohol consumption and pre-drinking, and mere measurement of pre-drinking behaviour, may be important in reducing pre-drinking alcohol consumption.

Caudwell et al. (2018) provided some speculation as to potential avenues for refining their intervention content and its application. First, autonomy-supportive strategies are usually delivered in face-to-face contexts, such as classrooms or conventional treatment environments (Ng et al., 2012; Teixera et al., 2020). It may be that more involvement with the research team (e.g. personalised correspondence providing the opportunity to clarify the participants' statements) could have better fostered a sense of autonomy support, and produced a detectable treatment effect (Wright, Dietze, Crockett, & Lim, 2016). In relation to the implementation intentions component of the intervention, participants were provided with the opportunity to select from prepared options, or write their own, with some participant-generated implementation intentions unlikely to be effective in achieving the intended behaviour (Caudwell et al., 2018). Conversely, participants in the combined condition who selected the completed implementation intentions may not have experience a sense of ownership over them nor a sense of personal relevance regarding them—both key components in the provision of autonomy support—which could have hindered the effectiveness of these plans. Though no significant differences in terms of reductions in alcohol consumption between experimenter-provided and self-generated implementation intentions have been observed, compliance may moderate the effectiveness of the latter (Armitage, 2009, Chap. 21).

Zamboanga et al. (2019) have also tested an intervention aimed at reducing the risk of excessive alcohol consumption and alcohol-related harm from pre-drinking, as well as drinking games, among college student athletes. The intervention adopted a randomised controlled design using an online intervention (myPlaybook). The intervention comprised three brief lessons, taking on average 12 minutes to complete, based on a range of behaviour change techniques (i.e. natural consequences, feedback and monitoring, comparison of behaviour, comparison of outcomes, and shaping knowledge). Participants completed these lessons at baseline, with the exception of the control group, who received the introductory lesson only. Participants were provided with a range of incentives to reward participation, were delivered email reminders, and were assessed at one- and four-month follow-up. Results indicated that the intervention had no effect on pre-drinking nor drinking game behaviour. Zamboanga et al. (2019) provided a brief summary of five intervention studies that target drinking games, four which do not appear to concern pre-drinking, with the exception of Borsari, Merrill, Yurasek, Miller, and Carey

(2016), who found no effect of brief advice or brief motivation intervention on mandated students' pre-drinking frequency at three, six, and nine months from baseline.

Limitations and Extensions of Pre-drinking Research

Several pre-drinking-specific inventories have been developed, many based directly, or loosely, on Cox and Klinger's (1988) motivational model of alcohol use. Generally, research supports motives that are consistent with positive anticipated affective responses, such as *social* and *enhancement* motives, which is consistent with the determinants of other forms of HED such as binge drinking. However, more idiosyncratic factors predict pre-drinking as well, including barriers, facilitation, and control-related elements. Other determinants have been identified, such as factors relating to cost (suggesting that one key motive for pre-drinking is drinking "less expensively"), and factors relating to impulsive processes such as implicit alcohol identity; although, the effects of these constructs have not been broadly studied. Moreover, research suggests considerable variability in the determinants across samples, indicating the imperative of exploring population-specific motives. For instance, Miller et al. (2015) have suggested that pre-drinking "reflects Australia's culture of determined drunkenness and requires serious, substantial, evidence-based interventions across a range of variables" (p. 11). It is important that research on this particular pattern of drinking is maintained, given that these patterns have been shown to influence and compound the deleterious effects HED in several countries. Similarly, research on pre-drinking could be broadened to incorporate similar patterns of alcohol consumption, such as side-loading (i.e. consuming previously procured alcohol within a licensed premise, or consuming alcohol when travelling between licensed premises) and back-loading (i.e. consuming alcohol after an event's conclusion), to determine if these behaviours are comparable in terms of risk and contextual determinants (O'Rourke et al., 2015).

Interventions aimed at reducing pre-drinking have been relatively limited in number and the evidence base is currently too small to make a definitive assessment of their effectiveness. Thus far, behaviour change interventions have been relatively ineffective (Borsari et al., 2016; Caudwell et al., 2018; Zamboanga et al., 2019). However, these studies did not specifically target the idiosyncratic beliefs identified in pre-drinking research, suggesting more intervention research is needed, particularly those drawing from the formative research reviewed earlier in this chapter. In particular, mixed-methods and qualitative approaches have shown that there may be more practical contextual factors that influence pre-drinking yet are not reflected in factor analytic approaches based on factor analyses alone, especially given that measures developed through factor analysis may have less relevance when applied to other national contexts.

Given the commonality observed between pre-drinking and general alcohol consumption motives, intervention strategies that have demonstrated efficacy in the broader HED and health behaviour change literature may have some utility in addressing pre-drinking specifically. Although ineffective in Caudwell et al. (2018), planning-based interventions have previously shown some promise in binge drinking (Murgraff, Abraham, & McDermott, 2007; Murgraff, White, & Phillips, 1996, see Chap. 21). Potentially, the influence of contextual dynamics inherent to the pre-drinking environment may be difficult to challenge with planning approaches, though further research is required to elucidate their effectiveness. For instance, pre-drinkers may find quantifying their alcohol consumption difficult (e.g. de Visser & Birch, 2012). Though this suggests that the implementation of plans to reduce pre-drinking alcohol consumption could be challenging, de Visser (2015) found that the provision of feedback on alcohol pouring tasks led to increased participant awareness of safe drinking guidelines and decreased alcohol consumption, relative to a "no feedback" condition. This may be a key finding to inform pre-drinking interventions, considering that pre-drinkers are comparatively unimpeded in their self-service and consumption of alcohol, as opposed to their service and consumption in licensed venues (Wells et al., 2009).

The influential enjoyment motives endorsed by pre-drinkers, and self-determined reasons for pre-drinking, present a considerable challenge for the development of effective health behaviour change interventions, yet there are some areas of research that may have utility in meeting this challenge. For example, research has shown that "next-day obligations" (e.g. work, sporting commitments) have considerable influence over drinking decisions, potentially due to the personal relevance of the obligation, and perceived immediacy of the consequences of drinking (Skidmore & Murphy, 2011). This may afford some potential to the use of decisional balance sheet—exercises that position the individual to consider the immediate and delayed positive and negative outcomes of pre-drinking (Foster, Neighbors, & Pai, 2015). Similarly, research has looked at drinking refusal self-efficacy as a factor that determines excessive alcohol consumption (Young, Connor, Ricciardelli, & Saunders, 2006). Given the excessive alcohol consumption that occurs during pre-drinking sessions, often leading being too drunk to leave the pre-drinking venue or unconsciousness (e.g. McCreanor et al., 2016), interventions that bolster drinking refusal self-efficacy may be successful in tempering excessive alcohol consumption during pre-drinking sessions, but research is need to confirm that social pressure to drink does not undermine the effectiveness of such interventions.

Though these additional intervention strategies have demonstrated efficacy in reducing alcohol consumption and binge drinking more broadly, care should be taken in extrapolating these findings to inform approaches to practices such as pre-drinking. The extensive research on determinants identified in the first sections of this chapter indicate pre-drinking as a specific case of risky HED with a specific profile of determinants that differ somewhat from other forms of excessive alcohol consumption. Identifying the psychological processes by which these strategies might influence pre-drinking, and systematically testing these intervention strategies in pre-drinking populations—perhaps complemented by existing effective behaviour change techniques—is warranted and an important avenue for future research. Concurrent research on the effects of government policy, legislation, and industry endeavours to protect individuals from alcohol-related harm and how this may precipitate behaviours such as pre-drinking is needed to ensure that risky alcohol consumption behaviours are not simply shifted to off-premise contexts.

Conclusion

The current chapter identified pre-drinking as a specific case of HED with deleterious effects on the health and safety of pre-drinking individuals and those around them, and substantive economic costs. As a specific form of alcohol consumption, there has been an increasing body of research exploring the determinants of pre-drinking, particularly those derived from theories of motivation and social cognition. The few interventions that have been developed to target pre-drinking behaviour to date appear relatively ineffective yet have signposted several important avenues for future research on pre-drinking interventions. Future pre-drinking research should aim to (1) adopt qualitative or mixed-methods approaches to ascertain the influential beliefs and determinants of pre-drinking behaviour within a given population, and reconcile these within existing health behaviour change theories to inform intervention development; (2) implement or modify existing behaviour change techniques either from the broader alcohol intervention literature or better-suited to the unique determinants of pre-drinking; and (3) inform public health measures that address the broader sociocultural factors that promote or precipitate pre-drinking behaviour.

References

Ajzen, I. (1991). The theory of planned behavior. *Organizational Behavior and Human Decision Processes, 50*(2), 179–211. https://doi.org/10.1016/0749-5978(91)90020-t

Armitage, C. J. (2009). Effectiveness of experimenter-provided and self-generated implementation intentions to reduce alcohol consumption in a sample of the general population: a randomized exploratory trial. *Health Psychology, 28*(5), 545–553. https://doi.org/10.1037/a0015984

Bachrach, R. L., Merrill, J. E., Bytschkow, K. M., & Read, J. P. (2012). Development and initial validation of a measure of motives for pregaming in college students. *Addictive Behaviors, 37*(9), 1038–1045. https://doi.org/10.1016/j.addbeh.2012.04.013

Borsari, B., Boyle, K. E., Hustad, J. T. P., Barnett, N. P., O'Leary Tevyaw, T., & Kahler, C. W. (2007). Drinking before drinking: Pregaming and drinking games in mandated students. *Addictive Behaviors, 32*(11), 2694–2705. https://doi.org/10.1016/j.addbeh.2007.05.003

Borsari, B., Merrill, J. E., Yurasek, A., Miller, M. B., & Carey, K. B. (2016). Does a brief motivational intervention reduce frequency of pregaming in mandated students? *Substance Use & Misuse*, 1–11. https://doi.org/10.3109/10826084.2016.1152494

Bush, K., Kivlahan, D. R., McDonell, M. B., Fihn, S. D., & Bradley, K. A. (1998). The AUDIT alcohol consumption questions (AUDIT-C): An effective brief screening test for problem drinking. *Archives of Internal Medicine, 158*(16), 1789. https://doi.org/10.1001/archinte.158.16.1789

Cameron, M. P., Roskruge, M. J., Droste, N., & Miller, P. G. (2018). Pre-drinking and the temporal gradient of intoxication in a New Zealand nightlife environment. *Journal of Studies on Alcohol and Drugs, 79*(1), 119–125. https://doi.org/10.15288/jsad.2018.79.119

Caudwell, K. M., & Hagger, M. S. (2014). Pre-drinking and alcohol-related harm in undergraduates: The influence of explicit motives and implicit alcohol identity. *Journal of Behavioral Medicine, 37*(6), 1252–1262. https://doi.org/10.1007/s10865-014-9573-6

Caudwell, K. M., & Hagger, M. S. (2015). Predicting alcohol pre-drinking in Australian undergraduate students using an integrated theoretical model. *Applied Psychology: Health and Well-Being, 7*(2), 188–213. https://doi.org/10.1111/aphw.12044

Caudwell, K. M., Keech, J. J., Hamilton, K., Mullan, B. A., & Hagger, M. S. (2019). Reducing alcohol consumption during pre-drinking sessions: Testing an integrated behaviour-change model. *Psychology & Health, 34*(1), 106–127. https://doi.org/10.1080/08870446.2018.1518527

Caudwell, K. M., Mullan, B., & Hagger, M. S. (2016). Combining motivational and volitional approaches to reducing excessive alcohol consumption in pre-drinkers: A theory-based intervention protocol. *BMC Public Health, 16*(45), 1–12. https://doi.org/10.1186/s12889-015-2648-7

Caudwell, K. M., Mullan, B., & Hagger, M. S. (2018). Testing an online, theory-based intervention to reduce pre-drinking alcohol consumption and alcohol-related harm in undergraduates: A randomized controlled trial. *International Journal of Behavioral Medicine, 25*(5), 592–604. https://doi.org/10.1007/s12529-018-9736-x

Chikritzhs, T. N., Dietze, P. M., Allsop, S. J., Daube, M. M., Hall, W. D., & Kypri, K. (2009). The 'alcopops' tax: Heading in the right direction. *Medical Journal of Australia, 190*(1), 294. https://doi.org/10.5694/j.1326-5377.2009.tb02415.x

Cooke, R., Dahdah, M., Norman, P., & French, D. P. (2016). How well does the theory of planned behaviour predict alcohol consumption? A systematic review and meta-analysis. *Health Psychology Review, 10*(2), 148–167. https://doi.org/10.1080/17437199.2014.947547

Cooper, M. L. (1994). Motivations for alcohol use among adolescents: Development and validation of a four-factor model. *Psychological Assessment, 6*(2), 117–128. https://doi.org/10.1037/1040-3590.6.2.117

Cox, W. M., & Klinger, E. (1988). A motivational model of alcohol use. *Journal of Abnormal Psychology, 97*(2), 168–180. https://doi.org/10.1037/0021-843X.97.2.168

de Visser, R. O. (2015). Personalized feedback based on a drink-pouring exercise may improve knowledge of, and adherence to, government guidelines for alcohol consumption. *Alcoholism: Clinical and Experimental Research, 39*(2), 317–323. https://doi.org/10.1111/acer.12623

de Visser, R. O., & Birch, J. D. (2012). My cup runneth over: Young people's lack of knowledge of low-risk drinking guidelines. *Drug and Alcohol Review, 31*(2), 206–212. https://doi.org/10.1111/j.1465-3362.2011.00371.x

Deci, E. L., & Ryan, R. M. (1985). *Intrinsic motivation and self-determination in human behaviour*. New York, NY: Plenum.

Doran, C. M., Hall, W., Shakeshaft, A. P., Vos, T., & Cobiac, L. (2010). Alcohol policy reform in Australia: What can we learn from the evidence? *Medical Journal of Australia, 192*(8), 468–470. http://www.ncbi.nlm.nih.gov.dbgw.lis.curtin.edu.au/

Ferris, J., Puljević, C., Labhart, F., Winstock, A., & Kuntsche, E. (2019). The role of sex and age on pre-drinking: An exploratory international comparison of 27 countries. *Alcohol and Alcoholism, 54*(4), 378–385. https://doi.org/10.1093/alcalc/agz040

Foster, D. W., Neighbors, C., & Pai, A. (2015). Decisional balance: Alcohol decisional balance intervention for heavy drinking undergraduates. *Substance Use & Misuse, 50*(13), 1717–1727. https://doi.org/10.3109/10826084.2015.1036883

Foster, J. H., & Ferguson, C. (2013). Alcohol 'pre-loading': A review of the literature. *Alcohol and Alcoholism, 49*(2), 213–226. https://doi.org/10.1093/alcalc/agt135

Gollwitzer, P. M. (1999). Implementation intentions: Strong effects of simple plans. *American Psychologist, 54*(7), 493. https://doi.org/10.1037/0003-066X.54.7.493

Gollwitzer, P. M., & Sheeran, P. (2006). Implementation intentions and goal achievement: A meta-analysis of effects and processes. *Advances in Experimental Social Psychology, 38*, 69–119. https://doi.org/10.1016/s0065-2601(06)38002-1

Hagger, M. S., & Chatzisarantis, N. L. D. (2009). Integrating the theory of planned behaviour and self-determination theory in health behaviour: A meta-analysis. *British Journal of Health Psychology, 14*(2), 275–302. https://doi.org/10.1348/135910708x373959

Hagger, M. S., Lonsdale, A. J., Hein, V., Koka, A., Lintunen, T., Pasi, H., … Chatzisarantis, N. L. D. (2012). Predicting alcohol consumption and binge drinking in company employees: An application of planned behaviour and self-determination theories. *British Journal of Health Psychology*, 1–29. https://doi.org/10.1111/j.2044-8287.2011.02043.x

Hallett, J., McManus, A., Maycock, B. R., Smith, J., & Howat, P. M. (2014). "Excessive drinking – an inescapable part of university life?" A focus group study of Australian undergraduates. *Open Journal of Preventive Medicine, 4*(7), 616–629. https://doi.org/10.4236/ojpm.2014.47071

Heckhausen, H. (1991). The rubicon model of action phases. In H. Heckhausen (Ed.), *Motivation and action*. New York, NY: Springer-Verlag.

Hofmann, W., Friese, M., & Wiers, R. W. (2008). Impulsive versus reflective influences on health behavior: A theoretical framework and empirical review. *Health Psychology Review, 2*(2), 111–137. https://doi.org/10.1080/17437190802617668

Howard, A. R., Albery, I. P., Frings, D., Spada, M. M., & Moss, A. C. (2019). Pre-partying amongst students in the UK: Measuring motivations and consumption levels across different educational contexts. *Substance Use & Misuse, 54*(9), 1519–1529. https://doi.org/10.1080/10826084.2019.1590414

Kahler, C. W., Strong, D. R., & Read, J. P. (2005). Toward efficient and comprehensive measurement of the alcohol problems continuum in college students: The brief Young adult alcohol consequences questionnaire. *Alcoholism: Clinical and Experimental Research, 29*(7), 1180–1189. https://doi.org/10.1097/01.ALC.0000171940.95813.A5

Koestner, R., Horberg, E., Gaudreau, P., Powers, T., Di Dio, P., Bryan, C., … Salter, N. (2006). Bolstering implementation plans for the long haul: The benefits of simultaneously boosting self-concordance or self-efficacy. *Personality and Social Psychology Bulletin, 32*(11), 1547–1558. https://doi.org/10.1177/0146167206291782

Kuntsche, E., & Kuntsche, S. (2009). Development and validation of the drinking motive questionnaire revised short form (DMQ–R SF). *Journal of Clinical Child & Adolescent Psychology, 38*(6), 899–908. https://doi.org/10.1080/15374410903258967

Kuntsche, E., Otten, R., & Labhart, F. (2015). Identifying risky drinking patterns over the course of Saturday evenings: An event-level study. *Psychology of Addictive Behaviors, 29*(3), 744–752. https://doi.org/10.1037/adb0000057

Kypri, K., Langley, J. D., Saunders, J. B., & Cashell-Smith, M. L. (2007). Assessment may conceal therapeutic benefit: Findings from a randomized controlled trial for hazardous drinking. *Addiction, 102*(1), 62–70. https://doi.org/10.1111/j.1360-0443.2006.01632.x

Labhart, F., Graham, K., Wells, S., & Kuntsche, E. (2013). Drinking before going to licensed premises: An event-level analysis of predrinking, alcohol consumption, and adverse outcomes. *Alcoholism: Clinical and Experimental Research, 37*(2), 284–291. https://doi.org/10.1111/j.1530-0277.2012.01872.x

Labhart, F., & Kuntsche, E. (2017). Development and validation of the predrinking motives questionnaire. *Journal of Applied Social Psychology, 47*(3), 136–147. https://doi.org/10.1111/jasp.12419

LaBrie, J. W., Hummer, J., Kenney, S., Lac, A., & Pedersen, E. (2011). Identifying factors that increase the likelihood for alcohol-induced blackouts in the prepartying context. *Substance Use & Misuse, 46*(8), 992–1002. https://doi.org/10.3109/10826084.2010.542229

LaBrie, J. W., Hummer, J. F., Pedersen, E. R., Lac, A., & Chithambo, T. (2012). Measuring college students' motives behind prepartying drinking: Development and validation of the Prepartying motivations inventory. *Addictive Behaviors, 37*(8), 962–969. https://doi.org/10.1016/j.addbeh.2012.04.003

LaBrie, J. W., & Pedersen, E. R. (2008). Prepartying promotes heightened risk in the college environment: An event-level report. *Addictive Behaviors, 33*(7), 955–959. https://doi.org/10.1016/j.addbeh.2008.02.011

Lindgren, K. P., Foster, D. W., Westgate, E. C., & Neighbors, C. (2013). Implicit drinking identity: Drinker + me associations predict college student drinking consistently. *Addictive Behaviors, 38*(5), 2163–2166. https://doi.org/10.1016/j.addbeh.2013.01.026

Livingston, M. (2012). Perceptions of low-risk drinking levels among Australians during a period of change in the official drinking guidelines. *Drug and Alcohol Review, 31*(2), 224–230. https://doi.org/10.1111/j.1465-3362.2011.00414.x

McCreanor, T., Lyons, A., Moewaka Barnes, H., Hutton, F., Goodwin, I., & Griffin, C. (2016). 'Drink a 12 box before you go': Pre-loading among young people in Aotearoa New Zealand. *Kōtuitui: New Zealand Journal of Social Sciences Online, 11*(1), 36–46. https://doi.org/10.1080/1177083X.2015.1037314

Mezquita, L., Ibáñez, M. I., Moya-Higueras, J., Villa, H., Arias, B., Fañanás, L., & Ortet, G. (2016). Psychometric properties of Drinking Motives Questionnaire-Revised (DMQ-R) in Spanish adolescents. *European Journal of Psychological Assessment, 34*(3), 145–153. https://doi.org/10.1027/1015-5759/a000319

Miller, P. G., & Droste, N. (2013). Alcohol price considerations on alcohol and illicit drug use in university students. *Journal of Alcoholism and Drug Dependence, 1*(2), 1–4. https://doi.org/10.4172/jaldd.1000109

Miller, P. G., Droste, N., Groot, F., Palmer, D., Tindall, J., Busija, L., … Wiggers, J. (2015). Correlates and motives of pre-drinking with intoxication and harm around licensed venues in two cities. *Drug and Alcohol Review, 35*(2), 177–186. https://doi.org/10.1111/dar.12274

Miller, P. G., Tindall, J., Sønderlund, A., Groombridge, D., Lecathelinais, C., Gillham, K., McFarlane, E., de Groot, F., Droste, N., Sawyer, A., Palmer, D., Warren, I., & Wiggers, J. (2012). *Dealing with Alcohol-Related Harm and the Night-Time Economy (DANTE): Final report* (Monograph Series No. 43). https://aic.gov.au/publications/ndlerfmonograph/monograph43

Murgraff, V., Abraham, C., & McDermott, M. (2007). Reducing Friday alcohol consumption among moderate, women drinkers: Evaluation of a brief evidence-based intervention. *Alcohol and Alcoholism, 42*(1), 37–41. https://doi.org/10.1093/alcalc/agl083

Murgraff, V., White, D., & Phillips, K. (1996). Moderating binge drinking: It is possible to change behaviour if you plan it in advance. *Alcohol and Alcoholism, 31*(6), 577–582. https://doi.org/10.1093/oxfordjournals.alcalc.a008193

Ng, J. Y. Y., Ntoumanis, M., Thøgersen-Ntoumani, C., Deci, E. L., Ryan, R. M., Duda, J. L., & Williams, G. C. (2012). Self-determination theory applied to health contexts. *Perspectives on Psychological Science, 7*(4), 325–340. https://doi.org/10.1177/1745691612447309

O'Rourke, S., Ferris, J., & Devaney, M. (2015). Beyond pre-loading: Understanding the associations between pre-, side-and back-loading drinking behavior and risky drinking. *Addictive Behaviors, 53*, 146–154. https://doi.org/10.1016/j.addbeh.2015.07.008

O'Neil, A. I., Lafreniere, K. D., & Jackson, D. L. (2016). Pre-drinking motives in Canadian undergraduate students: Confirmatory factor analysis of the Prepartying motivations inventory and examination of new themes. *Addictive Behaviors, 60*, 42–47. https://doi.org/10.1016/j.addbeh.2016.03.024

Pedersen, E. R. (2016). Using the solid research base on pregaming to begin intervention development: An epilogue to the special issue on pregaming. *Substance Use & Misuse, 51*, 1067–1073. https://doi.org/10.1080/10826084.2016.1187533

Pedersen, E. R., & LaBrie, J. W. (2007). Partying before the party: Examining prepartying behavior among college students. *Journal of American College Health, 56*(3), 237–245. https://doi.org/10.3200/JACH.56.3.237-246

Pilatti, A., & Read, J. P. (2018). Development and psychometric evaluation of a new measure to assess pregaming motives in Spanish-speaking young adults. *Addictive Behaviors, 81*, 134–142. https://doi.org/10.1016/j.addbeh.2018.01.019

Read, J. P., Merrill, J. E., & Bytschkow, K. (2010). Before the party starts: Risk factors and reasons for "pregaming" in college students. *Journal of American College Health, 58*(5), 461–472. https://doi.org/10.1080/07448480903540523

Riordan, B. C., Conner, T. S., Flett, J. A. M., Droste, N., Cody, L., Brookie, K. L., … Scarf, D. (2018). An intercept study to measure the extent to which New Zealand university students pre-game. *Australian and New Zealand Journal of Public Health, 42*(1), 30–34. https://doi.org/10.1111/1753-6405.12754

Room, R., & Livingston, M. (2009). Does it matter where the drinking is, when the object is getting drunk? *Addiction, 104*(1), 10–11. https://doi.org/10.1111/j.1360-0443.2008.02423.x

Rutledge, P. C., Bestrashniy, J. R. B. M., & Nelson, T. F. (2016). Problematic drinking among postgraduate students: Binge drinking, prepartying, and mixing alcohol with energy drinks. *Substance Use & Misuse, 51*(8), 972–982. https://doi.org/10.3109/10826084.2016.1152499

Skidmore, J. R., & Murphy, J. G. (2011). The effect of drink price and next-day responsibilities on college student drinking: A behavioral economic analysis. *Psychology of Addictive Behaviors, 25*(1), 57–68. https://doi.org/10.1037/a0021118

Slutske, W. S., Hunt-Carter, E. E., Nabors-Oberg, R. E., Sher, K. J., Bucholz, K. K., Madden, P. A. F., … Heath, A. C. (2004). Do college students drink more than their non-college-attending peers? Evidence from a population-based longitudinal female twin study. *Journal of Abnormal Psychology, 113*(4), 530–540. https://doi.org/10.1037/0021-843X.113.4.530

Teixera, P. J., Marques, M. M., Silva, M. N., Brunet, J., Duda, J., Haerens, L., … Hagger, M. S. (2020). A classification of motivation and behavior change techniques used in self-determination theory-based interventions in health contexts. *Motivation Science*. https://doi.org/10.1037/mot0000172

Wechsler, H., & Isaac, N. (1992). Binge' drinkers at Massachusetts colleges: Prevalence, drinking style, time trends, and associated problems. *The Journal of the American Medical Association, 267*(21), 2929–2931. https://doi.org/10.1001/jama.1992.03480210091038

Wells, S., Dumas, T. M., Bernards, S., Kuntsche, E., Labhart, F., & Graham, K. (2015). Predrinking, alcohol use, and breath alcohol concentration: A study of young adult bargoers. *Psychology of Addictive Behaviors, 29*(3), 683–689. https://doi.org/10.1037/adb0000065

Wells, S., Graham, K., & Purcell, J. (2009). Policy implications of the widespread practice of 'pre-drinking' or 'pre-gaming' before going to public drinking establishments – Are current prevention strategies backfiring? *Addiction, 104*(1), 4–9. https://doi.org/10.1111/j.1360-0443.2008.02393.x

Wright, C. J., Dietze, P. M., Crockett, B., & Lim, M. S. (2016). Participatory development of MIDY (Mobile intervention for drinking in young people). *BMC Public Health, 16*(1), 1–11. https://doi.org/10.1186/s12889-016-2876-5

Young, R. M., Connor, J. P., Ricciardelli, L., & Saunders, J. B. (2006). The role of alcohol expectancy and drinking refusal self-efficacy beliefs in university student drinking. *Alcohol and Alcoholism, 41*(1), 70–75. https://doi.org/10.1093/alcalc/agh237

Zamboanga, B. L., Merrill, J. E., Olthuis, J. V., Milroy, J. J., Sokolovsky, A. W., & Wyrick, D. L. (2019). Secondary effects of myPlaybook on college athletes' avoidance of drinking games or pregaming as a protective behavior strategy: A multisite randomized controlled study. *Social Science & Medicine, 228*, 135–141. https://doi.org/10.1016/j.socscimed.2019.02.016
Zamboanga, B. L., Schwartz, S., Ham, L., Borsari, B., & Van Tyne, K. (2010). Alcohol expectancies, pregaming, drinking games, and hazardous alcohol use in a multiethnic sample of college students. *Cognitive Therapy and Research, 34*(2), 124. https://doi.org/10.1007/s10608-009-9234-1

14

Strategies for Managing Alcohol Intake and Refusing Offers of Alcoholic Drinks

Dominic Conroy and Richard O. de Visser

Introduction

In this chapter we discuss literature addressing how people manage their alcohol intake, and what they do to refuse offers of alcoholic drinks. The relevant literature contains quantitative studies and qualitative studies, and the majority comes from the discipline of psychology. We first discuss the types of knowledge, motivation, and skills that are involved in individuals' adherence (or not) to guidelines for low-risk drinking. We then consider key psychological constructs relevant to considering how alcoholic drinks are resisted or refused. Having contextualised "managing alcohol intake" we will consider specific quantitative and qualitative studies of managing alcohol and refusing offers of alcoholic drinks. We conclude with a section designed to consider how the literature on managing alcohol intake and refusing alcoholic drinks might be extended in future research and how it might be best applied in policy and practice.

D. Conroy (✉)
School of Psychology, University of East London, London, UK
e-mail: d.conroy@uel.ac.uk

R. O. de Visser
Brighton and Sussex Medical School, University of Sussex, Falmer, UK
e-mail: r.o.devisser@bsms.ac.uk

R. Cooke et al. (eds.), *The Palgrave Handbook of Psychological Perspectives on Alcohol Consumption*, https://doi.org/10.1007/978-3-030-66941-6_14

Alcohol-Related Harms: Terminology, Guidelines, and Policies

As noted elsewhere in this collection, there is considerable evidence that higher levels of alcohol consumption are associated with various negative consequences for individuals' physical and psychological well-being, and for the harmonious functioning of society (Klingemann & Gmel, 2001; Weitzman, 2004; Rehm, 2011; GBD 2016 Alcohol Collaborators, 2018). Risks of alcohol can be understood in different ways. There are short-term risks of heavier alcohol consumption, including poisoning, accidents, injury, and being the perpetrator or victim of violence. There are also longer-term risks of greater alcohol consumption. In the long term, heavier alcohol consumption increases the risk of harm to many organ systems, including several types of cancer (e.g. Wittmann, Paulus, & Roenneberg, 2010; Nelson et al., 2013). Prolonged heavier alcohol consumption is also associated with a greater risk of poor psychological well-being (Weitzman, 2004; Wittmann et al., 2010). Given this evidence confirming the range and severity of potential harm, it is clear that if people decide to drink alcohol, then it is important for them to be encouraged to do so in moderation.

Various terms have been used to describe consuming alcohol in moderation—for example, "moderate drinking," "sensible drinking," and "low-risk drinking." In this chapter, we use the term "low-risk drinking." Moving on from that, advising people to engage in "low-risk drinking" draws attention to the question: What is "low-risk drinking"? To ensure that drinkers, health professionals, policy-makers and researchers are all able to communicate clearly about alcohol use, accurately measure alcohol use, and then estimate associations between levels of alcohol use and related harm, there is a need for a standardised language for describing alcohol intake. Many governments and government agencies have developed guidelines for low-risk drinking (referred to from this point as "guidelines"), which commonly include recommended daily and/or weekly maximum intake expressed as numbers of "standard drinks" or "units of alcohol" (Furtwängler & de Visser, 2013). However, there is wide variation in how different countries define standard drinks, and in the recommended daily and weekly intake maxima (Furtwängler & de Visser, 2013). That variation is important to note, but it is not the focus of this chapter. Instead, we are interested in whether and how people adhere to such low risk guidelines, and their strategies for "managing alcohol intake": that is, attempting to drink alcohol in moderation in the face of different pressures to drink.

Despite the existence and promotion of guidelines, many people exceed them. For example, one large-scale study in Canada—involving over 40,000 people aged 15 and over—found that 27% of drinkers did not comply with weekly guidelines, and that 39% of drinkers did not comply with daily intake guidelines (Zhao, Stockwell, & Thomas, 2015). Nationally representative data from Australia reveal that many drinkers consume alcohol above national guidelines in ways that place them at risk of harm over their lifetime and/or on a single drinking occasion (Australian Institute of Health and Welfare, 2017).

There are various ways to encourage people to drink less. Some of these are whole-population approaches specified in legislation that affect all drinkers (and non-drinkers): laws related to legal age for purchase and unsupervised consumption of alcohol, restrictions on alcohol marketing and pricing, regulation of trading hours for licensed premises, laws prohibiting sale of alcohol to drunk people, and so on. Drink-driving laws are another example of population-level approaches. Other approaches are designed to encourage people to make healthier choices about alcohol. These include public education and health promotion campaigns run by governments and non-government organisations which may use gain-framed messages to emphasise the benefits of drinking less and/or loss-framed messages to emphasise the harms that arise from drinking too much (Rothman & Salovey, 1997; Quick & Bates, 2010). There is a need to consider psychological and behavioural features of the various strategies used to encourage moderate drinking: these are addressed in the next section.

Psychological Components of Managing Intake and Refusing Alcohol

In this section we outline an established theoretical framework that can help formalise discussion of a general process (managing alcohol intake) and how that general process might play out in specific situations (e.g. refusing alcoholic drink offers). If individuals are to drink within government guidelines for alcohol intake, then they must understand what the guidelines are, and be motivated to adhere to them. They also need to possess a range of behavioural skills. Skills are required to adhere to government guidelines for alcohol intake, and further skills are required to resist temptations, expectations, or pressure to drink alcohol.

The Information-Motivation-Behavioural Skills (IMB) model is a straightforward statement that all three of its eponymous components

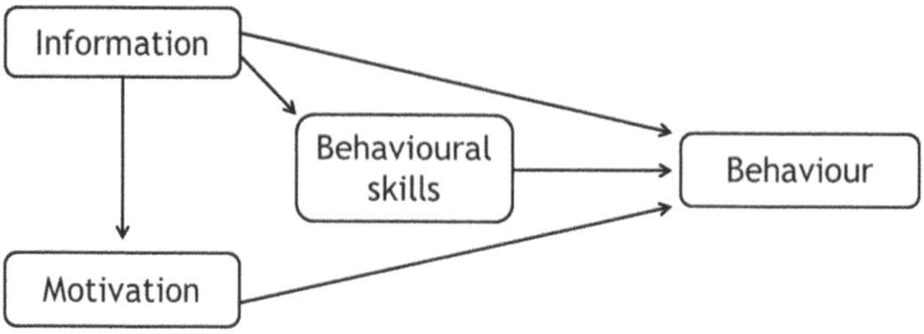

Fig. 14.1 Information-motivation-behavioural skills model. (Adapted from Fisher et al., 2003)

influence behaviour change (Fisher, Fisher, & Harman, 2003). The model is presented in Fig. 14.1. It proposes that knowledge is an important prerequisite for behaviour change: in the case of alcohol use, people cannot adhere to guidelines they do not know or do not understand. However, the model also argues that providing information is not enough, and it emphasises that people must be motivated to change their behaviour: in the context of alcohol use, many people know that heavy drinking leads to hangovers, but this knowledge in itself may not motivate them to change their behaviour. Providing information (or clarifying understanding) may induce motivation to change. For example, when a woman learns by how much she is exceeding government alcohol intake guidelines, she may be motivated to change her behaviour. The IMB argues that in addition to possessing accurate information and being motivated to change, a person must have the behavioural skills required to carry out the new pattern of behaviour. In some domains of health-related behaviour, the required skills may be easy to identify and few in number—for example, a person who learns that they are lactose intolerant will learn to read ingredient labels on packaged foodstuffs and ask staff in cafés or restaurants for information on ingredients. In the context of alcohol use, the required behavioural skills are greater in number and more diverse in nature: people must develop skills to manage their own desire or temptation to drink, they must learn how to space out their drinks and/or identify low-alcohol or alcohol-free alternatives, and they must learn how to respond to social expectations to drink, as well as more direct peer influences to drink. A key element of these skills is the ability to resist temptations, expectations, or pressure to drink alcohol. In the next two sections we apply the IMB to alcohol use, addressing each element with reference to relevant research.

Managing Alcohol Intake by Adhering to Guidelines for Low-Risk Drinking

Efforts to agree on standard drinks, and to agree recommended daily and weekly intake maxima are, as stated above, not the focus of this chapter. Our interest in this section is whether and how people use guidelines to manage their alcohol intake.

Information, Motivation, and Skills Relevant to Guidelines for Low-Risk Drinking

Information about guidelines appears to have reached most drinkers, but few have accurate knowledge of the guidelines (Coomber, Jones, Martino, & Miller, 2017; de Visser & Birch, 2012; de Visser, Brown, Cooke, Cooper, & Memon, 2017; McNally et al., 2019; Rosenberg et al., 2018;). Nor do many people feel familiar with the guidelines, and interestingly, self-reported familiarity with the guidelines is not a reliable indicator of actual knowledge of the guidelines (de Visser & Birch, 2012). One reason is that people tend to think of alcohol consumption in terms of glasses, bottles, and cans, rather than in units that do not always correspond with these measures. Qualitative research has also revealed that many people do not feel familiar with the guidelines despite being well aware of their existence, and that "units" or "standard drinks" are not intuitive or easy-to-use measures. For example, in a qualitative study of young people in the UK, one male interviewee noted: "I find the unit measurement actually quite cumbersome to work with in terms of judging what I am drinking," and a female participant said: "I find it quite hard to translate drinks to units. I kind of have looked into it and I always forget" (Furtwängler & de Visser, 2017b, p. 1705).

Motivation to adhere to guidelines can be conceptualised in various ways. One indicator is the perceived usefulness of the guidelines. Studies of students and non-student adults in the UK indicate that many drinkers do not perceive guidelines to be particularly useful (de Visser & Birch, 2012; de Visser, 2015; Lovatt et al., 2015; de Visser et al., 2017). In addition, daily recommended maxima are seen as irrelevant by those drinkers who tend not to drink every day, but instead engage in less frequent bouts of heavier drinking. Furthermore, drinkers tend not to be interested in changing their alcohol intake (de Visser, 2015; de Visser et al., 2017; Rosenberg et al., 2018). This unwillingness to change is perhaps more common among young adults—many of whom engage in heavy episodic drinking (HED) with the intention of getting drunk, and therefore perceive low daily intake guidelines as being irrelevant. For example, in one qualitative study, a male university student said:

> The thing is, you can drink within the recommended daily amount of units, but you don't get drunk on that. So socially it's almost a wasted enterprise. (Furtwängler & de Visser, 2017b, p. 1704)

Using more direct measures, quantitative studies have found that motivation to adhere to guidelines is low. In multivariate analyses among university students in the UK, Furtwängler and de Visser (2017a) found that stronger motivation to adhere to guidelines was predicted by greater conscientiousness, greater perceived usefulness of guidelines, greater familiarity with guidelines and less frequent drunkenness in the last month. As suggested by the IMB, this indicates that one way to increase motivation to adhere to guidelines would be to increase understanding of them, but that such efforts may not be effective for all drinkers.

Behavioural skills related to guidelines are multi-faceted. People must be able to: know or find the unit content of different packaged drinks; know the unit content of drinks they pour for themselves or are poured by others; and keep track of how many units they have consumed even in situations in which they may be becoming increasingly intoxicated. Research with samples of non-student adult drinkers in the UK indicates that many people lack these skills (e.g. Boniface, Kneale, & Shelton, 2013). For example, when people are asked to pour "usual drinks," they tend to pour volumes substantially larger than one "unit" or one "standard drink," and they tend to underestimate the unit content of the "usual drinks" that they pour (de Visser, 2015; de Visser & Birch, 2012). When asked to estimate the unit content of various drinks, students and non-student adults tend not to give accurate reports (de Visser, 2015; de Visser & Birch, 2012; de Visser et al., 2017). Furthermore, people tend not to be able to give accurate reports of their own alcohol intake. For example, Furtwängler and de Visser (2017a) asked a sample of university students to report exactly what they drank during their most recent drinking occasion, and then estimate the number of UK units this represented. The researchers then computed the actual number of units consumed based on students' reports of what they drank and compared these to the students' estimated. They found that only 31% of students gave estimates of unit intake that were within ±10% of their computed unit intake, and that 35% underestimated their alcohol intake by at least 10%. These findings show that people generally lack the skills required to accurately monitor their alcohol intake.

Enhancing Capacity to Adhere to Guidelines for Low-Risk Drinking

There is emerging evidence that interventions that address one or more elements of the IMB may increase people's capacity to adhere to guidelines. Although more generic (or less-focused) interventions may not produce significant intervention effects beyond greater awareness of guidelines (McNally et al., 2019), interventions more focused on how people use guidelines have been found to produce significant effects on antecedents of behaviour, and actual drinking behaviour. Two examples are summarised below.

In one intervention study in the UK, de Visser (2015) asked participants in the intervention group to pour their "usual drinks" of beer, wine, and spirits, and to estimate the unit content of each of them. Participants were also asked to pour what they thought were "units" of each of the three drink types. After the session, participants were provided with personalised feedback based on their performance in the drink pouring task, and their alcohol intake as reported in a questionnaire. The feedback reminded participants of government guidelines and the unit content of different drinks. It also indicated whether participants were drinking in excess of these guidelines. At two-month follow-up, the intervention group was compared to two other groups—people who did the drink pouring task but did not receive personalised feedback (this group allowed analyses of whether the drink pouring itself had an effect of the outcomes), and a control group which did not engage in the drink pouring task or get feedback on their alcohol intake. All participants had already completed a baseline survey that assessed their guideline-related knowledge and motivations as well as their patterns of alcohol use. Analyses revealed that the intervention produced several significant changes not observed in the other two groups: significant improvements in the accuracy of knowledge of the guidelines; significant reductions in alcohol units consumed per week; significant reductions in the number of days per week on which daily consumption maxima were exceeded. Although the intervention was successful in addressing both the "Information" and the "Behavioural skill" parts of the IMB model, it was rather resource-intensive given the time needed to conduct the pouring task and compile the personalised feedback. This suggested a need to identify and assess other means for helping people to better understand low-risk drinking guidelines and to calibrate their alcohol intake relative to such guidelines.

In a subsequent study, de Visser et al. (2017) assessed the impact of using glasses that were marked with the unit equivalent of different volumes of beer, wine, and spirit as well as statement of the guidelines. In the UK, such glasses are distributed by some local government public health teams as well as the industry-funded charity Drinkaware. All participants completed a baseline survey that assessed their guideline-related knowledge and motivations as well as their patterns of alcohol use. Participants assigned to the intervention group were given three of the plastic unit-marked glasses provide by Brighton & Hove City Council and asked to use them as much as possible for any alcoholic or non-alcoholic drinks. One month later, follow-up analyses comparing the intervention to a group control that only completed the baseline survey revealed that the intervention led to several significant changes: better knowledge of unit-based guidelines; better ability to estimate the unit content of various drinks; greater perceived usefulness of the guidelines; and more frequent counting unit intake. Unfortunately, the changes to alcohol intake observed following the drink-pouring feedback intervention were not found in this study. However, the fact that the glasses are relatively cheap suggests that they could be a useful part of broader efforts to increase people's capacity to drink according to guidelines for low-risk alcohol intake. It should be noted that more frequent use of the glasses was associated with larger changes in understanding and motivation. Furthermore, most participants were not concerned about changing their level of alcohol intake: the intervention may have been more effective among people who were already willing to change their behaviour.

Alternative strategies for enhancing people's capacity to adhere to guidelines include provision of information on labels on packaged alcohol products. In many countries, labels on packaged alcohol must contain specified information including its alcohol content by volume. For example, Regulation (EC) no. 110/2008 of the European Parliament and Council relates to labelling of spirits. However, if people are to adhere to guidelines stated in "units" or "standard drinks," then they may need specific information about "units" or "standard drinks" on labels. One Canadian study found that such information can help people to keep track of their alcohol intake relative to guidelines (Hobin et al., 2018). In that study, there was strong support for labels that included information about standard drink content of the container, and how this related to guidelines. Furthermore, providing labels that contained more information about standard drinks and guidelines was linked to participants' better ability to accurately monitor their alcohol intake relative to guidelines (see Chap. 19 for a detailed discussion of this topic).

The material discussed above is promising, but in any effort to motivate people to drink less, it must be acknowledged that drinkers commonly report strong motives for drinking—to aid socialising; for enhancement; to regulate emotions; to fit in—that may not be compatible by restricting intake to conform with guidelines (Cooper, 1994; Kuntsche, Knibbe, Gmel, & Engels, 2005). It is crucial to consider the importance to individuals of the motive to adhere to guidelines relative to the importance of these other motives.

Skills and Efficacy for Managing Alcohol Intake

In this chapter, we use the term "managing alcohol intake" to refer to the strategic management of alcohol consumption in the context of a range of pressures. These pressures may be internal (e.g. wanting to fit in), or external (e.g. being offered a drink). Strategic management can be understood to take place over different time scales. For example, management of alcohol intake could be explored over the course of an occasion (e.g. during a specific social event), or over a longer period (e.g. during a typical week). Research on managing these pressures is not novel: there is a long tradition of studies of how the temptation to drink might be successfully managed in people being treated for alcohol dependence (e.g. Marlatt & George, 1984; Hodgson, 1989; Solomon & Annis, 1990).

In contrast, research on managing alcohol intake from a public health promotion perspective is less prominent. This is perhaps surprising given the clear value of understanding how best to manage alcohol intake at the population level. However, the lack of emphasis on refusal/resistance strategies as a feature of public health promotion campaigns is also understandable given the degree of stigma associated with alcoholism and dependent drinking (Room, 2005; Schomerus et al., 2010; Hill & Leeming, 2014). Indeed, a health promotion approach geared towards managing drink intake might need to strike a fine line between bolstering drink management skills and not generating concern among individuals that they are stigmatised "problem drinkers."

Measurement of Drink Refusal Skills

As introduced above, literature on the ability to refuse alcoholic drinks had until the 1990s primarily focused on refusal skills in the context of controlled drinking and among individuals undergoing treatment for alcohol use disorders. This is evident in research designed to explore how social skills training may help individuals diagnosed with alcoholism to refuse alcoholic drinks in different situations (e.g. Foy, Miller, Eisler, & O'Toole, 1976).

Social Cognitive Theory (SCT: Bandura, 1986) has provided a useful framework for considering how skills relevant to resisting alcohol intake might be conceptualised and measured. Two key constructs in SCT have guided understanding of factors underpinning an individual's ability to manage alcohol intake: outcome expectancies and self-efficacy. Outcome expectancies are the positive and/or negative outcomes that an individual expects to be associated with a given behaviour. For example, an individual may expect alcohol use to be associated with positive outcomes such as having good time and/or negative outcomes such as behaving badly (Leigh & Stacy, 1993). Within the SCT, outcome expectancies are theorised to influence motivation to engage in the behaviour: if their balance of expectancies is more positive than negative, then a person will have greater motivation to drink. Self-efficacy refers to an individual's belief in their capacity to achieve particular goals. In the context of alcohol use self-efficacy can be conceptualised as belief in one's capacity to manage alcohol intake in specific situations and/or in general. SCT has formed the basis for measures of self-efficacy for refusing or resisting alcohol. We will now explore the emergence and application of some of these.

One way to operationalise self-efficacy for managing alcohol intake is "situational confidence," which refers to an individual's ability to resist alcohol in high risk situations. The Situational Confidence Questionnaire (SCQ: Annis, 1986) was developed and tested in several relapse prevention studies during the 1980s. The SCQ was configured to gauge individuals' skills in resisting triggers to drink posed by varied situations. These situational characteristics included emotions (e.g. unpleasant emotions, or conversely, pleasant times with others), physical sensation (e.g. physical discomfort), cognitive phenomena (e.g. urges and temptations), and interpersonal interactions (e.g. conflict with others, or social pressure to drink). Typically, the SCQ has been used in the context of substance dependence (Sandahl, Lindberg, & Rönnberg, 1990; Higgins, 1998). However, using a measure similar to the SCQ, a study of Chinese university students found that self-efficacy for alcohol self-regulation was related to mood, situational social pressures, and personal social pressures, and that students who possessed greater self-efficacy for alcohol self-regulation consumed alcohol less frequently (Ding, Newman, Buhs, & Shell, 2018).

Contemporary research includes many studies of the links between drink refusal skills and actual alcohol intake: some have focused on the general population, but many have been restricted to samples of university students. Much of this research has used measures other than the SCQ that have been derived directly from SCT. For example, the construct of Drink Refusal Self-Efficacy (DRSE: Baldwin, Oei, & Young, 1993) addresses capacity to manage alcohol intake in specific contexts. Usefully, the DRSE measure distinguishes between three different domains in which skills at refusing alcoholic drinks may be tested. The "Social pressure DRSE" sub-scale relates to skills for refusing alcohol under conditions of perceived or actual social pressure—for example, "I am able to refuse alcohol when someone offers me a drink." The "Emotional DRSE" sub-scale assesses the capacity to refuse alcohol under conditions of emotional strain—for example, "I am able to refuse alcohol when I am angry." The "Opportunistic DRSE" sub-scale relates to skills for refusing alcohol in circumstances in which there are opportunities to consume alcohol—for example, "I am able to refuse alcohol when I first arrive home". Psychometric studies have provided considerable support for the reliability and validity of various DRSE measures (Oei, Hasking, & Young, 2005; Young, Hasking, Oei, & Loveday, 2007; Patton et al., 2018).

A key strength of the DRSE scale is that it provides a comprehensive account of the various contextual demands that individuals may encounter. A further strength is that there is no assumption that DRSE is global and unitary. For example, an individual may have no problems refusing alcohol when put under pressure in social situations, but may struggle to resist alcohol at a time/place where they are used to drinking alcohol—that is, this person is high in Social pressure DRSE, but low in Opportunistic DRSE. Determining sub-scale differences has practical value as this might indicate the specific skills an individual might need to strengthen to become better able to manage their alcohol intake in different scenarios.

DRSE has been widely explored in clinical and general population samples. One focus of early work was to determine differential predictive effects of DRSE among different drinker types (Baldwin et al., 1993; Lee & Oei, 1993; Oei, Fergusson, & Lee, 1998; Lee, Oei, & Greeley, 1999). For example, in a study of regular drinking adults in the USA, Lee et al. (1999) found higher scores on all DRSE sub-scales among lighter drinkers than heavy drinkers. Since this time, evidence has accumulated to show that DRSE scores predict drinking behaviour across different cultural contexts (e.g. Oei & Jardim, 2007), and in specific samples including dependent drinkers (Schomerus et al., 2011). Other studies have drawn attention to the synergies between DRSE and other psychological constructs, with a particular focus on DRSE as a meditating factor in the relationship between personality and alcohol consumption. For example, a study of college students in the USA found that although alcohol-related problems were significantly more common among people who had lower scores on measures of conscientiousness and higher scores on measures of sensation-seeking, these links between personality variables and problematic drinking were weaker among those who had greater emotional and/or social pressure DRSE (Stevens, Littlefield, Blanchard, Talley, & Brown, 2016). In other research with undergraduates in the USA, the links between "drinking identity" (i.e. how identity-crucial an individual beliefs alcohol to be) and drinking practices were found to be partially mediated by both emotional DRSE and social pressure DRSE (Foster, Yeung, & Neighbors, 2014). Put another way, compared to other participants, people who reported that alcohol was central to their identity tended to drink more. However, if these people also had greater emotional and/or social DRSE, then the differences in alcohol intake were reduced. Further discussion of DRSE can be found in Chap. 4.

The Protective Behavioural Strategies scale (PBS: Martens et al., 2005) offers a different approach and an alternative framework for measuring capacity to manage alcohol intake or refuse drinks offers. The PBS originates from a harm reduction approach to alcohol consumption. Differing PBS measures have been used across studies but the range of protective behavioural strategies has commonly included: limiting alcohol consumption (e.g. stopping drinking at a predetermined time); specific drinking practices (e.g. avoiding drinking games); and reducing problems associated with alcohol consumption (e.g. refusing to travel in a car driven by someone who has been drinking). A recent comprehensive review drew attention to inconsistency between studies in terms of items included in PBS scales, and concerns about the psychometric properties of PBS measures (Pearson, 2013). Concerns that most PBS studies have been cross-sectional in design have been partly addressed in a study conducted in the USA that provided evidence that PBS sub-scales predict a range of negative alcohol-related consequences (e.g. social/interpersonal problems; poor self-care) at four- to six-week follow-up (Treloar, Martens, & McCarthy, 2015). An advantage of the PBS relative to other scales is its formulation of a broader range of context-related strategies relevant to understanding whether an individual is likely to be successful at refusing drinks.

Other refusal skills measures have been developed and empirically explored. For example, Shope et al.'s (1993) "refusal skill" scale placed emphasis on the tone and character of an individual's performance voice when refusing an alcoholic drink. This study focused on 14- to 19-year-old students in the USA, and data collection entailed participation in a brief acted out scene in which researchers would play the part of peers trying to pressure participants into drinking. Researcher ratings of how well the participant refused the offer to consume alcohol were then made. Some rating items were designed to gauge the convincingness of an individual's effort to refuse (e.g. "Overall, considering what was said, and how it was said, how convincing was the student's refusal"). Other ratings drew attention to features of tone (e.g. "How firm was the student's voice?"). Some items in Shope et al.'s (1993) scale act as non-verbal/postural proxies for refusal (e.g. "Did the student make eye contact?"). One clear advantage of this measurement approach is that it accommodates differing rater viewpoints about how successfully an individual had refused alcohol drinks. A second advantage is the focus on linguistic and paralinguistic information which may be relevant to the success of an individual's refusal behaviour. Clearly, recording this volume of information about drink refusal brings practical disadvantages (e.g. obtaining inter-coder agreement about the quality of a refusal performance) but the approach provides an important shift away from conceptualising "drink refusal skills" at the purely intra-individual of self-report measures.

Qualitative Exploration of Drink Refusal Skills

The discussion of drink refusal measures above highlighted how individuals might be rated differently on pre-defined criteria. These measures have provided a useful way of distinguishing between different types of drink refusal strategies, and they are useful in two ways: first, for identifying individuals who may lack skills in particular domains; and second, for guiding the development of interventions designed to enhance drink refusal skills (see below). However, quantitative approaches do not necessarily allow an understanding of the experience of successfully or unsuccessfully attempting to manage alcohol intake and/or refuse alcohol in specific situations.

Qualitative research has also contributed understanding of strategies involved in managing alcohol intake and refusing drinks by drawing attention to how features of talk and interaction might be involved in successfully refusing alcohol drinks. Qualitative studies have been particularly useful in highlighting the relational dynamics involved in refusing drinks (e.g. how pressure to drink might emerge during everyday conversation). In this sub-section we provide illustrations of how qualitative studies have helped enhance understanding of drink refusal skills.

Some qualitative studies have focused on particular samples of individuals (e.g. Bartram, Eliott, & Crabb, 2017; Conroy & de Visser, 2014). For example, Conroy and de Visser's (2014) UK-based research has provided insights into refusal strategies used by young adults who do not drink alcohol: some lifelong abstainers, and some who became non-drinkers more recently.

In-depth experiential interviews underscored key difficulties involved in successfully evading scrutiny over the decision not to drink while in the company of peers who do drink. Non-drinkers' accounts revealed that successfully managing drink offers could involve strategic switching between being direct (e.g. "No thanks, I don't drink alcohol") and being less direct by telling "white lies" (e.g. "I'm on antibiotics"). Interviewees also reported the importance of pre-emptive measures to close off rhetorical space for being pressured to drink or being pressured to give an account of oneself as a non-drinker. This is apparent in an extract from one of the interviews:

> I started to avoid drinking situations and going out with certain groups of people because I felt uncomfortable in those situations. A lot of the time I would give in to peer pressure and end up having a few drinks when I'd gone out with every intention not to. When I've quit smoking […] you know, just by sitting around other people smoking, or having people smoking, or people offering you a cigarette, it all puts pressure on you. (Conroy & de Visser, 2014, p. 545)

In this quote, Michelle identified various challenges faced by an individual when refusing to drink alcohol during a social situation. Speaking about her historical drinking practices, Michelle spoke to the particular vulnerability faced from the position of someone socially identifiable as a "moderate drinker" in a situation in that there will always be an expectation that they could drink more. Although moderate drinkers may face this pressure to drink, being identified as a non-drinker may mean being able to close down any perceived opportunities to be pressured to drink. Interviewees also referred to the value of having friends who are loyal and committed around them when refusing alcoholic drinks. These findings resonate with recent discussion of the reciprocal relationships between friendship quality and drinking practices (Conroy & MacLean, 2020).

Interventions to Enhance Drink Refusal Skills

Interventions designed to promote moderate drinking have sometimes been geared towards enhancing skills involved in managing alcohol intake or refusing drinks. In this section, we outline a selection of interventions that have employed drinks refusal measures.

Several studies in the health psychology literature have reported interventions involving mental imagery exercises designed to enhance motivation to drink in moderation (e.g. Conroy, Sparks, & de Visser, 2015; Hagger et al.,

2012). In such studies, people are encouraged to imagine and/or write about specific events, actions, or outcomes with the express purpose of increasing motivation toward a defined target action. For example, imagining and/or writing about specific strategies to be employed to successfully drink alcohol in moderation for the forthcoming week would be expected to increase motivation to drink in moderation. Conroy and Hagger (2018) conducted a systematic review of mental imagery interventions in the context of physical health behaviour, and Chap. 21 of this book addresses mental imagery interventions in the specific context of alcohol use. Here we outline the only study to have explored the impact of a "process" mental imagery exercise—that is, an intervention exercise specifically designed to encourage participants to imagine strategies that could be used to refuse alcohol (Conroy et al., 2015). In that study, university students were randomly allocated to a non-intervention control group, or a "process condition" in which they were directed to imagine and write about the strategies that they could use to reduce their alcohol intake during a situation involving alcohol consumption. Participants were then followed-up twice over a one-month period. The analyses revealed significant reductions in HED episodes among students in the process condition, but no such significant changes among the control group.

Other studies have included measures of drinks refusal (e.g. DRSE) as part of the measurement of capacity for refusing alcohol. For example, longitudinal studies of participants in the UK's "Dry January" have revealed that greater DRSE going into the one-month alcohol abstinence challenge is associated with a greater likelihood of completing the month of abstinence (de Visser, Robinson, & Bond, 2016). This is perhaps not surprising given the material covered above. However, abstinence challenges like Dry January also provide people with an opportunity to develop skills and confidence in managing potential opportunities to drink. Indeed, research has revealed that participants in Dry January experience increases in the social, emotional, and opportunistic domains of DRSE as well as improvements in general self-efficacy (de Visser et al., 2016; de Visser & Nicholls, 2020). Furthermore, research has also revealed positive feedback loops such that those who complete Dry January have larger improvements in DRSE than those who do not make it through the month without drinking. Structural equation modelling has shown that the observed increases in DRSE help to explain why people who successfully complete Dry January tend to drink less in the months following the end of the campaign (de Visser et al., 2016).

This material suggests that temporary abstinence challenges provide opportunities to develop skills and self-efficacy that persist. However, there is also emerging evidence that it is important to provide advice and support to people undertaking temporary abstinence challenges (de Visser & Nicholls, 2020). For example, Dry January provides people with a supported opportunity to develop and practice the skills required to resist temptation, expectation or pressure to drink. The website and other supporting material provide suggestions to help people through a one-month abstinence challenge: alcohol-free socialising, finding satisfying alcohol-free drinks, managing cravings and set-backs. In addition to providing tips and advice, it also contains motivating information about the likely benefits of not drinking for sleep, psychological well-being, energy levels, appearance, and personal finances.

Despite the large volume of studies employing measures of DRSE, very few have used the DRSE construct as a basis for delivering drink refusal training interventions. One exception to this is a study that provided a drink refusal skills training module as part of a 16-week combined behavioural intervention among 776 alcohol-dependent individuals in the USA (Witkiewitz, Donovan, & Hartzler, 2012). The intervention focused on enhancing drink refusal skills under conditions of social pressure and was tailored to each individual's social circumstances. Study findings revealed that compared to the control group, participants who received drink refusal skills training drank on significantly fewer days during treatment and up to one year following treatment. An alternative approach to enhancing DRSE is exemplified in ongoing work on school-based alcohol education in the UK. Based on earlier quantitative and qualitative research highlighting the influence of DRSE on secondary school students' alcohol use (de Visser et al., 2014; Graber et al., 2016), de Visser et al. (2015); de Visser, Graber, Abraham, Hart, and Memon, (2020) developed and evaluated interactive alcohol education sessions. The lessons focused on helping people to enhance their DRSE by developing skills and strategies to manage temptations, expectation, and pressure to drink. Although the programme was well-received by students and teachers, a small-scale trial revealed non-significant intervention effects on DRSE and alcohol use. Although there appears to be some promise in interventions focused on DRSE, there is a need to explore how to maximise the short- and long-term impact of drink refusal skills training, and to expand this into studies of the general population.

Proposing a Stage-Based Approach to Managing Alcohol Intake

The range of material covered in this chapter demonstrates the value of developing conceptual models and empirical evidence to enhance understanding of the information, motivation, and behavioural skills required to manage alcohol intake and to refuse alcohol. The empirical evidence discussed in this chapter clearly shows that people who are better informed, more motivated, and more highly skilled are less likely to consume alcohol in ways that are harmful to the health and well-being of themselves of others. However, if we want individuals to change their behaviour, then it is important to consider the processes through which behaviour change takes place.

Health psychology has offered several "processes of change" models that specify the different stages through which an individual would pass before longer-term behaviour change could be said to have occurred (e.g. Schwarzer, 1999). Process of change models include the "Transtheoretical Model" (TTM: Prochaska & DiClemente, 1984), the "Precaution Adoption Process Model" (PAPM: Weinstein, 1988) and the "Health Action Process Approach" (HAPA: Schwarzer & Luszczynska, 2008). The HAPA emphasises that health behaviours are adopted and maintained across distinctive motivational and volitional phases. It emphasises the importance of self-efficacy as an influential cognitive factor that is influential at all stages (Bandura 1986). The HAPA (Fig. 14.2) provides a useful theoretical and diagrammatic way of specifying how skills and capacities involved in refusing alcohol across situations cluster within particular stages. For example, "task self-efficacy"—incorporating DRSE and behavioural skills—would be required in order to deflect challenges to a decision not to drink alcohol during a specific social situation.

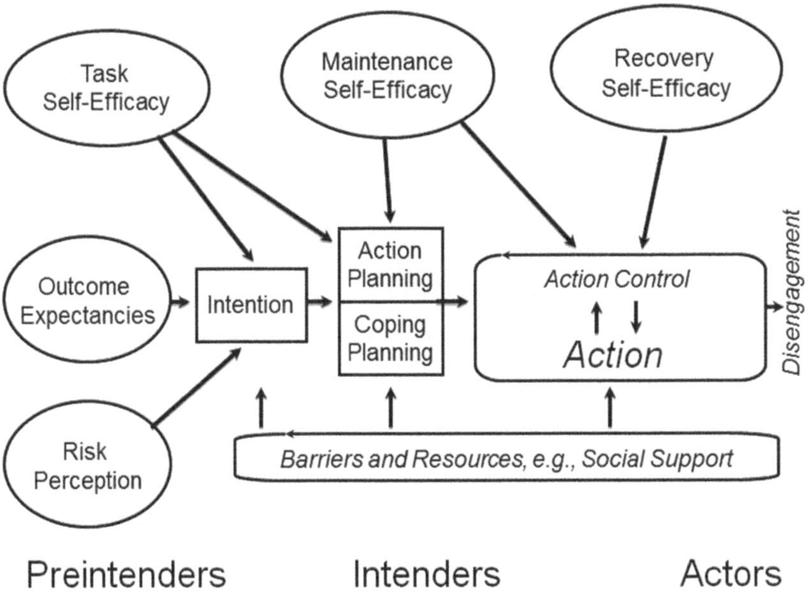

Fig. 14.2 Health action process approach. (Retrieved from http://www.hapa-model.de)

However, additional resources and skills would be required to maintain moderate drinking over a longer period: this is reflected in the construct "maintenance self-efficacy" and its associated skills. Furthermore, "recovery self-efficacy" and its associated skills would be required to resume moderate drinking or non-drinking after a setback or relapse. Recognising distinctions between these stage-specific psychological constructs is important because it demonstrates how different beliefs and skills may be required at each stage. Exploring distinct DRSE influences at each HAPA stage as an individual attempts to shift from habitual harmful drinking to habitual moderate alcohol consumption could be one avenue for future research. Stage models also help to explain why some people are able to initiate changes to their drinking in the short term, but fail to translate this into sustained longer-term behaviour change.

The HAPA usefully acknowledges temporally-orientated dimensions of SCT constructs. For example, it distinguishes between the influence of "maintenance self-efficacy" at the action planning phase and "recovery self-efficacy" at the action phase. This approach contrasts with many other health psychology models, which take a linear approach to predicting behaviour. The TTM—also referred to as the "Stages of Change" Model—takes this a step further by modelling behaviour change as a potentially cyclical process (Prochaska & DiClemente, 1984). The early part of the model is linear: people who are unaware of the need to change their unhealthy or risky behaviour are in the "pre-contemplation" stage. When people become aware of the need to change their behaviour, they enter the "contemplation" stage in which they weigh up the benefits and drawbacks of their current behaviour and of new patterns of behaviour. Those who decide that it is best to change then enter the "preparation" or "planning" stage in which they think about how they will enact their planned behaviour change. Once they are ready to change, people enter the "action" stage, and from here the linear model becomes (potentially) cyclical. People who are able to establish a new pattern of behaviour enter the "maintenance" stage. Those who are unable to establish a new pattern of behaviour and relapse to earlier behaviour may return to either (a) "contemplation"—in which they re-consider the benefits and drawbacks of behaviour change as well as their capacity to change, or (b) "planning"—in which they think about how they can better prepare themselves to enact their planned behaviour change.

We now revisit the IMB introduced earlier in this chapter. It provided a framework for encapsulating the different elements identified as relevant to "managing alcohol intake"—that is, holding accurate information, being motivated to change, and possessing the behavioural skills required to drink alcohol in moderation. There are some synergies between the TTM and the IMB. The "Information" part of the IMB could be likened to a shift from pre-contemplation to contemplation, the "Motivation" part of the IMB could be likened to a shift from contemplation to planning, and the "Behavioural skills" part of the IMB could be likened to the progression from planning to action and potential maintenance of behaviour change. The value of the TTM compared to many other psychological models of behaviour and behaviour change is that it explores and explains processes of change, and there is evidence for its value in explaining recovery from problematic alcohol use (Heather et al., 2009).

One limitation of the TTM (applicable to most stage-based and social-cognitive approaches) is the failure to account for less deliberative or unconsciously driven behaviour. Dual-process models overcome this issue by taking into account controlled and automatic process pathways underpinning drinking behaviour (Deutsch & Strack, 2006; Moss & Albery, 2009; Strack & Deutsch 2004). Such models acknowledge that in many cases, behaviour is influenced by reasoned action based on rational decision making, but they also emphasise that in many situations, behaviour is influenced by habitual patterns of behaviour and automatic responses triggered by situational cues and affective states. The extent to which behaviour is reasoned rather than automatic is determined by "boundary conditions," including emotional states and the modifying influence of intoxicants such as alcohol. In the case of alcohol use, much behaviour may be "habitual" at an individual or social level—for example, an after-work drink, a drink with dinner; celebration of milestones or transitions. Furthermore, intoxication tends to result in behaviour being influenced less by reasoned processes, and more by habitual processes or affective states. Dual-process models therefore acknowledge that the processes of change outlined above are influenced by people's habits, internal emotional states, and micro-social contexts. See Chap. 3 for further discussion of dual-process models as applied to drinking behaviours.

Discussion above has highlighted that encouraging longer-term behaviour change is likely to require success in addressing multiple relevant components (e.g. enhancing motivation, developing drink refusal skills). Discussion also emphasises the advantages of adopting a cyclical, stage-based approach to thinking about these features of managing alcohol intake—indeed, recognising that "the best-laid plans" may come unstuck may be critical to developing intake management skills that endure in the longer-term.

Conclusion

The material presented in this chapter has focused on research concerning managing alcohol intake in the context of wide-ranging pressures to drink. Understanding how alcohol intake is managed requires recognition of several distinct components: navigating guidelines for alcohol intake; acquiring and deploying the skills required to refuse alcohol; enhancing and maintaining motivation to drink moderately. Future work, including the application of stage-based models, could usefully expand on what is known by considering how best to support people to initiate and maintain changes to their alcohol intake.

References

Annis, H. M. (1986). *A relapse prevention model for the treatment of alcoholics.* New York, NY: Pergamon.

Australian Institute of Health and Welfare. (2017). *National drug strategy household survey 2016: Detailed findings* (Drug statistics series no. 31. Cat. No. PHE 214). Canberra, Australia: AIHW.

Baldwin, A. R., Oei, T. P., & Young, R. (1993). To drink or not to drink: The differential role of alcohol expectancies and drinking refusal self-efficacy in quantity and frequency of alcohol consumption. *Cognitive Therapy and Research, 17*, 511–530.

Bandura, A. (1986). Social foundations of thought and action: A social cognitive theory. Englewood Cliffs, NJ: Prentice-Hall.

Bartram, A., Eliott, J., & Crabb, S. (2017). 'Why can't I just not drink?' A qualitative study of adults' social experiences of stopping or reducing alcohol consumption. *Drug and Alcohol Review, 36*, 449–455.

Boniface, S., Kneale, J., & Shelton, N. (2013). Actual and perceived units of alcohol in a self-defined "usual glass" of alcoholic drinks in England. *Alcoholism: Clinical & Experimental Research, 37*, 978–983.

Conroy, D. & de Visser, R.O. (2014). Being a non-drinking student: an interpretative phenomenological analysis. *Psychology & Health, 29*, 536–551.

Conroy, D., Sparks, P., & de Visser, R.O. (2015). Efficacy of a non-drinking mental simulation intervention for reducing student alcohol consumption. *British Journal of Health Psychology, 20*, 688–707.

Conroy, D., & Hagger, M. S. (2018). Imagery interventions in health behavior: A meta-analysis. *Health Psychology, 37*(7), 668–679.

Conroy, D. E., & MacLean, S. (2020). Friendship and alcohol use among young adults: A cross-disciplinary perspective. In D. E. Conroy & F. Measham (Eds.), *Young Adult Drinking Styles: Current Perspectives on Research, Policy and Practice* (pp. 153–172). London, UK: Palgrave-Macmillan.

Coomber, K., Jones, S. C., Martino, F., & Miller, P. G. (2017). Predictors of awareness of standard drink labelling and drinking guidelines to reduce negative health effects among Australian drinkers. *Drug & Alcohol Review, 36*, 200–209. https://doi.org/10.1111/dar.12383

Cooper, M. L. (1994). Motivations for alcohol use among adolescents: Development and validation of a four-factor model. *Psychological Assessment, 6*, 117–128.

de Visser, R. O. (2015). Personalized feedback based on a drink-pouring exercise may improve knowledge of, and adherence to, government guidelines for alcohol consumption. *Alcoholism: Clinical & Experimental Research, 39*, 317–323.

de Visser, R. O., & Birch, J. D. (2012). My cup runneth over: Young people's lack of knowledge of low-risk drinking guidelines. *Drug & Alcohol Review, 31*, 206–212.

de Visser, R. O., Brown, C. E., Cooke, R., Cooper, G., & Memon, A. (2017). Using alcohol unit-marked glasses enhances capacity to monitor intake: Evidence from a mixed-method intervention trial. *Alcohol & Alcoholism, 52*, 206–212.

de Visser, R.O., Graber, R., Abraham, S.C.S., Hart, A., Memon, A. (2020). Resilience-based alcohol education: Developing an intervention; evaluating feasibility and barriers to implementation using mixed methods. *Health Education Research.*

de Visser, R. O., Graber, R., Hart, A., Abraham, C., Scanlon, T., Watten, P., & Memon, A. (2015). Using qualitative methods within a mixed-methods approach to developing and evaluating interventions to address harmful alcohol use among young people. *Health Psychology, 34*, 349–360.

de Visser, R. O., Hart, A., Abraham, C., Graber, R., Scanlon, T., & Memon, A. (2014). How alike are young non-drinkers, former-drinkers, low-risk drinkers, and hazardous drinkers? *Addictive Behaviors, 39*, 1258–1264.

de Visser, R. O., & Nicholls, J. (2020). Temporary abstinence during dry January: Predictors of success; impact on well-being and self-efficacy. *Psychology & Health, 35*, 1293–1305.

de Visser, R. O., Robinson, E., & Bond, R. (2016). Voluntary temporary abstinence from alcohol during "Dry January" and subsequent alcohol use. *Health Psychology, 35*, 281–289.

Deutsch, R., & Strack, F. (2006). Reflective and impulsive determinants of addictive behavior. In R. W. Wiers & A. W. Stacy (Eds.), *Handbook of implicit cognition and addiction* (pp. 45–57). London, UK: Sage.

Ding, L., Newman, I. M., Buhs, E. S., & Shell, D. F. (2018). Influence of peer pressure and self-efficacy for alcohol self-regulation on Chinese university physical education students' drinking behaviour. *Advances in Physical Education, 8*, 46–57.

Fisher, W. A., Fisher, J. D., & Harman, J. (2003). The information-motivation-Behavioral skills model: A general social psychological approach to understanding and promoting health behavior. In J. Suls & K. A. Wallston (Eds.), *Social psychological foundations of health and illness* (pp. 82–106). London, UK: Blackwell.

Foster, D. W., Yeung, N., & Neighbors, C. (2014). I think I can't: Drink refusal self-efficacy as a mediator of the relationship between self-reported drinking identity and alcohol use. *Addictive Behaviors, 39*, 461–468.

Foy, D. W., Miller, P. M., Eisler, R. M., & O'Toole, D. H. (1976). Social-skills training to teach alcoholics to refuse drinks effectively. *Journal of Studies on Alcohol, 37*, 1340–1345.

Furtwängler, N., & de Visser, R. O. (2017a). Motivation to adhere to unit-based guidelines for alcohol consumption and ability to do so is limited among university students. *Drugs: Education, Prevention and Policy, 24*, 418–425.

Furtwängler, N. A., & de Visser, R. O. (2017b). University students' beliefs about unit-based guidelines: A qualitative study. *Journal of Health Psychology, 22*, 1701–1711.

Furtwängler, N. A. F. F., & de Visser, R. O. (2013). Lack of international consensus in low risk drinking guidelines. *Drug & Alcohol Review, 32*, 11–18.

GBD 2016 Alcohol Collaborators. (2018). Alcohol use and burden for 195 countries and territories, 1990–2016: A systematic analysis for the Global Burden of Disease Study 2016. *Lancet, 392*, 1015–1035.

Graber, R., de Visser, R. O., Abraham, C., Memon, A., Hart, A., & Hunt, K. (2016). Staying in the 'sweet spot': A resilience-based analysis of the lived experience of low-risk drinking and abstention among British youth. *Psychology & Health, 31*, 79–99.

Hagger, M. S., Lonsdale, A., & Chatzisarantis, N. L. (2012). A theory-based intervention to reduce alcohol drinking in excess of guideline limits among undergraduate students. *British Journal of Health Psychology, 17*(1), 18–43.

Heather, N., Hönekopp, J., Smailes, D., & The UKATT Research Team. (2009). Progressive stage transition does mean getting better: A further test of the transtheoretical model in recovery from alcohol problems. *Addiction, 104*, 949–958.

Higgins, B. D. (1998). *Situational confidence, affect intensity and object relations in alcohol and cocaine-dependent men.* Unpublished doctoral dissertation, Columbia University, USA.

Hill, J. V., & Leeming, D. (2014). Reconstructing 'the alcoholic': Recovering from alcohol addiction and the stigma this entails. *International Journal of Mental Health & Addiction, 12*, 759–771.

Hobin, E., Vallance, K., Zuo, F., Stockwell, T., Rosella, L., Simniceanu, A., … Hammond, D. (2018). Testing the efficacy of alcohol labels with standard drink information and national drinking guidelines on consumers' ability to estimate alcohol consumption. *Alcohol & Alcoholism, 53*, 3–11.

Hodgson, R. J. (1989). Resisting temptation: A psychological analysis. *British Journal of Addiction, 84*, 251–257.

Klingemann, H., & Gmel, G. (Eds.). (2001). *Mapping the social consequences of alcohol consumption.* Dordrecht, The Netherlands: Kluwer.

Kuntsche, E., Knibbe, R., Gmel, G., & Engels, R. (2005). Why do young people drink? A review of drinking motives. *Clinical Psychology Review, 25*, 841–861.

Lee, N. K., & Oei, T. P. (1993). The importance of alcohol expectancies and drinking refusal self-efficacy in the quantity and frequency of alcohol consumption. *Journal of Substance Abuse, 5*, 379–390.

Lee, N. K., Oei, T. P., & Greeley, J. D. (1999). The interaction of alcohol expectancies and drinking refusal self-efficacy in high and low risk drinkers. *Addiction Research, 7*, 91–102.

Leigh, M. C., & Stacy, A. W. (1993). Alcohol outcome expectancies: Scale construction and predictive utility in higher order confirmatory models. *Psychological Assessment, 5*, 216–229.

Lovatt, M., Eadie, D., Meier, P. S., Li, J., Bauld, L., Hastings, G., & Holmes, J. (2015). Lay epidemiology and the interpretation of low-risk drinking guidelines by adults in the United Kingdom. *Addiction, 110*, 1912–1919.
Marlatt, G. A., & George, W. H. (1984). Relapse prevention: Introduction and overview of the model. *British Journal of Addiction, 79*, 261–273.
Martens, M. P., Ferrier, A. G., Sheehy, M. J., Corbett, K., Anderson, D. A., & Simmons, A. (2005). Development of the protective behavioral strategies survey. *Journal of Studies on Alcohol, 66*, 698–705.
McNally, K., Noonan, L. L., Cameron, M., Phillips, K., Baidoobonso, S., & Sabapathy, D. (2019). Public awareness of low-risk alcohol use guidelines. *Health Promotion Practice, 20*, 905–913.
Moss, A. C., & Albery, I. P. (2009). A dual-process model of the alcohol–behavior link for social drinking. *Psychological Bulletin, 135*, 516–530.
Nelson, D. E., Jarman, D. W., Rehm, J., Greenfield, T. K., Rey, G., Kerr, W. C., … Naimi, T. S. (2013). Alcohol-attributable cancer deaths and years of potential life lost in the United States. *American Journal of Public Health, 103*, 641–648.
Oei, T. P., Fergusson, S., & Lee, N. K. (1998). The differential role of alcohol expectancies and drinking refusal self-efficacy in problem and nonproblem drinkers. *Journal of Studies on Alcohol, 59*, 704–711.
Oei, T. P., Hasking, P. A., & Young, R. M. (2005). Drinking refusal self-efficacy questionnaire-revised (DRSEQ-R): A new factor structure with confirmatory factor analysis. *Drug and Alcohol Dependence, 78*, 297–307.
Oei, T. P., & Jardim, C. L. (2007). Alcohol expectancies, drinking refusal self-efficacy and drinking behaviour in Asian and Australian students. *Drug and Alcohol Dependence, 87*(2–3), 281–287.
Patton, K., Connor, J. P., Rundle-Thiele, S., Dietrich, T., Young, R. M., & Gullo, M. J. (2018). Measuring adolescent drinking-refusal self-efficacy: Development and validation of the drinking refusal self-efficacy questionnaire-shortened adolescent version (DRSEQ-SRA). *Addictive Behaviors, 81*, 70–77.
Pearson, M. R. (2013). Use of alcohol protective behavioral strategies among college students: A critical review. *Clinical Psychology Review, 33*, 1025–1040.
Prochaska, J. O., & DiClemente, C. C. (1984). *The transtheoretical approach: Towards a systematic eclectic framework*. Homewood, IL: Dow Jones Irwin.
Quick, B. L., & Bates, B. R. (2010). The use of gain- or loss-frame messages and efficacy appeals to dissuade excessive alcohol consumption …. *Journal of Health Communication, 15*, 603–628.
Rehm, J. (2011). The risks associated with alcohol use and alcoholism. *Alcohol Research & Health, 34*, 135–143.
Room, R. (2005). Stigma, social inequality and alcohol and drug use. *Drug & Alcohol Review, 24*, 143–155.
Rosenberg, G., Bauld, L., Hooper, L., Buykx, P., Holmes, J., & Vohra, J. (2018). New national alcohol guidelines in the UK: Public awareness, understanding and behavioural intentions. *Journal of Public Health, 40*, 549–556.
Rothman, A. J., & Salovey, P. (1997). Shaping perceptions to motivate healthy behavior: The role of message framing. *Psychological Bulletin, 121*, 3–19.

Sandahl, C., Lindberg, S., & Rönnberg, S. (1990). Efficacy expectations among alcohol-dependent patients: A Swedish version of the situational confidence questionnaire. *Alcohol & Alcoholism, 25*, 67–73.

Schomerus, G., Corrigan, P. W., Klauer, T., Kuwert, P., Freyberger, H. J., & Lucht, M. (2011). Self-stigma in alcohol dependence: consequences for drinking-refusal self-efficacy. *Drug and Alcohol Dependence, 114*(1), 12–17.

Schomerus, G., Lucht, M., Holzinger, A., Matschinger, H., Carta, M. G., & Angermeyer, M. C. (2010). The stigma of alcohol dependence compared with other mental disorders: A review of population studies. *Alcohol & Alcoholism, 46*, 105–112.

Schwarzer, R. (1999). Self-regulatory processes in the adoption and maintenance of health behaviors. *Journal of Health Psychology, 4*, 115–127.

Schwarzer, R., & Luszczynska, A. (2008). How to overcome health-compromising behaviors: The health action process approach. *European Psychologist, 13*, 141–151.

Shope, J. T., Copeland, L. A., Maharg, R., Dielman, T. E., & Butchart, A. T. (1993). Assessment of adolescent refusal skills in an alcohol misuse prevention study. *Health Education Quarterly, 20*(3), 373–390.

Solomon, K. E., & Annis, H. M. (1990). Outcome and efficacy expectancy in the prediction of post-treatment drinking behaviour. *British Journal of Addiction, 85*, 659–665.

Stevens, A. K., Littlefield, A. K., Blanchard, B. E., Talley, A. E., & Brown, J. L. (2016). Does drinking refusal self-efficacy mediate the impulsivity–problematic alcohol use relation? *Addictive Behaviors, 53*, 181–186.

Strack, F., & Deutsch, R. (2004). Reflective and impulsive determinants of social behavior. *Personality and Social Psychology Review, 8*, 220–247.

Treloar, H., Martens, M. P., & McCarthy, D. M. (2015). The protective behavioral strategies Scale-20: Improved content validity of the serious harm reduction subscale. *Psychological Assessment, 27*(1), 340–346.

Weinstein, N. D. (1988). The precaution adoption process. *Health Psychology, 7*(4), 355.

Weitzman, E. R. (2004). Poor mental health, depression, and associations with alcohol consumption, harm, and abuse in a national sample of young adults in college. *Journal of Nervous and Mental Disease, 192*, 269–277.

Witkiewitz, K., Donovan, D. M., & Hartzler, B. (2012). Drink refusal training as part of a combined behavioral intervention: Effectiveness and mechanisms of change. *Journal of Consulting and Clinical Psychology, 80*, 440.

Wittmann, M., Paulus, M., & Roenneberg, T. (2010). Decreased psychological well-being in late 'chronotypes' is mediated by smoking and alcohol consumption. *Substance Use & Misuse, 45*, 15–30.

Young, R. M., Hasking, P. A., Oei, T. P., & Loveday, W. (2007). Validation of the drinking refusal self-efficacy questionnaire—Revised in an adolescent sample (DRSEQ-RA). *Addictive Behaviors, 32*, 862–868.

Zhao, J., Stockwell, T., & Thomas, G. (2015). An adaptation of the yesterday method to correct for under-reporting of alcohol consumption and estimate compliance with Canadian low-risk drinking guidelines. *Canadian Journal of Public Health, 106*, e204–e209.

Section IV

Developmental Trajectories for Alcohol Use

15

Alcohol-Related Cognitions among Children Aged 2–12: Where Do They Originate From and How Do They Develop?

Megan Cook, Koen Smit, Carmen Voogt, and Emmanuel Kuntsche

Introduction

Research on alcohol consumption has often focused on adolescence, the period when initiation usually occurs and when there is an increased risk of harm due to experimentation. Despite consumption of alcohol before the age of 10 being rare, young children are nonetheless exposed to alcohol in the home, on television, for example, which has the potential to shape their knowledge, thoughts, and beliefs as well as their future drinking behaviour. Thus, by the time adolescents initiate alcohol consumption (in Australia in 2016, for example, this was approximately 16.1 years; Australian Institute of Health and Welfare, 2018), they already know what alcohol is, who is

M. Cook (✉) • E. Kuntsche
Centre for Alcohol Policy Research, La Trobe University, Melbourne, VIC, Australia
e-mail: m.cook@latrobe.edu.au; e.kuntsche@latrobe.edu.au

K. Smit
Centre for Alcohol Policy Research, La Trobe University, Melbourne, VIC, Australia

Behavioural Science Institute, Radboud University, Nijmegen, The Netherlands
e-mail: ksmit@trmibos.nl

C. Voogt
Trimbos Institute, Netherlands Institute of Mental Health, Utrecht, The Netherlands
e-mail: cvoogt@trmibos.nl

R. Cooke et al. (eds.), *The Palgrave Handbook of Psychological Perspectives on Alcohol Consumption*, https://doi.org/10.1007/978-3-030-66941-6_15

drinking it in what context, and how they expect it to affect them. This makes them aware of the external influences on consumption covered earlier in this book (see Chaps. 6, 7, 8, 9, and 10). During the late 1980s and early 1990s there were a number of studies in this area; however, a recent review of literature on children's alcohol-related knowledge, expectancies, and norms found that only 3 of the 17 included studies were conducted after the year 2000 (Voogt, Beusink, et al., 2017). A similar systematic review of children's alcohol-related knowledge, attitudes, and expectancies conducted between 2000 and 2017 found only 24 relevant studies (Jones & Gordon, 2017). This chapter will provide an overview of recent evidence concerning alcohol-related cognitions (knowledge, norms/attitudes, and expectancies), including from where they originate early in life and how they develop as children grow older, and will consider theoretical perspectives on the topic. Such an investigation of young children's alcohol-related cognitions is important because knowledge begins to be established before drinking is initiated; what children observe and learn about alcohol at a young age is formative and a crucial factor leading to future drinking behaviour (Jester et al., 2015).

What Do Children Know About Alcohol?

Alcohol-Related Knowledge

Children as young two years old demonstrate some knowledge about alcohol; young children can distinguish between alcoholic and non-alcoholic beverages based on smell (Mennella & Garcia, 2000), by using photographs (Kuntsche, Le Mével, & Zucker, 2016), or in a role-playing scenario involving grocery shopping (Dalton et al., 2005). For example, 62% of 120 children aged between two and six in the United States, role-playing as adults using props and dolls, bought alcohol as part of everyday groceries and 35% purchased both beer and wine, the two types of alcohol on offer (Dalton et al., 2005). Children were more likely to purchase alcohol if their parents drank alcohol at least monthly (Dalton et al., 2005).

Kuntsche and colleagues (2016) report in their study of children in French-speaking Switzerland that only 45% of three-year-olds were able to correctly identify beverages containing alcohol, which they conclude was no different from random choice[1] and suggests a limited knowledge of alcohol at this age.

[1] Random choice is the accidental chance of picking an alcoholic beverage. In this study, half of the beverages were alcoholic. A one sample t-test was used to determine whether choice was significantly above the 50% random choice.

Mennella and Garcia (2000) on the other hand were able to demonstrate that three-year-old children can distinguish alcoholic from non-alcoholic beverages based on smell. Among three- to six-year-olds, girls were found to more accurately identify the content and name of alcoholic beverages compared to boys (Kuntsche & Kuntsche, 2019). At four years old, children begin to show more nuanced knowledge of alcohol, for example, demonstrating that while adults can consume alcoholic beverages, children are restricted to non-alcoholic beverages (Kuntsche, Le Mével, & Zucker, 2016; Voogt, Beusink, et al., 2017). From five years onwards, children begin to show more sophisticated understandings of alcohol as a substance and its effects. For instance, they can identify short-term health risks and social harms from consumption, including that a 'drunk' person may 'walk strangely' (Valentine, Jayne, & Gould, 2014). From approximately 11 years, children can articulate—in response to open-ended interview questions about the physical effects of drinking large amounts of alcohol—some understanding of the depressant effects of alcohol on the brain, however many did not know that alcohol enters the bloodstream (Sigelman et al., 1999).

Studies have found that alcohol-related knowledge increases with age (Kuntsche, Le Mével, & Zucker, 2016; Kuntsche & Kuntsche, 2019), for example, false beliefs (e.g. alcohol causes trouble breathing) became less common over time among a sample of 6–12-year-olds in the United States (Bridges et al., 2003). However, this was not a consistent finding across all research; Jayne and Valentine (2017) concluded that among their sample of 5–12-year-olds from the United Kingdom there were no obvious patterns of knowledge in terms of gender or age.

Alcohol-Related Norms and Attitudes Towards Drinkers

Alcohol-related norms can be person-specific, for instance, who commonly consumes alcohol, or situation-specific, for example, when and where it is common to drink alcohol. Between three and six years of age, children possess some understanding of situation-specific alcohol-related norms, attributing alcohol consumption more often to adults at a party than when engaging in outdoor activities such as having a picnic (Kuntsche, Le Mével, & Zucker, 2016). From the age of five onwards, children have been shown to be aware of person-specific norms, for instance, that adults are more likely to consume alcohol than children and that males are more likely to consume alcohol than females and children (Kuntsche, Le Mével, & Zucker, 2016; Voogt, Otten, Kleinjan, Engels, & Kuntsche, 2017). Among more recent studies, only one revealed that girls had more knowledge of alcohol-related norms compared to boys, as they less often assigned alcoholic beverages to children compared to adults (Kuntsche, Le Mével, & Zucker, 2016; Voogt, Beusink, et al., 2017).

Finally, children's alcohol-related attitudes are a combination of beliefs, values, and feelings that influence individual responses to people, items, or situations (Velleman, 2009a). Attitudes can be implicit, activated automatically (see Chap. 3), or explicit, which require a level of introspection and are evaluated through self-report measures (Payne, Lee, Giletta, & Prinstein, 2016; see Chap. 2). Children's alcohol-related attitudes were assessed among three and eight years old (Mennella & Garcia, 2000; Mennella & Forestell, 2008), through odour-based tasks that examined hedonic responses to alcohol. Children identified pleasant or unpleasant odours through the attribution of a toy, either Big Bird (pleasant odours) or Oscar the Grouch (unpleasant). Another dimension of children's alcohol-related attitudes is children's acceptance of alcohol use behaviours. For example, whether sipping, which involves taking a small mouthful or a sample of a beverage (and in relation to alcohol often involves parents providing children with small tastes or sips out of their own glass), is wrong or not. Children's attitudes towards sipping are reported to become more positive between 11 and 12 years of age (Prins, Donovan, & Molina, 2011). Researchers hypothesise that this is the time when parents become less important and other sources of influence, such as friends and the media, begin to exert more influence (Prins et al., 2011).

Alcohol Expectancies

Alcohol Expectancies (AE) are personal beliefs about the consequences of substance use (Jones, Corbin, & Fromme, 2001). In Alcohol Expectancy Theory, individuals hold expectations of certain reinforcing effects that result as an outcome of behaviour (Goldman, Brown, & Christiansen, 1987; Jones et al., 2001; see Chap. 2). Expectancies operate as a function of long-term memory, impacting processes that govern both current and future behaviour. Expectancies can be considered explicit and assessed via questionnaires, or implicit and measured, for example, using an Implicit Association Task (IAT; see Smit et al., 2018; Thush & Wiers, 2007). AE are most commonly assessed through endorsement (agree/disagree) or perceived likelihood of an effect occurring (likely/unlikely). Subjective endorsement has been suggested as particularly important, as 'the more favourably people evaluate the impairment effects of drinking, the greater their overall alcohol use' (Jones et al., 2001, p. 62). However, simply having a certain expectancy or belief does not necessarily lead to behaviour (see Chap. 4 for a review of the evidence that AE predict consumption). Although an individual may hold a certain belief about the potential positive or negative effects of alcohol, they will only use a substance if they are motivated or desire to achieve that outcome (Cooper, Kuntsche, Levitt, Barber, & Wolf, 2016). Expectancies remain important as people who do not hold a certain belief or expectancy are unlikely to use alcohol to achieve that effect (Jones et al., 2001).

AE develop before children have had their first drinking experience. Expectancies are particularly important for young children, as a first-time drinker, with little to no direct experience, will be guided by their expectations of the effects of alcohol (Leigh, 1989). The theoretical processes thought to underlie the acquisition of AE at a young age (before alcohol initiation) are based on social learning principles (Bandura & Walters, 1977; Bandura, 1986; Campbell & Oei, 2010) and are shaped by environmental influences (discussed below). Predictors of adolescent alcohol use are divided into individual (e.g. alcohol-related cognitions, personality, genetic, and behavioural) and environmental (e.g. family, peers, and media) factors, with AE operating as mediators of the link between different individual and environmental predictors of alcohol use (Settles, Zapolski, & Smith, 2014; Treloar, Pedersen, & McCarthy, 2015; Banks & Zapolski, 2017; Smit et al., 2018).

Although the focus of this chapter is on recent research, it is important to first take a step back to briefly overview the work of Brown et al. (1980; Brown, Christiansen, & Goldman, 1987) on expectancies that began a long-documented association between adolescents' AE and alcohol use, which drives much of the present work. In the 1980s, expectancy research focused largely on positive expectancies associated with alcohol consumption; it wasn't until the 1990s that the predictive power of negative expectancies began to be explored in more depth. A simplistic explanation sees positive expectancies representative of motivation to consume and negative expectancies representative of motivation to restrain (Jones et al., 2001). In cross-sectional studies among adolescent and adult populations, positive expectancies have been found to predict alcohol use (Fromme, Stroot, & Kaplan, 1993; Leigh & Stacy, 1993) and have been suggested to predict successful treatment outcomes for problem drinking (Goldman, 1994). Dunn and Goldman (1996) found that the number and types of alcohol expectancy dimensions described for adults were also found for children. For example, alcohol expectancy dimensions can be conceptualised in terms of Russell's Circumplex Model of Affect (1980), created by crossing the dimensions of valence and activation

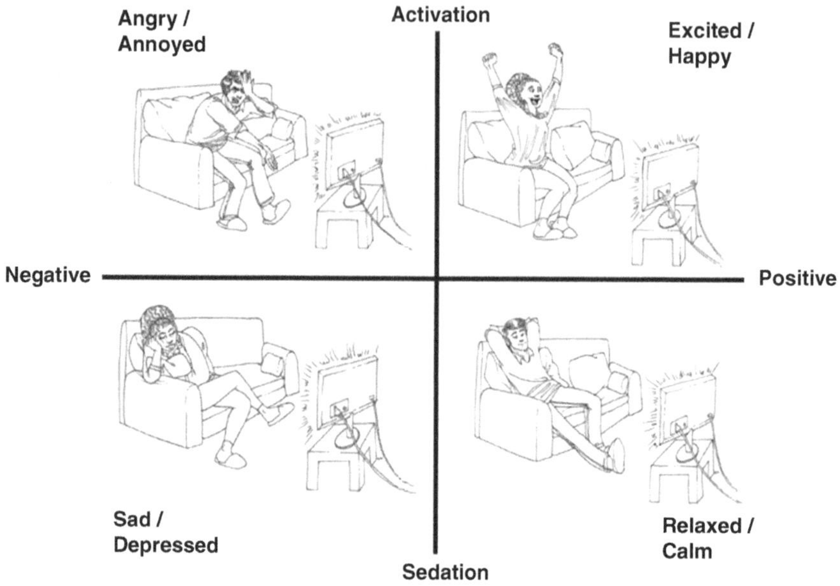

Fig. 15.1 Scenario examples from the AET in relation to the Circumplex Model of Affect. Note: Illustrations provided are examples. A wide range of emotions are represented for each person/gender in the full AE Task. The authors would like to thank Florian Labhart for writing the AET software; Caroline Tschumi for creating the AET drawings. (Kuntsche & Kuntsche, 2017)

(Wiers, 2008), resulting in four emotional categories: sedation positive, sedation negative, arousal positive, and arousal negative (see Fig. 15.1).

Children's Alcohol Expectancies

While some research has suggested that AE exist from the age of six (Jester et al., 2015; Mares, Stone, Lichtwarck-Aschoff, & Engels, 2015), other studies have suggested that by the age of four children already have certain AE and are able to recognise the emotional changes resulting from alcohol use (Donovan et al., 2004; Kuntsche, 2017; Voogt, Beusink, et al., 2017). Donovan et al. (2004) were able to demonstrate among three-year-olds that AE are precursors to alcohol use, significantly predicting early drinking onset. Similarly, using the Beverage Opinion Questionnaire, positive AE among six- to eight-year-olds have been shown to predict initiation and Heavy Episodic Drinking (HED; see Chap. 1) even nine years later (Jester et al., 2015). AE are predominantly negative in young children and endorsement of positive AE has been found to increase with age (Bridges et al., 2003; Chung, Hipwell,

Loeber, White, & Stouthamer-Loeber, 2008; Colder et al., 2014; Copeland, Proctor, Terlecki, Kulesza, & Williamson, 2014; Patrick, Wray-Lake, & Maggs, 2017), with the greatest shifts seeming to occur in the year after initiation or between 10 and 12 years (Donovan, Molina, & Kelly, 2009; Copeland et al., 2014; Smit et al., 2018). Studies assess AE using a variety of methods including open-ended interviews (Bridges et al., 2003), the Alcohol Expectancy Questionnaire-Adolescent (Copeland et al., 2014) or similarly structured questionnaires (Chung et al., 2008; Jester et al., 2015; Patrick et al., 2017), and IAT (Colder et al., 2014).

While positive AE have been found to increase with age, several studies have found that negative AE either remain stable over time (Bridges et al., 2003; Cameron, Stritzke, & Durkin, 2003; Colder et al., 2014) or slightly diminish with age. For instance, a study with Australian primary school children, aged between 8 and 12 years, found consistent negative and positive expectancies, rather than a predominance of one over the other (Cameron et al., 2003). Assessing three- to six-year-olds' knowledge of the emotional changes that result from alcohol consumption in Switzerland, Kuntsche (2017) found no significant age differences. Among six- to nine-year-olds from the Netherlands, Mares et al. (2015) found that older children in their sample held fewer positive expectancies and more negative expectancies. Colder et al. (2014) found that negative expectancies were still dominant at 10 years, but became more neutral during the transition to adolescence. While both expectancy theory and the results discussed suggest that more positive AE increase the likelihood to drink, the direction of causation of the association has been hypothesised to be reciprocal, whereby experiences also lead to changes in expectancies about the effects of alcohol (Slutske et al., 2002; Jester et al., 2015; Smit et al., 2018). See Table 15.1 for an overview of alcohol-related cognitions from 2 to 12, which demonstrates that many cognitions are first evident well before 7 years.

Acquisition of Alcohol-Related Cognitions: Theoretical Considerations

The theoretical processes thought to underlie the acquisition of alcohol-related cognitions are based on social learning principles and are shaped by environmental influences. It is important to state that the way young children learn about alcohol is no different from how they learn about any other concept or idea (Velleman, 2009b). Children learn many of the formative skills

Table 15.1 Age and alcohol-related cognitions

Age	Alcohol-related cognition operationalisation	Study (year)
2	Purchase alcohol in a shopping scenario[a]	Dalton et al. (2005)
3	Distinguish between alcoholic and non-alcoholic beverages using photographs and by odour[a] Knowledge of situation-specific alcohol-related norms[b] Accurately identify the content and name of alcoholic beverages[a]	Mennella and Garcia (2000) Kuntsche and Kuntsche (2019) Kuntsche, Le Mével, and Zucker (2016) Voogt, Otten et al. (2017)
4	Appreciation of gender-specific drinking norms[b] Understand the age restrictions on consumption[a] Recognise emotional changes resulting from alcohol use[c]	Kuntsche, Le Mével, & Zucker, 2016 Kuntsche (2017)
5	Identify short-term health risks and social harms[a] Communicate factual and negative information about alcohol[a] Knowledge of person-specific alcohol-related norms[b] Identify the name of alcoholic beverages based on their odour[a] Knowledge of how a drunk person may act[a]	Valentine et al. (2014) Hahn et al. (2000) Kuntsche, Le Mével, and Zucker (2016) Mennella and Forestell (2008)
6	Have explicit and mostly negative expectancies about the effects of alcohol[c] Believe alcohol will result in negative short-term outcomes[c]	Kuntsche, Le Mével, and Zucker (2016) Bridges et al. (2003)
7	****	
8	Boys are more likely than girls to identify alcohol[a] Boys are more likely than girls to intend to drink alcohol when older[b] Hold consistent negative and positive expectancies[c] Believe it is normal for mothers not to drink alcohol[b]	Andrews, Tildesley, Hops, Duncan, and Severson (2003) Cameron et al. (2003) Mares et al. (2015)
9	****	
10	****	
11	Alcohol behaviours (i.e. sipping) become more acceptable[b] Understand the depressant effects of alcohol on the brain[a]	Prins et al. (2011) Sigelman et al. (1999)
12	False beliefs about the effects of alcohol become less common[a]	Bridges et al. (2003)

Note: Cognitions reported in this table are reported at the age at which they first become evident, which of course may not be consistent for all children or consistent across all cultures. Cognitions are present at each stage afterwards and as discussed often become more nuanced with age

[a]Knowledge

[b]Norms and attitudes

[c]Expectancies

***In the studies reviewed between 2000 and 2019 no *new* cognitions have been found at this age and knowledge needed to perform or engage in a behaviour from an early age through modelling and observation of adults. Indeed, the mechanisms behind the acquisition of alcohol-related knowledge and many of the same theoretical processes, for example, Social Learning Theory (Bandura & Walters, 1977), socialisation (Donovan, 2016), and the Cognitive Model of Intergenerational Transference (Campbell & Oei, 2010), underlie general learning especially at a young age.

Social learning models of alcohol consumption hold that people form alcohol-related cognitions from their social and cultural environment. First, Social Learning Theory (SLT) postulates behaviours are learned through observation and subsequent modelling directly from parents and peers (primary social factors) and indirectly via, for example, the media (indirect reference groups) (Bandura & Walters, 1977; Bandura, 1986; Kobus, 2003). These influencers operate directly (e.g. through social reinforcement or sanctions) or indirectly (e.g. by influencing attitudes, norms, or beliefs) to affect alcohol use. When observing a behaviour, children form an idea about how to perform the behaviour, and what is achieved when the behaviour is performed (i.e. what the behaviour is good for). When an opportunity then arises to perform this behaviour, even years later, this knowledge is put into practice.

Second, socialisation is the fundamental process by which children learn about their culture and the expected behaviours of their society (Velleman, 2009a; Donovan, 2016). The core principles defined by SLT underlie primary socialisation theory which suggests four primary social contexts (family, media, peer clusters and school) through which norms and behaviours are learned (Kobus, 2003). This theory emphasises the relational bonds between social contexts that act as channels through which information is shared (Kobus, 2003). Finally, the Cognitive Model of Intergenerational Transference suggests that the observation of parental drinking habits contribute to what a child knows about alcohol (knowledge), its use in adult culture (norms), and what happens when alcohol is consumed (expectancies) (Campbell & Oei, 2010; Voogt, Beusink, et al., 2017). Like SLT, the Cognitive Model of Intergenerational Transference suggests that children will not immediately adopt the behaviours they see, but that children's cognitions mediate the behaviour; there may be a period of time between observation and modelling during which children process what they have seen, potentially in relation to other observed behaviour (Mares et al., 2015). According to these theoretical perspectives, alcohol use is considered as a learned response to the complex interaction of individual and environmental stimuli. These three theories all hold that behaviour is in some part learnt through observation. It is, however, the direct experience with a new behaviour (positive or negative) that determines whether it persists. Consequently, once children begin to have experience (i.e. consume alcohol themselves), observations of others consuming alcohol become less important (Kobus, 2003).

Influences on Alcohol-Related Cognitions

Family/Parental Influences (See Also Chap. 16)

One of the most commonly explored sources of children's knowledge of alcohol is the family and in particular parents. The effects of parenting on children's cognitions (and on behaviour) vary, depending on the age of the child, but consistently remain the most important pre-initiation influence. Evidence indicates that it is not parental drinking per se which has a direct impact on the alcohol-related cognitions, but rather young people's exposure to this consumption, that is, when parents or other adults drink alcoholic beverages in the *presence* of children and children see the consequences of their drinking (Smit et al., 2019). For example, drinking may occur when children are in bed or outside of the home, for example, after work, when children aren't around, compared to drinking at the dinner table when children are present (Voogt, Beusink, et al., 2017). Differences in children's exposure to observable behaviour and its consequences have been postulated as an explanation for the divergence in findings on children's alcohol-related cognitions (Voogt, Beusink, et al., 2017). In a Dutch study of 10–13-year-olds, exposure to parental drinking has been shown to mediate the relationship between parental alcohol use and pre-teen use (Smit et al., 2019). Among three- to six-year-olds, knowledge and alcohol-related norms (e.g. drinking being more common among men and at parties) were higher when parents drank frequently, at a higher quantity or during meals (Kuntsche & Kuntsche, 2019).

Additionally, exposure has been shown to have an impact not only on cognitions but on alcohol-related behaviour, for example, children's sipping of alcohol (Donovan & Molina, 2008, 2014; Jackson, Ennett, Dickinson, & Bowling, 2013). Sipping small amounts of alcohol—common practice among children aged between 6 and 12 years (Andrews et al., 2003; Zucker, Donovan, Masten, Mattson, & Moss, 2008; Jackson, Ennett, Dickinson, & Bowling, 2012)—is often viewed by parents as a controlled introduction to alcohol (Ward, Snow, & Aroni, 2010). As a first experience, sipping is often driven by adult's concern to ensure a supervised introduction to alcohol rather than being driven by children themselves (Ward et al., 2010). However, sipping alcoholic beverages by children and young adolescents instigates their curiosity about alcohol. This early drinking, including sips or tastes, has been shown to be connected to earlier and more harmful patterns of alcohol use in adolescence (Zucker et al., 2008; Donovan & Molina, 2011; Jackson, Barnett, Colby, & Rogers, 2015; Sharmin et al., 2017; Colder, Shyhalla, & Frndak, 2018). Despite its potential harm, it remains most common for sipping to occur in the home or family environment often attached to social or celebratory occasions, with few young children ever trying alcohol without their parents' knowledge (Andrews et al., 2003).

Adopting a socialisation perspective, Ennett et al. (2016) explored sipping as a powerful learning experience through which it may be instilled upon a child that drinking is an approved practice, setting a behavioural precedent. Briefly, more frequent parental alcohol consumption has been found to be associated with the belief that sipping by children is possibly protective and with less disapproval of their own children engaging in sipping of alcoholic beverages (Ennett, Jackson, Bowling, & Dickinson, 2013). Setting such a precedent may in turn make repeated and continued sipping more likely, particularly in the transition from childhood to adolescence. In a study conducted in the United States, at least one in five mothers thought of sipping as a deterrent to use through removing the 'forbidden fruit' appeal of alcohol and because children would not like the taste (Jackson et al., 2012). However, this remains contrary to other research suggesting children who had engaged in sipping by 10 years old were almost twice as likely to begin drinking before 15 (Donovan & Molina, 2011; Smit et al., 2018). Research from Australia on the supervised introduction to alcohol by parents found that 'there is no conclusive evidence that the consumption of sips of alcohol in early childhood is in the long-term, harmful or protective against alcohol-related problems in adult life and arguments to the contrary suggest correlation but not causation' (Ward et al., 2010, p. 274).[2]

It is important to note that the effects of sipping on future drinking behaviour may depend on cultural differences. On the one hand, in Southern European countries where light alcohol consumption is integrated into daily life, associated with food, and per capita consumption is relatively low (Room, 2010), sipping may not be associated with any long-term consequences—this experience cannot, necessarily, differentiate those who go on to misuse

[2] It is worth noting that researchers have raised concerns about using 'age at first drink' (a concept relied upon in many of these studies). For a discussion of the potential limitations, see Kuntsche, Rossow, et al. (2016).

alcohol from those who do not because it is norm for all children to sip alcohol. On the other hand, in cultures where HED is more prominent (e.g. Australia, the Netherlands, the Republic of Ireland, the United Kingdom), sipping might lead young people to become more curious about alcohol and because the norm for drinkers in these countries is to drink heavily, initiating curiosity in children may bring about long-term consequences as they seek to model normal drinking behaviour. Currently, there is a limited understanding of consequences of sipping as a function of cultural differences, especially because much international evidence excludes sips as a measure of consumption among younger participants (Donovan & Molina, 2008).

While research is still in its infancy, several studies have found associations between parental alcohol use and children's alcohol-related cognitions (Donovan & Molina, 2008; Voogt, Beusink, et al., 2017). In a UK study, children (aged 11) of parents with alcohol problems reported lower perceived risk of harm from drinking (Patrick et al., 2017). Observation of parental alcohol use was also found to predict positive AE among non-drinkers (12 years old) in Taiwan (Ting, Chen, Liu, Lin, & Chen, 2015). In Switzerland, replicating findings from earlier studies in the United States (Miller, Smith, & Goldman, 1990), children's AE were related to their parent's consumption, specifically children of heavy drinking parents developed stronger associations with negative effects of use (Kuntsche & Kuntsche, 2018). Recent research by Kuntsche and Kuntsche (2019) provides the first empirical evidence that children's knowledge of alcohol is associated with parental consumption as early as three years old. Research from the United Kingdom found that children were only able to correctly identify alcoholic beverages that their own parents or relatives drank, that is, those who existed in close proximity in children's social worlds (Valentine et al., 2014; Jayne & Valentine, 2017).

Some studies have identified gender differences in the association between parental alcohol use and offspring's alcohol-related cognitions. For instance, paternal alcohol use has been found to have a stronger association with children's expectancies compared to maternal alcohol use among 10-year-olds (Handley & Chassin, 2009; Pieters, Van, Engels, & Weirs, 2010), and in some cases this influence is stronger for boys (Handley & Chassin, 2009; Kuntsche & Kuntsche, 2018). To measure AE in young children, Mares et al. (2015) used the Berkeley Puppet Interview (BPI) which involves the use of two hand puppets. Children are asked whether they would agree with the positive or negative statements the puppets say, that is, 'adults become happy when they drink alcohol' or 'adults do not become happy when they drink alcohol'. Researchers found that among girls (mean age of eight years) more parental alcohol use was associated with less negative AE (Mares et al., 2015).

This study also found that mother's alcohol use was associated with less positive expectancies, while father's alcohol use was associated with more positive expectancies among the older children in their sample, potentially indicating (as suggested by the authors) that children believe it is non-normative for mothers to drink alcohol (Mares et al., 2015). However, much of the evidence on the relative impact of mothers versus fathers is somewhat mixed and many studies lack information on fathers' drinking, instead focusing only on mothers.

Parents often consider children under 12 years to be too young to know about or to begin learning about alcohol. Jayne and Valentine (2017) found that most parents of the children in their sample (aged 5–12) did not have rules relating to alcohol consumption, based on the assumption that children at this age do not engage in or are interested in alcohol consumption. However, as Valentine et al. (2014) suggest, the 'banal omnipresence' of alcohol in everyday life and particularly in familial spaces such as the home, mean parents are unintentionally modelling drinking to children, arguably from birth. Problematically, parents and other adults most commonly model the positive aspects of drinking to their children, and usually make sure to avoid demonstrating any negative consequences of drinking, including drinking to excess, meaning children are presented with a potentially very one-sided view of the effects (Jayne & Valentine, 2017). This suggestion is interesting when considering research on expectancies which shows that they are primarily negative at a young age (Kuntsche & Kuntsche, 2018). However, research has shown that alcohol dependence in parents is still associated with positive AE (Smit et al., 2018). While again these results may be related to children's perception of problematic drinking patterns, this suggests that the solution to the predominance of positive modelling may not just be increased negative modelling. Research has suggested that observation of problematic drinking patterns, that is, drunkenness, instead affects children's view of their parents as positive role models (Foster, Bryant, & Brown, 2017). Furthermore, the results presented here may be an example of the mixed information children receive from their immediate environment despite what parents report.

Other Considerations

As mentioned, parents are the primary influence on alcohol-related knowledge at a young age and while there are a range of others, the literature on these remains more limited. For example, extent of knowledge is inextricably interwoven with peer relationships. In saying this, peers are often far more influential for adolescents than for young children regarding alcohol consumption; as children move into adolescence, peer relationships generally become more important and all-encompassing (Patrick, Schulenberg, Maggs, & Maslowsky, 2016). For instance, peer alcohol use has been found to be associated with more positive AE among students aged 11–12 years (Ting et al., 2015). It may be interesting to consider whether during early childhood, children experience any peer effects, that is before the age of 10 if alcohol plays any role in peer interactions. Briefly, at this young age genetics play less of a role in influencing alcohol-related cognitions and behaviour, also becoming more important after 12 years once drinking has been initiated (Dick, 2011; Agrawal et al., 2012).

While many studies hypothesise the effect of media on the acquisition of alcohol-related knowledge, there is a notable absence of research formally investigating this relationship in young children. A study conducted in New Zealand by Casswell (1996) found that more than one-third of nine-year-olds cited television as a source of their knowledge, whereas in a recent study in Switzerland, no relationship was found between the frequency of television viewing per day and alcohol-related knowledge among three- to six-year-olds (Kuntsche & Kuntsche, 2019). However, the past 10 years have seen radical changes in the media landscape with increasing integration into our everyday lives, including social media—that is, Facebook and Instagram, streaming services, that is Netflix and YouTube—and the ubiquitous use of mobile phones and tablets. Researchers are only just beginning to explore what effect this may have generally, with a noticeable gap in relation to young children's developing alcohol-related cognitions between 2 and 12 years. It is briefly worth noting that research has suggested that any potential influence the media may exert can be offset through open communication and discussion promoting critical thinking about the messages being shown, and parental monitoring involving clear rules (Velleman, 2009a; Van den Eijnden, Van De Mheen, Vet, & Vermulst, 2011).

Limitations and Future Research Directions

There are several limitations to existing research on young children's alcohol-related cognitions. First, much of the evidence collected so far has been from cross-sectional study designs that restrict the causal conclusions that can be drawn (Voogt, Beusink, et al., 2017, see Chap. 2). In the literature reviewed in this chapter, there is a noticeable lack of evidence from large-scale epidemiological studies including children under 10 years (Zucker et al., 2008).

Furthermore—with the notable exception of Voogt, Otten, and colleagues (Voogt, Otten, et al., 2017)—evidence collected in these studies is primarily from non-representative and small convenience samples which enhances the risk of selection bias impairing external validity and generalisability. As a result, future research needs to focus on obtaining more representative samples (Voogt, Beusink, et al., 2017).

Another major limitation of the current research studies is the use of measures originally developed to assess adult cognitions, then adapted for college population groups and adolescents, and finally adapted again for children (Donovan, 2014). Such adaption ignores the fact that children are both different developmentally and articulate their experience of the world in individual ways to adults. In the past, the BPI was transferred from assessing children's general psychopathology (Stone et al., 2014) to assessing children's alcohol-related cognitions (Mares et al., 2015; Kuntsche & Kuntsche, 2017). However, the BPI was particularly burdensome for both child participants and researchers administering the task. Thus, researchers began to look for alternatives. Recently, several age-appropriate methods were developed specifically for young children, including the electronic Alcohol Beverages Task (eABT; Kuntsche, Le Mével, & Zucker, 2016) and the Alcohol Expectancy Task (AET; Kuntsche & Kuntsche, 2017), which have been validated as suitable for assessing alcohol-related cognitions among children. The AET, for example, overcomes limitations of previous measurement tools such as questionnaires, by using illustrated scenarios displayed on a tablet computer of people in everyday situational contexts displaying different emotional states (see Fig. 15.1). The tasks use of photographs of both alcoholic and non-alcoholic beverages avoids asking respondents potentially inappropriate questions that may encourage them to drink (Kuntsche & Kuntsche, 2017).

Studying young children provides opportunities for important insights including cross-generational perspectives, particularly as the experiences of adults and children vary immensely (Valentine et al., 2014). Research is often limited by adult views on what are children's best interests, which are suggested to be predicated on deterministic theories of child development and often result in the exclusion of children's own experiences of factors that impact on their life world (Valentine et al., 2014). It has been suggested that the lack of empirical first-hand evidence on young children's alcohol-related cognitions stems from the methodological constraints and challenges (and by extension we would also include ethical concerns) of engaging young children in research using traditional methods: that is, they cannot read or write proficiently, have limited language skills, and can be easily influenced by the interviewer or by the way questions are phrased (Kuntsche, Le Mével, & Zucker, 2016). Those age-appropriate methods available tend to be both financially and time costly requiring set-up, rely on recording, transcription, coding, and time intensive data entry into electronic databases for analysis (Kuntsche, Le Mével, & Zucker, 2016). Similar challenges in measurement at this age exist in trying to separate the impact of children's rapidly changing cognitive and language abilities from their cognitions (i.e. what is children's increasing capacity to articulate their knowledge as opposed to what is an increase or change in knowledge). In creating age-appropriate methodological approaches, such as the eABT and the AET discussed, researchers must negotiate these challenges.

Next to more age-appropriate measurements, it has been speculated that children learn about alcohol by overhearing adult conversations about alcohol and its effects (Kuntsche & Kuntsche, 2019). However, more research is needed to come to firmer conclusions in this respect. Moreover, researchers should also investigate the extent to which young children understand adult conversations of alcohol or are simply repeating what they have heard. Qualitative interviews with young children provide an opportunity to elicit such nuanced, first-hand, and detailed information. While recent developments in neutral and age-appropriate measurement tools have been made, such quantitative methods only tell half the story and we need to adopt and integrate qualitative methods, particularly among younger participants, to understand what young children know about alcohol, how young children conceptualise alcohol, and the origins of this knowledge. Furthermore, by engaging young people in research we can begin to confront and address young children's knowledge and the possible transition to problem-drinking patterns in meaningful ways that are acceptable to children. Although advocating for more evidence from children themselves, we acknowledge that evidence provided by parents (and other sources) are still required to build a comprehensive picture of the origins of children's alcohol-related cognitions (Kuntsche, Le Mével, & Zucker, 2016).

Finally, research is needed from different national and cultural contexts, as most of the studies reviewed in this chapter are from Anglophone and/or northern European countries (i.e. the Netherlands, Switzerland, the United Kingdom, the United States). This should include a more diverse range of countries and cultures including those across central, eastern, or southern European countries, lower-income countries, and those with a 'dry' alcohol culture (e.g. where alcohol is more restricted and less integrated into daily life; Room, 2010). For example, it would be interesting to explore what young children in India, which historically experiences high abstention rates among females (Benegal, 2005), know about alcohol. Future research may also wish to explore developmental trajectories, for example, what general knowledge is needed before alcohol-specific knowledge begins to develop, and whether norms and expectancies develop at the same time or whether one proceeds the other. Moreover, it is important to continue to investigate longitudinally whether the acquisition and development of alcohol-related cognitions in young children are predictive of alcohol use initiation in early adolescence and subsequent use in middle and late adolescence and (young) adulthood.

Conclusions

Taken together, the review presented in this chapter provides a compelling rationale for engaging in research with young children on their lived experience with alcohol. Examining alcohol from a child's perspective may allow us to see 'the world anew' as it were, providing new perspectives to an ostensibly enduring substance embedded in everyday practices. The development of alcohol-related cognitions is an ongoing process, in covering from age 2 to 12 we have only detailed a small portion of this trajectory, which will continue throughout adolescence and adulthood. It must be remembered that the way young children learn about alcohol and its use is no different from how they learn about any other concept or idea and it is important not to make alcohol out to be a special case. However, investigation of young children's alcohol-related cognitions is imperative, as what children observe and learn about alcohol at a young age is formative, and a crucial factor leading to future drinking behaviour. Finally, several important conceptual questions and an array of future research directions remain. Researchers should look to qualitative methods entwined with the adoption of a child-centred perspective, to begin to establish a more nuanced and wholesome picture of children's alcohol-related cognitions in the twenty-first century.

References

Agrawal, A., Freedman, N. D., Cheng, Y.-C., Lin, P., Shaffer, J. R., Sun, Q., … Cornelis, M. C. (2012). Measuring alcohol consumption for genomic meta-analyses of alcohol intake: Opportunities and challenges. *The American Journal of Clinical Nutrition, 95*(3), 539–547.

Andrews, J. A., Tildesley, E., Hops, H., Duncan, S. C., & Severson, H. H. (2003). Elementary school age children's future intentions and use of substances. *Journal of Clinical Child and Adolescent Psychology, 32*(4), 556–567.

Australian Institute of Health and Welfare. (2018). *Alcohol, tobacco & other drugs in Australia* (Cat. No: PHE 221). Canberra, Australia: Australian Government.

Bandura, A. (1986). *Social foundations of thought and action: A social cognitive theory*. Englewood Cliffs, NJ: Prentice-Hall, Inc..

Bandura, A., & Walters, R. H. (1977). *Social learning theory*. Englewood Cliffs, NJ: Prentice-hall.

Banks, D. E., & Zapolski, T. C. (2017). Racial differences in the link between alcohol expectancies and adolescent drinking. *Addictive Behaviors, 67*, 34–37.

Benegal, V. (2005). India: Alcohol and public health. *Addiction, 100*(8), 1051–1056.

Bridges, L. J., Sigelman, C. K., Brewster, A. B., Leach, D. B., Mack, K. L., Rinehart, C. S., & Sorongon, A. G. (2003). Cognitive predictors of children's attitudes toward alcohol and cocaine. *Journal of Child & Adolescent Substance Abuse, 12*(3), 19–44.

Brown, S. A., Christiansen, B. A., & Goldman, M. S. (1987). The alcohol expectancy questionnaire: An instrument for the assessment of adolescent and adult alcohol expectancies. *Journal of Studies on Alcohol, 48*(5), 483–491.

Brown, S. A., Goldman, M. S., Inn, A., & Anderson, L. R. (1980). Expectations of reinforcement from alcohol: Their domain and relation to drinking patterns. *Journal of Consulting and Clinical Psychology, 48*(4), 419–426.

Cameron, C. A., Stritzke, W. G., & Durkin, K. (2003). Alcohol expectancies in late childhood: An ambivalence perspective on transitions toward alcohol use. *Journal of Child Psychology and Psychiatry, 44*(5), 687–698.

Campbell, J. M., & Oei, T. P. (2010). A cognitive model for the intergenerational transference of alcohol use behavior. *Journal of Addictive Behaviours, 35*(2), 73–83.

Casswell, S. (1996). Alcohol use: Growing up and learning about drinking: Children in Dunedin in the 1980s. In P. A. Silva & W. R. Stanton (Eds.), *From child to adult: The Dunedin multidisciplinary health and development study* (pp. 206–224). Auckland, New Zealand: Oxford University Press.

Chung, T., Hipwell, A., Loeber, R., White, H. R., & Stouthamer-Loeber, M. (2008). Ethnic differences in positive alcohol expectancies during childhood: The Pittsburgh Girls Study. *Alcoholism: Clinical & Experimental Research, 32*(6), 966–974.

Colder, C., O'Connor, J. P., Read, R. D., Eiden, L. J., Lengua, L. W., Hawk, J., & Wieczorek, W. (2014). Growth trajectories of alcohol information processing and associations with escalation of drinking in early adolescence. *Psychology of Addictive Behaviours, 28*(3), 659–670.

Colder, C., Shyhalla, K., & Frndak, S. E. (2018). Early alcohol use with parental permission: Psychosocial characteristics and drinking in late adolescence. *Addictive Behaviors, 76*, 82–87.

Cooper, M. L., Kuntsche, E., Levitt, A., Barber, L. L., & Wolf, S. (2016). Motivational models of substance use: A review of theory and research on motives for using alcohol, marijuana, and tobacco. In K. J. Sher (Ed.), *The Oxford handbook of sub-*

stance use and substance use disorders (pp. 375–421). https://doi.org/10.1093/oxfordhb/9780199381678.013.017.

Copeland, A. L., Proctor, S. L., Terlecki, M. A., Kulesza, M., & Williamson, D. A. (2014). Do positive alcohol expectancies have a critical developmental period in pre-adolescents? *Journal of Studies on Alcohol and Drugs, 75*(6), 945–952.

Dalton, M. A., Bernhardt, A. M., Gibson, J. J., Sargent, J. D., Beach, M. L., Adachi-Mejia, A. M., ... Heatherton, T. F. (2005). Use of cigarettes and alcohol by preschoolers while role-playing as adults: "Honey, have some smokes". *Archives of Pediatrics & Adolescent Medicine, 159*(9), 854–859.

Dick, D. M. (2011). Developmental changes in genetic influences on alcohol use and dependence. *Child Development Perspective, 5*(4), 223–230.

Donovan, J. E. (2014). The burden of alcohol use: focus on children and preadolescents. *Alcohol Research: Current Reviews, 35*(2), 186–192.

Donovan, J. E. (2016). Child and adolescent socialization into substance use. In S. Brown & R. A. Zucker (Eds.), *The Oxford Handbook of Adolescent Substance Abuse.* Oxford University Press. https://doi.org/10.1093/oxfordhb/9780199735662.013.018

Donovan, J. E., Leech, S. L., Zucker, R. A., Loveland-Cherry, C. J., Jester, J. M., Fitzgerald, H. E., ... Looman, W. S. (2004). Really underage drinkers: Alcohol use among elementary students. *Alcoholism: Clinical and Experimental Research, 28*(2), 341–349.

Donovan, J. E., & Molina, B. S. (2008). Children's introduction to alcohol use: Sips and tastes. *Alcoholism: Clinical and Experimental Research, 32*(1), 108–119.

Donovan, J. E., & Molina, B. S. (2011). Childhood risk factors for early-onset drinking. *Journal of Studies on Alcohol and Drugs, 72*(5), 741–751.

Donovan, J. E., & Molina, B. S. (2014). Antecedent predictors of children's initiation of sipping/tasting alcohol. *Alcoholism: Clinical and Experimental Research, 38*(9), 2488–2495.

Donovan, J. E., Molina, B. S., & Kelly, T. M. (2009). Alcohol outcome expectancies as socially shared and socialized beliefs. *Psychology of Addictive Behaviors, 23*(2), 248–259.

Dunn, M. E., & Goldman, M. S. (1996). Empirical modeling of an alcohol expectancy memory network in elementary school children as a function of grade. *Experimental and Clinical Psychopharmacology, 4*(2), 209–217.

Ennett, S. T., Jackson, C., Bowling, J. M., & Dickinson, D. M. (2013). Parental socialization and children's susceptibility to alcohol use initiation. *Journal of Studies on Alcohol & Drugs, 74*(5), 694–702.

Ennett, S. T., Jackson, C., Choi, S., Hayes, K. A., Dickinson, D. M., & Bowling, J. M. (2016). A parenting program to promote an alcohol-free childhood: Influence on parents' readiness to prevent child sipping. *Journal of Studies on Alcohol & Drugs, 77*(2), 327–336.

Foster, J., Bryant, L., & Brown, K. (2017). *"Like sugar for adults": The effect of non-dependent parental drinking on children & families*. London, UK: Institute of Alcohol Studies.

Fromme, K., Stroot, E. A., & Kaplan, D. (1993). Comprehensive effects of alcohol: Development and psychometric assessment of a new expectancy questionnaire. *Journal of Psychological Assessment, 5*(1), 19–26.

Goldman, M. S. (1994). The alcohol expectancy concept: Applications to assessment, prevention, and treatment of alcohol abuse. *Applied and Preventive Psychology, 3*(3), 131–144.

Goldman, M. S., Brown, S. A., & Christiansen, B. A. (1987). Expectancy theory-thinking about drinking. In H. T. Blane & K. Leonard (Eds.), *Psychological theories of drinking and alcoholism* (pp. 181–226). New York, NY: Guilford Publications.

Hahn, E. J., Hall, L. A., Rayens, M. K., Burt, A. V., Corley, D., & Sheffel, K. L. (2000). Kindergarten children's knowledge and perceptions of alcohol, tobacco, and other drugs. *Journal of School Health, 70*(2), 51–55.

Handley, E. D., & Chassin, L. (2009). Intergenerational transmission of alcohol expectancies in a high-risk sample. *Journal of Studies on Alcohol and Drugs, 70*(5), 675–682.

Jackson, C., Ennett, S. T., Dickinson, D. M., & Bowling, J. M. (2012). Letting children sip: Understanding why parents allow alcohol use by elementary school–aged children. *Archives of Pediatrics and Adolescent Medicine, 166*(11), 1053–1057.

Jackson, C., Ennett, S. T., Dickinson, D. M., & Bowling, J. M. (2013). Attributes that differentiate children who sip alcohol from abstinent peers. *Journal of Youth & Adolescence, 42*(11), 1687–1695.

Jackson, K. M., Barnett, N. P., Colby, S. M., & Rogers, M. L. (2015). The prospective association between sipping alcohol by the sixth grade and later substance use. *Journal of Studies on Alcohol and Drugs, 76*(2), 212–221.

Jayne, M., & Valentine, G. (2017). 'It makes you go crazy': Children's knowledge and experience of alcohol consumption. *Journal of Consumer Culture, 17*(1), 85–104.

Jester, J. M., Wong, M. M., Cranford, J. A., Buu, A., Fitzgerald, H. E., & Zucker, R. A. (2015). Alcohol expectancies in childhood: Change with the onset of drinking and ability to predict adolescent drunkenness and binge drinking. *Addiction, 110*(1), 71–79.

Jones, B. T., Corbin, W., & Fromme, K. (2001). A review of expectancy theory and alcohol consumption. *Addiction, 96*(1), 57–72.

Jones, S. C., & Gordon, C. S. (2017). A systematic review of children's alcohol-related knowledge, attitudes and expectancies. *Preventive Medicine, 105*, 19–31.

Kobus, K. (2003). Peers and adolescent smoking. *Addiction, 98*, 37–55.

Kuntsche, E. (2017). "Do grown-ups become happy when they drink?" Alcohol expectancies among preschoolers. *Experimental and Clinical Psychopharmacology, 25*(1), 24–30.

Kuntsche, E., & Kuntsche, S. (2017). Development and initial validation of the alcohol expectancy task (AET). *Alcoholism: Clinical and Experimental Research, 41*(8), 1461–1470.

Kuntsche, E., & Kuntsche, S. (2018). Even in early childhood offspring alcohol expectancies correspond to parental drinking. *Drug & Alcohol Dependence, 183*, 51–54.

Kuntsche, E., & Kuntsche, S. (2019). Parental drinking and characteristics of family life as predictors of preschoolers' alcohol-related knowledge and norms. *Addictive Behaviors, 88*, 92–98.

Kuntsche, E., Le Mével, L., & Zucker, R. A. (2016). What do preschoolers know about alcohol? Evidence from the electronic Appropriate Beverage Task (eABT). *Addictive Behaviors, 61*, 47–52.

Kuntsche, E., Rossow, I., Engels, R., & Kuntsche, S. (2016). Is 'age at first drink' a useful concept in alcohol research and prevention? We doubt that. *Addiction, 111*(6), 957–965.

Leigh, B. C. (1989). In search of the seven dwarves: Issues of measurement and meaning in alcohol expectancy research. *Psychological Bulletin, 105*(3), 361–373.

Leigh, B. C., & Stacy, A. W. (1993). Alcohol outcome expectancies: Scale construction and predictive utility in higher order confirmatory models. *Psychological Assessment, 5*(2), 216–229.

Mares, S. H., Stone, L. L., Lichtwarck-Aschoff, A., & Engels, R. C. (2015). Alcohol expectancies in young children and how this relates to parental alcohol use. *Addictive Behaviors, 45*, 93–98.

Mennella, J. A., & Forestell, C. A. (2008). Children's hedonic responses to the odors of alcoholic beverages: A window to emotions. *Alcohol, 42*(4), 249–260.

Mennella, J. A., & Garcia, P. L. (2000). Children's hedonic response to the smell of alcohol: Effects of parental drinking habits. *Alcoholism: Clinical and Experimental Research, 24*(8), 1167–1171.

Miller, P. M., Smith, G. T., & Goldman, M. S. (1990). Emergence of alcohol expectancies in childhood: A possible critical period. *Journal of Studies on Alcohol, 51*(4), 343–349.

Patrick, M. E., Schulenberg, J. E., Maggs, J., & Maslowsky, J. (2016). Substance use and peers during adolescence and the transition to adulthood. In K. J. Sher (Ed.), *The Oxford handbook of substance use and substance use disorders*. https://doi.org/10.1093/oxfordhb/9780199381678.013.004.

Patrick, M. E., Wray-Lake, L., & Maggs, J. L. (2017). Early life predictors of alcohol-related attitudes among 11-year-old never drinkers. *Addictive Behaviors, 66*, 26–32.

Payne, B. K., Lee, K. M., Giletta, M., & Prinstein, M. J. (2016). Implicit attitudes predict drinking onset in adolescents: Shaping by social norms. *Health Psychology, 35*(8), 829–836.

Pieters, S., Van, d. V., Engels, R. C., & Weirs, R. W. (2010). Implicit and explicit cognitions related to alcohol use in children. *Addictive Behaviors, 35*, 471–478.

Prins, J. C., Donovan, J. E., & Molina, B. S. (2011). Parent-child divergence in the development of alcohol use norms from middle childhood into middle adolescence. *Journal of Studies on Alcohol and Drugs, 72*(3), 438–443.

Room, R. (2010). Dry and wet cultures in the age of globalization. *Salute e società, 9*(3), 229–238.

Russell, J. A. (1980). A circumplex model of affect. *Journal of Personality and Social Psychology, 39*(6), 1161–1178.

Settles, R. E., Zapolski, T. C., & Smith, G. T. (2014). Longitudinal test of a developmental model of the transition to early drinking. *Journal of Abnormal Psychology, 123*(1), 141–151.

Sharmin, S., Kypri, K., Khanam, M., Wadolowski, M., Bruno, R., & Mattick, R. P. (2017). Parental supply of alcohol in childhood and risky drinking in adolescence: Systematic review and meta-analysis. *International Journal of Environmental Research and Public Health, 14*(3), 287–304.

Sigelman, C. K., Silk, A., Goldberg, F., Davies, E. P., Dwyer, K. M., Leach, D., & Mack, K. (1999). Developmental differences in beliefs about how alcohol and cocaine affect behavior. *Journal of Applied Developmental Psychology, 20*(4), 597–614.

Slutske, W. S., Cronk, N. J., Sher, K. J., Madden, P. A., Bucholz, K. K., & Heath, A. C. (2002). Genes, environment and individual differences in alcohol expectancies among female adolescents and young adults. *Psychology of Addictive Behaviors, 16*(4), 308–317.

Smit, K., Otten, R., Voogt, C., Kleinjan, M., Engels, R., & Kuntsche, E. (2019). Exposure to drinking mediates the association between parental alcohol use and preteen alcohol use. *Addictive Behaviors, 87*, 244–250.

Smit, K., Voogt, C., Hiemstra, M., Kleinjan, M., Otten, R., & Kuntsche, E. (2018). Development of alcohol expectancies and early alcohol use in children and adolescents: A systematic review. *Clinical Psychology Review, 60*, 136–146.

Stone, L. L., van Daal, C., van der Maten, M., Engels, R. C., Janssens, J. M., & Otten, R. (2014). The Berkeley puppet interview: A screening instrument for measuring psychopathology in young children. *Child & Youth Care Forum, 43*(2), 211–225.

Thush, C., & Wiers, R. W. (2007). Explicit and implicit alcohol-related cognitions and the prediction of future drinking in adolescents. *Addictive Behaviors, 32*(7), 1367–1383.

Ting, T.-T., Chen, W. J., Liu, C.-Y., Lin, Y.-C., & Chen, C.-Y. (2015). Peer influences on alcohol expectancies in early adolescence: A study of concurrent and prospective predictors in Taiwan. *Addictive Behaviors, 40*, 7–15.

Treloar, H., Pedersen, S. L., & McCarthy, D. M. (2015). The role of expectancy in substance-abuse progression. In C. W. Lejuez & C. E. Kopetz (Eds.), *Addictions: A social psychological perspective* (pp. 120–147). New York, NY: Routledge.

Valentine, G., Jayne, M., & Gould, M. (2014). The proximity effect: The role of the affective space of family life in shaping children's knowledge about alcohol and its social and health implications. *Childhood, 21*(1), 103–118.

Van den Eijnden, R., Van De Mheen, D., Vet, R., & Vermulst, A. D. (2011). Alcohol-specific parenting and adolescents' alcohol-related problems: The interacting role of alcohol availability at home and parental rules. *Journal of Studies on Alcohol and Drugs, 72*(3), 408–417.

Velleman, R. (2009a). *How do children and young people learn about alcohol: A major review of the literature for the Joseph Rowntree Foundation.* York, UK: Joseph Rowntree Foundation.

Velleman, R. (2009b). *Influences on how children and young people learn about and behave towards alcohol: A review of the literature for the Joseph Rowntree Foundation (part one).* York, UK: Joseph Rowntree Foundation.

Voogt, C., Beusink, M., Kleinjan, M., Otten, R., Engels, R., Smit, K., & Kuntsche, E. (2017). Alcohol-related cognitions in children (aged 2–10) and how they are shaped by parental alcohol use: A systematic review. *Drug & Alcohol Dependence, 177*, 277–290.

Voogt, C., Otten, R., Kleinjan, M., Engels, R., & Kuntsche, E. (2017). Alcohol-related knowledge and alcohol-related norms in 4- to 6-year-olds—Evidence from the Dutch electronic appropriate beverage task. *Alcoholism: Clinical and Experimental Research, 41*(9), 1637–1647.

Ward, B., Snow, P., & Aroni, R. (2010). Children's alcohol initiation: An analytic overview. *Drugs: Education, Prevention and Policy, 17*(3), 270–277.

Wiers, R. W. (2008). Alcohol and drug expectancies as anticipated changes in affect: Negative reinforcement is not sedation. *Substance Use & Misuse, 43*(3–4), 429–444.

Zucker, R. A., Donovan, J. E., Masten, A. S., Mattson, M. E., & Moss, H. B. (2008). Early developmental processes and the continuity of risk for underage drinking and problem drinking. *Pediatrics, 121*(suppl 4), S252–S272.

16

Adolescent Perceptions of Alcohol Consumption: A Cultural Approach

Sara Rolando and Franca Beccaria

Introduction

Alcohol use among adolescents is a major social and public health issue in Western countries (WHO, 2018). Concern about young people's alcohol use had prompted a large number of quantitative studies of drinking practices and their correlates that have generated important knowledge: however, some important gaps in our knowledge remain. After explaining the main limitations with existing research, the present chapter suggests how a cultural approach focused on young people's attitude towards alcohol can help to bridge these gaps. This aim is pursued by drawing from the results of a large body of comparative qualitative studies that explored cultural differences in drinking between youth in Finland and Italy. After providing arguments for why these countries can be considered paradigmatic cases of traditional drinking cultures, the chapter elaborates on the role of these cultures in shaping the attitudes of young people towards drinking starting from early images of alcohol and related emotions that are formed during childhood. Then adolescents' conceptualisations of alcohol-related risks, addiction and Heavy Episodic Drinking (HED; see Chap. 1) and young adults' conceptualisation of appropriate and inappropriate drinking for young people and adults are analysed. At the end of the chapter the data

S. Rolando (✉) • F. Beccaria
Eclectica, Torino, Italy
e-mail: rolando@eclectica.it; beccaria@eclectica.it

R. Cooke et al. (eds.), *The Palgrave Handbook of Psychological Perspectives on Alcohol Consumption*, https://doi.org/10.1007/978-3-030-66941-6_16

presented are interpreted at the light of broader societal values and family relationships characterising different geographies, suggesting that a major emphasis on collective and familiar aims and responsibilities acts as a protective factor with regard to youth drinking.

Limitations with Existing Research on Youth Drinking

Because most of the research literature on young people's alcohol use has adopted a quantitative focus, this has produced a rather narrow picture of use that does not consider consumption in more holistic terms. A key limitation is that existing research in the field of youth drinking is based overwhelmingly on epidemiological and survey data which undervalue the users' perspective. This provides a rather narrow picture of alcohol use, because it is only discussed in terms of prevalence and health risk factors, rather than considering consumption in more holistic terms (see Chap. 1). Furthermore, the data are often deployed to increase social alarm—conveyed by mass media—by representing young people as a collective entity separate from adults, who are vulnerable, unconscious of risks, and passive in the face of external influences (Hellman, 2011; Beccaria & Rolando, 2015). Although large-scale studies do have the advantage of providing representative results which can be generalised, they necessarily rely on the theoretical framework of the researcher and do not go beyond what is seen as current knowledge of the determinants of the behaviour. In other words, they stay on the level of measurable constructs (see Chap. 4) and their correlations with drinking outcomes, such as consumption and harms, do not have the capacity to shed light on the often complex rationales of drinking practices because they do not give voice to individuals. This is a criticism that applies to all quantitative research, including quantitative studies of young people.

Another limitation with existing research studies is that most of the published research has been conducted in English-speaking countries (Allamani, Beccaria, & Einstein, 2017), in spite of well-documented significant cultural differences in alcohol use (see Chap. 7). This means that alcohol policy development may be influenced by evidence produced in these countries, based on the (often incorrect) assumption that it is universally valid (Allamani et al., 2017). Indeed, while a number of cross-national surveys, such as the European School Survey Project on Alcohol and Other Drugs (Kraus & Nociar, 2016), have been undertaken, these studies have been able to demonstrate variations in young people's use of alcohol between different countries and regions. However, they have been unable to adequately explain them because they have only collected quantitative data.

In contrast, qualitative data give voice to young people as actors and permit a focus on the meanings of alcohol consumption and the significant role that alcohol plays in their lives. Qualitative studies that include a focus on culture can deepen our understanding of the interplay between social and cultural factors and individual behaviour, but they are uncommon in the alcohol literature (Griffin, Bengry-Howell, Hackley, Mistral, & Szmigin, 2009; Measham & Østergaard, 2009). Even less common are comparative qualitative studies, despite these being particularly apt for highlighting the role of culture in regulating drinking, especially in terms of perceptions of acceptability and expectations around alcohol use (Brown, Creamer, & Stetson, 1987; Ahern, Galea, Hubbard, Midanik, & Syme, 2008). This lack of comparative qualitative studies may be due to the greater methodological complexity of such research (Tigerstedt & Törrönen, 2007). Only in recent years have the high-standard and rigorously comparative qualitative methods, such as the Reception Analytic Group Interview (RAGI), been developed (Sulkunen & Egerer, 2009; Törrönen, 2018). Based on the theory of images (Sulkunen, 2002, 2007), the RAGI technique entails the use of pictures/clips as stimuli to be freely discussed by participants. A few written questions are used: these do not investigate personal experiences directly but ask for an interpretation of the situation (e.g. what is happening in the scene and what might happen after). The interviewer is expected to intervene as little as possible in order to minimise her/his influence, thereby enhancing comparability across groups (Sulkunen & Egerer, 2009).

Based on these premises, the present chapter discusses the results of a body of comparative qualitative studies (Rolando, Beccaria, Tigerstedt, & Törrönen, 2012; Hellman & Rolando, 2013; Katainen & Rolando, 2014; Rolando & Katainen, 2014; Rolando, Törrönen, & Beccaria, 2014) conducted mainly in Italy and Finland, and representing paradigmatic cases of southern and northern youth drinking cultures (Tigerstedt & Törrönen, 2007). For more information about the methodology of the studies to which this chapter refers to, please see Rolando (2015).

Cross-Cultural Analyses of Adolescents and Alcohol

Differences between Northern and Southern European drinking cultures have been studied since the 1970s (Sulkunen, 1976; Mäkelä, Room, Single, Sulkunen, & Walsh, 1981). Initially the focus was on total per capita consumption, rate of abstinence and frequency of drunkenness, but later studies added a focus on alcohol control policies and regulations (Allamani, Beccaria, & Voller 2010; Beccaria & Prina, 1996). The northern/southern dichotomy was developed from the evidence that although overall per capita alcohol consumption was higher in southern wine-producing countries, such as Italy, Spain and Portugal, alcohol-related problems including violence and deaths attributable to acute alcohol poisoning were higher in northern countries, such as the Nordic countries and the UK. This was interpreted on the basis of the predominant drinking styles; while wine consumption was integrated into daily life in Southern Europe, beer or spirits were mainly used as intoxicant during weekends and on special occasions in Northern Europe (Bye & Rossow, 2010; Mäkelä, Tigerstedt, & Mustonen, 2012). Another way of describing this difference would be to say that southern countries have 'wet' drinking cultures in which alcohol is part of everyday life, whereas northern countries have 'dry' drinking cultures in which alcohol use is not part of everyday life, but is instead part of 'time out' (Room & Mäkelä, 2000; Room, 2010; Savic, Room, Mugavin, Pennay, & Livingston, 2016). Further discussion of the utility of such categorisations is included in Chap. 7.

Some features of northern and southern drinking cultures have changed considerably over recent decades because of oppositional drinking trends that have commonly been interpreted as part of an international globalisation of alcohol consumption (Järvinen & Room, 2007; Bjarnason, 2010). For example, Fig. 16.1 illustrates convergence in per capita annual alcohol consumption in Italy and Finland resulting from marked declines in alcohol intake in Italy and more modest increases in alcohol intake in Finland. However, it is worth noticing that the same socio-economic changes (such as increasing urbanisation and industrialisation) have influenced alcohol use in opposite ways in the two countries (Beccaria et al., 2010). Furthermore, we must consider that neither changes in levels of consumption nor changes in beverage preferences necessarily indicate that drinking styles are becoming more similar (Beccaria et al., 2010).

Indeed, despite the overall consumption levels becoming closer, differences in alcohol-related risks persist. According to the WHO's Global Information

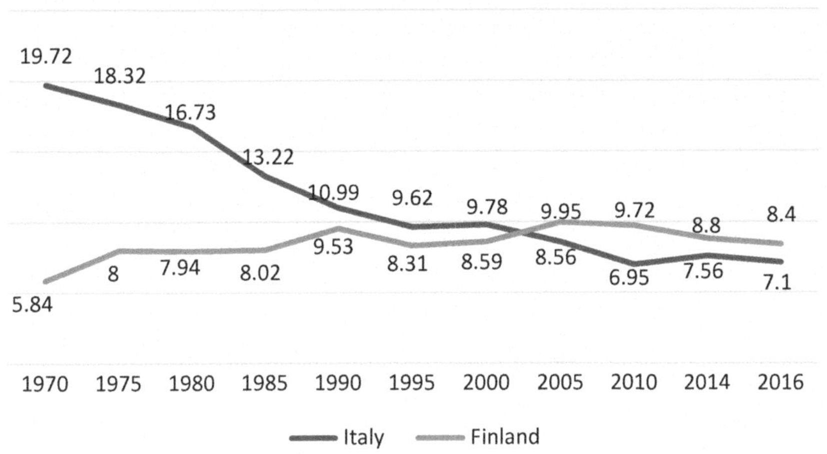

Fig. 16.1 Alcohol recorded per capita consumption (L/year, pop. 15+). (Source: Global Information System on Alcohol and Health (GISAH), 2019)

System on Alcohol and Health (2019), in 2016, there were differences in indicators of problematic drinking among those aged 15+ years:

(i) the prevalence of HED (defined as consuming at least 60 g of pure alcohol on at least one occasion in the past 30 days) was 39% in Finland compared to 33% in Italy; (ii) 12-month prevalence of alcohol use disorders was 9% in Finland compared to 1% in Italy; (iii) 12-month prevalence of alcohol dependence was 5% in Finland compared to 1% in Italy. Cross-national differences in alcohol consumption are also observable among young people: among those aged 15–19 years, the prevalence of HED was 52% in Finland and 45% in Italy. Furthermore, the international Health Behaviour in School-Aged Children (HBSC) survey shows that although there has been a marked decline in alcohol consumption, there is still a noticeable gap between Italian and Finnish adolescents' drunkenness rates (Inchley, Currie, Vieno, Torsheim, et al., 2018). Although the gap in consumption patterns appears to be reducing—partly because of a recent increase of the proportion of abstainers among young people in northern countries (Norström & Svensson, 2014; Raninen, Livingston, & Leifman, 2014; Kraus et al., in press)—the data also continue to suggest that there are still two different youth drinking patterns or cultures in Europe (Järvinen & Room, 2007). These patterns map onto the dry/wet categorisation referred to (and critiqued) in other chapters in this collection (Chap. 7). The first pattern or culture is apparent in the Nordic countries and the UK and is characterised by more positive expectations of drinking consequences, a propensity towards HED drinking, and a greater prevalence of alcohol use disorders. The second pattern or culture is typical of

Mediterranean countries, including Italy, Spain and Portugal, and is characterised by higher per capita consumption, but less HED and a lower prevalence of alcohol use disorders (Currie et al. 2012). Another finding from cross-national surveys is that the southern youth drinking culture is characterised by less HED and episodes of 'drunkenness'. This gap has been interpreted by three explanations: (1) a lower amount of actual consumption: (2) greater inhibition about heavy drinking; and (3) a more 'extreme' negative meaning attributed to drunkenness (Room, 2010; Beccaria, Petrilli, & Rolando, 2015). Taking into account persisting different between-country data—despite the apparent recently converging trends—it has been argued that they can be explained by the different cultural positions of drinking in the two countries, with the main feature being public attitudes towards drunkenness (Beccaria et al., 2010).

However, the aim in this chapter is not to argue for, or to refute, the thesis of convergence, but to instead use comparative data to better understand the role of drinking culture in shaping attitudes towards alcohol among young people. Indeed, alcohol consumption choices aim at drawing symbolic boundaries, which are socially rather than individually constructed and negotiated (Lamont & Molnár, 2002; Törrönen & Maunu, 2005). In pursuing this aim, the transitional nature of youth will be taken into account (Neve, Lemmens, & Drop, 2000; Beccaria & Scarscelli, 2007), by following how perceptions are modelled during the whole socialisation process, starting from early images of alcohol that are formed during childhood, and modified during the approach to adulthood.

Early Images of Alcohol

It is well established that young people develop expectations towards alcohol long before they drink themselves, and that these beliefs influence alcohol consumptions later in adolescence and adulthood (Velleman, 2009). These first images of alcohol are maybe the most persistent, since they are strongly related to perceptions and values attached to alcohol in a specific society (Velleman, 2009). It is striking, therefore, that this topic has not been given much attention in research (Törrönen & Rolando, 2018; Jayne & Valentine, 2016, see Chap. 15).

To address this gap in the literature, we conducted a cross-cultural qualitative study in Finland and Italy. Data were derived from 16 group interviews with a total of 190 participants aged 17–70. The sample was divided into four age[1] groups (young people, young adults, middle-age adults, older adults) and gender (Rolando et al., 2012; Törrönen & Rolando, 2018) to allow analysis of cohort effects and sex differences. Analysis of transcripts of group interviews focused on interviewees' recall of, and reflections on, their childhood experiences of family members' drinking. Group members were encouraged to articulate expressively and concretely what kinds of emotional response they developed towards alcohol consumption in specific situations (Törrönen & Rolando, 2018). No great differences were observed across different cohorts. This suggests that first memories related to alcohol use are quite stable over time, more so than actual behaviours or drinking styles. However, there were some evidences of cross-cultural differences.

In Italy, most of the interviewees could not even remember the very first time they realised adults were drinking, since alcohol was an ordinary and daily presence on the table, like water: it did not, therefore, arouse particular curiosity or emotions in children. The most recurrent narrative, present in all cohorts, was related to ordinary meal drinking with family members and relatives, as Claudio (male adult) said:

> I remember that a big bottle of wine was always present on the table. My grandfather, my father, my mother and almost all my relatives always had wine with the meal. (Törrönen & Rolando, 2018: 228)

Another recurrent narrative—which became increasingly apparent in the accounts of younger cohorts—referred to drinking in festive situations, where alcohol was linked to positive meanings and to positive emotions, like in the case of a young woman:

> I come from a very pleasure-loving family. [...] I remember that there were a lot of friends who came to meet us. I have always related [drinking] to good natured moments. (Törrönen & Rolando, 2018: 228)

Italian interviewees also recounted recollections related to the winemaking process, noting that it was not rare—especially in the past—that children were involved in helping adults to pick grapes or to bottle wine. These memories were also related to positive feelings, again dealing with good family interactions and pride in belonging to the family's traditions. Finally, some Italian interviewees—all of them older adults—gave accounts associated with negative emotions. They referred to the frightening behaviour of some male family

[1] Because different age ranges were used for groups in Italy (17–20; 37–40; 52–55; 67–70) and Finland (17–24; 25–32; 41–48; 57–64) we refer to group names to allow for comparison.

members who had been drinking. However, they expressed tolerance of this behaviour, emphasising that the violent or aggressive behaviour was due to alcohol, not the person's personal attitudes.

In contrast, Finnish interviewees described experiences in what may be considered an opposite order of relevance. The most prevalent Finnish master narrative concerned heavy drinking at home, typically attributed to fathers, as in Saku's (male, adult) account below. These kinds of memories were often associated with negative emotions such as anxiety and fear, even when the adults described were not considered alcohol dependent:

> My father was not an alcoholic. He drank seldom but when he drank he became very aggressive. He had long good periods but when the time for drinking came I needed to lurk and was even afraid for a couple of days, that nothing bad would happen. (Törrönen & Rolando, 2018: 230)

Another recurrent element of Finnish interviewees' recollections related to celebrations and festive situations, which again typically referred to intoxicated adults. These could either entail positive emotions for children, such as having fun, or entail negative emotions related to the fear of being a target of aggression or violence, as in the case of Lauri, a young Finnish man:

> I remember that I was afraid of my uncle every Midsummer. He always drank himself stupid and was somewhat aggressive. I remember hiding from him. (Törrönen & Rolando, 2018: 231)

The third most common narrative in the Finnish interviews was about moderate routine drinking at home, attributed mainly to fathers' rituals of relaxed drinking such as during sauna or when watching TV. These memories did not have clear links to positive or negative emotions in the participants' recollections, because moderate drinking did not affect adults' behaviours. What is interesting is that even when reporting positive or neutral recollections, most of the Finnish interviewees felt it necessary to specify that the situation was perceived as 'safe', thereby indicating a general tendency to evaluate drinking outcomes in terms of risk. In contrast to the Italian data, drinking with meals did not emerge as a recurrent feature within the Finnish accounts. However, when it did, it was related to positive emotions like closeness to parents and good-natured enjoyment.

First Drinks

When talking about youth drinking and related risk factors, the age of onset is considered a major risk factor, and there is a common agreement that the later first drinking occurs, the less likely it is that risky consumption styles and alcohol-related problems will develop—for a review, see Velleman (2009). Internationally, recommendations for alcohol intake suggest postponing the onset of drinking as much as possible, forbidding the use of alcohol in the domestic sphere (Van der Vorst et al. Van Der Vorst, Engels, Meeus, Deković, & Van Leeuwe, 2005; Dalton et al., 2006) and especially parental supply (Chan et al., 2018; Mattick et al., 2018). However, a small number of available studies conducted in the Mediterranean countries have found contrasting results, indicating that early contact with alcohol drinking in the family context can have a protective influence, fostering more moderate use and reducing the risk of excessive drinking during adolescence (Simons-Morton, 2004; Bonino, Cattelino, & Ciairano, 2005; Bellis et al., 2007; Strunin et al., 2010). This may be due to young people modelling the behaviour of their parents, who are drinking moderately themselves (see Chap. 15 for more on how observing parents drinking can inform beliefs about consumption). Furthermore, a systematic review pointed out that a causal relationship between parental supply of alcohol and risky drinking in adolescence cannot be inferred due to methodological limitations, particularly the fact that most studies do not distinguish sips from whole drinks (Sharmin et al., 2017). Comparative qualitative research is therefore very useful to explain this contrasting evidence, by showing how different cultural aspects of drinking shape the perceptions of children and adolescents.

One example of the value of comparative cross-cultural qualitative research into first personal experiences with alcohol was based on data collected as described above in relation to early images of alcohol in Italy and Finland (Beccaria et al., 2010; Rolando et al., 2012). The analysis revealed some similarities, but also some important differences. First, it demonstrated how the term 'first drink'—considered a key indicator in surveys—can assume very different meanings to young people living in different cultures. In Italy—despite the decrease in daily drinking over recent decades (Allamani & Prina, 2007)—it was found that the first contact with alcohol was usually with wine, and typically occurred under parental supervision and with parental permission. It usually consisted of a small taste that some may not even consider 'real' consumption or 'sip'. The first 'real' drink generally took place after several years of a 'training period' during which children were allowed, on special occasions, to participate in a family toast. This kind of managed introduction to alcohol emerged in most interviewees' accounts as not particularly exciting and not arousing strong emotions because it was taken for granted and a normal part of growing up. For the same reason it was not easy for Italian interviewees to reconstruct their 'real' first drink, although it was easy for them to imagine how it would have gone. This is a typical account, provided by a boy belonging to the 17–20-year-old cohort: '*My first memory was at New Year's Eve, perhaps. The bottom of the glass of champagne. I must have been maybe seven or eight*' (Rolando et al., 2012, p. 206). Italian interviewees generally associated participating in a family celebration by taking part in a family toast with pleasant feelings and positive images strictly connected to family traditions and ties.

Only a small minority of Italian participants (5 out of 102) reported that their first tastes of alcohol occurred outside of the family context, instead being shared with friends or peers. Those who reported that their first drinks occurred outside of family occasions were all teenagers who did not have an opportunity to taste alcohol with their parents because their families did not drink daily during meals. In some cases, this kind of first experience led to intoxication. In contrast, the most commonly spread narrative about first experiences entailed a progressive approach to drinking which seldom involved intoxication, neither in the case of older generations nor the younger ones. In the case of adults and elderly interviewees, the first 'real' drink occurred as the natural outcome of a period of increasingly significant tasting and the beginning of regular and moderate consumption during meals within the family context. For the younger interviewees, the first 'real' drink tended to occur with friends or peers outside of the home and independently from meals, typically in pubs or bars.

The accounts of Finnish interviewees contrasted with those of Italian interviewees. In Finland, the vast majority of interviewees—across all age cohorts—recalled their first drinking experiences as an important and memorable event, which occurred outside home and without parental knowledge (thereby taking on a transgressive meaning). In addition, in many cases, the first drink also resulted in the first experience of drunkenness, as indicated by one female interviewee: '*I remember that I first tasted only about two bottles of beer, and then we were supposed to be completely pissed*' (Rolando et al., 2012, p. 207). Among the younger participants, there were a few accounts about more permissive parents letting their children drink small volumes of alcoholic beverages at home with the aim of reducing their overall consumption. However, according to the participants' recollections, the outcome may not have been that wished for by parents because what was supposed to be drinking under parental supervision easily became 'preloading'—that is, beginning drinking at home before going out to drink more (Foster & Ferguson, 2013; see Chap. 13):

> I remember when parents agreed to buy my friends and me a bottle of cider each [...] To us, we had just supplied ourselves with some extra alcohol, but my parents imagined that our drinking stopped after those two bottles. (Rolando et al., 2012, p. 207)

To sum up the comparison between the two countries and drinking cultures: in Italy drinking onset was gradual, every day or ordinary, and either integrated with family habits—in the case of older generations—or celebrated with parents on some special occasions—in the case of younger generations. In Finland, on the contrary, the first contact with alcohol was kept separate from adults' drinking, often overlapped with the first drunkenness, and assumed a transgressive meaning.

Adolescents' Understanding of Acceptable Drinking, Risk and Drunkenness

Given that most young adolescents have not yet started drinking themselves, it could be that they perceive alcohol within a general framework, picked up from public debate or from school, more restrictive and focused on risk and harms (Scheffels, Moan, & Storvoll, 2016; Simonen et al., 2017). Indeed, it has been argued that, on the one hand, those who are not yet involved in drinking practices tend to be more critical towards excessive drinking (Padget, Bell, Shamblen, & Ringwalt, 2006). On the other hand, during adolescence risk-taking plays an important role in identity-making processes (Bonino et al., 2005), so that most adolescents, sooner or later, experiment with drinking and excessive drinking: first drunkenness can assume the role of a rite of passage, recounted as mythical experiences that reinforce belonging to the peer group (Beccaria & Sande, 2003).

To get a deeper understanding of adolescents' perceptions of alcohol, it is therefore useful to analyse their expectations: that is, how they conceptualise acceptable drinking and risks. This is what was done in a comparative study involving a total of 105 pupils aged 13–16 in group discussions in Finland and Italy (Hellman & Rolando, 2013). The study analysed how participants discussed a beer commercial portraying a situation in which social drinking norms were broken. The commercial depicted a romantic date setting resulting in the young woman's disappointment because the man does not pay attention to her expectations (sitting and drinking together) but focuses exclusively on his very individual pleasure of drinking. This male's character behaviour was harshly criticised by Italian pupils, both boys and girls, who condemned the use of alcohol solely addressed to personal pleasure and satisfaction without attention to others' expectations and needs. The reference to 'drinking just for the sake of it' emerged as a recurrent concept, blamed by interviewees as revealing as a lack of social responsibility and sign of immaturity:

> There's the woman who drinks to celebrate something, in an elegant refined way, she doesn't drink for the sake of it, while the man drinks to have a drink, for the sake of it; this also shows, for example, that young people drink not to celebrate something, simply for the sake of it, to have a drink with friends, to have a laugh, to joke. (Hellman & Rolando, 2013, p. 54)

In addition, they framed the male character's (lack of) agency in a broader set of informal broken rules related to the company (with a woman you cannot drink as you do it with friends), to the choice of beverage (champagne is more suited to a date than a drink of beer) and to the way of drinking (drinking from the bottle is not proper). These responses drew attention to a whole repertoire of rules for drinking that were highly detailed according to the situation (e.g. not to drink on empty stomach, not to drink alone, not to drink and drive). In contrast, Finnish adolescents did not judge the man's behaviour as breaking any specific social drinking norms. However, identifying the comic strand, they emphasised it, by imagining that both characters would get completely drunk at the end of the evening. In contrast with Italian interviewees, within their comments, there were no references to proper versus improper ways of drinking, and the only core issue they focused on when negotiating the scene was the level of intoxication. Taking for granted that drunkenness is the natural outcome of drinking, many observed that the man portrayed was not '*really real drinking*', since it was '*only drinking a bit*' (Hellman & Rolando, 2013, p. 56). Furthermore, his drinking was recognised as a reason for itself, even enabling the drinker to achieve his goals in terms of increased self-esteem and fun.

Another cross-cultural study, this time comparing Italy and Norway, based on 40 group discussions involving a total of 89 adolescents aged 15–16, focused on their perceptions and conceptualisations of alcohol-related risks, particularly addiction (Rolando & Katainen, 2014). The group discussions were stimulated by showing participants a set of clips portraying youth drinking situations taken from movies. On the one hand, a number of similarities were found in the data. For example, drinking alone and drinking because of personal problems were considered by participants in both countries to be very risky practices and uncommon among young people. On the other hand, cultural variations emerged consisting of a more nuanced, detailed and contextualised conceptual framework evident among the Italian participants, who distinguished several level of risk based on situations, beverages and ways of drinking. In the responses of Italian participants, references to their family drinking rules and habits were recurrent, as well as the notion that the family was a key element in problematic drinking and alcoholism. Indeed, for the vast majority of Italian participants, the real cause of addiction was considered to be rooted in family dysfunction and life context (e.g. deprivation, lack of education), and the worst consequence of alcohol dependence was considered to be being unable to take care of their own family. Nevertheless, they recognised that the risk is also intrinsic in alcohol as a specific substance with additive properties, as pointed out by one female participant:

> After a while alcohol is addictive, so that if in the beginning you drink and sometimes get drunk, and sometimes you can be stupid [it's fine] ... but if you always do it it's dangerous. (Rolando & Katainen, 2014, p. 196)

In contrast, Finnish adolescents attributed alcohol addiction to personal shortcomings and problems: risks were little discussed only with reference to drinking because of sadness or other negative emotions:

> If she becomes accustomed to that, I mean, if she thinks that drinking helps with all her troubles, then she could become [an alcoholic]. (Rolando & Katainen, 2014, p. 198)

From the accounts of Finnish participants, the general pattern to emerge was that the risks are not inherent in alcohol itself or the context of drinking, but that risks arise because of the drinker's lack of competence to engage in responsible drinking. Therefore, if one drinks in the 'right' way—a concept that actually was not much elaborated—and for the 'right' reasons, then he/she runs no risk of become addicted.

Based on the same dataset, a third study focused on Finnish and Italian adolescents' understandings of HED, with the aim of comparing its association with different concepts of self-control (Katainen & Rolando, 2015). The analysis revealed a cultural variation in the definition of control. Again, Italian participants displayed a more problem-oriented approach and discussed many factors that can influence young people's capacity of control: some of these main factors were internal/individual, such as lack of experience and negative emotions, whereas others were more external and related to peer pressure or to the strength of alcoholic drinks (varying based on the specific beverage).

Finnish pupils also referred to external factors. In particular, they underlined the importance of drinking for having fun and drinking on their own will as protective factors. However, they put more emphasis on the drinker's individual competence than their Italian counterparts. According to them, therefore, having fun with friends was a legitimate and relatively unproblematic behaviour, even in the case of heavy drinking (which was seen as self-evident when partying with friends). According to most of the Italian interviewees, on the contrary, the opinion prevailed that heavy drinking entails risks in any case when it concerns minors. It was generally taken for granted that approaching adulthood, young people become more moderate in their alcohol consumption, and tend to quit drinking to get drunk:

> When you grow up you become smarter, whereas when you are in high school… some don't, but I know some people who will say, for instance: 'I go out on Saturday night to get drunk.' (Katainen & Rolando, 2015, p. 12)

Furthermore, two different conceptions of self-control related to HED emerged in the two countries: for Finnish participants, self-control related to the ability of managing the right level of intoxication, whereas for Italian participants, it related to the ability to avoid getting drunk (see Chap. 1 for more on subjective definitions of stages of intoxication). There was a common agreement around this aim, which was put into relation with the will of not to become a burden to friends and not to experience negative outcome, as one Italian male adolescent:

> You don't have to necessarily get drunk, you've just to drink the right amount, so you have fun with friends, you don't throw up and you're OK. (Katainen & Rolando, 2015, p. 8)

Approaching Adulthood: Perceptions of Adult Drinking

The transitional nature of youth is largely overlooked in the public debate around young people's drinking. The main international surveys, such as ESPAD and HBSC, as well as other smaller cross-national studies, often compare data on teenagers' alcohol consumption in different locations, without comparing them with those of adults in the same locations, and without acknowledging that most people, once they enter adulthood, usually limit their alcohol use (Beccaria & Scarscelli, 2007; Fillmore, 1988; Neve et al., 2000).

To fully address how to understand youth drinking, it is therefore very useful to compare adolescents' and young adults' perceptions about what, in a specific culture, is socially defined as acceptable and proper drinking in different life stages. Based on the same cross-generational data set used to analyse recollections about first images and first drinking (Beccaria et al., 2010), we conducted another comparative study of 17–20-year-olds in Italy and 17–24-year-olds in Finland. The study focused on how young adults conceptualised appropriate and inappropriate drinking for young people and adults. The discussion was facilitated by the presentation of pictures depicting adults and young people in their 20s in several drinking situations (Rolando et al., 2014). The study applied the concept of 'boundary work' as analytical and theoretical concept, assuming that symbolic boundaries used by people to judge behaviours in terms of 'normal' or 'deviant' are shaped by cultural repertoires and socially negotiated rather than individual constructs (Lamont, 2000; Törrönen & Maunu, 2005). When discussing the picture stimuli, the Italian young adult participants recognised clear boundaries between appropriate and inappropriate drinking with reference to a broad repertoire of drinking patterns. These resembled the informal norms of the traditional Italian drinking culture, such that drinking during the day is inappropriate, that spirits are more dangerous than wine, and that drinking while eating is better than drinking separately from meals. Furthermore, these social norms were attributed to both young people and adults, thereby showing that young people share with adults a range of drinking patterns. A typical example was the habit of 'doing aperitifs', a recent drinking practice which consists of drinking a glass of wine or another beverage while eating snacks or more elaborate cooked food, before (or more commonly) instead of dinner. According to participants, especially female participants, this is a normal and quite ordinary setting for both adults and young people. So too was drinking while on a date and drinking wine at dinner, especially at restaurants:

> I would see it [the scene] exactly with my boyfriend, I mean, going out and having dinner with your boyfriend, or as an aperitif. When I go out for dinner with my boyfriend I always drink wine. (Rolando et al., 2014, p. 232)

In addition, it emerged from the participants' accounts that they also engaged in situations where young people and adults drink together: one example of such situations was family gatherings.

The unique boundary between youth and adult drinking emerging from the Italian participants' discussions was related to drunkenness. In line with studies focused on drinking trajectories (Beccaria & Scarscelli, 2007) and on HED (Beccaria et al., 2015), Italian participants considered intoxication to be an expected and accepted part of young people's drinking repertoires, but not part of adults' drinking repertoires. Drunkenness was thus not blameworthy if it is occurring during youth, but it was interpreted as deviant behaviour if it occurred among adults. For example, one Italian young woman gave the following commenting on a picture portraying a man passed out sleeping on the table:

> Not adults. My dad I've never seen him in this way. But this set made of a bottle, cigarettes and a table at home reminds me a lot of evenings. (Rolando et al., 2014, p. 242)

In contrast to Italian respondents, Finnish interviewees did not associate any picture showing adults drinking with their own drinking experiences. This indicates that they perceived adults' drinking situations and drinking practices as separate from their own. Furthermore, they did not describe clear boundaries between proper and improper drinking styles when discussing the picture stimuli—neither with reference to young people nor to adults. Indeed, when discussing drinking styles, their point of reference was always individual aims and desires rather than social norms or others' expectations.

All of the Finnish participants' comments about pictures revolved around whether the situation was more likely to lead to light drinking or HED, with the latter option more frequently supported. In other words, intoxication emerged as a constant topic and reference frame when discussing drinking styles, independently from the drinkers' age. This suggests that drinking to drunkenness was seen as typical for both young people and adults in Finland. For instance, when commenting on the drunken man lying on the table, common reactions were '*This is my father*' or '*This is a typical Saturday*' (Rolando et al., 2014, p.245). However, at the same time, this common habit did not result in a bridge between generations because adult drinking situations were never associated with youth drinking but perceived as 'others'. Indeed, young people's heavy drinking was also interpreted as transgressing adults' expectations of appropriate behaviour. As a result, paradoxically, on the one hand, youth drinking in Finland seems to serve as a means to oppose the formal drinking norms, but—due to the ambiguity of adults' messages—it also reproduces the intoxication-oriented tradition (Törrönen & Rumeliotis 2014; Härkönen, 2013).

Towards a Broader Interpretation of Youth Drinking

From a cultural perspective, the alcohol socialisation process is the fundamental means through which a society transmits to new generations shared attitudes and beliefs about drinking and drunkenness (Velleman, 2009). As is the case for many other processes of children's social learning (Bandura & McClelland, 1977), parental observation and modelling assume a crucial role in shaping children's relationship with alcohol (see Chap. 15). The first difference between Mediterranean meal-drinking and Scandinavian intoxication-oriented drinking cultures emerges therefore at this early stage, as the first image captured from the social context differently conditions the children's emotional relationship with alcohol (Törrönen & Rolando, 2018). In the Italian interviewees' retrospective accounts of their first contact with drinking, children's socialisation to drinking was commonly positioned either in everyday life or festive moderate drinking linked to meals. The first type of drinking was associated with neutral emotions; the second type with positive emotions. In contrast, Finnish interviewees' accounts of first memories of alcohol were related most frequently either to heavy domestic drinking or to festive drinking situations (often involving drunkenness). In both of these situations, positive and negative emotions emerged—with the negative emotions linked to fear of adults changing their behaviour when they were under the influence of alcohol. Solitary drinking was not present in Italian interviewees' recollections—drinking was always recalled as a shared social activity. In contrast, in Finnish interviewees' accounts there was more space for solitary drinking (Törrönen and Härkönen 2016).

Later on in the alcohol socialisation process, parents in the two countries/cultures have different influences on the actual drinking practices of their children as a result of different patterns of involvement in their children's first tastes of alcohol. Italian interviewees described how parents choose to take an active role in the socialisation process, by gradually introducing children to alcohol in the home. This was in stark contrast to the accounts of Finnish interviewees, whose accounts revealed that young people's first contact with alcohol typically happens outside of the home, is hidden from parents, and thereby has or acquires a transgressive meaning (Rolando et al., 2012; Maunu and Simonen 2010). It may be the case that in other countries parents feel less powerful to influence their children's drinking (Rolando et al., 2014; Velleman, 2009; Järvinen & Østergaard, 2009, see Chap. 17), but their relinquishment of influence—combined with ambivalent behaviours—is also reflected in a durable separation of young people's experiences from adults. Indeed, the pattern of closeness versus distance between Finnish and Italian young people and adults seems to persist in the two countries until adulthood, shaping very different perceptions about drinking—and particularly drunkenness (Rolando et al., 2014).

Italian adolescents' perceptions of alcohol followed the traditional social norms of the 'wet' Mediterranean drinking cultures, entailing a broad repertoire of drinking styles and a negative attitude towards intoxication: intoxication was socially tolerated in youth but not in adulthood. In contrast, Finnish adolescents' perceptions of alcohol did not refer to any shared drinking norms between young people and adults, and intoxication was a constant reference point—and almost taken for granted across various situations. Although in line with the general drinking culture, this is clearly not the result of an alcohol socialisation process consciously and actively enacted by adults, but rather the outcome of a certain degree of ambivalence, not only linked to alcohol properties but also linked to the fact that parents' recommendations and formal norms clash with social behaviours.

Adolescents' perceptions of consumption reflect not only the specificities of the drinking culture but also more general societal values. It is well known that family cohesion, communication and supervision have a protective effect with respect to young people's risky drinking (Velleman, Templeton, & Copello 2005). Accordingly, the recurrent references to family and others' expectations in young Italians' discourses support the hypothesis that Italian familism (Saraceno, 2000) has had a protective effect on youth drinking (Rolando, 2015; Rolando & Beccaria 2018), as observed also in relation to Mexican youth (Strunin et al., 2013, 2015). Mediterranean familism is a special kind of collectivistic culture defined by Dwairy (2002) as (an ideal type of) a sociocultural system in which individuals are expected to accomplish social and familial norms, values and roles. Conversely, an individualistic culture encourages children to develop independent and autonomous personalities (Dwairy, 2002). In collectivistic/familistic cultures, such as Italian society, collective/family aims prevail over individual ones and interpersonal responsibilities are emphasised over individual rights, so that people tend to adapt their behaviours to the context rather than to personal disposition (Dwairy,

2002; Triandis, 1995). In contrast, in individualistic cultures, such as Finland, individual aims and personal fulfilment are prioritised.

Italian and Finnish adolescents' perceptions about drinking and the risks of drinking seem to fit with this categorisation, which was introduced in alcohol studies to explain the differences emerged among adolescents' alcohol images in five European countries (Hellman et al. 2010). As explained above, other people's expectations were a constant point of reference in Italians' accounts about their decision-making processes about whether and how to drink, and thereby limiting drinking. In contrast, in the Finnish accounts, attention to interpersonal responsibilities did not emerge, whereas personal fulfilment and individual tastes were often emphasised (Hellman & Rolando, 2013). This pattern also influences the perception of risky drinking, which is highly individualised among Finnish adolescents who maintain that a competent drinker can easily manage alcohol without running risks independently from external circumstances and factors, thereby shaping more positive attitudes towards heavier, and potentially risky, drinking. This feature could provide an explanation of why evidence about the impact of self-efficacy is inconsistent, depending on which aspect of it is under observation (McKay et al., 2012). Indeed, this concept includes not only the ability to resist peer pressure (so-called drink-refusal self-efficacy; see Chap. 4) but also the belief of being able to handle alcohol, which in turn may lead to overlooking the risks related to the context and to alcohol's intrinsic addiction properties (Rolando & Katainen, 2014). Heavy drinking can therefore become a way of testing and demonstrating the individual's ability to manage the right level of intoxication, as seems to have happened in Finland for many generations (Härkönen, 2013).

The individualistic-collectivistic pattern could therefore provide an explanation for the major propensity to drunkenness and risky drinking of northern young people (Järvinen & Room, 2007). Anyway, if we assume this perspective, we cannot avoid acknowledging that the global 'individualisation' process (Beck, 2000; Beck & Beck-Gernsheim, 2002) represents a challenge for all western society, which should be taken into consideration with reference to all risk behaviours.

Conclusion

The chapter argues that to fully understand adolescent perceptions of drinking, it is important to look at such perceptions as a product of a process of meaning-making that begins in childhood and evolves throughout adolescence and emerging adulthood, and that this process is highly influenced by the surrounding drinking culture. Taking Finland and Italy as paradigmatic examples of southern/'wet' and northern/'dry' youth drinking cultures, the bulk of studies presented in this chapter suggests a possible coherent explanation of why culture-specific differences in attitudes towards drinking and intoxication persist among European young people despite the apparent process of homogenisation of drinking practices. Finally, it suggests that these differences, related to adolescents' perceptions of alcohol, have to be interpreted also in the view of broader societal values concerning the emphasis on individual versus societal/family aims and responsibilities, the latter assuming a protective role.

References

Ahern, J., Galea, S., Hubbard, A., Midanik, L., & Syme, S. L. (2008). "Culture of drinking" and individual problems with alcohol use. *American Journal of Epidemiology, 167*, 1041–1049.

Allamani, A., Beccaria, F., & Einstein, S. (2017). A commentary on the limits of alcoholic beverage policies. *Alcohol and Alcoholism, 52*, 706–714.

Allamani, A., Beccaria, F., & Voller, F. (2010). The puzzle of Italian drinking: Trends in alcohol consumption, harms and policy: Italy 1990–2010. *Nordic Studies on Alcohol and Drugs, 27*, 465–478.

Allamani, A., & Prina, F. (2007). Why the decrease in consumption of alcoholic beverages in Italy between the 1970s and the 2000s? Shedding light on an Italian mystery. *Contemporary Drug Problems, 34*, 187–197.

Bandura, A., & McClelland, D. C. (1977). *Social learning theory* (Vol. 1). Prentice Hall: Englewood cliffs.

Beccaria, F., Petrilli, E., & Rolando, S. (2015). Binge drinking vs. drunkenness. The questionable threshold of excess for young Italians. *Journal of Youth Studies, 18*(7), 823–838.

Beccaria, F., & Prina, F. (1996). Le dimensioni culturali e sociali dell'alcol [Cultural and social dimensions of alcohol]. In A. Moiraghi Ruggenini (Ed.), *Alcologia*. Milano, Italy: Masson.

Beccaria, F., & Rolando, S. (2015). The Italian politics of alcohol: The creation of a public arena at the end of the 20th century. *International Journal of Drug Policy, 26*, 662–669.

Beccaria, F., & Sande, A. (2003). Drinking games and rite of life projects: A social comparison of the meaning and functions of young people's use of alcohol during the rite of passage to adulthood in Italy and Norway. *Young, 11*, 99–119.

Beccaria, F., & Scarscelli, D. (2007). Life cycles and changes in alcoholic beverage consumption: Research project & theoretical frame work. *Contemporary Drug Problems, 34*, 287–298.

Beccaria F. (ed.), Prina F., Rolando S., Simonen J., Tigerstedt C., Torronen J. (2010). *Alcol e generazioni. Cambiamenti di stile e stili in cambiamento [Alcohol and generations. Changes in style and changing styles in Italy and Finland]*. Milano: Carrocci.

Beck, U. (2000). *The Brave New World of Work*. Cambridge: Polity Press.

Beck, U., & Beck-Gernsheim, E. (2002) *Individualization: Institutionalized Individualism and Its Social and Political Consequences*. London: Sage.

Bellis, M. A., Hughes, K., Morleo, M., Tocque, K., Hughes, S., Allen, T., … Fe-Rodriguez, E. (2007). Predictors of risky alcohol consumption in schoolchildren and their implications for preventing alcohol-related harm. *Substance Abuse Treatment, Prevention, and Policy, 2*, 15.

Bjarnason, T. (2010). *A European alcohol youth culture? Convergent and divergent trends in adolescent alcohol consumption 1995–2007*. Nordic Alcohol and Drug Researchers Assembly, Reykjavik. Conference presentation.

Bonino, S., Cattelino, E., & Ciairano, S. (2005). *Adolescents and risk. Behaviors, functions and protective factors*. Milan, Italy: Springer-Verlag.

Brown, S. A., Creamer, V. A., & Stetson, B. A. (1987). Adolescent alcohol expectancies in relation to personal and parental drinking patterns. *Journal of Abnormal Psychology, 96*(2), 117.

Bye, E. K., & Rossow, I. (2010). The impact of drinking pattern on alcohol-related violence among adolescents: An international comparative analysis. *Drug and Alcohol Review, 29*, 131–137.

Chan, G. C., Leung, J., Kelly, A. B., Connor, J., Edward, S., Hall, W., … Patton, G. (2018). Familial alcohol supply, adolescent drinking and early alcohol onset in 45 low and middle income countries. *Addictive Behaviors, 84*, 178–185.

Dalton, M., Adachi-Mejia, A., Longacre, M., Titus Ernstoff, L., Gibson, J., Martin, S., … Beach, M. (2006). Parental rules and monitoring of children's movie viewing associated with children's risk for smoking and drinking. *Pediatrics, 118*, 1932–1942.

Dwairy, M. 2002. Foundations of Psychosocial Dynamic Personality Theory of Collective People. *Clinical Psychology Review, 22*(3), 345–362. https://doi.org/10.1016/S0272-7358(01)00100-3.

Fillmore, K. M. (1988). Alcohol use across the life course. In *Alcohol use across the life course* (pp. IX–121).

Foster, J. H., & Ferguson, C. (2013). Alcohol 'pre-loading': A review of the literature. *Alcohol and Alcoholism, 49*, 213–226.

Global Information System on Alcohol and Health (GISAH). (2019). Data Repository retrivable on https://apps.who.int/gho/data/node.main.GISAH.

Griffin, C., Bengry-Howell, A., Hackley, C., Mistral, W., & Szmigin, I. (2009). Every time I do it I absolutely annihilate myself': Loss of (self)-consciousness and loss of memory in young people's drinking narratives. *Sociology, 43*, 457.

Härkönen, J. (2013). *Not a wet generation but a wet nation: The dynamics of change and stasis in the Finnish drinking culture from 1968–2008*. Tampere, Finland: Juvenes Print – Finnish University Print. https://helda.helsinki.fi/bitstream/handle/10138/38905/harkonen_dissertation.pdf?sequence=1

Hellman, M. (2011). Studying young recipients of alcohol marketing – Two research paradigms and their possible consolidation. *Nordic Studies on Alcohol and Drugs, 28*, 415–431.

Hellman, M., & Rolando, S. (2013). Collectivist and individualist values traits in Finnish and Italian adolescents' alcohol norms. *Drugs and Alcohol Today, 13*(1), 51–59.

Inchley, J., Currie, D., Vieno, A., Torsheim, T., et al. (2018). *Adolescents alcohol-related behaviours: Trends and inequalities in the WHO European region 2002–2014*. Copenhagen, Denmark: WHO Regional Office for Europe.

Järvinen, M., & Østergaard, J. (2009). Governing adolescent drinking. *Youth & society, 40*(3), 377–402.

Järvinen, M., & Room, R. (2007). Conclusion: Changing drunken component or reducing alcohol-related harm. In M. Järvinen & R. Room (Eds.), *Youth drinking cultures* (pp. 161–174). Aldershot, UK: Ashgate.

Jayne, M., & Valentine, G. (2016). *Childhood, family, alcohol*. London, UK: Routledge.

Katainen, A., & Rolando, S. (2014). Adolescents' understandings of binge drinking in Southern and Northern European contexts – Cultural variations of 'controlled loss of control'. *Journal of Youth Studies, 18*(2), 151–166. https://doi.org/10.1080/13676261.2014.933200

Katainen, A., & Rolando, S. (2015). Adolescents' understandings of binge drinking in Southern and Northern European contexts–cultural variations of 'controlled loss of control'. *Journal of Youth Studies, 18*(2), 151–166.

Kraus, L., & Nociar, A. (2016). *ESPAD report 2015: results from the European school survey project on alcohol and other drugs*. European Monitoring Centre for Drugs and Drug Addiction.

Kraus, L., Room, R., Livingston, M., Pennay, A., Holmes, J., & Törrönen, J. (in press). Long waves of consumption or a unique social generation? Exploring recent declines in youth drinking. *Addiction Research & Theory, 28*(3), 183–193.

Lamont, M. (2000). *The dignity of working men: Morality and the boundaries of race, class, and immigration*. Cambridge, MA: Harvard University Press.

Lamont, M., & Molnár, V. (2002). The study of boundaries in the social sciences. *Annual Review of Sociology, 28*, 167–195.

Mäkelä, K., Room, R., Single, E., Sulkunen, P., & Walsh, B. (1981). *Alcohol, society, and the state: I. A Comparative Study of Alcohol Control*. Toronto, Canada: Addiction Research Foundation.

Mäkelä, P., Tigerstedt, C., & Mustonen, H. (2012). The Finnish drinking culture: Change and continuity in the past 40 years. *Drug and Alcohol Review, 31*, 831–840.

Mattick, R. P., Clare, P. J., Aiken, A., Wadolowski, M., Hutchinson, D., Najman, J., … Vogl, L. (2018). Association of parental supply of alcohol with adolescent drinking, alcohol-related harms, and alcohol use disorder symptoms: A prospective cohort study. *The Lancet Public Health, 3*(2), e64–e71.

McKay, M. T., Sumnall, H. R., Cole, J. C., & Percy, A. (2012). Self-esteem and self-efficacy: Associations with alcohol consumption in a sample of adolescents in Northern Ireland. *Drugs: education, prevention and policy, 19*(1), 72–80.

Measham, F., & Østergaard, J. (2009). The public face of binge drinking: British and Danish young women, recent trends in alcohol consumption and the European binge drinking debate. *Probation Journal, 56*, 415–434.

Neve, R. J., Lemmens, P. H., & Drop, M. J. (2000). Changes in alcohol use and drinking problems in relation to role transitions in different stages of the life course. *Substance Abuse, 21*, 163–178.

Norström, T., & Svensson, J. (2014). The declining trend in Swedish youth drinking: Collectivity or polarization? *Addiction, 109*, 1437–1446.

Padget, A., Bell, M., Shamblen, S., & Ringwalt, C. (2006). Does learning about the effects of alcohol on the developing brain affect children's alcohol use? *Prevention Science, 7*, 293–302.

Raninen, J., Livingston, M., & Leifman, H. (2014). Declining trends in alcohol consumption among Swedish youth—Does the theory of collectivity of drinking cultures apply? *Alcohol and Alcoholism, 49*, 681–686. https://doi.org/10.1093/alcalc/agu045

Rolando, S. (2015). *Images of alcohol in the transition to adulthood: Comparing different geographies: Examples from Italy and Finland.* Helsinki, Finland: Unigrafia.

Rolando, S., & Beccaria, F. (2018). Young people and drinking in Italy: The good side of familism. *Journal of Modern Italian Studies, 23*(1), 93–107.

Rolando, S., Beccaria, F., Tigerstedt, C., & Törrönen, J. (2012). First drink: What does it mean? The alcohol socialization process in different drinking culture. *Drugs: Education, Prevention, and Policy, 19*, 201–212.

Rolando, S., & Katainen, A. (2014). Images of alcoholism among adolescents in individualistic and collectivistic geographies. *NAD-Nordic Studies on Alcohol and Drugs, 31*, 189–205.

Rolando, S., Törrönen, J., & Beccaria, F. (2014). Boundaries between adult and youth drinking as expressed by young people in Italy and Finland. *Young, 22*, 227–252.

Room, R. (2010). Culture 'asciutte' e culture 'bagnate' nell'epoca della globalizzazione. *Salute e Società, 9*, 231–240.

Room, R., & Mäkelä, K. (2000). Typologies of the cultural position of drinking. *Journal of Studies on Alcohol, 61*(3), 475–483. https://doi.org/10.15288/jsa.2000.61.475

Saraceno, C. 2000. Being Young in Italy: The Paradoxes of a Familistic Society. *The European Journal of Social Quality, II*(2), 120–132.

Savic, M., Room, R., Mugavin, J., Pennay, A., & Livingston, M. (2016). Defining "drinking culture": A critical review of its meaning and connotation in social research on alcohol problems. *Drugs: Education, Prevention and Policy, 23*, 270–282. https://doi.org/10.3109/09687637.2016.1153602

Scheffels, J., Moan, I. S., & Storvoll, E. E. (2016). Everything in moderation? A mixed methods study on perceptions of parents' drinking in the presence of children. *Nordic Studies on Alcohol and Drugs, 33*, 551–566.

Sharmin, S., Kypri, K., Khanam, M., Wadolowski, M., Bruno, R., & Mattick, R. (2017). Parental supply of alcohol in childhood and risky drinking in adolescence: Systematic review and meta-analysis. *International Journal of Environmental Research and Public Health, 14*(3), 287.

Simonen, J., Törrönen, J., Tigerstedt, C., Scheffels, J., Moan, I. S., & Karlsson, N. (2017). Do teenagers' and parents' alcohol-related views meet? – Analyzing focus group data from Finland and Norway. *Drugs: Education, Prevention & Policy*. Early Online: 1–9. https://doi.org/10.1080/09687637.2017.1337725.

Simons-Morton, B. (2004). Prospective association of peer influence, school engagement, drinking expectancies, and parent expectations with drinking initiation among sixth graders. *Addictive Behaviors, 29*, 299–309.

Strunin, L., Díaz-Martínez, A., Díaz-Martínez, L. R., Kuranz, S., Hernández-Ávila, C. A., García-Bernabé, C. C., & Fernández-Varela, H. (2015). Alcohol use among Mexican youths: Is familismo protective for moderate drinking? *Journal of Child and Family Studies, 24*(2), 309–316.

Strunin, L., Lindeman, K., Tempesta, E., Ascani, P., Anav, S., & Parisi, L. (2010). Familial drinking in Italy: Harmful or protective factors? *Addiction Research and Theory, 18*, 344–358.

Strunin, L., Martínez, A. D., Díaz-Martínez, L. R., Heeren, T., Kuranz, S., Winter, M., … Solís-Torres, C. (2013). Parental monitoring and alcohol use among Mexican students. *Addictive Behaviors, 38*, 2601–2606.

Sulkunen, P. (1976). Drinking patterns and the level of alcohol consumption: An international overview. In R. J. Gibbons (Ed.), *Research advances in alcohol and drugs problems* (Vol. 3, pp. 223–281). New York, NY: Wiley.

Sulkunen, P. (2002). Between culture and nature. Intoxication in cultural studies of alcohol and drug use. *Contemporary Drug Problems, 29*, 253–276.

Sulkunen, P. (2007). Images of addiction: Representations of addictions in films. *Addiction Research and Theory, 15*(6), 543–559.

Sulkunen, P., & Egerer, M. (2009). Reception analytical group interview. A short introduction and manual. *Research Reports*, 260.

Tigerstedt C., Törrönen J. (2007). *Comparative research strategies and changes in drinking cultures.* SoRAD – Forskningsrapport nr 45.

Törrönen, J. (2018). Using vignettes in qualitative interviews as clues, microcosms or provokers. *Qualitative Research Journal, 18*, 276–286.

Törrönen, J., & Maunu, A. (2005). Going out, sociability, and cultural distinctions. *Nordic Studies on Alcohol and Drugs, 22*, 25–43 (English Supplement).

Törrönen, J., & Rolando, S. (2018). Safe and unsafe drinking situations through children's eyes: Comparing recalled childhood emotions regarding family members' drinking from Italy and Scandinavia. *Childhood, 25*, 220–236.

Törrönen, J., & Roumeliotis, F. (2014). Masculinities of drinking as described by Swedish and Finnish age-based focus groups. *Addiction Research & Theory, 22*, 126–136.

Triandis, H. C. (1995). *Individualism and Collectivism*. Boulder, CO: Westview.

Van Der Vorst, H., Engels, R. C., Meeus, W., Deković, M., & Van Leeuwe, J. (2005). The role of alcohol-specific socialization in adolescents' drinking behaviour. *Addiction, 100*, 1464–1476.

Velleman, R. (2009). *Influences on how children and young people learn about and behave towards alcohol: A review of the literature for the Joseph Rowntree Foundation* (part one). Available at http://www.jrf.org.uk/sites/files/jrf/children-alcohol-use-partone.pdf

Velleman, R. D., Templeton, L. J., & Copello, A. G. (2005). The role of the family in preventing and intervening with substance use and misuse: a comprehensive review of family interventions, with a focus on young people. *Drug and alcohol review, 24*(2), 93–109.

WHO. (2018). *Adolescent alcohol-related behaviours: Trends and inequalities in the WHO European region, 2002–2014*. Geneva, Switzerland: WHO.

17

Parental Communication About Alcohol Consumption

Alexandra Sawyer, Nigel Sherriff, and Lester Coleman

Introduction

This chapter begins by providing a general overview of alcohol use in adolescence and the role parents play in shaping adolescents' alcohol use. Next, there follows a summary of current research on parental communication about alcohol, focusing on the content and frequency of alcohol-specific conversations and how these are associated with adolescent alcohol use. The chapter moves on to present findings from a recent study where in-depth interviews were carried out with adolescents aged 15–17 years exploring conversations they have had with their parents about alcohol. These included the style of conversations, triggers to conversations about alcohol, topics conveyed during conversations, and effectiveness of these conversations. The chapter ends by outlining implications for how best to support parents in having conversations with young people.

Alcohol Use in Adolescence

Adolescence is a peak period for the initiation and use of substances, and many adolescents experiment with or consume alcohol regularly (Petit, Kornreich, Verbanck, Cimochowska, & Campanella, 2013; Degenhardt,

A. Sawyer (✉) • N. Sherriff • L. Coleman
School of Health Sciences, University of Brighton, Brighton, UK
e-mail: a.sawyer@brighton.ac.uk; n.s.sherriff@brighton.ac.uk

R. Cooke et al. (eds.), *The Palgrave Handbook of Psychological Perspectives on Alcohol Consumption*, https://doi.org/10.1007/978-3-030-66941-6_17

Stockings, Patton, Hall, & Lynskey, 2016). Alcohol misuse in young people continues to be a key public health priority with the World Health Organization's (WHO's) global strategy to reduce the harmful use of alcohol including a specific focus on young people (World Health Organization, 2010). Whilst a range of factors influence alcohol use, including genetic, family, and peer influences, and also wider social (see Chap. 9), environmental (see Chap. 10), and legislative contexts (see Chap. 1), there is an increasing awareness of the role that parents can have in the development of their children's drinking behaviour through processes such as modelling, supervision, and parent-child communication (see Chap. 15). In particular, research suggests that good parental communication is an effective strategy to help young people develop and sustain a healthy relationship with alcohol (Ryan, Jorm, & Lubman, 2010; Carver, Elliott, Kennedy, & Hanley, 2017). In this chapter, 'parents' refer to the primary caregivers of young people in the home. In addition to biological and adoptive parents, main caregivers may include kinship (e.g. grandparents), foster, and other types of caregivers.

Recent data suggests that alcohol use amongst young people in the United Kingdom (UK) is declining; results from the *Smoking, Drinking and Drug Use Among Young People in England (SDD) Surveys* show that between 2003 and 2014 there was a steady decline in the number of 11- to 15-year-olds who reported drinking alcohol (NHS Digital, 2017). Additionally, a recent WHO report highlights the UK as one of the countries with the largest reduction of weekly alcohol consumption in young people between 2002 and 2014 (Inchley et al., 2018). Although the reasons for this decline are not well understood (Pape, Rossow, & Brunborg, 2018), it is thought that improvements in parenting—defined as parents who are less likely to drink in front of their children, less likely to approve of their children drinking, more likely to know their children's whereabouts and activities, and have warmer and closer relationships with their children—and economic factors which reduce the affordability of alcohol are the most likely factors to account for this decline (Institute of Alcohol Studies, 2016; Pape et al., 2018). Furthermore, in a recent study researchers analysed data from almost 10,000 young people aged 16–24 years collected as part of the annual Health Survey for England. They found that between 2005 and 2015 the numbers of 16- to 24-year-olds who described themselves as non-drinkers rose from 18% to 29% (Ng Fat, Shelton, & Cable, 2018). The authors concluded that abstaining from alcohol was becoming 'more mainstream' amongst young people, who view drunkenness as less acceptable.

Despite this decline, alcohol use amongst young people in the UK is still common; 44% of pupils aged 11–15 surveyed in the 2018 SDD survey reported that they had ever drunk an alcoholic drink (NHS Digital, 2019).[1] The same prevalence was reported in the 2016 survey (NHS Digital, 2017). Overall, 10% of the surveyed school pupils said they had drunk alcohol in the last week. As expected, alcohol consumption was related to age; 14% of 11-year-olds reported having had an alcoholic drink compared with 70% of 15-year-olds. Nine per cent of all pupils said they had drunk in the last four weeks, and for 15-year-olds this was 22%. Alcohol consumption is higher amongst 16- and 17-year-olds; the 2016 Health Survey for England reported that almost two-thirds (64%) of 17-year-old boys and almost one-half (48%) of girls drink on a weekly basis (Public Health England, 2016). Furthermore, alcohol consumption amongst young people in the UK is also high compared to other European countries. For instance, results from the European Survey Project on Alcohol and Drugs (Hibell et al., 2012) show that the UK is consistently classified as a high prevalence country for underage alcohol use.[2]

Results from the What About YOUth survey (Health and Social Care Information Centre, 2015) show that alcohol consumption is more prevalent amongst certain groups of young people—young people from a white background were more likely to have an alcoholic drink compared to those from a black and minority ethnic background (72% versus 27%). Furthermore, patterns of drinking also varied by deprivation level—young people in the least deprived areas were more likely to have had an alcoholic drink (66%) and to be regular drinkers (8%) compared to those in the most deprived areas (44% and 4%, respectively). Finally, the SDD survey analysed factors associated with drinking in the last week and the strongest associations were age, recent drug use, smoking, drinkers at home, white ethnicity, truancy, and parents who do not discourage drinking (NHS Digital, 2019).

There is unequivocal evidence that frequent drinking and drunkenness is associated with adverse psychological, social, and physical health consequences, including brain damage, academic failure, violence, injuries, and unprotected sexual intercourse (Perkins, 2002; Hingson, Zha, & Weitzman, 2009). The most recent SDD survey showed that commonly reported consequences from drinking were felt ill or sick (40%), vomited (23%), had an argument (18%), damaged clothes or other items (17%), and lost money or other items (17%) (NHS Digital, 2019). One study used data from the WHO's Global Burden of Disease study (Murray & Lopez, 1996) to estimate cause-specific disability-adjusted life years (DALYs) for young people aged

[1] In 2016 the question used to establish whether a pupil had drunk alcohol changed, meaning the results from the 2016 and 2018 surveys are not comparable with previous years.

[2] The UK was not included in the more recent 2015 European Survey Project on Alcohol and Drugs report.

10–24. This analysis reported that alcohol represents one of the main risk factors for DALYs (7% of DALYs) (Gore et al., 2011), with the contribution of other risk factors to disease that normally start in adolescence such as smoking, low physical activity, and overweight/obesity only emerged in mid-to-late adulthood. These findings suggest that alcohol use in adolescence may have a substantial impact in later life. There is also evidence to suggest that early initiation of alcohol use is associated with greater likelihood of more frequent use and substance misuse problems (Morean, Corbin, & Fromme, 2012; Ohannessian, Finan, Schulz, & Hesselbrock, 2015). For example, findings from a large epidemiological survey showed that young people who consume alcohol before the age of 15 are reported to be four times more likely to meet the criteria for alcohol dependence at some point in their lives (Grant & Dawson, 1997). These findings suggest that public health strategies should focus on adolescent drinking as a priority (Gore et al., 2011); delaying and decreasing alcohol use remains an important public health issue (although see Chap. 16 for a discussion of how cultural differences in drinking impact on age of onset) and there is a need to explore factors that influence alcohol-related behaviours and beliefs among young people.

Young people report different reasons for drinking alcohol. A systematic review of 82 studies reported that most young people reported drinking alcohol for social (e.g. drinking to be sociable) or enhancement motives (e.g. drinking to have fun) (Kuntsche, Knibbe, Gmel, & Engels, 2005). In comparison, only a few young people reported drinking for coping motives (e.g. drinking to forget problems) or conformity motives (e.g. drinking to fit in). See Chap. 4 this volume for more on drinking motives. There was evidence to suggest that social motives were associated with moderate alcohol use, enhancement motives with heavy drinking, and coping motives with alcohol-related problems. Alcohol expectancies, or beliefs about how alcohol might impact one's behaviour, are widely recognised as one of the strongest predictors of alcohol use in adolescents (Boyd, Sceeles, Tapert, Brown, & Nagel, 2018). A recent review of 43 studies looked at the development of alcohol expectancies over time found that alcohol expectancies become more positive over time, with more positive alcohol expectancies (i.e. alcohol will result in positive experiences and outcomes) in adolescence and more negative alcohol expectancies in childhood (Smit et al., 2018). Research consistently suggests that adolescents with positive alcohol expectancies are more likely to drink alcohol frequently (Montes et al., 2017) and display more problematic drinking patterns (Cable & Sacker, 2008). Adolescent alcohol expectancies have also been shown to influence long-term patterns of alcohol use. For example, a large longitudinal study found that positive alcohol expectancies in adolescence were strong predictors of alcohol use up to 20 years later (Patrick, Wray-Lake, Finlay, & Maggs, 2010). For more on alcohol expectancies, see Chap. 4.

Research suggests that parents can influence the development of alcohol expectancies. In particular, studies have shown that parental alcohol use and dependency as well as visible alcohol-related consequences can increase positive alcohol expectancies in adolescents (Smit et al., 2018). In addition to having a direct impact on alcohol use, alcohol expectancies are considered important mediators of the relationship between environmental and individual factors and alcohol use. For example, some studies have shown that parental alcohol use was related to adolescents' alcohol use through alcohol expectancies (Epstein, Griffin, & Botvin, 2008).

Parental Communication About Alcohol

Parents are considered to play a crucial role in shaping young people's relationship with alcohol. This is reflected in government policy guidelines from around the world which recognise parents as an important influence of their children's alcohol-related attitudes and behaviours. For example, government guidelines from Australia (National Health and Medical Research Council (NHMRC), 2009), Canada (Canadian Centre on Substance Use and Addiction, 2018), New Zealand (Health Promotion Agency, 2011), and the UK (Donaldson, 2009), as well as the European Union (Steffens & Sarrazin, 2016), all identify parents as key stakeholders in the prevention of adolescent alcohol misuse (Yap, Cheong, Zaravinos-Tsakos, Lubman, & Jorm, 2017). Such guidelines state that young people should not drink alcohol until the age of 15 and adolescents under the age 18 should delay alcohol use as long as possible. For example, the UK guidelines (Donaldson, 2009) state, "*If young people aged 15 to 17 years consume alcohol it should always be with the guidance of a parent or carer in a supervised environment*". It is notable, however, that these guidelines were published over a decade ago and since then there have been changes to UK adult drinking guidelines (Department of Health, 2016) and a reduction in the proportion of young people drinking alcohol (NHS Digital, 2017), suggesting an update of these guidelines is urgently needed.

Research on family influences on alcohol consumption suggests a number of factors are likely to influence young people's drinking. Two systematic reviews (Ryan et al., 2010; Yap et al., 2017) of parenting strategies associated with adolescent alcohol use reported several strategies that were related to lower levels of adolescent drinking: parental modelling (adolescents learning drinking behaviours by observing their parents); parental monitoring (parents' knowledge of their child's activities, whereabouts, and friends); parental involvement (parents and child doing activities together, such as hobbies, chores, watching television); and good parent-child relationship quality.

Parent-child communication is being increasingly explored as an important influence on adolescent alcohol-related behaviours and beliefs for a number of reasons. For one thing, communication is viewed as an important quality of good parenting; for another, communication is a modifiable factor which can be easily incorporated into family-based interventions aimed at reducing excessive adolescent alcohol consumption. Communication is defined as verbal and non-verbal interactions that convey information (Boone & Lefkowitz, 2007) and is multidimensional. The dimensions of communication include not only its frequency, quality, and content but also the strategy it represents such as discussion or asking questions (Boone & Lefkowitz, 2007). Open communication, which refers to the ability to share feelings, approach difficult topics, and ask for help (Riesch, Anderson, & Krueger, 2006), is considered as high-quality communication and talking frequently is assumed to be a characteristic of good family functioning.

Alcohol-specific communication is defined as a direct conversation between an adult and their child regarding alcohol use (Reimuller, Hussong, & Ennett, 2011). Verbal communication is viewed as the most direct way for parents to express their thoughts, rules, and concerns about alcohol to their children (Ennett, Bauman, Foshee, Pemberton, & Hicks, 2001). Reports of alcohol-specific conversations vary between studies; however, as might be expected, parents are more likely to speak about alcohol with older children. For example, one study found that on average at 13 years of age, 43% of children reported having conversations with their parents about alcohol (Miller-Day, 2002). At 18 years of age, this increased to 93% (Miller-Day, 2008). These findings are consistent with a previous qualitative study, where young people reported that communication with parents about alcohol started becoming more open later in adolescence (Jacob, Macarthur, Hickman, & Campbell, 2016). Drinkaware[3] recently surveyed over 1000 UK adults who had a child aged 13–17 as well as more than 500 of their children about young people's drinking behaviours (Drinkaware, 2017). Most young people (88%) said their parents had spoken to them about alcohol which was corroborated by the parents with 87% saying that they had spoken to their child about

[3]The Drinkaware Trust is a UK-wide alcohol education charity, established through an agreement between the UK government and the alcohol industry. It is funded largely by voluntary and unrestricted donations from UK alcohol producers, retailers, and supermarkets.

alcohol. It was also found that most parents began having alcohol-related conversations when their child was around 14 years old, around the time when many young people start drinking; the latest SDD survey suggests that 70% of 15-year-olds have had an alcoholic drink (NHS Digital, 2019).

Parents talk about a range of alcohol-related topics with their children. Frequently discussed topics include alcohol use rules such as a total ban on alcohol use or being allowed to drink alcohol at home in the presence of parents (Ennett et al., 2001; Van Der Vorst, Burk, & Engels, 2010; Abar, Morgan, Small, & Maggs, 2012); information regarding the negative consequences that will result from drinking alcohol such as the health impacts and dangers of drink-driving (Ennett et al., 2001; Sherriff, Cox, Coleman, & Roker, 2008; Boyle & Boekeloo, 2009); and harm reduction strategies (i.e. not drinking quickly, limiting intake, not leaving a drink unattended) (Miller-Day & Dodd, 2004; Abar et al., 2012).

A recent study which involved interviews with 48 parents across the UK provides further insight into the topics most discussed by parents with their children aged between 15 and 17 years (Sawyer, Coleman, Cooke, Hodgson, & Sherriff, 2018). Parents discussed a range of short- and long-term effects associated with alcohol consumption including hangovers, increased vulnerability to assault, effects on behaviour (e.g. lower inhibitions), dangers of drinking alcohol (e.g. drink-driving), and impact of drinking on physical (such as damage to organs) and mental health (e.g. addiction). The most common topics discussed by parents focused on sensible drinking topics such as not drinking too much/avoiding Heavy Episodic Drinking (HED; see Chap. 1), being aware of their limits, strengths of different types of alcohol, alternating between alcoholic and non-alcoholic drinks, and the importance of not mixing drinks. Views on how to stay safe when drinking were also common in parents' accounts. Messages that parents tried to convey included drinking water and eating before drinking, not leaving drinks unattended/avoiding drink spiking, keeping their mobile phone charged, calling parents if there are any problems, staying with reliable friends, and drinking in a safe environment. Overall, there was an understanding that a parent may not always be aware what their child is doing, therefore, it was seen as important that they provide information so that if their child does drink, they do so safely and sensibly.

Research suggests that parents rarely talk about the perceived positive impacts of alcohol with their children. One study found that although parents did talk about the perceived benefits of alcohol, such as making it easier to talk to people, they were discussed much less in comparison to other topics such as the possible negative health, social, and academic consequences

(Menegatos, Lederman, & Floyd, 2016). Ironically, as Cook et al. (Chap. 15) show, this is the opposite of how parents behave with regard to alcohol consumption in front of their children; parents routinely shield their (young) children from the negative effects alcohol might have on them. However, another study found that some parents thought that alongside the negative impacts of alcohol it was also important to convey that drinking can be a normal part of adult life if used sensibly and in moderation (Sherriff et al., 2008).

Overall, the literature shows that most parents feel comfortable talking to their children about alcohol (Sherriff et al., 2008; Sawyer et al., 2018). Findings from the Drinkaware 2016 questionnaire found that nearly all parents surveyed said they felt 'very comfortable' or 'fairly comfortable' talking to their child about drinking alcohol (95%), with only 4% of parents reporting that they felt 'uncomfortable' (Drinkaware, 2017). However, it is important to recognise that there might be a respondent bias in this survey—those parents who feel more comfortable talking to their children may have been more likely to complete the survey. Some differences in levels of comfort were observed according to the gender of the parent. For example, mothers reported feeling more comfortable discussing alcohol with their children compared to fathers (73% of women saying they are 'very comfortable' compared to 58% of men). This is consistent with other research, which suggests that mothers are more likely to initiate conversations about alcohol with their children compared to fathers (Van Der Vorst, Engels, Meeus, Deković, & Van Leeuwe, 2005; Van Der Vorst et al., 2010). This finding may also reflect the well-established finding that men drink more alcohol, on average, than women, meaning that men might feel less comfortable discussing drinking with their children than women due to embarrassment or regrets about their own behaviour.

Although parents generally report feeling comfortable talking about alcohol with their children, some parents report that their knowledge is lacking on certain topics such as units of alcohol, legal issues around alcohol and young people, alcohol dependency, and types of alcohol that young people drink, which can make it difficult for them to talk about these topics (Sherriff et al., 2008; Sawyer et al., 2018). Challenges in starting conversations and concerns about providing inconsistent messages have also been highlighted as areas of difficulty by parents (Sherriff et al., 2008).

The importance of parent-child alcohol-specific communication is based on the assumption that open conversations about alcohol with adolescents strengthens family relationships which increases the ability of families to protect their children from alcohol use and also reduce the taboo associated with alcohol at the same time (Van Der Vorst et al., 2010). However, the empirical literature tends to report inconsistent findings regarding the relationship between parent-child communication and adolescent alcohol consumption. Whilst some studies show that more frequent alcohol-specific communication is protective and related to lower levels of adolescent drinking (Highet, 2005; Miller-Day & Kam, 2010), other studies have shown that communicating more frequently about alcohol is associated with elevated levels of alcohol use in young people (Spijkerman, van den Eijnden, & Huiberts, 2008; Van Der Vorst et al., 2010; van den Eijnden, van de Mheen, Vet, & Vermulst, 2011).

Recent analysis of the 2016 Drinkaware questionnaire (Drinkaware, 2017), which included responses from 561 matched parent-child pairs, explored how different types of parent-child conversations (i.e. gentle reminder, formal sit-down conversation, triggered conversations, practical advice, and providing information) were associated with young people's (13–17 years) alcohol-related behaviour (measured by whether they had ever drunk an alcoholic drink) and harmful outcome (whether they had ever vomited as a result of drinking alcohol) (Jones et al., 2020). Findings showed that most types of conversations were associated with a higher probability of having drunk alcohol or having vomited, with weak evidence for only one type of conversation, that is, providing information, being associated with a reduced risk. The authors discuss the possible role of reactance in explaining this relationship, where health promotion messages may be perceived as restricting or threatening freedom which can prompt health impairing behaviours in an attempt to regain that freedom (Brehm & Brehm, 1981). It is also possible that talking about alcohol might trigger adolescents' curiosity about alcohol and therefore encourage them to drink (Jones et al., 2020).

Several studies of alcohol-specific communication between parents and adolescents suggest more complex associations between frequency of conversations and adolescent drinking behaviours. For example, there is evidence to suggest that more frequent conversations may be more beneficial in families where parents have a problem with alcohol. This was explored in one study which found that parents with alcohol problems communicated more frequently with their child about alcohol, which in turn was related to less excessive adolescent drinking and fewer alcohol-related problems (Mares, van der Vorst, Engels, & Lichtwarck-Aschoff, 2011). Similarly, another study reported that more frequent conversations about alcohol were associated with more negative perceptions about alcohol (e.g. HED is very dangerous) for those children who had already used alcohol or had friends who used alcohol (Brittner, Pugh, Soren, Richter, & Stockwell, 2018).

A recent review found that communication specifically about substance use was related to lower levels of alcohol, tobacco, and drug use in adolescence (Carver et al., 2017). However, the authors concluded that having frequent conversations with adolescents about alcohol use is not enough: conversations need to be of high quality. For example, three studies included in the review found that frequency of communication was indirectly protective against alcohol, tobacco, and cannabis use, *only* when combined with high-quality conversations, defined as those that display mutual understanding and respect between parent and child (Koning, van den Eijnden, & Vollebergh, 2014). Parents in another study also highlighted the importance of listening to and actively involving children in any conversations about alcohol (Sawyer et al., 2018). An open and honest conversation with children about alcohol was also highlighted as important not only to demystify alcohol but also to demonstrate that parents are comfortable talking about alcohol, which consequently may make children at ease when discussions occur (Sawyer et al., 2018).

Therefore, it seems that high-quality conversations which are open and two way are critical factors in the relationship between alcohol-specific communication and adolescent alcohol use (Carver et al., 2017). In contrast, young people can find being lectured about their drinking threatening and this approach can be less effective in promoting moderate consumption (Carver et al., 2017). Indeed, researchers suggest that to more fully understand the influence of parent communication on young people's drinking outcomes, measures should be taken that assess both the frequency of communication and the content of the conversations to explore the style of communication (e.g. relaxed versus formal sit-down style) and the types of messages (e.g. rule based, health messages) that are being communicated and how these are differentially related to adolescent alcohol use (Miller-Day & Kam, 2010). Finally, it has been suggested that high-quality conversations are facilitated by high levels of parent-child connectedness (Carver et al., 2017), which has been defined as "*the quality of the emotional bond between parent and child and by the degree to which this bond is both mutual and sustained over time*" (Lezin, Rolleri, Bean, & Taylor, 2004, p. 6). Specifically, when parent-child connectedness is high, communication is open, frequent, and adolescents feel comfortable. This implies that parents should also be provided with support around promoting high levels of connectedness to improve the quality of their communication about alcohol with their adolescents.

How Do Young People Perceive Parental Conversations About Alcohol?

Findings from the most recent SDD survey found that the majority of young people (77%) considered their parents to be a source of helpful information about drinking alcohol (NHS Digital, 2019). Studies suggest that young people value the conversations they have with parents about alcohol and one study on young people's risky drinking reported that young people would like more discussions with their parents about alcohol (Coleman & Cater, 2005). As discussed above, parents are not always sure how to start and approach conversations about alcohol. Furthermore, many prevention programmes encourage parent-child alcohol-specific communication to reduce young people's alcohol use. However, advice rarely indicates what parents should say to young people when they do discuss the topic (Reimuller et al., 2011). This is especially important as there is some evidence to suggest that alcohol-related conversations without guidance can actually have negative effects; Van der Vorst and colleagues found that when parents who did not regularly communicate with their child attempted to communicate the dangers of alcohol consumption, their efforts to discourage problem drinking actually increased their adolescent's desire to drink (Van Der Vorst et al., 2010). Therefore, broad suggestions for parents to talk to their child about alcohol may be counterproductive. In order to be able to provide evidence-based recommendations to parents it is important to examine the types of alcohol-related conversations that young people themselves find most helpful.

A recent study with 48 parents and 16 young people from across the UK aimed to understand how parental conversations influence alcohol-related attitudes and behaviours of their 15- to 17-year-old children (Sawyer et al., 2018). An important part of this study was to explore how alcohol-related conversations were perceived by young people. Relatively little research has focused on young people's perspectives around parental influences on patterns of alcohol use and fewer studies have directly explored alcohol-related communication from the young person's perspective: in particular, how conversations were initiated, what topics were spoken about, and how messages were conveyed, as well as young people's perceptions of the most useful conversations. To address these gaps in the literature, Sawyer et al. (2018) interviewed 16 young people, 8 males and 8 females, three were aged 15, seven were aged 16, and six were aged 17. All of the young people were either in college or in school in the UK. In terms of experience with alcohol, whilst all the young people interviewed had consumed alcohol on at least one occasion, the majority exhibited infrequent and low levels of drinking, and even rarer occasions of drunkenness. Where drunkenness had occurred, this tended to be an isolated occasion, such as at a party. As such, in reviewing these findings it is important to consider that perceptions of conversations may differ with a sample of young people who are more frequent and heavier drinkers.

Young people in this study generally reported drinking at three different levels. Firstly, a few young people reported tasting/drinking alcohol on one or two occasions and, from this, were not tempted to drink more regularly, commonly put off by general disinterest or taste. A further proportion reported slightly more experience, with alcohol confined to special events such as New Year's Eve or family gatherings. For the sample of young people as a whole, this was the most common drinking experience. A smaller proportion of young people reported drinking more frequently up to a couple of times a week and two young people recalled experiences of being affected by alcohol or being drunk. However, being drunk was a rare event that did not lead to more regular episodes of drunkenness. The majority of alcohol consumption occurred at home or at parties in the presence of adults, although a smaller proportion reported drinking away from their or other's parents. This is consistent with the 2018 SDD survey, which found that those children who drank alcohol mostly drank with their parents (66%) and were most likely to drink alcohol in their own home (66%), someone else's home (41%), or at parties with friends (40%) (NHS Digital, 2019). These findings emphasise the important role that parents can play in shaping young people's alcohol-related attitudes and behaviours. For those young people who had rarely drunk alcohol, the most common explanation was a dislike of the experience, the anticipated effects, and conflict with other activities. The next section presents the young people's findings under the following headings: (i) Triggers to conversations; (ii) Topics conveyed during conversations; and (iii) Effectiveness of conversations.

Triggers to Conversations

All the young people reported that conversations were exclusively 'in passing' and never a formal 'sit-down' conversation. This type of conversation was most appreciated by young people due to its informal and casual nature. In comparison, a more formal, lecture style of conversation was viewed as a less effective way of talking about alcohol as this can be more intimidating.

> Usually we don't really have sit down conversations and stuff, usually you're out and about doing stuff or walking the dog. (17-year-old female)

> I think for some people it would be easier [to talk about alcohol] in passing because some people would find it hard to have like a sit-down conversation because they'd find that quite intimidating. (15-year-old female)

An important part of Sawyer et al.'s (2018) study was to explore how conversations about alcohol were initiated. Overall, young people recalled that conversations were raised more often by their parents than themselves. A range of different strategies were used by parents to start such an open and 'in passing' conversation about alcohol. However, the most frequent trigger to a conversation about alcohol was just before a child went out for the night or was attending a party, where the parent perceived that alcohol might be available. The typical conversation in these circumstances, mentioned by the majority of young people, tended to be short and direct about being sensible. For these instances it was evident that no specific details were relayed about being sensible, implying that children understood what this meant from previous conversations.

> Not an awful lot, just if I go to a party they will say 'don't drink too much, be sensible, know your limits'. (16-year-old male)

On other occasions, if the conversation about a party occurred sometime prior to the event, then this allowed for a lengthier dialogue.

> The first time that they [parents] knew I was going out to a party…and that there was going to be alcohol there, we spoke about it and how to just make sure that I'm responsible with it. (15-year-old female)

A further trigger to alcohol-related discussions were parents becoming aware of their child's peers having started drinking. This influence from other people also extended to the drinking behaviour of relatives. For two of the young people interviewed, their relatives were heavy drinkers, which presented an opportunity for parents to talk about alcohol more frequently.

> My grandpa was debatably an alcoholic, so we've had discussions about that, so I've seen the negative consequences of it. I guess I've learnt through that, but we've definitely had conversations about how that can be really bad and stuff, but not necessarily directly about alcohol, more in the context of my grandpa. (17-year-old female)

Social media was viewed as an important source of information about alcohol for some of the young people interviewed in this study. However, it was also used as a means of facilitating dialogue between children and their parents about alcohol. For example, one young person described how her father shared information about the negative effects of alcohol that he had seen on social media.

> Whenever my dad sees things on Facebook he will come and show me…I think he has shown me some stuff on alcohol…what it does to your digestive system and what happens to it when it's in your stomach and it's quite interesting when he shows me. (15-year-old female)

Young people reported getting information about alcohol from school, which also presented an opportunity for their parents to start a conversation about alcohol with them. For example, one young person recalled how her parents discussed alcohol when it was known that a conversation in school had occurred or had been covered in a related lesson.

> I think probably they did speak about it with me when I came home from school. Having said that I'd had a conversation about it at school, and then they've gone over it again just to reiterate it and clarify what their opinion was. (17-year-old female)

As further context around starting the conversations, young people reported favourably on hearing about their parents' own experiences. This ties in with the general respect children had about the experiences of their parents who were seen to authenticate the information transferred. The quote below reflects the understanding that young people have about the greater number of experiences parents have had compared to themselves, and also the value attached to real-life examples.

> It'd be really difficult not to be able to [talk to your parents] because I think it's a really important part because obviously they've had much more experience with everything. (15-year-old female)

The value of the parental experience was further exemplified by one young person's unfortunate experience which then led him to trust his parents in the future.

They suggested drinking spirits straight was not a good idea and I ignored them, and then I got drunk, and I found that was quite unpleasant so I follow that [advice] now. I realised they are probably right, I should let them tell me what they know, instead of just doing my own thing. (16-year-old male)

Beyond the specific conversation-starters, any triggering of conversation was also considered to have a better impact if it was at a suitable time or place. In particular, young people expressed favour towards conversations at a relaxed time such as over dinner.

Probably at home, so maybe in the evening, probably at the weekend when I'm less busy, yeah generally fairly relaxed kind of time. (15-year-old male)

We normally talk about it over dinner because that's when we're all sitting down together as a family and all talk about stuff. (15-year-old female)

Topics Conveyed During Conversations

Given the sample's limited drinking and experience of drunkenness, these discussions (and the way they were triggered) can be considered on the whole to be effective in terms of harm reduction. As is to be expected, the information represented in these conversations was diverse. The main topic area reported by the young people were ways to drink sensibly and limit the effects, which was expressed in several ways. As for most topics, young people's interviews tended to either express their harm reduction behaviours and techniques or draw on the specific conversation with their parents that led to this. The more general chats lack specific detail implying that they are short-cut comments typical of the brief words of advice just prior to going out (e.g. to a party). These are highlighted in the quotes below where the young people recall being given general advice about being aware of their limit.

Well sort of, just they tell me just to know your limit and make sure you don't go over it. (16-year-old female)

Drink slowly and know your limit, and also I suppose to know your limit, you have to find your limit and doing that in a fairly safe environment. (15-year-old male)

A range of more specific strategies used to limit the effects of alcohol were also described such as having water in between drinks or drinking soft drinks, avoiding drinking spirits neat, avoiding mixing drinks, and eating a full meal beforehand. Alternating alcohol with water and drinking alcohol with food are recommended by the Low Risk (Chap. 1) Drinking Guidelines (Department of Health, 2016) of ways to reduce short-term risks from single occasion drinking sessions. However, avoiding mixing drinks and avoiding drinking spirits neat are absent from these guidelines, suggesting these are examples of 'folk wisdom' rather than scientifically proven strategies to reduce risks from alcohol.

> It's probably more the fact that they were saying obviously warning not to mix spirits and cider and that, and to stick to the cider or vodka. (17-year-old female)

> If I'm going to drink alcohol, I'll eat before because I've learnt that drinking alcohol and then eating afterwards is not good for your body, because teachers have said stories about their friends drinking alcohol and eating afterwards and just being sick everywhere. (16-year-old male)

Again, focusing on avoiding the short-term impacts, one person mentioned avoiding the dangers of spiked drinks.

> I keep my phone with me and I always take my drink with me wherever I go so I don't leave it…Just about making sure that you open your own drink and making sure that you know it's not been spiked, and not going over your limit. (16-year-old female)

Aside from limiting the effects of alcohol, additional, more isolated comments included legal issues regarding drunkenness such as drunk and disorderly and the dangers of drink-driving (both in a legal and safety sense).

> Laws like don't drink and drive and things like that. (17-year-old male)

Although the majority of the conversations were about the short-term consequences and ways to avoid these, two young people also mentioned they had had conversations about the longer-term health dangers and alcohol addiction.

> It was the immediate effects of getting drunk and the fact that it can…I don't know exactly, I just know that it can cause damage, internal damage if you're drinking too much, you can become addicted. (15-year-old male)

A further conversation arose about general vulnerability, and this conversation is a good example of how this information was translated in an open and 'in passing' manner whilst out on a dog walk.

> My dad did have a conversation with me the other week, we were on a dog walk, and talked about uni and stuff, and he said, 'you be careful about what other people can do to you when you're drunk'. So, I know to be sensible with it, and people can put stuff in your drinks, especially at university, when you're a bit older, because at our age I think you're quite safe, because you're usually at friends' houses, and parents are often there, and yeah but as you get older. (17-year-old female)

Young people also noted that the conversation topics had become more informative as they had grown older as their parents recognised that they were more likely to be in situations where alcohol was the norm, which is consistent with previous research (Jacob et al., 2016).

> ...with me getting older, I have noticed they [chats about alcohol] are becoming more frequent...I'd say mainly my parents raise the topic. (16-year-old female)

This emphasises the fact that conversations about alcohol are rarely static within this age group and are likely to change depending on the age of the child. Finally, although from a small sub-sample, it was possible that there was some emerging evidence of a gender match in the conversations where boys preferred to talk to their dad and girls to their mum.

> My mum...I [female] don't know I guess I have a strong relationship with her, I just find it easier to talk with. (17-year-old female)

> Yes, generally if I've [male] got a problem as well about alcohol I'll talk to my dad instead of my mum, because of that experience that he has. (16-year-old male)

Effectiveness of These Conversations

It is difficult to reach firm conclusions over the effectiveness of parental conversations about alcohol in reducing young people's alcohol misuse based on the data from this study. However, beyond noting the low levels of drinking generally within this young person sample, positive inferences can be drawn in two ways. Firstly, young people's judgement over their knowledge and awareness around alcohol and its potential consequences. For the few young people who provided information in this area, the majority (but not all—see later in this section for knowledge gaps) considered themselves sufficiently knowledgeable about alcohol.

> It depends what you mean by successful, I mean, I've taken the information on board. (16-year-old male)

Secondly, the majority of young people in this study demonstrated an ability to avoid alcohol or drink in moderation.

> I've always listened to their [parents] advice and not drink excessively, I don't go out, I don't drink to get drunk or have fun, I just drink socially, so I don't want to get myself drunk. (16-year-old male)

> I know when to stop, I know what would happen if I did it too often and too much and know the limits of what can and what can't be done safely with it. (17-year-old female)

In further evidence of effective conversations, the quote below shows one of the closest links between parental conversations and positive outcomes. In this example, a young person was learning from her mum when attending the same event and trusting her advice throughout. An instance of a conversation whilst drinking was a rare occurrence in this sub-sample, but this example illustrates the issues of positive modelling, respecting the child's independence, and the child valuing her parent's advice.

> As I said at my party, it was have another drink and be like really bad or not, and I'd be like, 'mum, shall I have another drink?' And she'd be like, 'no', and I'm okay that's fine. It's like she can see when I'm at my limit and obviously I can feel that as well, but I'll ask her and she'll tell me, 'no don't drink anymore'. (17-year-old female)

However, it is also worth noting that young people were aware of some gaps in their knowledge and expressed a desire to find out more information about alcohol in certain areas. Some of these were identified as specific gaps of information, although excluded from these examples are areas where young people 'don't know what they don't know'.

> I know a bit about units but I'm not that confident in it…I think I know like how dangerous it could be if you let it get to measures, but I mean I don't really know much about it. (15-year-old female)

The two quotes below show examples of knowledge gaps which are more abstract and are likely to require more detailed conversations or drinking experience, such as understanding one's own limit. Frequent conversations young people report having with their parents is about sticking to their limit, but this can be problematic if the extent of this limit is unknown or may change through time or depending on whether they have taken measures to influence their limit (e.g. eating beforehand).

> I guess [more information] like finding your own limit, I haven't found mine yet. (16-year-old female)

> Probably slightly, I could choose to have that [more about alcohol] discussion, yeah…Probably the effects that it has, and maybe…, maybe why people drink…Yes because I suppose lots of people do it for lots of different reasons, so why they drink, why other people drink. (15-year-old male)

A further example of a gap in knowledge was young people wanting to know about the different types of alcohol, particularly how they differ in strength.

> I don't necessarily feel like I need any more information, but maybe more generally the types of alcohol there are and which ones are the really strong spirits and which ones aren't…So it'd just be better to know them more and which ones are stronger and that you should probably stay away from more. (16-year-old female)

Finally, one young person revealed she had limited knowledge about alcohol and did not receive much advice from her parents. This example reflects a contrast to the majority of other young people's experiences in this study. She explained this by the nature of her relationship with her parents compounded by her father's use of alcohol. This shows that a fundamental feature underpinning effective dialogue about alcohol is the nature of the parent-child relationship.

> We're not the sort of, we [with mum] don't have the relationship where she'd talk to me about things like that…I don't see my dad as much and because he's got quite a weird relationship with alcohol, I don't know, we don't really talk about it as much…No, they've never really offered me any information. (16-year-old female)

Later on in the conversation with this adolescent, the possibility that her perceived lack of knowledge may increase her chance of experiencing alcohol-related harm because she admitted she often drinks before going out is discussed.

> Yeah not an insane amount, but I definitely do it [drink before going out], especially if I'm with friends and we're getting ready. (16-year-old female)

In summary, Sawyer et al.'s (2018) data suggests that young people value having conversations with their parents about alcohol, consistent with previous research. Alcohol-related conversations were generally viewed as being 'in passing' and rarely a formal sit-down conversation; this more relaxed, informal, style of conversation was viewed favourably and considered more effective than being lectured at. The timing of conversations was also important to young people, having a greater impact if they were at a suitable time or place and when everyone was relaxed. These findings provide further support for the importance of high-quality conversations where young people feel listened to and able to contribute equally (Carver et al., 2017). It has been suggested that conversations that are rule based and involve discussions of parents' own alcohol use are not effective in reducing alcohol-related harm, whereas open conversations that discuss the health implications are more effective (Carver et al., 2017). In Sawyer et al.'s study, the most commonly discussed topics were around sensible drinking and limiting the effects of alcohol, and much fewer conversations were around rule-setting. Conversations mainly focused on the short-term consequences associated with drinking alcohol. Interviews with parents in this same study suggested that topics which focus on the short-term dangers of alcohol are thought to be more memorable and therefore have more of an impact on young people compared to longer-term effects (e.g. addiction). Parents discussed their own 'real life' experiences and the young people in this study appeared to find it helpful to hear about these stories. Although young people generally considered themselves knowledgeable about alcohol, some noted they wanted more information in certain areas such as how to find their 'limit', different types and strengths of alcohol, and units of alcohol. Although this was a small study, it provided an in-depth insight into the participant's perceptions of the conversations they have with their parents about alcohol, which has previously been lacking in the literature. The findings can be used to guide evidence-based recommendations for parents to support conversations they have with their older children about alcohol.

Conclusions

This chapter shows that parental communication about alcohol can play an important role in shaping young people's alcohol-related attitudes and behaviours. However, when exploring the relationship between alcohol-specific conversations and alcohol use in young people it is important to look beyond the frequency of conversations. For example, the content and quality of conversations, as well as the drinking behaviours of peers and family members, are likely to influence the association between parental communication and young people's alcohol use. It is important that researchers continue to explore *how* parents talk about alcohol, *what* parents talk about, and *how* young people (especially those who drink heavily) perceive these conversations. Future studies on how to approach and conduct such conversations could identify factors common to all these conversations.

References

Abar, C. C., Morgan, N. R., Small, M. L., & Maggs, J. L. (2012). Investigating associations between perceived parental alcohol-related messages and college student drinking. *Journal of Studies on Alcohol and Drugs, 73*(1), 71–79. https://doi.org/10.15288/jsad.2012.73.71

Boone, T. L., & Lefkowitz, E. S. (2007). Mother-adolescent health communication: Are all conversations created equally? *Journal of Youth and Adolescence, 36*(8), 1038–1047. https://doi.org/10.1007/s10964-006-9138-2

Boyd, S. J., Sceeles, E. M., Tapert, S. F., Brown, S. A., & Nagel, B. J. (2018). Reciprocal relations between positive alcohol expectancies and peer use on adolescent drinking: An accelerated autoregressive cross-lagged model using the NCANDA sample. *Psychology of Addictive Behaviors, 32*(5), 517–527. https://doi.org/10.1037/adb0000371

Boyle, J., & Boekeloo, B. (2009). The association between parent communication and college freshmen's alcohol use. *Journal of Drug Education, 39*(2), 113–131. https://doi.org/10.2190/DE.39.2.a

Brehm, S. S., & Brehm, J. W. (1981). *Psychological reactance: A theory of freedom and control.* New York: Academic Press.

Brittner, M. R., Pugh, B., Soren, K., Richter, L., & Stockwell, M. S. (2018). Frequency of parent-adolescent alcohol-specific communication and adolescent perceptions of alcohol. *Clinical Pediatrics, 57*(11), 1332–1339. https://doi.org/10.1177/0009922818779220

Cable, N., & Sacker, A. (2008). Typologies of alcohol consumption in adolescence: Predictors and adult outcomes. *Alcohol and Alcoholism, 43*(1), 81–90. https://doi.org/10.1093/alcalc/agm146

Canadian Centre on Substance Use and Addiction. (2018). *Canada's low-risk alcohol drinking guidelines.* Retrieved from https://www.ccsa.ca/sites/default/files/2019-03/2012-Canada-Low-Risk-Alcohol-Drinking-Guidelines-Brochure-en_0.pdf

Carver, H., Elliott, L., Kennedy, C., & Hanley, J. (2017). Parent–child connectedness and communication in relation to alcohol, tobacco and drug use in adolescence: An integrative review of the literature. *Drugs: Education, Prevention and Policy, 24*(2), 119–133. https://doi.org/10.1080/09687637.2016.1221060

Coleman, L., & Cater, S. (2005). Underage 'binge' drinking: A qualitative study into motivations and outcomes. *Drugs: Education, Prevention and Policy, 12*(2), 125–136. https://doi.org/10.1080/0968763051233132352l

Degenhardt, L., Stockings, E., Patton, G., Hall, W. D., & Lynskey, M. (2016). The increasing global health priority of substance use in young people. *The Lancet Psychiatry, 3*(3), 251–264.

Department of Health. (2016). *UK Chief Medical Officers' Alcohol Guidelines Review: Summary of the proposed new guidelines.* Retrieved from https://www.gov.uk/government/publications/alcohol-consumption-advice-on-low-risk-drinking

Donaldson, L. (2009). *Guidance on the consumption of alcohol by children and young people.* A report by the chief medical officer. Retrieved from https://pdfs.semanticscholar.org/31a3/8b3f7b981c462ac17b65ea1e7a9daa1e2e06.pdf?_ga=2.85106073.1237593046.1584973437-143633635.1584973437

Drinkaware. (2017). *Teenage drinking and the role of parents and guardians: Findings from Drinkaware Monitor –2016.* Retrieved from https://www.drinkaware.co.uk/research/our-research-and-evaluation-reports/drinkaware-monitor-2016/

Ennett, S. T., Bauman, K. E., Foshee, V. A., Pemberton, M., & Hicks, K. A. (2001). Parent-child communication about adolescent tobacco and alcohol use: What do parents say and does it affect youth behavior? *Journal of Marriage and Family, 63*(1), 48–62. https://doi.org/10.1111/j.1741-3737.2001.00048.x

Epstein, J. A., Griffin, K. W., & Botvin, G. J. (2008). A social influence model of alcohol use for inner-city adolescents: Family drinking, perceived drinking norms, and perceived social benefits of drinking. *Journal of Studies on Alcohol and Drugs, 69*(3), 397–405. https://doi.org/10.15288/jsad.2008.69.397

Gore, F. M., Bloem, P. J., Patton, G. C., Ferguson, J., Joseph, V., Coffey, C., … Mathers, C. D. (2011). Global burden of disease in young people aged 10-24 years: A systematic analysis. *Lancet, 377*(9783), 2093–2102. https://doi.org/10.1016/s0140-6736(11)60512-6

Grant, B. F., & Dawson, D. A. (1997). Age at onset of alcohol use and its association with DSM-IV alcohol abuse and dependence: Results from the national longitudinal alcohol epidemiologic survey. *Journal of Substance Abuse, 9*, 103–110. https://doi.org/10.1016/s0899-3289(97)90009-2

Health and Social Care Information Centre. (2015). *Health and wellbeing of 15-year-olds in England – Main findings from the what about youth? survey 2014*. Retrieved from https://digital.nhs.uk/data-and-information/publications/statistical/health-and-wellbeing-of-15-year-olds-in-england/main-findings%2D%2D-2014

Health Promotion Agency. (2011). *Low-risk alcohol drinking advice*. Retrieved from http://www.alcohol.org.nz/help-advice/advice-on-alcohol/low-risk-alcohol-drinking-advice

Hibell, B., Guttormsson, U., Ahlström, S., Balakireva, O., Bjarnason, T., Kokkevi, A., & Kraus, L. (2012). *The 2011 ESPAD report – Substance use among students in 36 European countries*. Retrieved from http://www.espad.org/sites/espad.org/files/The_2011_ESPAD_Report_FULL_2012_10_29.pdf

Highet, G. (2005). Alcohol and cannabis: Young people talking about how parents respond to their use of these two drugs. *Drugs: Education, Prevention and Policy, 12*(2), 113–124. https://doi.org/10.1080/09687630412331315125

Hingson, R. W., Zha, W., & Weitzman, E. R. (2009). Magnitude of and trends in alcohol-related mortality and morbidity among U.S. college students ages 18–24, 1998–2005. *Journal of Studies on Alcohol and Drugs, 16*, 12–20. https://doi.org/10.15288/jsads.2009.s16.12

Inchley, J. C., Currie, D. B., Vieno, A., Torsheim, T., Ferreira-Borges, C., Weber, M., … Breda, J. (2018). *Adolescent alcohol-related behaviours: Trends and inequalities in the WHO European region, 2002–2014*. Copenhagen: WHO Regional office for Europe.

Institute of Alcohol Studies. (2016). *Why are young people drinking less?* Retrieved from http://www.ias.org.uk/uploads/pdf/IAS%20reports/rp22072016.pdf

Jacob, N., Macarthur, G. J., Hickman, M., & Campbell, R. (2016). A qualitative investigation of the role of the family in structuring young people's alcohol use. *European Journal of Public Health, 26*(1), 102–110. https://doi.org/10.1093/eurpub/ckv123

Jones, A. M., Sawyer, A., Huber, J. W., Coleman, L., Dunne, N., & Sherriff, N. (2020). Parent-child conversations associated with alcohol-related risk behaviours in young people (13–17 years) in the UK: a cross-sectional study. *BMJ Open, 10*(6), e033171. https://doi.org/10.1136/bmjopen-2019-033171

Koning, I. M., van den Eijnden, R. J., & Vollebergh, W. A. (2014). Alcohol-specific parenting, adolescents' self-control, and alcohol use: A moderated mediation model. *Journal of Studies on Alcohol and Drugs, 75*(1), 16–23. https://doi.org/10.15288/jsad.2014.75.16

Kuntsche, E., Knibbe, R., Gmel, G., & Engels, R. (2005). Why do young people drink? A review of drinking motives. *Clinical Psychology Review, 25*(7), 841–861. https://doi.org/10.1016/j.cpr.2005.06.002

Lezin, N., Rolleri, L. A., Bean, S., & Taylor, J. (2004). *Parent-child connectedness: Implications for research, interventions, and positive impacts on adolescent health*. Retrieved from http://recapp.etr.org/recapp/documents/research/litreview.pdf

Mares, S. H. W., van der Vorst, H., Engels, R. C. M. E., & Lichtwarck-Aschoff, A. (2011). Parental alcohol use, alcohol-related problems, and alcohol-specific attitudes, alcohol-specific communication, and adolescent excessive alcohol use and alcohol-related problems: An indirect path model. *Addictive Behaviors, 36*(3), 209–216. https://doi.org/10.1016/j.addbeh.2010.10.013

Menegatos, L., Lederman, L. C., & Floyd, K. (2016). When parents talk about college drinking: An examination of content, frequency, and associations with students' dangerous drinking. *Health Communication, 31*(3), 287–298. https://doi.org/10.1080/10410236.2014.948709

Miller-Day, M. (2002). Parent-adolescent communication about alcohol, tobacco, and other drug use. *Journal of Adolescent Research, 17*(6), 604–616. https://doi.org/10.1177/074355802237466

Miller-Day, M. (2008). Talking to youth about drugs: What do late adolescents say about parental strategies? *Family Relations, 57*(1), 1–12. https://doi.org/10.1111/j.1741-3729.2007.00478.x

Miller-Day, M., & Dodd, A. H. (2004). Toward a descriptive model of parent-offspring communication about alcohol and other drugs. *Journal of Social and Personal Relationships, 21*(1), 69–91. https://doi.org/10.1177/0265407504039846

Miller-Day, M., & Kam, J. A. (2010). More than just openness: Developing and validating a measure of targeted parent-child communication about alcohol. *Health Communication, 25*(4), 293–302. https://doi.org/10.1080/10410231003698952

Montes, K. S., Witkiewitz, K., Andersson, C., Fossos-Wong, N., Pace, T., Berglund, M., & Larimer, M. E. (2017). Trajectories of positive alcohol expectancies and drinking: An examination of young adults in the US and Sweden. *Addictive Behaviors, 73*, 74–80. https://doi.org/10.1016/j.addbeh.2017.04.021

Morean, M. E., Corbin, W. R., & Fromme, K. (2012). Age of first use and delay to first intoxication in relation to trajectories of heavy drinking and alcohol-related problems during emerging adulthood. *Alcoholism, Clinical and Experimental Research, 36*(11), 1991–1999. https://doi.org/10.1111/j.1530-0277.2012.01812.x

Murray, C., & Lopez, A. (1996). Quantifying the burden of disease and injury attributable to ten major risk factors. In C. Murray & A. Lopez (Eds.), *The global burden of disease: A comprehensive assessment of mortality and disability from diseases, injuries, and risk factors in 1990 and projected to 2020* (pp. 295–324). Cambridge, MA: Harvard University Press.

National Health and Medical Research Council (NHMRC). (2009). *Australian guidelines to reduce health risks from drinking alcohol.* Retrieved from https://www.nhmrc.gov.au/about-us/publications/australian-guidelines-reduce-health-risks-drinking-alcohol

Ng Fat, L., Shelton, N., & Cable, N. (2018). Investigating the growing trend of non-drinking among young people; analysis of repeated cross-sectional surveys in England 2005–2015. *BMC Public Health, 18*(1), 1090. https://doi.org/10.1186/s12889-018-5995-3

NHS Digital. (2017). *Smoking, drinking and drug use among young people in England 2016.* Retrieved from https://digital.nhs.uk/data-and-information/publications/statistical/smoking-drinking-and-drug-use-among-young-people-in-england/2016

NHS Digital. (2019). *Smoking, drinking and drug use among young people in England 2018.* Retrieved from https://digital.nhs.uk/data-and-information/publications/statistical/smoking-drinking-and-drug-use-among-young-people-in-england/2018

Ohannessian, C. M., Finan, L. J., Schulz, J., & Hesselbrock, V. (2015). A long-term longitudinal examination of the effect of early onset of alcohol and drug use on later alcohol abuse. *Substance Abuse, 36*(4), 440–444. https://doi.org/10.1080/08897077.2014.989353

Pape, H., Rossow, I., & Brunborg, G. S. (2018). Adolescents drink less: How, who and why? A review of the recent research literature. *Drug and Alcohol Review, 37*(Supplement 1), S98–S114. https://doi.org/10.1111/dar.12695

Patrick, M. E., Wray-Lake, L., Finlay, A. K., & Maggs, J. L. (2010). The long arm of expectancies: Adolescent alcohol expectancies predict adult alcohol use. *Alcohol and Alcoholism, 45*(1), 17–24. https://doi.org/10.1093/alcalc/agp066

Perkins, H. W. (2002). Surveying the damage: A review of research on consequences of alcohol misuse in college populations. *Journal of Studies on Alcohol (Supplement 14)*, 91–100. https://doi.org/10.15288/jsas.2002.s14.91

Petit, G., Kornreich, C., Verbanck, P., Cimochowska, A., & Campanella, S. (2013). Why is adolescence a key period of alcohol initiation and who is prone to develop long-term problem use?: A review of current available data. *Socioaffective Neuroscience & Psychology, 3*(1), 21890.

Public Health England. (2016). *Data intelligence summary: Alcohol consumption and harm among under 18 year olds.* Retrieved from https://assets.publishing.service.gov.uk/government/uploads/system/uploads/attachment_data/file/542889/Alcohol_consumption_and_harms_in_under_18s.pdf

Reimuller, A., Hussong, A., & Ennett, S. T. (2011). The influence of alcohol-specific communication on adolescent alcohol use and alcohol-related consequences. *Prevention Science, 12*(4), 389–400. https://doi.org/10.1007/s11121-011-0227-4

Riesch, S. K., Anderson, L. S., & Krueger, H. A. (2006). Parent–child communication processes: Preventing children's health-risk behavior. *Journal for Specialists in Pediatric Nursing, 11*(1), 41–56. https://doi.org/10.1111/j.1744-6155.2006.00042.x

Ryan, S. M., Jorm, A. F., & Lubman, D. I. (2010). Parenting factors associated with reduced adolescent alcohol use: A systematic review of longitudinal studies. *The Australian and New Zealand Journal of Psychiatry, 44*(9), 774–783. https://doi.org/10.1080/00048674.2010.501759

Sawyer, A., Coleman, L., Cooke, R., Hodgson, L., & Sherriff, N. (2018). Understanding conversations about alcohol between parents and their 15-17 year olds: A qualitative study. *BMC Public Health, 18*(1). https://doi.org/10.1186/s12889-018-5525-3

Sherriff, N., Cox, L., Coleman, L., & Roker, D. (2008). Communication and supervision of alcohol in the family: Parental perspectives. *Children and Society, 22*(5), 370–382. https://doi.org/10.1111/j.1099-0860.2007.00116.x

Smit, K., Voogt, C., Hiemstra, M., Kleinjan, M., Otten, R., & Kuntsche, E. (2018). Development of alcohol expectancies and early alcohol use in children and adolescents: A systematic review. *Clinical Psychology Review, 60*, 136–146. https://doi.org/10.1016/j.cpr.2018.02.002

Spijkerman, R., van den Eijnden, R. J., & Huiberts, A. (2008). Socioeconomic differences in alcohol-specific parenting practices and adolescents' drinking patterns. *European Addiction Research, 14*(1), 26–37. https://doi.org/10.1159/000110408

Steffens, R., & Sarrazin, D. (2016). *Guidance to reduce alcohol-related harm for young people – Background paper*. Retrieved from http://www.rarha.eu/Resources/Deliverables/Lists/Work%20Package%205/Attachments/20/RARHA.WP5.T3.YoungPeople.pdf

van den Eijnden, R. J., van de Mheen, D., Vet, R., & Vermulst, A. D. (2011). Alcohol-specific parenting and adolescents' alcohol-related problems: The interacting role of alcohol availability at home and parental rules. *Journal of Studies on Alcohol and Drugs, 72*(3), 408–417. https://doi.org/10.15288/jsad.2011.72.408

Van Der Vorst, H., Burk, W. J., & Engels, R. C. (2010). The role of parental alcohol-specific communication in early adolescents' alcohol use. *Drug and Alcohol Dependence, 111*(3), 183–190. https://doi.org/10.1016/j.drugalcdep.2010.03.023

Van Der Vorst, H., Engels, R. C., Meeus, W., Deković, M., & Van Leeuwe, J. (2005). The role of alcohol-specific socialization in adolescents' drinking behaviour. *Addiction, 100*(10), 1464–1476. https://doi.org/10.1111/j.1360-0443.2005.01193.x

World Health Organization. (2010). *Global strategy to reduce the harmful use of alcohol*. Retrieved from https://www.who.int/substance_abuse/activities/gsrhua/en/

Yap, M. B. H., Cheong, T. W. K., Zaravinos-Tsakos, F., Lubman, D. I., & Jorm, A. F. (2017). Modifiable parenting factors associated with adolescent alcohol misuse: A systematic review and meta-analysis of longitudinal studies. *Addiction, 112*(7), 1142–1162. https://doi.org/10.1111/add.13785

18

Adolescent Alcohol Use and Development: Layered Ecological Contexts and Agents for Change

Kathryn L. Modecki, Lisa Buckley, and Kyra Hamilton

Introduction

Alcohol use among adolescents is relatively common, and risky levels of alcohol use among teenagers remains a pressing issue worldwide. Peer, school, and social environments can influence risky levels of alcohol use among adolescents and can exert both a protective and risk effect. In this chapter, we describe risky drinking during adolescence and highlight developmental issues which make alcohol use a major cause for concern during this formative developmental period. Next, guided by a protective and risk theoretical framework and drawing on the empirical literature in developmental, health, and

K. L. Modecki (✉)
Menzies Health Institute Queensland, School of Applied Psychology, Griffith University, Brisbane, QLD, Australia

School of Psychology & Exercise Science, Murdoch University, Murdoch, WA, Australia
e-mail: k.modecki@griffith.edu.au

L. Buckley
School of Public Health, The University of Queensland, Herston, QLD, Australia
e-mail: l.buckley@uq.edu.au

K. Hamilton
Menzies Health Institute Queensland, School of Applied Psychology, Griffith University, Brisbane, QLD, Australia
e-mail: kyra.hamilton@griffith.edu.au

R. Cooke et al. (eds.), *The Palgrave Handbook of Psychological Perspectives on Alcohol Consumption*, https://doi.org/10.1007/978-3-030-66941-6_18

social psychology, we examine the role of developmental hazards and protective assets for risky alcohol use across adolescent environments. In particular, we consider identity, peer contexts and social norms, and school climate and supports as contexts for enhancing youth assets and preventing or mitigating adolescents' risky drinking. We conclude the chapter with a summary of directions forward.

For many young people, alcohol is their 'drug of choice', and for adolescents, in particular, alcohol use remains a critical issue (Miech et al., 2019).[1] In the U.S. alone, underage drinking among young people aged 16–20 is tied to more than 4000 deaths per year and more than 110,000 emergency room visits for injuries related to alcohol (CDCP, 2018). In national high-school-based surveys, roughly 30% of adolescents report having drunk alcohol in the past month and 17% report having been a passenger in a vehicle driven by someone who had consumed alcohol (Kann et al., 2018). Not only does adolescents' drinking place them at physical risk for harm, adolescents are more likely to drink to excess, which in and of itself is associated with problems including higher rates of school absence, unplanned and unsafe sexual activity, memory problems, and drug use (CDCP, 2018; NIAAA, 2017). Further, adolescents who engage in early substance use are at especially high risk for disorder, and youth who first use alcohol at age 14 or younger are at five times increased risk for substance use disorder in their lifetime relative to adolescents whose first use is at age 21 or older (SAMSHA, 2009).

One of the major challenges for practitioners and scholars in targeting change in excessive adolescent drinking is that numerous contexts for intervention—peers, school, social norms—which transmit connection and support, can, by the same token, serve to catalyse risk (Chung, Creswell, Bachrach, Clark, & Martin, 2018). As a result, harnessing the promise of these many, layered contexts as mechanisms for prevention and reduction of risky alcohol use arguably requires improved conceptualization of youths' developmental mandate as they experience each of these elements (Tolan, Guerra, & Kendall, 1995). In this chapter, we draw on developmental, health, and social psychology research to provide an overview of these adolescent realms, including identity, peer relationships, social contexts, and school connection and support, and how these impact youths' experiences (Fig. 18.1). With a brief overview of the developmental features of this period of rapid biological,

[1] Given our focus on developmental features of problematic drinking, this chapter discusses adolescence (ages 12–18) as the primary age group of interest. However, because young adulthood (ages 19–21) is also a time of heavy drinking (which has been well catalogued via university-based samples) and scholars at times refer to this period as 'late adolescence' we denote these references via the more generic term of 'young people'.

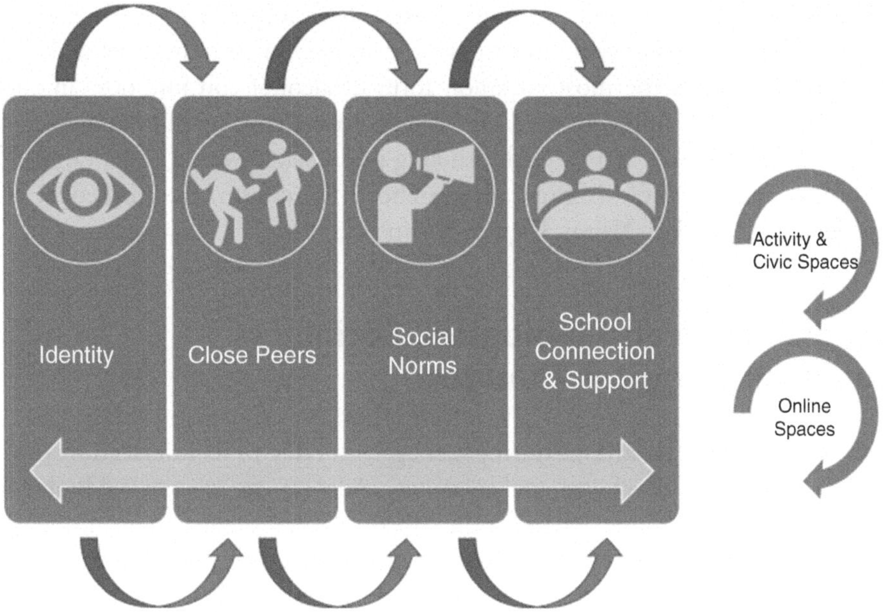

Fig. 18.1 Contexts for adolescent intervention

psychological, and social change, we consider how these various realms can transmit risk and conversely, how they might be drawn upon in the service of adolescent health, namely, prevention and reduction of risky alcohol use.

Adolescent Alcohol Use

Adolescents are more likely to engage in Heavy Episodic Drinking (HED; see Chap. 1) relative to other age groups and, when they do so, they are more likely to experience alcohol-related harms (CDCP, 2018; Macht, Crews, & Vetreno, 2020). That said, at present there is not one single, consistently applied definition of 'risky drinking'. Most international agencies (e.g. in the U.S., the U.K., and Australia) suggest no consumption or delaying alcohol consumption is safest for adolescents (NIAAA, 2017; NHMRC, 2020). There is also recognition that adolescent consumption is less frequent but often of greater quantity on a single occasion than for adults; thus, they are more likely to engage in HED (CDCP, 2018). Here, HED is defined as an episode of high-volume alcohol consumption. In Australia, current guidelines suggest adults who consume four standard drinks or more on any day are at an elevated risk of harm (NHMRC, 2020). Other definitions of HED reflect blood alcohol content

(BAC) reached, for example, having a BAC above 0.08 g/dL (NIAAA, 2017), again reflecting consumption in a single setting. Regardless of how defined (see Chap. 1), HED is the most common form of alcohol consumption among adolescents. For example, in the U.S. 90% of alcohol consumed by adolescents is via HED (NIAAA, 2017). Such drinking is associated with a wider range of problems and most of alcohol's adverse effects (Hamilton, Keech, Peden, & Hagger, 2018; Miller, Naimi, Brewer, & Jones, 2007).

Adolescence and Biological, Social, and Psychological Changes

HED is especially hazardous during teenage years due to its intersection with a critical period of developmental sensitivity. Adolescence is a time of biological and cognitive change, when limbic subcortical areas (nucleus accumbens) are generally mature and fully networked, yet adolescents' top-down prefrontal areas, including basal ganglia, remain under-networked and in need of fine-tuning (Casey, Getz, & Galvan, 2008). As a result, the limbic areas are arguably more efficient, and these areas are also highly sensitive to detecting motivationally and emotionally relevant cues within adolescents' environment (Casey & Jones, 2010). This transitional developmental phase means that adolescents face a more difficult time placing the metaphorical brakes on their behaviour than do children or adults, particularly within social and emotionally laden contexts that 'pull' from the reward systems (Modecki, 2009; Shulman & Cauffman, 2014). While prefrontal cortical and subcortical regions continue to be refined, with maturity and related experience, youths' cognitive control mechanisms come online more rapidly and efficaciously so that by young adulthood, individuals benefit from a more balanced system of reward-drive relative to cognitive control (Modecki, 2016; Shulman et al., 2016).

Importantly, puberty also brings with it a social repositioning towards peers. Adolescent relationships reorient away from parents and towards same-aged friends and friendship groups. Developmental research likewise shows a pattern of heightened susceptibility to peer influence (Modecki, 2008; Monahan, Steinberg, Cauffman, & Mulvey, 2009). This susceptibility to peers is, in part, attributable to the rising importance of friendships and social identities, as youth seek to explore new contexts and settings outside of adult purview. In fact, it is developmentally normative for youth to explore novel settings and, simultaneously, to 'try out' different social identities, as a means to find their 'fit' and figure out 'who' they may, or may not, want to be (Modecki, Blomfield Neira, & Barber, 2018).

While social settings are a key element of adolescents' identity development, social contexts themselves can present as a risk factor for adolescent problem behaviour (see Chap. 9 for more on social contexts). An emerging body of research likewise points to the potency of peers' mere presence in adolescent risk taking (Chein, Albert, O'Brien, Uckert, & Steinberg, 2011). Particularly when youth are surrounded by individuals participating in behaviours that are riskier than their own, adolescents have been shown to engage in heightened risk taking (Centifanti, Modecki, MacLellan, & Gowling, 2016) as well as when they are in the presence of a peer (stranger) who displays risk-accepting norms (Bingham et al., 2016). They also show differences in rates of risk taking under particular social/emotional contexts such as experiencing social rejection (Simons-Morton et al., 2019). Findings from functional magnetic resonance imaging (fMRI) studies indicate that social contexts characterized by the presence of peers may be especially activating for the motivational emotional neural systems associated with adolescent sensation seeking (Crone & Dahl, 2012). Furthermore, such neurological processing during social-emotional tasks is complicated by adolescents' wider socio-economic experiences (Buckley, Broadley, & Cascio, 2019).

Given the ongoing psychological and neurological changes that occur across adolescence, not only are youth especially sensitive to social and affective rewards in tandem with relatively sluggish control systems, this time of developmental sensitivity also translates to a heightened susceptibility to substance addiction, including alcohol disorders (Casey & Jones, 2010). In fact, adolescence brings a 'perfect storm' of neurological drive towards reward and associated risk, and a systemic malleability that can beget a trajectory of longer-term problems (Steinberg, 2007). For example, patterns of elevated alcohol and marijuana use in adolescence appear to suppress age-typical increases in psychosocial maturity (e.g. increased emotional temperance and resistance to peer influence) from adolescence to young adulthood (Chassin et al., 2010). Further too, a review of studies of adolescents' alcohol and marijuana use point to diminished attention, processing speed, spatial skills, learning, memory, and problem solving (Bava & Tapert, 2010). Parallel changes have likewise been observed in brain functions and structures, including prefrontal, cerebellum, and hippocampus volume and atypical patterns of activation (Bava & Tapert, 2010). Thus, endeavours to prevent, delay, or attenuate adolescent alcohol use, especially risky use, can be especially consequential not only for youth health and well-being, but for their longer-term developmental course.

Layered Contexts as Settings for Change

Given co-occurring biological, psychological, and social changes that accompany adolescence, which put youth at developmental risk for alcohol use and misuse, a parallel, developmentally informed framework that addresses this susceptibility and considers corresponding opportunities for enhancing supports is critical for prevention and intervention. In this chapter, we assert that programmes which take advantage of multiple, developmentally salient contexts are especially useful for effective adolescent intervention. With 90% of evidence-based behavioural and mental health interventions not yet used in public or private sphere, taking best advantage of youth development and associated settings in real-world contexts makes intuitive sense (Eddy, Reid, & Fetrow, 2000). In fact, mobilizing the potency of youth identity, peer relationships, social contexts, and school norms and support as mediating mechanisms for prevention arguably represents a best bet for stemming alcohol use during adolescence. Next we outline these different components of a developmentally salient framework.

Identity

Adolescent identity development is an essential element of the transitional phase between childhood and adulthood. Thus, youth are 'trying out' different conceptualizations of themselves and who they want to represent to the outside world. Positive identity development during adolescence sets the stage for enhanced outcomes during young adulthood, including health and educational attainment (Marsh & O'Mara, 2008). When adolescents' identity crystallizes in a manner that enhances their sense of their own capacities across various life domains (social, academic) this has rippling positive effects on their emotional and physical well-being. Yet, by young adulthood (19–21 years of age), when individuals' sense of self leans towards identity 'experimentation' and feeling 'in between', this transitional self-concept is subsequently associated with heavier drinking (Gates, Corbin, & Fromme, 2016). This is especially the case among adolescents coming to understand their cultural and ethnic identity. For example, among recently immigrated Mexican American youth, cultural identity confusion predicts more positive attitudes towards alcohol use (Grigsby et al., 2018) and is associated with growth in positive alcohol expectancies (Oshri et al., 2014; see Chap. 4). As a result, to the extent that adolescents are able to try on different prosocial identities, including experimenting with who they are and their positive norms and values, this bodes well for their reduced alcohol experimentation and risky alcohol use (McCabe, Modecki, & Barber, 2016; Drane, Modecki, & Barber, 2017). Here, school-based after school settings, positive school peers, and positive adult role models are all thought to contribute to positive identity exploration and associated reductions in adolescents' alcohol-related risk (Modecki, Barber, & Eccles, 2014).

In addition to self-identity transitions and confusions affecting alcohol use, holding behavioural identities may also play a role in risky drinking behaviours. In identity theory (Stryker, 1968), the self is considered reflexive; it can categorize itself in particular ways in relation to other social categories, thus forming an identity through a process of self-categorization or identification. An individual can hold multiple identities that make up their self-concept, and these are thought to be organized into a hierarchy according to the most valued self-identities; the more salient the self-identity, the more likely the individual will act in line with the identity (Stryker, 1968). For example, if an individual identifies strongly as a person who drinks alcohol, drinking alcohol will form an important part of their self-concept and, in turn, this 'drinker identity' will influence future actions to engage in drinking alcohol (see also Chap. 11). Thus, self-identity is germane for young people when the individual values the role of being a drinker and considers this an important part of their self-concept. A body of research has shown support for the role of self-identity on a range of behaviours (Rise, Sheeran, & Hukkelberg, 2010), including alcohol use in young adults (Connor, Warren, Close, & Sparks, 2006).

However, it is important to note that identity is not a unitary construct, and in line with dual process models (Hagger, Gucciardi, Turrell, & Hamilton, 2019; Hagger & Hamilton, 2020; Strack & Deutsch 2004), personal identities are proposed to comprise a conscious, explicit component and a non-conscious, implicit component. The former, explicit identity is consistent with reflective, deliberative thinking and usually measured by self-report examining whether an individual endorses a certain identity. The latter, implicit identity, is consistent with reactive, automatic thinking and usually measured using implicit association tests which use semantic strength of word pairings as indicators of implicit identity (Greenwald, Nosek, & Banaji, 2003; Lindgren, Foster, Westgate, & Neighbors, 2013). In the context of alcohol consumption, research has shown that implicit alcohol associations, in particular drinking identity, predicts risky drinking behaviour (Lindgren, Ramirez, Olin, & Neighbors, 2016; Caudwell, Keech, Hamilton, Mullan, & Hagger, 2019; Hamilton, Gibbs, Keech, & Hagger, 2019) and, more worrisome, future risk of alcohol use disorder (Lingren et al. 2016). In a recent study examining both explicit and implicit drinker identity, only explicit identity was found to predict hazardous drinking (Tatnell, Loxton, Modecki, & Hamilton, 2019). Taken together, these findings may suggest that some young people are more likely to engage in risky drinking as a consequence of an implicit process, while others' decisions are determined by reasoned process.

In a bid to tie prevention science to positive development concepts of identity development (e.g. Modecki et al., 2018), several recent interventions have demonstrated that bolstering youths' identity progression as a protective, micro-intervention process holds promise for reducing externalizing behaviour (Eichas et al., 2010). For instance, the Changing Lives Program has shown evidence for positive development as a putative mediator of reductions in problems, via decreases in internalizing behaviours. Other approaches using micro-interventions to target internalizing challenges have themselves shown good early evidence, using daily texting to enhance mediating processes of change (Kivity & Huppert, 2016). Emphasizing positive identity development, whether broadly in relation to gender, sexual, and ethnic identity and self-concept, or more narrowly (and relatedly) in relation to self-typologies (e.g. 'the behaviours I will or will not or do or do not engage in'), is a modifiable feature of adolescent development that is gaining traction across various prevention arenas (Eichas, Montgomery, Meca, & Kurtines, 2017).

It is also worth highlighting that identity is inextricably linked to wider social structures (Terry, Hogg, & White, 1999). As a result, role identity or self-identity is not only a key feature of behaviour, it is also closely tied to social influence. Thus, it is not only adolescents' identity development which acts as a contributor to alcohol use, also contributing are the social implications of risky alcohol behaviour in relation to adolescents' identity with specific roles, which are socially prescribed and embedded within social contexts such as the peer and school unit.

Peer Pressure and Approval

Developmentally, adolescents are especially attuned to peer approval and susceptibility to peer influence plays an outsized role in youth risky decision making, including risky drinking (Drane et al., 2017). There is a considerable body of research showing actual peer alcohol use and perceived peer alcohol use is associated with adolescent's use, including school-based peers. Having peers and friends who consume alcohol is associated with both the initiation and continued use of alcohol (Leung, Toumbourou, & Hemphill, 2014). Further, having friends who engage in other risky behaviours is associated with greater likelihood of alcohol use (Clark, Nguyen, & Belgrave, 2011).

Prominent social psychological theories, such as the theory of planned behaviour (Ajzen, 1991), point to the salience of perceived social approval from important others for enhanced behavioural outcomes. For behaviours that lend themselves to social approval, such as alcohol use, beliefs held about the pressure from important others to perform or not to perform a behaviour (i.e. subjective norms; Ajzen, 1991) and perceptions of important others' own behavioural performance (i.e. descriptive norms; Rivis & Sheeran, 2003) are known to influence individuals' motivations and, therefore, their actions. Meta-analytic research has shown support for the role of such normative influence in predicting positive intentions to consume alcohol, with intentions, in turn, shown to predict greater drinking behaviour (Cook, Dahdah, Norman, & French, 2016; see also Chaps. 2 and 21, this volume).

That said, peer influence and approval is not directed only towards antisocial behaviours. While the negative influence of peers has been extensively studied, prosocial peers can play an active and protective role in reducing the likelihood of alcohol use. For example, the availability of prosocial peers in a students' social network is protective, including identifying no or few friends who consume alcohol (Maxwell, 2002). Further, experimental research shows that adolescent decision making in the presence of relatively more prosocial peers works to pull them towards better outcomes such as less risk taking (Centifanti et al., 2016).

Notably, intervention efforts to bolster adolescents' resistance to peer pressure have demonstrated enhanced skills in delaying and refusing peers (Wolfe, Crooks, Chiodo, Hughes, & Ellis, 2012). However, enhanced resistance to peer influence has not generally emerged as a successful mediator for reduced alcohol involvement. Rather, involvement with prosocial peers and their associated norms and values appears to be an especially fruitful path to protect youth against risky alcohol use.

Additionally, adolescents value and report that they directly intervene to reduce the risk taking and alcohol use of their friends (Buckley, Chapman, Sheehan, & Reveruzzi, 2014) although this varies across adolescence, with younger adolescents and older adolescents most likely to intervene to stop friends' drinking compared with mid-adolescents (Flannagan, Flay, and Galley, 1998). Those adolescents who report that they do intervene are more likely to have social environments that support intervening, including their peers, parents, and school, as well as having positive expectations and confidence to intervene (Buckley, Chapman, Sheehan, & Cunningham, 2012;

Chapman, Buckley, Reveruzzi, & Sheehan, 2014). Some research suggests that having more protective resources (e.g. social supports and prosocial models at home, school, and with friends as well as social control and self-efficacy) can predict intervening in friends' risk taking up to a year later (whereas having few risk factors is not predictive; see Buckley & Chapman, 2016).

Wider Social Networks and Group Norms

Of course, peer relationships represent a subset of wider social networks that influence adolescents' beliefs and behaviour. The broader peer and school environments carry social influences, which also impact adolescents' alcohol use. Thus, beyond close social pressures, social contexts and their accompanying positive attitudes and expectations regarding alcohol use and modelling of drinking behaviour contribute to initiation and escalation in youth drinking (Griffith and Botvin 2010). Reflecting the fact that youth are cloaked in a wider network of attitudes, norms, and behaviours, change in descriptive norms has been shown to mediate the relation between drinking with peers and later alcohol use (Brooks-Russell, Simons-Morton, Haynie, Farhat, & Wang, 2014), and some of the most potent intervention effects on subsequent alcohol use have been demonstrated in relation to changing peer or group norms (Cimini et al., 2009).

In contrast to subjective and descriptive norms, group norms refer to prescriptions, whether explicit or implicit, regarding the appropriate attitudes and behaviours of a member of a specific group within a specific context (White, Hogg, & Terry, 2002). In fact, social identity theorists (Turner, Hogg, Oakes, Reicher, & Wetherell, 1987; Hogg & Abrams, 1988) would assert that the normative influence from an ingroup with whom youth identify is an especially powerful determinant of group members' behaviour. Accordingly, individuals' motivation to act is more likely when there is normative support from a relevant group for performing the behaviour and for attitudes towards the given behaviour than without ingroup support (Terry & Hogg, 1996). Group norms therefore influence individuals' decisions as the individual, based on observing other members, seeks to act in a manner similar with their ingroup, thus achieving categorization as a group member (Turner et al., 1987; Hogg & Abrams, 1988). Research in risky drinking has found support for these predictions, showing that the norms of a behaviourally relevant reference group (i.e. friends and peers) predicted intentions to engage in HED, especially for young people who identified strongly with the reference group (Johnson & White, 2003).

However, interventions aimed at altering social norms have met with mixed success. Social campaigns on university campuses which attempt to alter perceived norms around heavy alcohol use have largely proven unsuccessful (Wechsler et al., 2003), whereas social norm change with young people via social networking sites (SNS) is showing potential promise (Ridout & Campbell, 2014). Further, a meta-analysis of brief alcohol interventions finds distinct differences in effectiveness of component interventions (component modules which can be added or subtracted based on intervention aims; Collins et al., 2014; Guerra, Modecki, & Cunningham, 2014) between adolescents (high schoolers) and late adolescents/young adults (university-based individuals). In this case, adolescent (but not young adult) programmes which included norm-referencing as a key mediator are amongst the most effective (Tanner-Smith & Lipsey, 2015).

School Connection and Social Support

School Connection

Although to some degree encompassed in the above discussion of peer influence and group norms, it is worth characterizing the specific roles of school connection and social support in relation to adolescent alcohol involvement. While parents remain important influences on adolescents' decisions and behaviours (see Chaps. 15, 16, and 17), as youth develop and progress towards young adulthood, relationships outside the home become increasingly important. Teachers, school staff, and young people spend large amounts of time together, but their relevance goes beyond simply the relationships with individuals—it includes feelings of commitment and bonds to the school institution (Pittman & Richmond, 2007).

Conceptually, there have been many ways of understanding the influence of the school relationships and the school environment on adolescents' alcohol use. For example, Libbey (2004) identified some of the numerous terms to conceptualize school relationships, including support, attachment, bonding, connectedness, engagement, involvement, and climate. The U.S. National School Climate Council likewise recommends an encompassing definition of patterns of experiences of school life, reflecting norms, goals, values, teaching, organization structure, and relationships. Relationships include connections among students, teachers, and staff; feelings of commitment to the school; and community connections. Thus, there is a conceptual overlap between group norms and school connection in which theories of school connectedness, engagement, and bonding suggest that students who are engaged with their school will avoid acting outside school norms. That is, connected students are theorized to have a 'stake' in conforming to the school values and correspondingly align with such values (Hawkins, Catalano, & Miller, 1992). Thus, with a bond or close tie to the school and associated extracurricular settings, students regulate their alcohol use to the perceived norms and values of limited use (McCabe et al., 2016).

For instance, connection to school helps bolster academic identity (and vice versa) and multiple aspects of the school relationship predict alcohol use, reflecting protective factors for reducing the likelihood of use. As one example, Li and Lerner (2011) found that sense of school membership was a significant predictor of lower likelihood of substance use, and in a survival analysis predicted later and reduced substance use risk (Li et al., 2011). Blum and Ireland (2004) also found alcohol use was less likely for those higher on school connectedness, which in their data was a stronger protective factor than family and other adult connections. Likewise, Chapman and colleagues report associations between school connectedness and alcohol-related injuries. Employing a comprehensive measure of school connectedness and the sense of belonging associated with their school, adolescents' school connectedness was associated with reduced likelihood of alcohol-related injuries and increased willingness to look-out for and protect close friends from alcohol-related harms (Chapman, Buckley, Sheehan, Shochet, & Romaniuk, 2011; Chapman et al., 2014).

The benefits of positive school relationships on consumption have also been observed longitudinally. An increase in school connectedness through high school has been found to predict a lower likelihood of HED (Weatherson et al., 2018). Additional longitudinal research has identified developmental periods during which school factors are most protective of reduced likelihood of consumption, and when change signals risk (Fleming, Catalano, Haggerty, & Abbott, 2010). Illustratively, both early levels and change in school bonding during middle school predict later alcohol use—indicating that school bonds and their directional trajectory are especially important for protecting children as they enter periods of high risk for alcohol use. Indeed, higher levels of school connectedness have also been shown to delay initiation of alcohol use. Specifically, greater school connectedness appears to be particularly relevant for initial alcohol engagement, though once initiated and possibly entrenched, connections and relationships at school may have less direct relevance (Dornbusch, Erickson, Laird, & Wong, 2001). Similarly, considering school relationships in terms of teacher support, higher support has been linked with lower likelihood of initiation of alcohol use, but perceived teacher support appears to have little effect on the reduction of frequency (McNeely & Falci, 2004).

Social Support

Also related to school connection, but worthy of its own consideration, is a sense of social support from others as a protective element for adolescent alcohol use, especially continued use in response to stressors and challenges. Illustratively, social development models highlight components of attachment (e.g. close emotional ties) and commitment (e.g. investment to the school) in association with decreased alcohol use (Lonczak et al., 2001). Similarly, Stage-Environment Fit theory proposes that adolescents' alcohol use results, in part, from a mismatch between perceived needs and opportunities (Eccles et al., 1993). Accordingly, adolescents lose motivation and interest and their behaviour becomes less aligned with school norms if their social environment does not meet their needs.

The protective nature of support is also seen with a broad conceptualization of school 'community'. That is, Battistich and Hom (1997) defined relationships with school in terms of a 'caring community'. This was reflected in care, support, shared norms, and involvement. Students in schools with higher scores as a caring community had a lower likelihood of drug use (alcohol, cigarettes, and marijuana). In this case, teachers may be especially likely to show support and concern for students, enabling adolescents to approach them and seek help. Adolescents also take cues from their teachers who in turn can provide positive messaging around limiting or avoiding alcohol use. As one example, Buckley, Chapman, Sheehan, and Cunningham (2012) found that greater support from teachers was associated with the confidence to intervene and protect friends' who were drinking.

Wider supportive relationships may, in fact, be protective against the initiation of alcohol use as well as adolescents' use of alcohol to cope with problems later down the line. For example, parental support acts as a stress-buffering effect in relation to adolescents' substance use; high supports both dampen effects of adolescent risk factors and enhance effects of their protective factors (Wills & Cleary, 1996). More broadly, research has shown that social support from different sources, such as family members and friends, significantly and positively influences young people's drinking decisions (e.g. Bonnie et al., 2004).

Conclusion

In this chapter, we have briefly outlined some of the key developmentally salient features of the teenage years and how these can increase vulnerabilities in relation to risky alcohol use. In turn, we have sought to draw attention to positive prospects for prevention of alcohol initiation and escalations in HED across the teenage years. In order to be effective with adolescents, any intervention seeking to mitigate or prevent risky drinking must be developmentally informed. Looking to the future, harnessing our increasing developmental understanding of adolescence for enhanced prevention and intervention (e.g. Conrod, Castellanos, & Mackie, 2008) should be at the forefront of new endeavours and modifications of existing intervention programmes aimed at reducing alcohol use in young people. Further too, policy makers and practitioners might look to novel, developmentally important contexts which help youth thrive in other capacities (i.e. activity participation, youth mentoring programmes, civic engagement) as other potential best bets for preventing alcohol use and associated problems (e.g. Modecki et al., 2018). Finally, some of the most exciting new opportunities for reaching adolescents in their natural contexts and providing support and information for preventing problematic alcohol use are found online, whether via social media channels, online information, or via prosocial online spaces and meeting boards (i.e. Duvenage et al., 2019). All told, early prevention and intervention are critical for preventing adolescent alcohol use and mitigating risky drinking trajectories. Zeroing-in on contexts and settings where youth naturally spend time and taking advantage of opportunities to render peers, classmates, teachers, and parents into 'change agents' are unequivocal best bets for cost-effective early investments.

References

Ajzen, I. (1991). The theory of planned behavior. *Organizational Behavior and Human, Decision Processes, 50*, 179–211.

Battistich, V., & Hom, A. (1997). The relationship between students' sense of their school as a community and their involvement in problem behaviors. *American Journal of Public Health, 87*(12), 1997–2001.

Bava, S., & Tapert, S. F. (2010). Adolescent brain development and the risk for alcohol and other drug problems. *Neuropsychology Review, 20*(4), 398–413.

Bingham, C. R., Simons-Morton, B. G., Pradhan, A. K., Li, K., Shope, J. T., Almani, F., … Albert, P. S. (2016). Peer passenger norms and pressure: Experimental effects on simulated driving among teenage males. *Transportation Research Part F: Traffic Psychology & Behaviour, 41*, 124–137.

Blum, R. W., & Ireland, M. (2004). Reducing risk, increasing protective factors: Findings from the Caribbean youth health survey. *Journal of Adolescent Health, 35*(6), 493–500.

Bonnie, R. J., O'Connell, M. E., & National Research Council. (2004). Developmental and environmental influences on underage drinking: A general overview. In *Reducing underage drinking: A collective responsibility*. Washington, DC: National Academies Press (US).

Brooks-Russell, A., Simons-Morton, B., Haynie, D., Farhat, T., & Wang, J. (2014). Longitudinal relationship between drinking with peers, descriptive norms, and adolescent alcohol use. *Prevention Science, 15*(4), 497–505.

Buckley, L., Broadley, M., & Cascio, C. (2019). Socio-economic status and the developing brain in adolescence. *Child Neuropsychology, 25*, 859–884.

Buckley, L., & Chapman, R. (2016). Characteristics of adolescents who intervene to stop the risky and dangerous behavior of their friends. *Accident Analysis & Prevention, 88*, 187–193.

Buckley, L., Chapman, R., Sheehan, M., & Cunningham, L. (2012). Keeping friends safe: A prospective study examining early adolescent's confidence and support networks. *Education Studies, 38*, 373–381.

Buckley, L., Chapman, R., Sheehan, M., & Reveruzzi, B. (2014). In their own words: Adolescents strategies to prevent friend's risk taking. *Journal of Early Adolescence, 34*(4), 539–561.

Buckley, L., Reveruzzi, B., Dingli, K., Chapman, R. L., & Sheehan, M. (2020). Skills for Preventing Injury in Youth: Evaluating Change in Adolescent Alcohol Use, Violence, and Road-Related Injuries. *Youth & Society*. https://doi.org/10.1177/0044118X20914171.

Casey, B. J., Getz, S., & Galvan, A. (2008). The adolescent brain. *Developmental Review, 28*(1), 62–77.

Casey, B. J., & Jones, R. M. (2010). Neurobiology of the adolescent brain and behavior: Implications for substance use disorders. *Journal of the American Academy of Child & Adolescent Psychiatry, 49*(12), 1189–1201.

Caudwell, K. M., Keech, J. J., Hamilton, K., Mullan, B. A., & Hagger, M. S. (2019). Reducing alcohol consumption during pre-drinking sessions: Testing an integrated behaviour-change model. *Psychology & Health, 34*(1), 106–227.

Centers for Disease Control and Prevention. (2018). *Underage drinking fact sheet, 2018*. Atlanta, GA: US Department of Health and Human Services, Centers for Disease Control and Prevention.

Centifanti, L. C. M., Modecki, K. L., MacLellan, S., & Gowling, H. (2016). Driving under the influence of risky peers: An experimental study of adolescent risk taking. *Journal of Research on Adolescence, 26*(1), 207–222.

Chapman, R. L., Buckley, L., Reveruzzi, B., & Sheehan, M. (2014). Injury prevention among friends: The benefits of school connectedness. *Journal of Adolescence, 37*(6), 937–944.

Chapman, R. L., Buckley, L., Sheehan, M. C., Shochet, I. M., & Romaniuk, M. (2011). The impact of school connectedness on violent behavior, transport risk-taking behavior, and associated injuries in adolescence. *Journal of School Psychology, 49*(4), 399–410.

Chassin, L., Dmitrieva, J., Modecki, K., Steinberg, L., Cauffman, E., Piquero, A. R., … Losoya, S. H. (2010). Does adolescent alcohol and marijuana use predict suppressed growth in psychosocial maturity among male juvenile offenders? *Psychology of Addictive Behaviors, 24*(1), 48.

Chein, J., Albert, D., O'Brien, L., Uckert, K., & Steinberg, L. (2011). Peers increase adolescent risk taking by enhancing activity in the brain's reward circuitry. *Developmental Science, 14*(2), F1–F10.

Chung, T., Creswell, K. G., Bachrach, R., Clark, D. B., & Martin, C. S. (2018). Adolescent binge drinking: Developmental context and opportunities for prevention. *Alcohol Research: Current Reviews, 39*(1), 5.

Cimini, M. D., Martens, M. P., Larimer, M. E., Kilmer, J. R., Neighbors, C., & Monserrat, J. M. (2009). Assessing the effectiveness of peer-facilitated interventions addressing high-risk drinking among judicially mandated college students. *Journal of Studies on Alcohol and Drugs, Supplement, 16*, 57–66.

Clark, T. T., Nguyen, A. B., & Belgrave, F. Z. (2011). Risk and protective factors for alcohol and marijuana use among African-American rural and urban adolescents. *Journal of Child & Adolescent Substance Abuse, 20*(3), 205–220.

Collins, L. M., Trail, J. B., Kugler, K. C., Baker, T. B., Piper, M. E., & Mermelstein, R. J. (2014). Evaluating individual intervention components: Making decisions based on the results of a factorial screening experiment. *Translational Behavioral Medicine, 4*(3), 238–251.

Connor, M., Warren, R., Close, S., & Sparks, P. (2006). Alcohol consumption and the theory of planned behavior: An examination of the cognitive mediation of past behavior. *Journal of Applied Social Psychology, 29*, 1676–1704.

Conrod, P. J., Castellanos, N., & Mackie, C. (2008). Personality-targeted interventions delay the growth of adolescent drinking and binge drinking. *Journal of Child Psychology and Psychiatry, 49*(2), 181–190.

Cook, R., Dahdah, M., Norman, P., & French, D. (2016). How well does the theory of planned behaviour predict alcohol consumption? A systematic review and meta-analysis. *Health Psychology Review, 10*, 148–167. https://doi.org/10.1080/17437199.2014.947547

Crone, E. A., & Dahl, R. E. (2012). Understanding adolescence as a period of social–affective engagement and goal flexibility. *Nature Reviews Neuroscience, 13*(9), 636.

Dornbusch, S. M., Erickson, K. G., Laird, J., & Wong, C. A. (2001). The relation of family and school attachment to adolescent deviance in diverse groups and communities. *Journal of Adolescent Research, 16*(4), 396–422.

Drane, C. F., Modecki, K. L., & Barber, B. L. (2017). Disentangling development of sensation seeking, risky peer affiliation, and binge drinking in adolescent sport. *Addictive Behaviors, 66*, 60.

Duvenage, M., Uink, B. N., Zimmer-Gembeck, M. J., Barber, B. L., Donovan, C. L., & Modecki, K. L. (2019). Ambulatory assessment of adolescent coping: It's a complicated process. *Journal of Research on Adolescence, 29*(3), 578–594.

Eccles, J. S., Midgley, C., Wigeld, A., Buchanan, C. M., Reuman, D., & Flanagan, C. (1993). The impact of stage-environment on young adolescents experiences in schools and in families. *American Psychologist, 48*, 90–101.

Eddy, J. M., Reid, J. B., & Fetrow, R. A. (2000). An elementary school-based prevention program targeting modifiable antecedents of youth delinquency and violence: Linking the interests of families and teachers (LIFT). *Journal of Emotional and Behavioral Disorders, 8*(3), 165–176.

Eichas, K., Albrecht, R. E., Garcia, A. J., Ritchie, R. A., Varela, A., Garcia, A., … Jaccard, J. (2010). Mediators of positive youth development intervention change: Promoting change in positive and problem outcomes? *Child & Youth Care Forum, 39*(4), 211–237.

Eichas, K., Montgomery, M. J., Meca, A., & Kurtines, W. M. (2017). Empowering marginalized youth: A self-transformative intervention for promoting positive youth development. *Child Development, 88*(4), 1115–1124.

Fleming, C. B., Catalano, R. F., Haggerty, K. P., & Abbott, R. D. (2010). Relationships between level and change in family, school, and peer factors during two periods of adolescence and problem behavior at age 19. *Journal of Youth and Adolescence, 39*(6), 670–682.

Gates, J. R., Corbin, W. R., & Fromme, K. (2016). Emerging adult identity development, alcohol use, and alcohol-related problems during the transition out of college. *Psychology of Addictive Behaviors, 30*(3), 345.

Greenwald, A. G., Nosek, B. A., & Banaji, M. R. (2003). Understanding and using the implicit association test: I. an improved scoring algorithm. *Journal of Personality and Social Psychology, 85*(2), 197–216. https://doi.org/10.1037/0022-3514.85.2.197

Grigsby, T. J., Forster, M., Meca, A., Zamboanga, B. L., Schwartz, S. J., & Unger, J. B. (2018). Cultural stressors, identity development, and substance use attitudes among Hispanic immigrant adolescents. *Journal of Community Psychology, 46*(1), 117–132.

Guerra, N., Modecki, K., & Cunningham, W. (2014). *Developing social-emotional skills for the labor market: The PRACTICE model* (World Bank Policy Research Working Paper, 7123).

Hagger, M. S., Gucciardi, D. F., Turrell, A. S., & Hamilton, K. (2019). Self-control and health-related behaviour: The role of implicit self-control, trait self-control, and beliefs in self-control. *British Journal of Health Psychology, 24*, 764–786. https://doi.org/10.1111/bjhp.12378

Hagger, M. S., & Hamilton, K. (2020). Changing behaviour using integrated theories. In M. S. Hagger, L. Cameron, K. Hamilton, N. Hankonen, & T. Lintunen

(Eds.), *Handbook of behavior change* (pp. 208–224). New York, NY: Cambridge University Press.

Hamilton, K., Gibbs, I., Keech, J. J., & Hagger, M. S. (2019). Reasoned and implicit processes in heavy episodic drinking: An integrated dual process model. *British Journal of Health Psychology*. Advanced online publication. https://doi.org/10.1111/BJHP.12401

Hamilton, K., Keech, J. J., Peden, A., & Hagger, M. S. (2018). Alcohol use, aquatic injury, and unintentional drowning: A systematic review. *Drug and Alcohol Review, 37*, 752–773. https://doi.org/10.1111/dar.12817

Hawkins, J. D., Catalano, R. F., & Miller, J. Y. (1992). Risk and protective factors for alcohol and other drug problems in adolescence and early adulthood: Implications for substance abuse prevention. *Psychological Bulletin, 112*(1), 64.

Hogg, M. A., & Abrams, D. (1988). *Social identification: A social psychology of intergroup relations and group processes*. London, UK: Routledge.

Johnson, K., & White, K. (2003). Binge-drinking: A test of the role of group norms in the theory of planned behaviour. *Psychology & Health, 18*, 63–77. https://doi.org/10.1080/0887044021000037835

Kann, L., McManus, T., Harris, W. A., Shanklin, S. L., Flint, K. H., Queen, B., … Lim, C. (2018). Youth risk behavior surveillance—United States, 2017. *MMWR Surveillance Summaries, 67*(8), 1.

Kivity, Y., & Huppert, J. D. (2016). Does cognitive reappraisal reduce anxiety? A daily diary study of a micro-intervention with individuals with high social anxiety. *Journal of Consulting and Clinical Psychology, 84*(3), 269.

Leung, R. K., Toumbourou, J. W., & Hemphill, S. A. (2014). The effect of peer influence and selection processes on adolescent alcohol use: A systematic review of longitudinal studies. *Health Psychology Review, 8*(4), 426–457.

Li, Y., & Lerner, R. M. (2011). Trajectories of school engagement during adolescence: Implications for grades, depression, delinquency, and substance use. *Developmental Psychology, 47*(1), 233.

Libbey, H. P. (2004). Measuring student relationships to school: Attachment, bonding, connectedness, and engagement. *Journal of School Health, 74*(7), 274–283.

Lindgren, K. P., Foster, D. W., Westgate, E. C., & Neighbors, C. (2013). Implicit drinking identity: Drinker+me associations predict college student drinking consistently. *Addictive Behaviours, 38*(5), 2163–2166. https://doi.org/10.1016/j.addbeh.2013.01.026

Lindgren, K. P., Ramirez, J. J., Olin, C. C., & Neighbors, C. (2016). Not the same old thing: Establishing the unique contribution of drinking identity as a predictor of alcohol consumption and problems over time. *Psychology of Addictive Behaviors, 30*(6), 659–671. https://doi.org/10.1037/adb0000195

Lonczak, H. S., Huang, B., Catalano, R. F., Hawkins, J. D., Hill, K. G., Abbott, R. D., … Kosterman, R. (2001). The social predictors of adolescent alcohol misuse: A test of the social development model. *Journal of Studies on Alcohol, 62*(2), 179–189.

Macht, V., Crews, F. T., & Vetreno, R. P. (2020). Neuroimmune and epigenetic mechanisms underlying persistent loss of hippocampal neurogenesis following adolescent intermittent ethanol exposure. *Current Opinion in Pharmacology, 50*, 9–16.

Marsh, H. W., & O'Mara, A. (2008). Reciprocal effects between academic self-concept, self-esteem, achievement, and attainment over seven adolescent years: Unidimensional and multidimensional perspectives of self-concept. *Personality and Social Psychology Bulletin, 34*(4), 542–552.

Maxwell, K. A. (2002). Friends: The role of peer influence across adolescent risk behaviors. *Journal of Youth and Adolescence, 31*(4), 267–277.

McCabe, K. O., Modecki, K. L., & Barber, B. L. (2016). Participation in organized activities protects against adolescents' risky substance use, even beyond development in conscientiousness. *Journal of Youth and Adolescence, 45*(11), 2292–2306.

McNeely, C., & Falci, C. (2004). School connectedness and the transition into and out of health-risk behavior among adolescents: A comparison of social belonging and teacher support. *Journal of School Health, 74*(7), 284–292.

Miech, R. A., Johnston, L. D., O'Malley, P. M., Bachman, J. G., Schulenberg, J. E., & Patrick, M. E. (2019). *Monitoring the future national survey results on drug use, 1975–2018: Volume I, secondary school students*. Ann Arbor, MI: Institute for Social Research, The University of Michigan. Available at http://monitoringthefuture.org/pubs.html#monographs

Miller, J. W., Naimi, T. S., Brewer, R. D., & Jones, S. E. (2007). Binge drinking and associated health risk behaviors among high school students. *Pediatrics, 119*(1), 76–85.

Modecki, K. L. (2008). Addressing gaps in the maturity of judgment literature: Age differences and delinquency. *Law and Human Behavior, 32*(1), 78.

Modecki, K. L. (2009). "It's a rush": Psychosocial content of antisocial decision making. *Law and Human Behavior, 33*(3), 183–193.

Modecki, K. L. (2016). Do risks matter? Variable and person-centered approaches to adolescents' problem behavior. *Journal of Applied Developmental Psychology, 42*, 8–20.

Modecki, K. L., Barber, B. L., & Eccles, J. S. (2014). Binge drinking trajectories across adolescence: For early maturing youth, extra-curricular activities are protective. *Journal of Adolescent Health, 54*(1), 61–66.

Modecki, K. L., Blomfield Neira, C., & Barber, B. L. (2018). Finding what fits: Breadth of participation at the transition to high school mitigates declines in self-concept. *Developmental Psychology, 54*(10), 1954.

Monahan, K. C., Steinberg, L., Cauffman, E., & Mulvey, E. P. (2009). Trajectories of antisocial behavior and psychosocial maturity from adolescence to young adulthood. *Developmental Psychology, 45*(6), 1654.

National Institute on Alcohol Abuse, & Alcoholism. (2017). *Underage drinking*. US Department of Health and Human Services. Downloaded from: https://www.niaaa.nih.gov/publications/brochures-and-fact-sheets/underage-drinking

NHMRC (2020). Australian Guidelines to Reduce Health Risks from Drinking Alcohol. National Health and Medical Research Council, Australian Research Council and Universities Australia. Commonwealth of Australia, Canberra.

Oshri, A., Schwartz, S. J., Unger, J. B., Kwon, J. A., Des Rosiers, S. E., Baezconde-Garbanati, L., … Villamar, J. A. (2014). Bicultural stress, identity formation, and alcohol expectancies and misuse in Hispanic adolescents: A developmental approach. *Journal of Youth and Adolescence, 43*(12), 2054–2068.

Pittman, L. D., & Richmond, A. (2007). Academic and psychological functioning in late adolescence: The importance of school belonging. *The Journal of Experimental Education, 75*(4), 270–290.

Ridout, B., & Campbell, A. (2014). Using Facebook to deliver a social norm intervention to reduce problem drinking at university. *Drug and Alcohol Review, 33*(6), 667–673.

Rise, J., Sheeran, P., & Hukkelberg, S. (2010). The role of self-identity in the theory of planned behavior. *Journal of Applied Social Psychology, 40*, 1085–1105. https://doi.org/10.1111/j.1559-1816.2010.00611.x

Rivis, A., & Sheeran, P. (2003). Descriptive norms as an additional predictor in the theory of Planned Behaviour: A meta-analysis. *Current Psychology, 22*, 218–233.

SAMSHA. (2009). *Results from the 2008 national survey on drug use and health: National findings*. Rockville, MD: Office of Applied Studies, DHHS.

Shulman, E. P., & Cauffman, E. (2014). Deciding in the dark: Age differences in intuitive risk judgment. *Developmental Psychology, 50*(1), 167.

Shulman, E. P., Smith, A. R., Silva, K., Icenogle, G., Duell, N., Chein, J., & Steinberg, L. (2016). The dual systems model: Review, reappraisal, and reaffirmation. *Developmental Cognitive Neuroscience, 17*, 103–117.

Simons-Morton, B., Bingham, R., Li, K., Hu, C., Buckley, L., Falk, E., & Shope, J. (2019). The effect of teenage passengers on simulated risky driving among teenagers: A randomized trial. *Frontiers in Psychology, 10*, 923.

Steinberg, L. (2007). Risk taking in adolescence: New perspectives from brain and behavioral science. *Current Directions in Psychological Science, 16*(2), 55–59.

Strack, F., & Deutsch, R. (2004). Reflective and impulsive determinants of social behavior. *Personality and Social Psychology Review, 8*(3), 220–247.

Stryker, S. (1968). Identity salience and role performance: The relevance of symbolic interaction theory for family research. *Journal of Marriage and the Family, 30*, 558–564.

Tanner-Smith, E. E., & Lipsey, M. W. (2015). Brief alcohol interventions for adolescents and young adults: A systematic review and meta-analysis. *Journal of Substance Abuse Treatment, 51*, 1–18.

Tatnell, D. G., Loxton, N. J., Modecki, K., & Hamilton, K. (2019). Testing a model of reward sensitivity, implicit and explicit drinker identity, and hazardous drinking. *Psychology & Health, 34*(12), 1407–1420. https://doi.org/10.1080/08870446.2019.1606221

Terry, D. J., & Hogg, M. A. (1996). Group norms and the attitude-behavior relationship: A role for group identification. *Personality and Social Psychology Bulletin, 22*, 776–793.

Terry, D. J., Hogg, M. A., & White, K. M. (1999). The theory of planned behaviour: Self-identity, social identity and group norms. *British Journal of Social Psychology, 38*(3), 225–244.

Tolan, P. H., Guerra, N. G., & Kendall, P. C. (1995). A developmental ecological perspective on antisocial behavior in children and adolescents: Toward a unified risk and intervention framework. *Journal of Consulting and Clinical Psychology, 63*(4), 579.

Turner, J. C., Hogg, M. A., Oakes, P. J., Reicher, S. D., & Wetherell, M. S. (1987). *Rediscovering the social group: A self-categorisation theory*. Oxford, UK: Blackwell.

Weatherson, K. A., O'Neill, M., Lau, E. Y., Qian, W., Leatherdale, S. T., & Faulkner, G. E. (2018). The protective effects of school connectedness on substance use and physical activity. *Journal of Adolescent Health, 63*(6), 724–731.

Wechsler, H., Nelson, T. E., Lee, J. E., Seibring, M., Lewis, C., & Keeling, R. P. (2003). Perception and reality: A national evaluation of social norms marketing interventions to reduce college students' heavy alcohol use. *Journal of Studies on Alcohol, 64*(4), 484–494.

White, K. M., Hogg, M. A., & Terry, D. J. (2002). Improving attitude-behavior correspondence through exposure to normative support from a salient ingroup. *Basic and Applied Social Psychology, 24*, 91–103.

Wills, T. A., & Cleary, S. D. (1996). How are social support effects mediated? A test with parental support and adolescent substance use. *Journal of Personality and Social Psychology, 71*(5), 937.

Wolfe, D. A., Crooks, C. V., Chiodo, D., Hughes, R., & Ellis, W. (2012). Observations of adolescent peer resistance skills following a classroom-based healthy relationship program: A post-intervention comparison. *Prevention Science, 13*(2), 196–205.

Section V

Interventions to Reduce Alcohol Consumption

19

Alcohol Labelling: Evidence for Product Information Interventions

Anna K. M. Blackwell, Natasha Clarke, Emily Pechey, and Angela S. Attwood

Introduction

Alongside unhealthy diet, tobacco use and physical inactivity, the harmful use of alcohol is one of four key behavioural risk factors for non-communicable diseases. However, product labelling regarding the content of alcoholic drinks, and the potential health harms associated with their consumption, falls behind that of food and tobacco. Firstly, this chapter reviews product labelling of alcohol drink content, including energy (i.e. calories), standard drinks (known as *units* in the UK), and low-risk drinking guidelines. Currently, the provision of this information is limited across many countries, public knowledge is similarly poor, and it has received little research attention. We argue that addressing the absence of this information for consumers is an important target for both research and policy, and we consider how these labels could be optimised. Secondly, we review the growing body of evidence for the inclusion of health warning labels on alcohol products and the impact of message content

A. K. M. Blackwell (✉) • A. S. Attwood
School of Psychological Science, University of Bristol, Bristol, UK
e-mail: anna.blackwell@bristol.ac.uk; angela.attwood@bristol.ac.uk

N. Clarke • E. Pechey
Department of Public Health and Primary Care, University of Cambridge, Cambridge, UK

R. Cooke et al. (eds.), *The Palgrave Handbook of Psychological Perspectives on Alcohol Consumption*, https://doi.org/10.1007/978-3-030-66941-6_19

and framing, as well as the use of images, on their effectiveness among different drinking demographics. Evidence is explored for the potential impact on alcohol-related knowledge, attitudes, and behaviour of different labelling strategies. Finally, we consider barriers and facilitators regarding the successful evaluation, and potential implementation, of alcohol product labelling.

Labelling of Consumer Products

> Citizens have the right to obtain relevant information on the health impact, and in particular on the risks and consequences related to harmful and hazardous consumption of alcohol, and to obtain more detailed information on added ingredients that may be harmful to the health of certain groups of consumers. (European Commission, 2006)

Many countries require food labelling of ingredients and nutritional content to provide dietary information (e.g. Food Standards Agency, 2018. Tobacco health warning labelling is also common and has been effective for increasing knowledge, perceptions of harm, and smoking cessation (Hammond, 2011). However, the information required on alcohol labels varies globally and alcohol labelling often falls below the standards mandated for food (World Health Organization, 2017). The way alcoholic products are currently labelled minimises consumers' ability to make informed choices about the amount they drink or the potential health-related impact of different products.

Alcohol products sold outside of licensed premises require basic information to be presented on labels, such as the alcohol by volume of the product, and common allergens, although, in contrast to food products, alcohol labels generally do not include nutritional information (e.g. ingredients, calories). Some countries (e.g. the UK) provide health information through voluntary industry-led schemes. However, these labels often lack features to draw consumers' attention (Petticrew et al., 2016), and industry-led health information in the form of responsibility messages, such as "*Enjoy Heineken Responsibly*", more closely resemble marketing slogans (Farke, 2011). While some countries mandate health warnings (e.g. the US), these messages are often small and text only. Policy makers have raised concerns about lack of access to consumer information; however, regulatory change is slow. A rapid evidence review of the effectiveness of alcohol control policies in England included *provision of information and education* as one of seven different policy areas for reducing alcohol-related harm (Burton et al., 2017). The review identified the role of education for addressing consumers' right to information. However, evaluations of existing alcohol labelling suggest that it is not sufficient for changing drinking behaviour, in part due to the reliance on these voluntary schemes and poorly implemented mandatory schemes (Burton et al., 2017).

The Content of Alcohol Products: Energy Labelling

At the most basic level, consumers should have access to information that allows them to identify their energy intake from food and drinks as well as the amount of alcohol in drink products. Studies of food labelling interventions have demonstrated that strategies such as traffic light labelling, guideline daily amounts, and energy information on menus can increase selection of healthier food options (Cecchini & Warin, 2016; Crockett et al., 2018). However, approximately three out of four countries do not require basic consumer information (i.e. calories, additives) on alcohol labels (World Health Organization, 2018b). For example, in the European Union, alcoholic drinks are exempt from legislation that requires ingredients and nutritional information to be listed on food and soft drinks (EU Regulation 1169/2011). In 2017, the European Commission reviewed this exemption and gave the alcohol industry an opportunity to develop a self-regulatory proposal to address this absence of information. In 2018, the industry responded with a proposal to provide information either on labels or online. The proposal was considered inadequate by health advocates and, as of 2019, was under review by the Commission.

The discrepancy between nutritional labelling on alcoholic drinks and all other food and drinks is mirrored within the research literature. There has been a striking lack of research on the potential impact of nutritional alcohol labelling on alcohol-related attitudes and consumption (Burton et al., 2017) considering that alcohol accounts for almost a tenth (8.4%) of the total energy intake of UK drinking adults and the rates of obesity are increasing (Public Health England, 2016a, 2016b). Alcohol contains 7.1 kilocalories per gram: second only to fat (9 kcal/g) as the most energy dense foodstuff (World Health Organization, 2017). This is particularly important given that global obesity rates have almost tripled since the 1970s (World Health Organization, 2018c), and the impact of alcohol consumption on the liver is synergistic with being overweight (Hart, Morrison, Batty, Mitchell, & Davey Smith, 2010). A survey of over 2000 adults in the UK by the Royal Society for Public Health (2014) found that the majority underestimated the calorie content of beer and wine. In contrast, in Attwood, Blackwell, and Maynard's (2019) survey of 1499 UK drinkers it was found that, on average, respondents overestimated calories in alcoholic drinks; however, there was a large variation in estimates highlighting that drinkers' knowledge of calories in alcohol is poor.

Previous studies of calorie alcohol labelling suggest it may have little impact on behaviour; Bui, Burton, Howlett, and Kozup (2008) found wide variation in calorie estimates among a sample of university students, as reported elsewhere, but also increased intentions to consume wine and spirits in response to accurate information, suggesting that nutritional information could lead to more favourable evaluations of certain products. A laboratory study by Maynard et al. (2017) looking at the effects of a single exposure to calorie information on acute drinking behaviour (i.e. ad libitum consumption) found that calorie information had no impact on consumption. However, calorie details were provided alongside other text-based statements and single exposure to information with limited saliency may not be sufficient to change behaviour (see Chap. 14). Qualitative responses from mostly undergraduate student participants reported that they may be more likely to reduce food intake than alcohol intake, highlighting potential unintended consequences of providing calorie information on alcohol labels.

Understanding the calorie content of alcoholic drinks is an important target, which could be achieved through improved product labelling. However, further research is needed to determine how to increase attention to, and understanding of, nutritional labelling. In addition, exploration of the unintended consequences of presenting calorie information is required, the potential for which should not be seen as a reason to withhold information but highlights the importance of implementing nutritional labelling alongside alcohol-related health messages and broader alcohol education (Martin-Moreno et al., 2013).

The Content of Alcohol Products: Standard Drinks and Low-Risk Drinking Guidelines

Understanding or monitoring alcohol intake can be difficult for consumers as the strength (alcohol by volume: ABV) and size of alcoholic drinks vary depending on drink type (beer, wine, spirits) and purchase location (i.e. on licensed premises, off-licensed premises). For example, there is 10 ml of pure alcohol in a single measure (25 ml) of a 40% ABV spirit, like whisky, compared to 34 ml of pure alcohol in a large glass (250 ml) of 13.5% ABV wine (see Chap. 1). Many countries have established a *standard drink* measure to represent a fixed amount of pure alcohol; however, this amount varies across countries, and not all countries use the term *standard drink.* For example, in the UK, the term *unit* is used instead and the two drinks above contain 1.0 and 3.4 units respectively (1 unit = 10 ml pure alcohol) (National Health Service, 2018); whereas, in the US they contain 0.6 and 1.9 standard drinks (1 standard drink = 17.7 ml pure alcohol) (National Institute on Alcohol Abuse and Alcoholism, 2019). The modal amount of pure alcohol in a standard drink across 37 countries that use such a definition is 12.5 ml (range 10-25 ml), consistent with the World Health Organization (WHO) definition (Kalinowski & Humphreys, 2016). Several countries have established daily and/or weekly low-risk drinking guidelines (see Chap. 1) to support consumers to monitor their drinking based on a number of standard drinks or units. However, the low-risk guideline amount also varies widely across the 37 countries, ranging 122.5–350 ml per week for men and women, often with a higher guideline amount for men (Kalinowski & Humphreys, 2016). The lack of international consensus prevents consistent labelling of products (Furtwængler & de Visser, 2013).

The use of units as a measure of alcoholic intake was introduced in the UK in 1987. In 2009, 90% of people said that they were aware of measuring alcohol in this way but there was confusion regarding the number of units in different types of alcohol, and people rarely used units to monitor their drinking (ONS, 2010). The Alcohol Pledge, part of the Responsibility Deal agreement between the UK government and alcohol industry (Department of Health, 2011), aimed to address this issue through the provision of standard drinks and low-risk drinking guidelines on alcohol labels. A systematic review of the labelling agreement found that unit labelling could support drinkers to understand alcohol strength (Knai, Petticrew, Durand, Eastmure, & Mays, 2015). The review found less support for behaviour change and suggested that measures were needed to educate consumers on the meaning of units. However, an assessment of the industry-led labels found that they often fell below best practice: information was generally small and on the reverse of products (Petticrew et al., 2016), which undermined their effectiveness.

Psychological research has repeatedly shown that adolescents and young adults are confused as to what counts as a unit of alcohol. For example, de Visser and Birch (2012) found in samples of school children and university students that most underestimated the number of units in alcoholic drinks, poured measures much larger than unit, and familiarity with units was not related to accuracy of pouring (see Chap. 1 for more on this issue). Research with Australian and Canadian drinkers has shown that standard drink labelling can improve accuracy in estimating alcohol content and consumption compared to ABV labelling (Hobin et al., 2018; Osiowy, Stockwell, Zhao, Thompson, & Moore, 2015; Stockwell, Blaze-Temple, & Walker, 1991a), including pouring accuracy (Stockwell, Blaze-Temple, & Walker, 1991b), which is important for monitoring consumption. There is some concern that standard drink labelling could facilitate the selection of higher strength drinks (Jones & Gregory, 2009). However, Osiowy et al. (2015) found that drinkers were more likely to suggest they would use this information to stay below the drink-driving limit and believed they would be helpful for staying within low-risk drinking guidelines.

The UK low-risk drinking guidelines were updated in 2016 to recommend that both men and women do not regularly consume more than 14 units per week (i.e. 140 ml of pure alcohol). This amount was based on evidence that drinking at, or above, this level equates to a 1% likelihood of alcohol-related mortality (Department of Health, 2016). Stevely et al. (2018) considered the value of low-risk drinking guidelines in relation to the COM-B model of behaviour change (Michie, van Stralen, & West, 2011), which proposes that behaviour results from the interaction of capability (physical or psychological), opportunity (environmental or social), and motivation (automatic or reflective). The following elements were identified as relevant to the effectiveness of the low-risk drinking guidelines for changing behaviour: consumer knowledge of guidelines, skills to monitor drinking, access to information, and intention to drink within the recommended amount (see Chap. 14). Their study, based on a large, cross-sectional survey of UK adults between November 2015 and January 2017, found that reported exposure to the updated guidelines, alongside increased capability and opportunity to change, was not maintained over time after their release. In 2017, analysis of alcohol labels found that only 1 in over 300 included the updated information (Alcohol Health Alliance, 2017).

It is perhaps not surprising that in the year following their release only around one in ten people knew the UK guideline amount for men and women (Rosenberg et al., 2017; Attwood et al., 2019). Focus groups with UK drinkers highlighted limited understanding of the meaning of low-risk drinking guidelines, in terms of how they relate to personal levels of risk, and drinkers often struggled with the validity of a universal guideline amount despite wide variation in age, weight, and underlying health (Attwood et al., 2019). Poor communication of both standard drinks and low-risk drinking guidelines has meant that they lack meaning and usefulness for consumers. In 2014, over 10 million UK adults regularly consumed more than 14 units per week (Public Health England, 2016b), and inadequate communication may mean that people are unaware of how much they drink and their relative risk of harm. Furthermore, alcohol-related mortality is greater among more deprived socio-economic groups, and awareness of low-risk guidelines is lower (Rosenberg et al., 2017), potentially widening health inequalities in alcohol-related harm. Stevely et al. (2018) suggested that limited large-scale, well-designed, theory-based promotion may partly explain the low impact of drinking guidelines to change behaviour. Increased awareness would facilitate drinkers' ability and motivation to adhere to the low-risk guidelines.

The Content of Alcohol Products: Optimising the Impact of Labels

Drinkers must identify the energy content and number of standard drinks they consume, to accurately monitor intake, and understand the extent to which their consumption differs from the guidelines, for this information to effectively support decision making. The evidence demonstrates the potential for alcohol-related health information interventions to improve knowledge and awareness, but the implementation strategies need to be evidence-based and designed to maximise effectiveness (Burton et al., 2017). A systematic review of evidence for standard drink labelling (Wettlaufer, 2018) highlighted the importance of label saliency, including size and placement. A number of recommendations exist, including placing labels in a standard location, parallel to the base, attracting attention through the use of bold text and in bordered boxes (Eurocare, 2012), on a contrasting colour background (Laughery, Vaubel, Young, Brelsford, & Rowe, 1993), with health information covering at least one-third of the product label and nutritional information and standard drink information appearing alongside health warnings (Anderson et al., 2013). However, there is a lack of evidence to inform the presentation of alcohol content and low-risk drinking guideline information to maximise understanding and utility.

Blackwell, Drax, Attwood, Munafò, and Maynard's (2018) online study of UK drinkers asked participants to estimate the number of drinks they could consume before reaching the low-risk guideline amount (i.e. 14 units). Participants were presented with novel labels (i.e. units in drinks: number of standard drinks per serving as a proportion of the guideline amount) made faster, more accurate responses compared to those shown industry standard labels (i.e. total number of units in container and/or ABV). Providing information per serving in the context of the drinking guidelines may be critical to enable effective monitoring of drinking, which has been lacking to date (see Chap. 20 for more on how monitoring can inform alcohol interventions). Focus groups with Canadian adults support these findings: drinkers identified the need to have standard drink and guideline information on labels to effectively monitor and modify their consumption (Vallance et al., 2017). They also felt that a combination of different presentation styles, including pictograms and simple charts, would be useful, for attracting attention and providing clear information, which was considered particularly important for people with low literacy, and that labels should be larger, or at least bold and on the front of products to increase salience.

Improving consumer knowledge may not be sufficient for changing behaviour, on which unconscious processes can have a great influence (Marteau, Hollands, & Fletcher, 2012), but it may be an important basis for action (Anderson et al., 2013). Behaviour change in terms of population-level reductions in drinking may take time and operate downstream of changes in knowledge; therefore, it is important that studies measure knowledge as a key indicator of success, and likely mediator of behavioural outcomes. Furthermore, providing information about the content of alcohol products addresses a key consumer right for making informed decisions about products bought and consumed. Comprehensive alcohol labelling strategies also need to communicate the range of health, as well as social and economic, harms associated with consumption. In the next section, we discuss how alcohol-related harms could be presented on alcoholic product and the impact on alcohol-related knowledge, attitudes, intentions, and behaviours of different health warning labels.

The Harms Associated with Alcohol Consumption: Health Warning Labels

Despite alcohol consumption being among the top ten global risk factors for disease (Forouzanfar et al., 2016), only one in four countries requires the inclusion of information about alcohol-related harms on alcohol labels—in some cases based on voluntary agreements with industry (e.g. Chile, Japan, and the UK) (World Health Organization, 2018a). The nature of labelling requirements varies widely between countries. Some messages are general (e.g. "*drink in moderation*"—Argentina; "*avoid excessive alcohol consumption*"—Brazil) and specific messages often refer to either the risks of drinking whilst pregnant (e.g. "*Consumption of alcohol beverages during pregnancy, even in small amounts, can have serious consequences for the child's health*"—France), underage drinking (e.g. "*Sale to and consumption by persons under 18 years of age is prohibited*"—Mozambique), or drink-driving (e.g. "*Consumption of alcohol is injurious to health. Be safe – don't drink and drive*"—India) (see Fig. 19.1 for examples from the US and UK). A few countries specify a broader range of messages (e.g. in Kenya alcohol products must display at least two health warnings from a selection) and formatting requirements (e.g. warnings must cover 10% of the surface in Ecuador and 40% in Uzbekistan) (IARD, 2019). Only seven countries require the rotation of warning messages (World Health Organization, 2018b), despite recommendations from the field of tobacco labelling that specify the need to rotate warnings as the impact of repeated messages tends to decrease over time (Hammond, 2009).

Existing product labels can increase awareness of alcohol-related harms, but evidence suggests they do not change behaviour (Tim Stockwell, 2006; Wilkinson & Room, 2009). There are increasing worldwide calls for better alcohol product labels—from researchers, public health bodies, and the public—that clearly describe the harms associated with alcohol consumption (World Health Organization, 2010, 2017). However, there is a lack of consensus on the content or form of message that might be most effective. The next section reviews the evidence for the effectiveness of alcohol-related health warning labels including the influence of message content and framing, the use of images, as well as individual differences. Importantly, evidence on objective drinking outcomes is limited and the majority of studies focus on influencing surrogate outcomes, such as perceptions, intentions, or hypothetical situations, that may not impact on actual consumption.

Health Warning Label Message Content and Framing

The majority of recent research has examined health warning labels that communicate long-term health risks, such as diabetes, mental illness, heart

GOVERNMENT WARNING: (1) According to the Surgeon General, women should not drink alcoholic beverages during pregnancy because of the risk of birth defects. (2) Consumption of alcoholic beverages impairs your ability to drive a car or operate machinery, and may cause health problems.

UK
Unit
Per
25ml
UK
Units
For further health
information visit
drinkaware.co.uk
18+

Fig. 19.1 Existing health warnings from the US and UK

disease, cancer, brain damage, liver damage, and liver disease (Wigg & Stafford, 2016; Stafford & Salmon, 2017; Jongenelis, Pratt, Slevin, & Pettigrew, 2018; Sillero-Rejon et al., 2018; Clarke et al., 2020). Long-term health messages can decrease consumption intentions and increase perceptions of disease risk (Jongenelis et al., 2018). Messages focusing on cancer can increase risk perceptions (Chen & Yang, 2015), may increase awareness and prompt conversations about alcohol-related cancer risk (Miller, Ramsey, Baratiny, & Olver, 2016), and are considered by the public to be believable, convincing, and personally relevant (Pettigrew et al., 2014). In addition, cancer warnings can decrease drinking intentions (Pettigrew et al., 2016), arouse negative emotions (Pechey et al., 2020), and are more likely to make people want to drink less compared to other health conditions (Attwood et al., 2019; Winstock, Holmes, Ferris, & Davies, 2019). Messages referring to the increased risk of cancer related to alcohol consumption are of particular interest given these encouraging findings as well as current low levels of public awareness of the link between alcohol consumption and cancer (Scheideler & Klein, 2018). Health warning labels communicating the acute effects of alcohol are less common, but message content includes arrests, road accidents, alcohol-induced vomiting, acne, poor interpersonal choices, and risks of drinking during pregnancy. Findings indicate short-term health messages can also reduce drinking intentions (Collymore & McDermott, 2015; Krischler & Glock, 2015; Sillero-Rejon et al., 2018).

Health message framing can be an important factor in message effectiveness. There is accumulating evidence that specific cancer messages (e.g. bowel cancer) may have increased impact on awareness and consumption intentions compared to general cancer messages (Pettigrew et al., 2014; Miller et al., 2016; Pettigrew et al., 2016). Specific health warnings are rated as more believable and have higher ratings of perceived alcohol-related disease risk than general health warnings (Blackwell et al., 2018). An online study measuring responses to 21 pictorial health warning labels found that specific liver and bowel cancer labels were rated as more negatively arousing and decreased desire to consume an alcoholic drink compared to general cancer labels (Pechey et al., 2020).

There are mixed findings as to whether framing a message positively or negatively is most effective. Some research indicates that negatively framed health warning labels (i.e. stressing the negative impact of heavy drinking) have a greater influence and can reduce motivation to drink alcohol compared to positively framed health warning labels (i.e. stressing the rewards of drinking less) (Jarvis & Pettigrew, 2013; Blackwell et al., 2018). In contrast, Previte, Russell-Bennett, and Parkinson (2015) demonstrated that positively framed value propositions more strongly influenced the processing of an alcohol moderation message than negatively framed propositions. Another study found no differences in positively and negatively framed labels on intentions to reduce consumption or attitudes towards alcohol prevention (Quick & Bates, 2010). The wording of a statement can also produce differential effects. Health warning labels using terms that stress causality such as *causes* and *increases your risk of* are judged as more convincing and believable than *can cause* (Pettigrew et al., 2014). However, studies measuring the impact of different message types on objective consumption outcomes are required before firm conclusions can be drawn on their effectiveness.

Pictorial Health Warning Labels

Pictorial health warning labels, with an image representing an adverse health effect, alongside a text statement, are mandated on tobacco packaging in many countries. There is a substantial body of evidence demonstrating their impact on a range of effectiveness outcomes including cessation-related behaviours (Hammond, 2011), with evidence indicating labels which produce negative emotions are most effective (Cho et al., 2018). This is demonstrated by a greater effect of graphic pictorial warnings than text-only warnings (Hammond, 2011; Noar et al., 2015; Brewer et al., 2016). A review of alcohol labelling studies highlighted caution when generalising results from tobacco labelling studies to alcohol, and identified a weak current evidence base for both text and pictorial health warning labels (Hassan & Shiu, 2018).

One laboratory study showed that intentions to reduce and quit consumption were higher following exposure to pictorial health warning labels (e.g. "*Alcohol causes fatal liver cancer*" alongside image of diseased liver) compared to control, but that these ratings were similar to text-only health warning labels (Wigg & Stafford, 2016). Using the same labels, it was found that pictorial and text-only health warning labels were equally as effective in reducing the speed of drinking compared to no label in a laboratory study—albeit in a small sample of female undergraduate students (Stafford & Salmon, 2017). An online study using a hypothetical selection measure found that pictorial labels can decrease the likelihood of choosing alcohol compared to no labels and text-only labels, in a sample of 6024 participants (Clarke et al., 2020). Hassan and Shiu (2018) highlighted in their review that research is required to assess different levels of *graphicness* similar to that undertaken in tobacco control (e.g. Kees, Burton, Andrews, & Kozup, 2010). Initial findings indicate that highly severe images (e.g. an image of someone injured from a car accident) are perceived as more effective and result in increased motivation to drink less compared to moderately severe images (e.g. an image of someone drinking while driving) (Sillero-Rejon et al., 2018).

The tobacco literature suggests that labels which produce negative emotions are most effective (Cho et al., 2018), but it is not yet clear whether the same mechanism applies to alcohol. Pictorial labels inducing disgust have been shown to be just as, or even more, potent as fear-inducing labels and researchers have recommended that they warrant the same attention (Collymore & McDermott, 2015). Conversely, pictorial labels also have the potential to evoke defensive reactions, which may impact their potential effectiveness. Defensive reactions include avoidance of warnings—not attending to them (Maynard et al., 2014)—or opposing them through reactance behaviours—a negative response to the labels (Hall et al., 2016). Avoidance and reactance are more likely with more severe pictorial labels compared to moderately severe labels (Sillero-Rejon et al., 2018). However, tobacco research suggests that defensive reactions do not necessarily indicate a lack of effectiveness (Osman, Thrasher, Yong, Arillo-Santillán, & Hammond, 2017). Further research should consider the overall goal of alcohol product labelling (i.e. drinking within the low-risk guidelines) compared to tobacco control (i.e. cessation), when evaluating message reactions and identifying the most appropriate label message or image to use.

Individual Differences in Response to Health Warning Labels

Individuals are more likely to accept a warning message if they view it as relevant to them (Thomson, Vandenberg, & Fitzgerald, 2012; Winstock et al., 2019). Message relevance may vary according to individual differences including gender, age, drinking patterns, and familiarity with alcohol products, which are discussed in turn below.

Gender has been highlighted as an important factor to consider in label design and implementation (Hassan & Shiu, 2018). For example, Jarvis and Pettigrew (2013) found that drink-driving messages were most impactful for female drinkers and messages about health effects on the brain most impactful for male drinkers. The only study to date assessing the impact of pictorial health warning labels on alcohol consumption rate was in a female-only sample (Stafford & Salmon, 2017), and the findings need to be replicated in a broader drinking population.

Alcohol-related outcome expectancies change across a person's lifespan. Young people tend to discount the future compared to older individuals, often making decisions based on short-term consequences (Steinberg & Scott, 2003); therefore, health warning labels that demonstrate short-term risks may be more effective for younger people than those emphasising long-term effects (Leigh & Stacy, 2004). Labels addressing positive alcohol-related outcomes have been shown to impact young adults more than health-related warnings (Krischler & Glock, 2015). In a sample of 40 students, labels that contradicted positive *social* alcohol expectancies (i.e. *"Alcohol leads to problems with other people"*) were more effective than health warning labels (Glock & Krolak-Schwerdt, 2013). Findings from a focus group study with students in Australia suggested that labels could be effective for younger drinkers if they were more noticeable and relevant through referencing short-term effects of alcohol consumption, as long-term effects are more easily dismissed at earlier life stages (Jones & Gregory, 2010). Differences in label effectiveness according to age are particularly important to consider as a key limitation of previous lab-based studies is the use of young, mainly student populations. Future research should aim to include a wide range of participants who are representative of broad drinking populations especially given recent trends showing a decline in adolescent drinking (Pape, Rossow, & Brunborg, 2018).

Reactions and responses to health warning labels may also differ by individual alcohol consumption levels as well as brand knowledge and preference. Krischler and Glock (2015) suggest labels stating outcome expectancies may be more effective in heavier drinkers, as heavier drinkers emphasise the positive outcomes related to alcohol consumption (Reich & Goldman, 2005). Jarvis and Pettigrew (2013) used choice modelling to demonstrate that negatively framed messages have the greatest influence on the higher alcohol consuming classes. However, in a large online study an existing Australian label failed to influence high-risk drinkers (Coomber, Jones, Martino, & Miller, 2016), although this could be due to familiarity with the label. Initial findings from eye-tracking studies show a focus on branding compared to warnings on labels (Kersbergen & Field, 2017). In addition, individuals can correctly identify warnings at a higher rate for plain packaged alcohol (Al-Hamdani & Smith, 2017). Similarly to branding, preferences for different types of alcohol drive choice behaviour and processing of warnings statements may differ by drink type (Jarvis, Pettigrew, & Olaru, 2015).

In summary, the evidence demonstrates that there is not a one-size-fits-all approach; however, with the right design, labels may be a promising avenue for future policy and research aiming to reduce the harms associated with excessive alcohol consumption. Broadly speaking, any health message should be serious, using simple, clear, and unambiguous language (Thomson et al., 2012). Based on the existing evidence, specific, negatively framed health messages emphasising long-term health risks may have the most potential, but many studies include measures of intentions or risk perceptions, which do not necessarily translate to actual behaviour, and very few include objective consumption behaviours. Therefore, evidence on actual consumption and in real-world settings is required before such conclusions can be confirmed.

Implementation of Alcohol Product Labelling

Policy makers and health advocates have been discussing the need for more consumer information on labels for many years (European Commission, 2006; World Health Organization, 2010; Eurocare, 2014). The alcohol industry presents a challenge to progressing both legislative changes and the delivery of quality research necessary to inform policy. Some of the challenges of introducing evidence-based labelling interventions are discussed in this section, alongside possible alternative or complementary approaches to facilitate the availability of the health information that consumers urgently need.

Barriers to Implementation of Health Warning Labels

The alcohol industry can be a huge obstacle to the overall effectiveness of alcohol labelling on drinking attitudes and behaviour, as well as the progress of field research to evaluate the impact of new labelling strategies. Alcohol-related cues and environmental contexts are significant drivers of positive alcohol-related cognitions (Monk, Pennington, Campbell, Price, & Heim, 2016), and harm messages are battling with the pro-drinking environment and alcohol marketing. In real-world settings, it is likely that labels will be less attended to than in controlled research settings (Kersbergen & Field, 2017; Pham, Rundle-Thiele, Parkinson, & Li, 2017).

> There is extensive alcohol marketing with comparatively few messages focused on the potential harms associated with alcohol. It is recommended that governments collaborate with multiple stakeholders to maximize the preventive impact of restrictions on alcohol marketing and advertising, and a broader implementation of alcohol warning messages. (Wettlaufer, Cukier, & Giesbrecht, 2017)

Field studies are notoriously more difficult to run in any research area; however, the controversial nature of health warning labels, alongside the influence of the alcohol industry, makes conducting field studies to test these labels almost impossible. This is well illustrated by a recent attempt in Yukon, Canada (Stockwell, Solomon, O'Brien, Vallance, & Hobin, 2020). This study collaborated with a local supermarket to have real alcohol products in store display health warning labels in order to test their effects on alcohol purchasing. However, within four weeks of beginning data collection, the study was halted due to pressure from national alcohol organisations (Institute for Alcohol Studies, 2018). The study has now been allowed to continue, without the cancer-related warning labels (Government of Yukon, 2018). In addition, public information provided by the alcohol industry in relation to alcohol-related harms has been shown to be distorted, through omission, misrepresentation of risk, and distraction from certain risk messages, which highlights the need to prohibit industry involvement in policy development or delivery (Petticrew, Maani Hessari, Knai, & Weiderpass, 2018).

Alcohol Product Labelling as Part of a Broader Approach

Qualitative interviews and focus groups with stakeholders and drinkers in the UK and Canada have highlighted the importance of placing alcohol labelling interventions within broader approaches to reduce alcohol-related harm, including education to support understanding of alcohol content, low-risk guidelines, and relative personal risk of harm (Vallance et al., 2017; Attwood et al., 2019). In addition to product labelling, information should be available on other materials (e.g. beer mats, glassware, and posters) where product labels are not always visible (e.g. when drinks are served in a glass in bars and restaurants), as well as in non-drinking spaces (e.g. public transport) to maximise exposure to information. Changes to product labelling may require lengthy legislative changes and there may be opportunities to introduce alcohol-related health communication more readily through alternative methods, offering greater exposure across a range of contexts. This may be an important first step for improving knowledge and changing attitudes, which are necessary precursors to behaviour change.

A Phased Approach to Introducing Alcohol Product Labelling

Any proposals for alcohol labelling interventions should first consider the purpose and short-, medium-, or long-term goals. Public knowledge of alcohol content, low-risk guidelines, and specific alcohol-related harms remains low and there are continuing beliefs surrounding the positive effects of alcohol, specifically moderate wine consumption (German & Walzem, 2000); therefore, addressing health literacy is a key priority. Over time, increased exposure to information could influence people's attitudes towards alcohol as a potentially harmful product and beliefs about personal risk of harm. In an online study with 5528 participants, assessing 21 different pictorial health warning labels, acceptability for pictorial health warning labels was low, with only three health warning labels rated as acceptable (Pechey et al., 2020). However, it is important to note that acceptability of a policy often increases after it has been implemented (Reynolds, Pilling, & Marteau, 2018). In the case of alcohol health warning labels, low acceptability may be due to a lack of awareness of the links between alcohol and health conditions. Increased awareness of the health impacts of alcohol consumption, particularly the link with cancer, can lead to increased support for policies (Bates et al., 2018; Weerasinghe et al., 2020). Thus, with increased communication on alcohol health risks, there may be increased acceptability.

A phased approach to health warning labelling could first implement more acceptable label formats, such as presenting risk information in tabular and bar graph format, which have both been shown to increase perceived likelihood of cancer risk from heavy episodic drinking (see Chap. 1 for a definition) compared to text-only labels (Chen & Yang, 2015). The inclusion of more contentious strategies such as pictorial health warning labels could be implemented subsequently, as part of a longer-term plan. Any evaluation of labelling strategies should also follow this phased approach so that knowledge and understanding are key early outcomes of effectiveness before examining behaviour.

Conclusions

There is currently a dearth of accessible alcohol-related health information necessary for consumers to make informed choices about their alcohol intake. Reliance to date on inconsistently implemented voluntary schemes, poorly designed educational campaigns, and minimal communication of guidelines, in the context of pervasive alcohol marketing and increased availability of alcohol, may explain the limited success of existing information provision to reduce alcohol consumption. Further research is needed to identify how to optimise labelling to support consumer understanding of personal consumption, and relative risk of health harms, and to assess the impact of labelling on objective drinking outcomes over longer-term periods. The inclusion of alcohol content information (i.e. calorie and standard drinks) in the context of low-risk guidelines may be useful for promoting understanding and monitoring of alcohol intake, enabling comparisons across alcohol products so that consumers can opt for lower alcohol strength or calorie drinks, and understanding the harms of excessive alcohol consumption. The impact of alcohol health warning labels is likely to vary depending on personal context and individual drinking habits, but based on the existing evidence, specific, negatively framed health messages emphasising long-term health risks may have the most potential. Alcohol product labelling interventions may impact drinkers' capability and motivation to control drinking behaviour, which are fundamental requirements of successful behaviour change—see COM-B model of behaviour change (Michie et al., 2011). While information alone may not be sufficient to drive behaviour change, particularly in the short term, it may be a necessary precursor to change; therefore, alcohol product labelling may be an important component of a broader strategy to reduce alcohol-related harm.

References

Alcohol Health Alliance UK. (2017). *Right to know: Are alcohol labels giving consumers the information they need?* Retrieved from London, UK: http://ahauk.org/wp-content/uploads/2017/08/Right-to-Know-AHA-August-2017.pdf

Al-Hamdani, M., & Smith, S. M. (2017). Alcohol health-warning labels: Promises and challenges. *Journal of Public Health, 39*(1), 3–5. https://doi.org/10.1093/pubmed/fdx010

Anderson, W., Gilmore, S. I., Bauld, L., Bellis, M., Brown, K. A., Drummond, C., … Parsons, H. (2013). Health first: An evidence-based alcohol strategy for the UK. Retrieved from Alcohol Health Alliance, UK: https://ahauk.org/resource/health-first-an-evidence-based-alcohol-strategy-for-the-uk/

Attwood, A. S., Blackwell, A. K. M., & Maynard, O. M. (2019). *Alcohol harms and product labelling: What, who and how?* Bristol, UK: University of Bristol Tobacco and Alcohol Research Group.

Bates, S., Holmes, J., Gavens, L., de Matos, E. G., Li, J., Ward, B., … Buykx, P. (2018). Awareness of alcohol as a risk factor for cancer is associated with public support for alcohol policies. *BMC Public Health, 18*(1), 688. https://doi.org/10.1186/s12889-018-5581-8

Blackwell, A. K. M., Drax, K., Attwood, A. S., Munafò, M. R., & Maynard, O. M. (2018). Informing drinkers: Can current UK alcohol labels be improved? *Drug and Alcohol Dependence, 192*, 163–170. https://doi.org/10.1016/j.drugalcdep.2018.07.032

Brewer, N. T., Hall, M. G., Noar, S. M., Parada, H., Stein-Seroussi, A., Bach, L. E., … Ribisl, K. M. (2016). Effect of pictorial cigarette pack warnings on changes in smoking behavior a randomized clinical trial. *JAMA Internal Medicine, 176*(7), 905–912. https://doi.org/10.1001/jamainternmed.2016.2621

Bui, M., Burton, S., Howlett, E., & Kozup, J. (2008). What am I drinking? The Effects of Serving Facts Information on Alcohol Beverage Containers. *Journal of Consumer Affairs, 42*(1), 81–99. https://doi.org/10.1111/j.1745-6606.2007.00095.x

Burton, R., Henn, C., Lavoie, D., O'Connor, R., Perkins, C., Sweeney, K., … Sheron, N. (2017). A rapid evidence review of the effectiveness and cost-effectiveness of alcohol control policies: An English perspective. *The Lancet, 389*(10078), 1558–1580. https://doi.org/10.1016/S0140-6736(16)32420-5

Cecchini, M., & Warin, L. (2016). Impact of food labelling systems on food choices and eating behaviours: A systematic review and meta-analysis of randomized studies., *17*(3), 201–210. https://doi.org/10.1111/obr.12364

Chen, Y., & Yang, Z. J. (2015). Message formats, numeracy, risk perceptions of Alcohol-attributable cancer, and intentions for binge drinking among college students. *Journal of Drug Education, 45*(1), 37–55. https://doi.org/10.1177/0047237915604062

Cho, Y. J., Thrasher, J. F., Yong, H. H., Szklo, A. S., O'Connor, R. J., Bansal-Travers, M., … Borland, R. (2018). Path analysis of warning label effects on negative emotions and quit attempts: A longitudinal study of smokers in Australia, Canada, Mexico, and the US. *Social Science and Medicine, 197*, 226–234. https://doi.org/10.1016/j.socscimed.2017.10.003

Clarke, N., Pechey, E., Mantzari, E., Blackwell, A. K. M., De-loyde, K., Morris, R., … Hollands, G. J. (2020). Impact of health warning labels communicating the risk of cancer on alcohol selection: An online experimental study. *Addiction*. https://doi.org/10.31234/osf.io/rv2p6

Collymore, N. N., & McDermott, M. R. (2015). Evaluating the effects of six alcohol-related message frames on emotions and intentions: The neglected role of disgust. *Journal of Health Psychology, 21*(9), 1907–1917. https://doi.org/10.1177/1359105314567910

Coomber, K., Jones, S. C., Martino, F., & Miller, P. G. (2016). Predictors of awareness of standard drink labelling and drinking guidelines to reduce negative health effects among Australian drinkers. *Drug and Alcohol Review*. https://doi.org/10.1111/dar.12383

Crockett, R. A., King, S. E., Marteau, T. M., Prevost, A. T., Bignardi, G., Roberts, N. W., … Jebb, S. A. (2018). Nutritional labelling for healthier food or non-alcoholic drink purchasing and consumption. *Cochrane Database of Systematic Reviews, 2*. https://doi.org/10.1002/14651858.CD009315.pub2

de Visser, R. O., & Birch, J. D. (2012). My cup runneth over: Young people's lack of knowledge of low-risk drinking guidelines. *Drug and Alcohol Review, 31*(2), 206–212. https://doi.org/10.1111/j.1465-3362.2011.00371.x

Department of Health. (2011). *Public health responsibility deal: Alcohol pledges*. Retrieved from https://responsibilitydeal.dh.gov.uk/alcohol-pledges/

Department of Health. (2016). *UK chief medical officers' alcohol guidelines review: Summary of the proposed new guidelines*. Retrieved from https://assets.publishing.service.gov.uk/government/uploads/system/uploads/attachment_data/file/489795/summary.pdf

Eurocare. (2012). *Eurocare library of health warning labels*. Retrieved from http://www.eurocare.org/resources/eurocare_papers_and_publications

Eurocare. (2014). *What's not on the bottle? Eurocare reflections on alcohol labelling*. Retrieved from Brussels, Belgium: http://www.eurocare.org/resources/policy_issues/labelling

European Commission. (2006). *Communication from the commission to the council, the European parliament, the European economic and social committee and the committee of the regions: An EU strategy to support member states in reducing alcohol related harm*. Retrieved from https://eur-lex.europa.eu/legal-content/EN/TXT/?uri=celex:52006DC0625

Farke, W. (2011). *Health warnings and responsibility messages on alcoholic beverages – A review of practices in Europe*. Retrieved from Mainz, Germany. http://www.eurocare.org/eu_projects/protect

Food Standards Agency. (2018). *Packaging and labelling. How to label your food packaging products and the legal requirements that you have to follow as a food business*. Retrieved from https://www.food.gov.uk/business-guidance/packaging-and-labelling

Forouzanfar, M. H., Afshin, A., Alexander, L. T., Anderson, H. R., Bhutta, Z. A., Biryukov, S., … Murray, C. J. L. (2016). Global, regional, and national comparative risk assessment of 79 behavioural, environmental and occupational, and metabolic risks or clusters of risks, 1990–2015: A systematic analysis for the global burden of disease study 2015. *The Lancet, 388*(10053), 1659–1724. https://doi.org/10.1016/S0140-6736(16)31679-8

Furtwængler, N. A. F. F., & de Visser, R. O. (2013). Lack of international consensus in low-risk drinking guidelines. *Drug and Alcohol Review, 32*(1), 11–18. https://doi.org/10.1111/j.1465-3362.2012.00475.x

German, J. B., & Walzem, R. L. (2000). The health benefits of wine. *Annual Review of Nutrition, 20*, 561–593. https://doi.org/10.1146/annurev.nutr.20.1.561

Glock, S., & Krolak-Schwerdt, S. (2013). Changing outcome expectancies, drinking intentions, and implicit attitudes toward Alcohol: A comparison of positive

expectancy-related and Health-related Alcohol warning labels. *Applied Psychology. Health and Well-Being, 5*(3), 332–347. https://doi.org/10.1111/aphw.12013
Government of Yukon. (2018). *Northern territories alcohol study to resume*. Retrieved from http://www.gov.yk.ca/news/18-027.html
Hall, M. G., Sheeran, P., Noar, S. M., Ribisl, K. M., Bach, L. E., & Brewer, N. T. (2016). Reactance to health warnings scale: Development and validation. *Annals of Behavioral Medicine*. https://doi.org/10.1007/s12160-016-9799-3
Hammond, D. (2009). *Tobacco labelling & packaging toolkit: A guide to FCTC Article 11*. Retrieved from https://www.who.int/fctc/guidelines/article_11.pdf
Hammond, D. (2011). Health warning messages on tobacco products: A review. *Tobacco Control, 20*(5), 327–337. https://doi.org/10.1136/tc.2010.037630
Hart, C. L., Morrison, D. S., Batty, G. D., Mitchell, R. J., & Davey Smith, G. (2010). Effect of body mass index and alcohol consumption on liver disease: Analysis of data from two prospective cohort studies. *BMJ, 340*. https://doi.org/10.1136/bmj.c1240
Hassan, L., & Shiu, E. (2018). A systematic review of the efficacy of alcohol warning labels: Insights from qualitative and quantitative research in the new millennium. *Journal of Social Marketing, 8*(3), 333–352. https://doi.org/10.1108/JSOCM-03-2017-0020.
Hobin, E., Vallance, K., Zuo, F., Stockwell, T., Rosella, L., Simniceanu, A., … Hammond, D. (2018). Testing the efficacy of Alcohol labels with standard drink information and National Drinking Guidelines on consumers' ability to estimate Alcohol consumption. *Alcohol and Alcoholism, 53*(1), 3–11. https://doi.org/10.1093/alcalc/agx052
IARD, (2019). *Health warning labeling requirements*. London, UK: International Alliance for Responsible Drinking. Retrieved from http://iardwebprod.azurewebsites.net/science-resources/detail/Health-Warning-Labeling-Requirements
Institute for Alcohol Studies. (2018). *Can't handle the proof*. Retrieved from http://www.ias.org.uk/Blog/Cant-handle-the-proof.aspx
Jarvis, W., & Pettigrew, S. (2013). The relative influence of alcohol warning statement type on young drinkers' stated choices. *Food Quality and Preference, 28*(1), 244–252. https://doi.org/10.1016/j.foodqual.2012.08.011
Jarvis, W., Pettigrew, S., & Olaru, D. (2015). *Alcohol warning statement effectiveness under different alcohol category conditions*. Paper presented at the ideas in marketing: Finding the new and polishing the old, Cham.
Jones, S. C., & Gregory, P. (2009). The impact of more visible standard drink labelling on youth alcohol consumption: Helping young people drink (ir)responsibly? *Drug and Alcohol Review, 28*(3), 230–234. https://doi.org/10.1111/j.1465-3362.2008.00020.x
Jones, S. C., & Gregory, P. (2010). Health warning labels on alcohol products – The views of Australian university students. *Contemporary Drug Problems, 37*. https://doi.org/10.1177/009145091003700106

Jongenelis, M., Pratt, I. S., Slevin, T., & Pettigrew, S. (2018). Effectiveness of warning labels at increasing awareness of Alcohol-related cancer risk among heavy drinkers. *Journal of Global Oncology, 4*(supplement 2), 4s–4s. https://doi.org/10.1200/jgo.18.28900.

Kalinowski, A., & Humphreys, K. (2016). Governmental standard drink definitions and low-risk alcohol consumption guidelines in 37 countries. *Addiction, 111*(7), 1293–1298. https://doi.org/10.1111/add.13341

Kees, J., Burton, S., Andrews, J. C., & Kozup, J. (2010). Understanding how graphic pictorial warnings work on cigarette packaging. *Journal of Public Policy & Marketing, 29*(2), 265–276. https://doi.org/10.1509/jppm.29.2.265

Kersbergen, I., & Field, M. (2017). Alcohol consumers' attention to warning labels and brand information on alcohol packaging: Findings from cross-sectional and experimental studies. *BMC Public Health, 17*(1), 123. https://doi.org/10.1186/s12889-017-4055-8

Knai, C., Petticrew, M., Durand, M. A., Eastmure, E., & Mays, N. (2015). Are the public Health responsibility Deal alcohol pledges likely to improve public health? An evidence synthesis. *Addiction, 110*(8), 1232–1246. https://doi.org/10.1111/add.12855

Krischler, M., & Glock, S. (2015). Alcohol warning labels formulated as questions change alcohol-related outcome expectancies: A pilot study. *Addiction Research & Theory, 23*(4), 343–349. https://doi.org/10.3109/16066359.2015.1009829

Laughery, K. R., Vaubel, K. P., Young, S. L., Brelsford, J. W., & Rowe, A. L. (1993). Explicitness of consequence information in warnings. *Safety Science, 16*. https://doi.org/10.1016/0925-7535(93)90025-9

Leigh, B. C., & Stacy, A. W. (2004). Alcohol expectancies and drinking in different age groups. *Addiction, 99*(2), 215–227. https://doi.org/10.1111/j.1360-0443.2003.00641.x

Marteau, T. M., Hollands, G. J., & Fletcher, P. C. (2012). Changing human behavior to prevent disease: The importance of targeting automatic processes. *Science, 337*(6101), 1492. https://doi.org/10.1126/science.1226918

Martin-Moreno, J. M., Harris, M. E., Breda, J., Moller, L., Alfonso-Sanchez, J. L., & Gorgojo, L. (2013). Enhanced labelling on alcoholic drinks: Reviewing the evidence to guide alcohol policy. *European Journal of Public Health, 23*(6), 1082–1087. https://doi.org/10.1093/eurpub/ckt046

Maynard, O. M., Attwood, A. S., O'Brien, L., Brooks, S., Hedge, C., Leonards, U., & Munafò, M. R. (2014). Avoidance of cigarette pack health warnings among regular cigarette smokers. *Drug and Alcohol Dependence, 136*, 170–174.

Maynard, O. M., Langfield, T., Attwood, A. S., Allen, E., Drew, I., Votier, A., & Munafò, M. R. (2017). No impact of calorie or unit information on ad libitum Alcohol consumption. *Alcohol and Alcoholism, 53*(1), 12–19. https://doi.org/10.1093/alcalc/agx066%J

Michie, S., van Stralen, M. M., & West, R. (2011). The behaviour change wheel: A new method for characterising and designing behaviour change interventions. *Implementation Science, 6*, 42. https://doi.org/10.1186/1748-5908-6-42

Miller, E. R., Ramsey, I. J., Baratiny, G. Y., & Olver, I. N. (2016). Message on a bottle: Are alcohol warning labels about cancer appropriate? *BMC Public Health, 16*(1), 1–10. https://doi.org/10.1186/s12889-016-2812-8

Monk, R. L., Pennington, C. R., Campbell, C., Price, A., & Heim, D. (2016). Implicit Alcohol-related expectancies and the effect of context. *Journal of Studies on Alcohol and Drugs, 77*(5), 819–827.

National Health Service. (2018). *Alcohol units*. Retrieved from https://www.nhs.uk/live-well/alcohol-support/calculating-alcohol-units/

National Institute on Alcohol Abuse and Alcoholism. (2019). *What is a standard drink?* Retrieved from https://www.niaaa.nih.gov/alcohol-health/overview-alcohol-consumption/what-standard-drink

Noar, S. M., Hall, M. G., Francis, D. B., Ribisl, K. M., Pepper, J. K., & Brewer, N. T. (2015). Pictorial cigarette pack warnings: A meta-analysis of experimental studies. *Tobacco Control*. https://doi.org/10.1136/tobaccocontrol-2014-051978

ONS. (2010). *Opinions survey report no. 42. Drinking: adults' behaviour and knowledge in* 2009. Retrieved from Newport: UK: http://webarchive.nationalarchives.gov.uk/20151014031149/http://www.ons.gov.uk/ons/rel/lifestyles/drinking%2D%2Dadult-s-behaviour-and-knowledge/2009-report/index.html

Osiowy, M., Stockwell, T., Zhao, J., Thompson, K., & Moore, S. (2015). How much did you actually drink last night? An evaluation of standard drink labels as an aid to monitoring personal consumption. *Addiction Research & Theory, 23*(2), 163–169.

Osman, A., Thrasher, J. F., Yong, H.-H., Arillo-Santillán, E., & Hammond, D. (2017). Disparagement of health warning labels on cigarette packages and cessation attempts: Results from four countries. *Health Education Research, 32*(6), 524–536. https://doi.org/10.1093/her/cyx065%J

Pape, H., Rossow, I., & Brunborg, G. S. (2018). Adolescents drink less: How, who and why? A review of the recent research literature. *Drug and Alcohol Review, 37*, S98–S114.

Pechey, E., Clarke, N., Mantzari, E., Blackwell, A. K. M., De-loyde, K., Morris, R., … Hollands, G. J. (2020). Image-and-text health warning labels on alcohol and food: Potential effectiveness and acceptability. *BMC Public Health, 20*, 376.

Petticrew, M., Douglas, N., Knai, C., Durand, M. A., Eastmure, E., & Mays, N. (2016). Health information on alcoholic beverage containers: Has the alcohol industry's pledge in England to improve labelling been met? Addiction, 111(1), 51–55. doi:https://doi.org/10.1111/add.13094.

Petticrew, M., Maani Hessari, N., Knai, C., & Weiderpass, E. (2018). How alcohol industry organisations mislead the public about alcohol and cancer. *Drug and Alcohol Review, 37*(3), 293–303. https://doi.org/10.1111/dar.12596

Pettigrew, S., Jongenelis, M., Chikritzhs, T., Slevin, T., Pratt, I. S., Glance, D., & Liang, W. (2014). Developing cancer warning statements for alcoholic beverages. *BMC Public Health, 14*(1), 786. https://doi.org/10.1186/1471-2458-14-786

Pettigrew, S., Jongenelis, M. I., Glance, D., Chikritzhs, T., Pratt, I. S., Slevin, T., … Wakefield, M. (2016). The effect of cancer warning statements on alcohol consumption intentions. *Health Education Research, 31*(1), 60–69. https://doi.org/10.1093/her/cyv067

Pham, C., Rundle-Thiele, S., Parkinson, J., & Li, S. (2017). Alcohol warning label awareness and attention: A multi-method study. *Alcohol and Alcoholism, 53*(1), 39–45. https://doi.org/10.1093/alcalc/agx087

Previte, J., Russell-Bennett, R., & Parkinson, J. (2015). Shaping safe drinking cultures: Evoking positive emotion to promote moderate-drinking behaviour. *International Journal of Consumer Studies, 39*(1), 12–24. https://doi.org/10.1111/ijcs.12146

Public Health England. (2016a). *National diet and nutrition survey: Results from years 5 and 6 (combined) of the rolling programme (2012/2013–2013/2014).* Retrieved from https://www.gov.uk/government/statistics/ndns-results-from-years-5-and-6-combined

Public Health England. (2016b). *The public health burden of alcohol and the effectiveness and cost-effectiveness of alcohol control policies. An evidence review.* Retrieved from https://www.gov.uk/government/uploads/system/uploads/attachment_data/file/583047/alcohol_public_health_burden_evidence_review.pdf

Quick, B. L., & Bates, B. R. (2010). The use of gain- or loss-frame messages and efficacy appeals to dissuade excessive Alcohol consumption among college students: A test of psychological reactance theory. *Journal of Health Communication, 15*(6), 603–628. https://doi.org/10.1080/10810730.2010.499593

Reich, R. R., & Goldman, M. S. (2005). Exploring the alcohol expectancy memory network: The utility of free associates. *Psychology of Addictive Behaviors, 19*(3), 317–325. https://doi.org/10.1037/0893-164x.19.3.317

Reynolds, J. P., Pilling, M., & Marteau, T. M. (2018). Communicating quantitative evidence of policy effectiveness and support for the policy: Three experimental studies. *Social Science and Medicine, 218*, 1–12. https://doi.org/10.1016/j.socscimed.2018.09.037

Rosenberg, G., Bauld, L., Hooper, L., Buykx, P., Holmes, J., & Vohra, J. (2017). New national alcohol guidelines in the UK: Public awareness, understanding and behavioural intentions. *Journal of Public Health*, 1–8. https://doi.org/10.1093/pubmed/fdx126

Royal Society for Public Health. (2014). *Increasing awareness of 'invisible' calories from alcohol.* Retrieved from https://www.rsph.org.uk/uploads/assets/uploaded/979245d2-7b5d-4693-a9b3fb1b98b68d76.pdf

Scheideler, J. K., & Klein, W. M. P. (2018). Awareness of the link between alcohol consumption and cancer across the world: A review. *Cancer Epidemiology,*

Biomarkers & Prevention, 27(4), 429–437. https://doi.org/10.1158/1055-9965.EPI-17-0645%J

Sillero-Rejon, C., Attwood, A. S., Blackwell, A. K. M., Ibáñez-Zapata, J. A., Munafò, M. R., & Maynard, O. M. (2018). Alcohol pictorial health warning labels: The impact of self-affirmation and health warning severity. *BMC Public Health, 18*(1), 1403. https://doi.org/10.1186/s12889-018-6243-6

Stafford, L. D., & Salmon, J. (2017). Alcohol health warnings can influence the speed of consumption. *Journal of Public Health, 25*(2), 147–154. https://doi.org/10.1007/s10389-016-0770-3

Steinberg, L., & Scott, E. S. (2003). Less guilty by reason of adolescence: Developmental immaturity, diminished responsibility, and the juvenile death-penalty. *American Psychologist, 58*(12), 1009–1018. https://doi.org/10.1037/0003-066x.58.12.1009

Stevely, A. K., Buykx, P., Brown, J., Beard, E., Michie, S., Meier, P. S., & Holmes, J. (2018). Exposure to revised drinking guidelines and 'COM-B' determinants of behaviour change: Descriptive analysis of a monthly cross-sectional survey in England. *BMC Public Health, 18*(1), 251. https://doi.org/10.1186/s12889-018-5129-y

Stockwell, T. (2006). *A review of research into the impacts of Alcohol warning labels on attitudes and behaviour*. Victoria BC, Canada: Centre for Addictions Research of BC University of Victoria.

Stockwell, T., Blaze-Temple, D., & Walker, C. (1991a). A test of the proposal to label containers of alcoholic drink with alcohol content in standard drinks. *Health Promotion International, 6*(3), 207–215.

Stockwell, T., Blaze-Temple, D., & Walker, C. (1991b). The effect of 'standard drink' labelling on the ability of drinkers to pour a 'standard drink'. *Australian Journal of Public Health, 15*(1), 56–63.

Stockwell, T., Solomon, R., O'Brien, P., Vallance, K., & Hobin, E. (2020). Cancer warning labels on Alcohol containers: A consumer's right to know, a Government's responsibility to inform, and an Industry's power to thwart. *Journal of Studies on Alcohol and Drugs, 81*, 284–292.

Thomson, L. M., Vandenberg, B., & Fitzgerald, J. L. (2012). An exploratory study of drinkers views of health information and warning labels on alcohol containers. *Drug and Alcohol Review, 31*(2), 240–247. https://doi.org/10.1111/j.1465-3362.2011.00343.x

Vallance, K., Romanovska, I., Stockwell, T., Hammond, D., Rosella, L., & Hobin, E. (2017). "We have a right to know": Exploring consumer opinions on content, design and acceptability of enhanced Alcohol labels. *Alcohol and Alcoholism, 53*(1), 20–25. https://doi.org/10.1093/alcalc/agx068%J

Weerasinghe, A., Schoueri-Mychasiw, N., Vallance, K., Stockwell, T., Hammond, D., McGavock, J., … Hobin, E. (2020). Improving knowledge that Alcohol can cause cancer is associated with consumer support for alcohol policies: Findings from a real-world alcohol labelling study. *International Journal of Environmental Research and Public Health, 17*(2), 398.

Wettlaufer, A. (2018). Can a label help me drink in moderation? A review of the evidence on standard drink labelling. *Substance Use and Misuse, 53*(4), 585–595. https://doi.org/10.1080/10826084.2017.1349798

Wettlaufer, A., Cukier, S. N., & Giesbrecht, N. (2017). Comparing Alcohol marketing and Alcohol warning message policies across Canada. *Substance Use and Misuse, 52*(10), 1364–1374. https://doi.org/10.1080/10826084.2017.1281308

Wigg, S., & Stafford, L. D. (2016). Health warnings on alcoholic beverages: Perceptions of the health risks and intentions towards alcohol consumption. *PLoS One, 11*(4), e0153027.

Wilkinson, C., & Room, R. (2009). Warnings on alcohol containers and advertisements: International experience and evidence on effects. *Drug and Alcohol Review, 28*. https://doi.org/10.1111/j.1465-3362.2009.00055.x

Winstock, A. R., Holmes, J., Ferris, J. A., & Davies, E. L. (2019). Perceptions of alcohol health warning labels in a large international cross-sectional survey of people who drink Alcohol. *Alcohol and Alcoholism*. https://doi.org/10.1093/alcalc/agz099

World Health Organization. (2010). *Global strategy to reduce harmful use of alcohol*. Retrieved from https://www.who.int/substance_abuse/activities/gsrhua/en/

World Health Organization. (2017). *Alcohol labelling: A discussion document on policy options*. Retrieved from https://www.eurocare.org/media/GENERAL/docs/reports/2017wh07alcohollabellingfullv2.pdf

World Health Organization. (2018a). *Global health observatory data repository: Health warning labels on alcohol containers by country*. Retrieved from https://apps.who.int/gho/data/view.main.55920

World Health Organization. (2018b). *Global status report on alcohol and health 2018*. Retrieved from https://www.who.int/substance_abuse/publications/global_alcohol_report/en/

World Health Organization. (2018c). *Obesity and overweight*. Retrieved from http://www.who.int/news-room/fact-sheets/detail/obesity-and-overweight

20

Electronic Brief Personalised Feedback Interventions for Alcohol Use

Bridgette M. Bewick, Robert C. Dempsey, John McAlaney, and Helen F. Crosby

Introduction

Developing and implementing effective interventions to prevent and intervene with harmful alcohol use remains imperative if the global burden of alcohol-related harms is to be reduced and the lives of those affected improved. Excessive alcohol consumption remains a significant public health problem. Worldwide, three million deaths every year are attributed to the harmful use of alcohol (World Health Organization (WHO), 2018). Harmful use is linked to 200 health conditions, including liver disease, cardiovascular diseases, and poor mental health (WHO, 2018). The misuse of alcohol has

B. M. Bewick (✉)
School of Medicine, University of Leeds, Leeds, UK
e-mail: b.m.bewick@leeds.ac.uk

R. C. Dempsey
Department of Psychology, Manchester Metropolitan University, Manchester, UK
e-mail: r.dempsey@mmu.ac.uk

J. McAlaney
Faculty of Science and Technology, Bournemouth University, Bournemouth, UK
e-mail: jmcalaney@bournemouth.ac.uk

H. F. Crosby
School of Social and Health Sciences, Leeds Trinity University, Leeds, UK
e-mail: h.crosby@leedstrinity.ac.uk

R. Cooke et al. (eds.), *The Palgrave Handbook of Psychological Perspectives on Alcohol Consumption*, https://doi.org/10.1007/978-3-030-66941-6_20

negative health and social consequences for the individual and wider society. The WHO aims to cut the harmful use of alcohol by 10% by 2025 (WHO, 2018). Recent evidence suggests this target is unlikely to be met; instead, it appears that annual consumption of alcohol globally is on the increase (Manthey et al., 2019).

Brief alcohol interventions offer one means of intervening to reduce and avoid harmful alcohol use. Brief interventions generally include a focus on individuals' beliefs and attitudes, their self-efficacy, and a focus on how an individual's behaviour or attitude compares to other people's (Kaner & Bewick, 2011). Brief alcohol interventions differ in their mode of delivery, intervention content, and duration. For example, they may be delivered in a single (e.g. Acuff et al., 2019) or multiple sessions (e.g. Liu et al., 2011), on an individual (e.g. Carey, Carey, Maisto, & Henson, 2006) or group basis (e.g. Kenney, Napper, LaBrie, & Martens, 2014). They may include personalised normative feedback (e.g. Wilke, Mennicke, Howell, & Magnuson, 2014), motivational interviewing (e.g. Daeppen et al., 2011), or cognitive behavioural therapy (e.g. Marques & Formigoni, 2001). Despite growing evidence for the effectiveness of brief alcohol interventions for reducing harmful alcohol use (Angus, Latimer, Preston, Li, & Purshouse, 2014; Kaner et al., 2009; Platt et al., 2016), their impact on the prevalence of harmful alcohol use is unexpectedly low (Riper et al., 2018). In part this is due to the challenge of successfully implementing brief alcohol interventions. Traditional, human-supported brief alcohol interventions can be costly, labour intensive, and difficult to implement on a large-scale (Carey, Scott-Sheldon, Carey, & DeMartini, 2007). Electronic brief alcohol interventions may address some of these challenges. The aim of this chapter is to review the intervention content, evidence base, effectiveness, future challenges, and opportunities associated with the use of electronic brief interventions for alcohol.

Electronic Brief Alcohol Interventions

The development of the ubiquitous internet affords an opportunity for scalability of electronic brief alcohol interventions, and their availability continues to increase over time (Riper et al., 2011). Time has also seen an increase in the quality of studies, with a marked increase in studies using randomised controlled trials (Cunningham, Khadjesari, Bewick, & Riper, 2010). Electronic brief alcohol interventions provide several opportunities that are difficult to deliver with offline equivalents. For example, they are able to deliver interventions in ways that can be tailored to the individual and reactive to their beliefs and behaviours. This differs from other forms of public health intervention that are more static or passive in nature. For example, a mass media campaign to reduce harmful alcohol consumption through the use of posters and television adverts relies on the targeted individuals being exposed to intervention messages by passing by the poster locations or watching television during the selected television adverts. Even if a mass media campaign saturates the media channels of the target population, there are likely to be periods of time in which individuals will not encounter those media messages. This is largely outside of the control of the organisation or researchers who are delivering the intervention. Similarly, an individually targeted brief alcohol intervention typically requires a relatively high degree of commitment from the target population, such as attendance at a physical location or a fixed time window in which their participation must occur. Whilst this may be simpler to achieve in settings where individuals can to a degree be compelled to take part in activities or when dedicated time can be allocated for an activity this is not always feasible. Electronic brief alcohol interventions provide opportunities to overcome many of these obstacles, by enabling interventions to be delivered in a schedule and format that is set by the researcher or health organisation. This is especially the case if the electronic brief intervention is delivered or facilitated by smartphones, given the ubiquity of smartphone ownership in developed countries and the high frequency with which a typical smartphone user checks their device each day (Deloitte, 2018).

Personalised Feedback

One active ingredient of many electronic brief alcohol interventions is personalised feedback (Prosser, Gee, & Jone, 2018). The tailoring or personalisation of feedback is usually based on user characteristics (e.g. gender; Pedersen, Parast, Marshall, Schell, & Neighbors, 2017) or self-reported behaviour and attitudes (e.g. number of drinks consumed; Ridout & Campbell, 2014). Personalised feedback has been identified by the National Institute on Alcohol Abuse and Alcoholism (NIAAA) as being a component of the most effective strategies to reduce harmful alcohol consumption on college campuses (NIAAA, 2015). Personalised feedback may be effective for several reasons. People are driven to determine how we compare to those around us (Festinger, 1954). Personalised feedback can offer an approximation of how our alcohol consumption compares to others. In the case of social norms-based personalised feedback it may explicitly quantify how one's alcohol use compares to their peers (Dempsey, McAlaney, & Bewick, 2018). People are motivated to seek out both positive and negative social information (Taylor, Bomyea, & Amir, 2010), which can be inferred from any personalised feedback that we may receive about our individual alcohol use. Alcohol use is an example of a behaviour that can be viewed by individuals as both a positive or negative social behaviour (e.g., Chap. 1, Sher, Bartholow, & Nanda, 2001) and, as such, individuals may engage with personalised feedback because they have an expectation of receiving either negative or positive social information.

The process of personalising the response means face-to-face delivery of personalised feedback is resource intensive because it involves asking individuals to report their past alcohol consumption before comparing this to gender-specific, population-level norms, and then feeding back to individuals how their consumption compares to these norms. As a result, it was not initially feasible to deliver human-generated personalised feedback on a larger scale or population level. Thus, at first personalised feedback interventions were only available in person for those accessing specialist services (Borsari & Carey, 2000). Technological advances mean personalised feedback can now be generated and sent automatically to larger groups of participants who may access their feedback more remotely. Complex algorithms instantly take information provided by the user and generate increasingly nuanced personalised feedback based on gender-specific population-level norms. For example, Bewick, Trusler et al. (2008) used data from a previous, university-wide, survey to inform feedback provided to university students in their intervention. Personalised feedback can be delivered as a standalone intervention or integrated with other active ingredients and behaviour change techniques, such as other motivational and self-regulatory interventions described in Chap. 21.

Evidence for Electronic Personalised Feedback Interventions

Population

Providing an aid for early identification, prevention, and intervention, electronic personalised feedback interventions are almost always targeted at individuals with problematic, or at risk of developing problematic drinking behaviour. Electronic personalised feedback interventions are particularly attractive for use in populations where help-seeking behaviour is relatively low, for example, college or university students (Wechsler et al., 2002), emergency department patients (Suffoletto et al., 2015), and military personnel (Miller, DiBellow, Carey, & Pederson, 2018; Pemberton et al., 2011). Electronic personalised interventions are not a substitute for more intensive interventions required to address alcohol dependence. The low-intensity nature of electronic brief alcohol interventions that include personalised feedback render them appropriate for being delivered population-wide—for example, in a workplace (e.g. Doumas & Hannah, 2008).

The majority of studies investigating the effectiveness of electronic brief alcohol interventions that include personalised feedback or electronic personalised interventions have targeted high school (e.g. Ganz et al., 2018) and college/university students (e.g. Bewick et al., 2010; LaBrie et al., 2013). This evidence spans heterogeneous populations, including students from Brazil (Bedendo, Ferri, de Souza, Andrade, & Noto, 2019), Canada (e.g. Thompson, Burgess, & MacNevin, 2018), Germany (e.g. Ganz et al., 2018), New Zealand (e.g. Kypri, Saunders, & Gallagher, 2003), Sweden (e.g. Bendtsen, Bendtsen, Karlsson, White, & McCambridge, 2015), the United Kingdom (e.g. Bewick et al., 2010), and the United States (e.g. Neighbors et al., 2019; Strohman et al., 2016). The research literature has also paid particular attention to subpopulations of students who may be at higher risk for problematic alcohol use, including first-year students (e.g. Doumas & Andersen, 2009), student athletes (e.g. Doumas, Haustveit, & Coll, 2010), mandated college students (e.g. Dunn, Fried-Somerstein, Flori, Hall, & Dvorak, 2019), and students studying abroad (e.g. Pedersen, Neighbors, Atkins, Lee, & Larimer, 2017).

Delivery Mode

Early variants of electronic personalised feedback interventions delivered relatively static content using CD-ROM or PC installed software (Carey, Carey, Maisto, & Henson, 2009). These interventions were quickly superseded by interventions delivered via email and the World Wide Web (e.g., Doumas & Hannah, 2008); the latter now constitutes the majority of electronic personalised feedback interventions tested today. We are, however, seeing the rise of electronic personalised feedback interventions using text messages (e.g. Bernstein et al., 2018; Suffoletto et al., 2015), social networking media (e.g. Facebook; Ridout & Campbell, 2014), and smartphone applications (e.g. Bertholet, Godinho, & Cunningham, 2019; Crane, Garnett, Michie, West, & Brown, 2018). Such approaches reflect the fact that some individuals prefer to receive and complete interventions on their mobile phone or smartphone as opposed to completing an intervention using a desktop or laptop computer.

Duration of Intervention Test

Electronic brief alcohol interventions that include personalised feedback and electronic personalised feedback interventions vary substantially in the length of time users are expected to invest in the intervention. Some interventions are designed as very brief single sessions (e.g. Bewick, Trusler et al. 2008), and others deliver a series of interactions over a relatively brief period of time (e.g. two sets of text messages delivered over two days apart; Suffoletto et al., 2015). Some electronic brief alcohol interventions that include personalised feedback ask users to follow an entirely automated modular programme (e.g. Guillemont et al., 2017; Ingersoll et al., 2018). In a recent superiority randomised control trial, an effective electronic screening and brief intervention that included electronic personalised normative feedback was as effective as an extended internet intervention (Cunningham et al., 2017).

Intervention Content

Electronic personalised feedback interventions, by their very nature, always include some form of alcohol-related personalised feedback. The electronic personalised feedback interventions delivered to date have, however, varied in their use of normative or comparative feedback (e.g. to others' alcohol behaviour or attitudes), the inclusion of additional therapeutic interventions to promote behaviour change, and the targeting of a range of health-related behaviours in addition to alcohol use. Many electronic personalised feedback interventions also incorporate self-monitoring into their intervention design, both of which are established as effective techniques for behaviour change (National Institute for Health and Care Excellence (NICE), 2014).

Interventions based solely on personalised feedback often include personalised normative feedback (e.g. Neighbors et al., 2015). Personalised normative feedback includes information on both the individual's own drinking behaviour/attitude and information on how that behaviour/attitude compares to those in a salient peer group. Electronic personalised normative feedback can be tailored to specific norms, in terms of sex, ethnicity, and other more-context specific social norms (such as affiliation with student societies, e.g. LaBrie et al., 2013). These norms can be descriptive or injunctive norms (McAlaney, Bewick, & Hughes, 2011). Descriptive norms refer to how frequent or common a behaviour is believed to be, such as the perception that an individual has about how frequently and heavily their peers drink alcohol. Injunctive norms refer to beliefs about attitudes, such as if an individual believes their peers to be supportive of drinking alcohol to the point of drunkenness (see Chap. 4 for more on descriptive and injunctive norms). Personalised feedback interventions that do not include these normative comparisons are also available. Such interventions present a summary of the users' own behaviour/attitude without presenting any comparative norms. They may also include information on consequences and behaviour modification techniques.

Personalised feedback is sometimes integrated into electronic brief alcohol interventions that include components from other therapeutic principles (i.e. integrated interventions). A recent review of brief interventions for alcohol use concluded that integrated interventions (that included personalised feedback) were more effective than standalone electronic personalised feedback interventions (Riper et al., 2018); Riper et al.'s review excluded student and pregnant populations and also excluded studies that included low-risk drinkers.

While many electronic brief alcohol interventions that include personalised feedback/electronic personalised feedback interventions target drinking behaviour as experienced on a 'regular' day there is a body of evidence seeking to understand if targeting particular events or occasions could be effective in reducing alcohol-related harms. For example, one could target students who are about to turn 21 years of age (e.g. Bernstein et al., 2018) or those attending Mardi Gras (e.g. Buckner, Neighbors, Walukevich-Dienst, & Young, 2019).

The majority of electronic brief alcohol interventions that include personalised feedback/electronic personalised feedback interventions have alcohol as their only behavioural target. It is however possible to deliver e-interventions that target multiple behaviours. For example, Parekh, King, Boyle, and Vandelanotte (2014) created a computer-tailored intervention that included personalised feedback for diet, smoking, alcohol, physical activity, and body mass index. Aharonovich, Stohl, Cannizzaro, and Hasin (2017) investigated the effectiveness of an intervention to reduce non-injection drug and alcohol use for people living with HIV. The extent to which theoretical underpinnings informed the development of personalised feedback interventions might explain the diversity in intervention targets, messages, and effectiveness.

Theoretical Underpinnings

The normative feedback component of electronic personalised normative feedback interventions is designed to promote change in behaviour and/or attitudes by correcting misperceptions commonly held by heavier consumers of alcohol (Dempsey et al., 2018; McAlaney et al., 2011) consistent with the social norms approach proposed by Perkins and Berkowitz (1986). The greater the misperception between an individual's own behaviour/attitude and the perceived behaviour/attitude of others the more likely the individual is to engage in that behaviour or conform to that perceived attitude (e.g., Neighbors, Dillard, Lewis, Bergstrom, & Neil, 2006). There is extensive evidence that these misperceptions exist for alcohol use and across other health-related behaviours (for a brief review see Dempsey et al., 2018). Electronic personalised feedback aims to challenge these misperceptions, and the implicit social pressure to engage in heavier alcohol use, by highlighting the discrepancy between individual's perceptions and the actual reported norms for that behaviour amongst a relevant social group through personalised feedback (e.g. other student peers at the same university, other employees in your organisation). Reducing this misperception gap, or 'self-other' discrepancy, is considered to be the mechanism underlying many social norms-focused electronic personalised normative feedback interventions (Dempsey et al., 2018). The normative comparison in electronic personalised normative feedback is theorised to motivate heavy drinkers to re-evaluate their use of alcohol and thereby alter their behaviour (Agostinelli & Miller, 1994). Evidences of intervention effects being mediated by changes in perceptions of peer drinking (e.g. Dempsey et al., 2018; Doumas et al., 2010) lend support to this theoretical explanation of how electronic personalised normative feedback interventions work.

It should, however, be noted that many electronic brief alcohol interventions are not explicitly based on an established theoretical model in terms of their development or evaluation, and many provide limited information about their underlying theoretical basis (Miller, Meier, Lombardi, & Leffingwell, 2015; Tebb et al., 2016). Having a clear underpinning theory to electronic personalised normative feedback interventions is important as it accommodates an understanding of what works in an intervention and why (Tebb et al., 2016), facilitates efforts to replicate intervention findings, and also allows for further theory refinement, although many published electronic personalised normative feedback interventions do not attempt the latter (Garnett et al., 2018).

Effectiveness of Electronic Brief Alcohol Interventions with Personalised Feedback

The effectiveness of electronic personalised normative feedback for alcohol use appears to vary according to the specific alcohol use behaviours and setting under scrutiny. By far the most widely studied group in relation to the effectiveness of electronic personalised normative feedback for alcohol use are college or university students, who represent a clearly identifiable social group, who often report excessive alcohol consumption (Davoren, Demant, Shiely, & Perry, 2016), and who can be easily targeted for intervention. There is a growing evidence base for the effectiveness of electronic brief alcohol interventions that include personalised feedback and electronic personalised feedback interventions for modifying student drinking behaviour (Prosser et al., 2018). There are studies that show that interventions are not always successful, however, including a recent paper by Davies, Lonsdale, Hennelly, Winstock, and Foxcroft (2017) that reported no effect of receiving a digital intervention containing personalised feedback on risky drinking in a sample of university students. Hence, there is a need to advance our understanding of how best to target and to tailor these interventions because relatively little is known about what works best and for whom. It may be that, for university students, some interventions are more effective when delivered early on in their university careers (i.e. during freshman/first and sophomore/second years; Strohman et al., 2016). It is known that alcohol consumption varies over university careers, with data from Bewick, Mulhern, et al. (2008) showing that consumption decreases from first year to second year and then further in the final year, while data from Ferrer, Dillard, and Klein (2012) showed that freshmen students' drank more in the first semester than the second semester and followed a similar pattern in their sophomore year. Research to identify patterns of consumption among university students at different points of their academic careers can be used to inform the delivery of interventions (see Chap. 21 for more on this issue).

Multiple studies also suggest that electronic brief alcohol interventions including personalised feedback may be more effective for students who are high-risk drinkers (e.g. Doumas, Esp, Flay, & Bond, 2017). Text message-based electronic personalised normative feedback interventions have also been found to be effective in college student populations. Students who received personalised feedback and interactive text messaging reported significantly greater reductions in likelihood of driving after drinking and a reduction in the number of drinks consumed before driving (Teeters, Soltis, & Murphy, 2018).

Outside university and college campuses, outcomes for workplace-focused electronic personalised normative feedback interventions focused on employee alcohol use have been more mixed. Some studies suggest promising outcomes if recruitment and retention of users can be achieved (e.g. Brendryen, Johansen, Duckert, & Nevsvag, 2017; Pemberton et al., 2011). Other evidence suggests low-intensity electronic personalised feedback interventions are not effective in occupational settings (e.g. Khadjesari, Freemantle, Linke, Hunter, & Murray, 2015). While studies support the feasibility and safety of delivering electronic personalised feedback interventions in an occupational setting, one of the main barriers to successful implementation remains recruitment and retention of users (Brendryen et al., 2017). The relatively low number of trials in occupational settings, combined with the heterogeneity of workplaces and interventions, makes it difficult to draw firm conclusions on the likely effectiveness of electronic personalised feedback interventions in workplace settings.

Results from electronic personalised normative feedback interventions delivered in healthcare settings are also mixed; Johnson et al. (2018) reported no significant effect of an electronic personalised normative feedback intervention delivered to hospital outpatients with hazardous and harmful levels of drinking. Qualitative interviews suggested that participants did not believe their drinking was problematic and expressed a preference for face-to-face treatment by a general practitioner rather than electronic interventions (Johnson et al., 2018). Text message delivered electronic feedback that aimed to increase awareness of drinking intentions and promote goal-setting and goal attainment in order to reduce harmful alcohol use was effective in young adults attending US emergency departments (Suffoletto et al., 2012). The positive intervention effects remained at a nine-month follow-up. The authors concluded that the SMS interactive dialogue intervention was more effective, and importantly more acceptable for this population, than the traditional emergency department setting phone call 'boosters' (e.g. Donovan et al., 2015). This provides an illustration of where electronic personalised feedback interventions could provide an effective alternative to more resource-intensive human-delivered low-level interventions.

Comparatively fewer studies have tested the use of electronic personalised normative feedback interventions at the general population level despite their potential to reach large numbers of the population. One study attempted to recruit participants via an email advertising campaign, with those who were identified as drinking at hazardous levels invited to enrol in a study that included an evaluation of an electronic brief alcohol intervention which incorporated personalised feedback (Guillemont et al., 2017). The study struggled to retain participants, with almost 70% of those allocated to the intervention arm of the study lost to follow-up before completion of baseline. Of those that completed the study, there was evidence that the electronic brief alcohol intervention had a positive impact on weekly alcohol intake and excessive drinking. While promising, these results should be treated with caution due to the high rate of loss to follow-up.

Electronic personalised normative feedback interventions can be targeted towards and personalised for users based on existing alcohol consumption patterns, event-specific drinking behaviours, and/or specific social groups or individuals living or working in a particular geographical location. There is evidence to suggest that electronic personalised normative feedback interventions can be effective in improving alcohol-related outcomes amongst heavier consumers of alcohol, such as heavy drinking first-year intercollegiate athletes (e.g. Doumas et al., 2010) and nightclub patrons classified as high risk (Sanchez & Sanudo, 2018). Targeting electronic personalised normative feedback interventions to those about to encounter a high-risk situation for harmful alcohol use (e.g. a 21st birthday party) can also be an effective strategy (Bernstein et al., 2018), especially for those at higher risk for harmful alcohol consumption.

Given electronic brief alcohol interventions and electronic personalised feedback interventions are often disseminated population-wide (e.g. to all students at a university, to all nightclub patrons), concerns have been raised for the potential for such interventions to have a negative effect on those abstaining from alcohol or drinking at relatively low levels: the so-called boomerang effect (Schultz, Nolan, Cialdini, Goldstein, & Griskevicius, 2007). Worthy of particular scrutiny are personalised normative feedback interventions that could alert participants to their drinking below 'the norm' leading to increases in consumption. A USA study, designed specifically to investigate the existence of the boomerang effect, found no such effect thereby suggesting that personalised normative feedback is not harmful for lighter drinkers (Prince, Reid, Carey, & Neighbors, 2014). Rather, it appears that electronic personalised normative feedback for lighter drinkers and abstainers from alcohol use may have a protective effect against increases in future alcohol use (e.g. Larimer et al., 2007).

While there is growing evidence of the effectiveness of electronic brief alcohol interventions that include personalised feedback for reducing alcohol behaviours, it is not clear if targeting multiple behaviours at once undermines or not the effectiveness of electronic brief alcohol interventions that include personalised feedback/electronic personalised feedback interventions. While some studies report significant improvements in alcohol intake (e.g. Aharonovich et al., 2017; Parekh et al., 2014) others found no significant improvement (e.g. Kypri & McAnally, 2005).

Challenges Associated with Electronic Brief Alcohol Interventions

Whilst there has been a rapid growth in the use of and sophistication of electronic personalised feedback interventions which aim to improve alcohol use outcomes, there remain a number of challenges for the field to address. Despite the growing evidence base for electronic brief alcohol interventions that include personalised feedback and electronic personalised feedback interventions, there remains a relative paucity of information on what motivates individuals to engage with these online programmes under voluntary conditions (Ganz et al., 2018). Studies in the general population often struggle to recruit, retain, and engage participants (e.g. Bertholet et al., 2019; Guillemont et al., 2017), and similar issues with participant attrition have been noted amongst university student samples (Foxcroft, Moreira, Almeida Santimano, & Smith, 2015). If we are to realise the potential for electronic personalised feedback interventions to contribute to reducing the global burden of alcohol misuse we must advance our understanding of how to successfully engage individuals with such interventions.

Studies evaluating the effectiveness of electronic personalised feedback interventions typically focus on the immediate or short-term effects of feedback on alcohol use, with few investigating the longer-term effects of electronic personalised feedback interventions (e.g. Neighbors et al., 2010). Given the typically brief and time-limited nature of personalised normative feedback, it may be additional top-up or booster administrations of brief feedback that are required to maintain positive changes in alcohol use over the medium-to-longer term.

By necessity, many personalised feedback interventions include self-report assessments and self-monitoring components. There remain concerns around the use of self-report data when evaluating the effectiveness of alcohol interventions in general, and those that include personalised feedback and electronic personalised normative feedback (e.g. Dempsey et al., 2018). The field would benefit from the development of objective measures of alcohol use that are widely available, cost-effective, and can be easily integrated into electronic personalised normative feedback interventions. It is likely that self-assessment/self-monitoring is an active ingredient of some personalised feedback interventions (e.g. Bewick et al., 2013; Marley, Bekker, & Bewick, 2016), although the finding of significant reactivity to assessment is not consistent across all trials (e.g. Suffoletto et al., 2015). It may be that where assessment leads to successful self-monitoring, the effect of electronic brief alcohol interventions/

electronic personalised normative feedback interventions is being underestimated. The field would benefit from the inclusion of four-group trial designs, which feature intervention and control groups which receive, or do not receive, baseline assessments (Solomon, 1949), allowing for the potential effects of baseline assessments on behaviour change to be accounted for.

Concerns have also been raised of the potential for personalised feedback to result in a self-report bias due to social desirability. This self-report bias could, it is argued, account partially/solely for the reported reductions in drinking/drinking-related behaviour associated with interventions that include personalised feedback (Cunningham & Wong, 2013).

Future Directions for Research

The development of web-based technologies has enabled the delivery of more personalised feedback interventions for alcohol use, and the increasing sophistication of mobile technologies provides opportunities to extend complexity and reach. Devices, such as smartphones, that are used to deliver electronic brief alcohol interventions have grown increasingly powerful and are able to record a wide range of user data. This data includes not only the direct usage of the device but also other information such as the physical movement of the individual and their geographic location. With regard to alcohol use, for example, it could be possible to use smartphone data to determine how often an individual visits bars, and if so which friends or work colleagues they are most likely to do so with. This type of data collection can occur in the background and requires no effort by the individual, other than providing the initial permissions for this data to be shared with researchers or health experts. This has the potential for opening up new areas of personalised feedback. For example, a system could be created to message an individual when they have spent a certain amount of time in a bar. By working with the individual this message could be personalised to a goal that they set themselves—for instance, a request that they be sent an intervention message suggesting they may wish to go home if the system detects that they have been in a bar for more than two hours. Taken further, such systems could link to other information available through the individual's smartphone. For example, any financial transaction relating to the purchase of alcohol by use of a credit or debit card could be blocked once the individual has spent a predetermined amount of money on alcohol on a night out. Such an approach is already being trialled in relation to problem gambling (Monzo, 2018).

Personalised feedback can also be delivered using systems that not only react to individual behaviour but also predict future states of behaviour through the use of machine learning and artificial intelligence. This approach has been used to predict future suicide attempts with a relatively high degree of accuracy (Walsh, Ribeiro, & Franklin, 2017). For alcohol use e-interventions, the application of machine learning and artifical intelligences may be able to detect when there is about to be an escalation in alcohol consumption, or when an individual may be about to place themselves in a dangerous situation as a result of drunkenness and send personalised feedback to the individual. More routinely, the system could learn the alcohol consumption practices of the individual and identify exactly when to send personalised feedback messages that are the most likely to have a beneficial impact. A system such as this could operate 24 hours a day and take action in the absence of any human operator, although this is not to say that such systems should be left completely unsupervised by human experts.

Conclusion

Electronic personalised feedback interventions are under-utilised in general population samples despite evidence they are effective when delivered to college or university student samples. Web-based personalised feedback interventions have facilitated greater personalisation of feedback towards specific target groups—often based on personalised normative feedback. Research is needed to develop the theory base for these interventions, thus making it difficult to identify active ingredients and effective treatment mechanisms. Advances in mobile technology and the internet-of-things hold promise for the development of more sophisticated interventions and the collection of alcohol-related behaviours in addition to self-report measures. Realising the potential for new technologies to increase the effectiveness and successful implementation of personalised feedback will allow us to intervene early and thereby contribute to a reduction in the global burden of alcohol-related harms and improve the lives of those affected.

References

Acuff, S. F., Voss, A. T., Dennhardt, A. A., Borsari, B., Martens, M. P., & Murphy, J. G. (2019). Brief motivational interventions are associated with reductions in alcohol-induced blackouts among heavy drinking college students. *Alcoholism: Clinical and Experimental Research, 43*, 988–996.

Agostinelli, G., & Miller, W. R. (1994). Drinking and thinking: How does personal drinking affect judgments of prevalence and risk. *Journal of Studies on Alcohol, 55*, 327–337.

Aharonovich, E., Stohl, M., Cannizzaro, D., & Hasin, D. (2017). HealthCall delivered via smartphone to reduce co-occurring drug and alcohol use in HIV-infected adults: A randomized pilot trial. *Journal of Substance Abuse Treatment, 83*, 15–26.

Angus, C., Latimer, N., Preston, L., Li, J., & Purshouse, R. (2014). What are the implications for policy makers? A systematic review of the cost-effectiveness of screening and brief interventions for alcohol misuse in primary care. *Frontiers in Psychiatry, 5*, 114.

Bedendo, A., Ferri, C. P., de Souza, A. A. L., Andrade, A. L. M., & Noto, A. R. (2019). Pragmatic randomized controlled trial of a web-based intervention for alcohol use among Brazilian college students: Motivation as a moderating effect. *Drug and Alcohol Dependence, 199*, 92–100.

Bendtsen, P., Bendtsen, M., Karlsson, N., White, I. R., & McCambridge, J. (2015). Online alcohol assessment and feedback for hazardous and harmful drinkers: Findings from the AMADEUS-2 randomised controlled trial of routine practice in Swedish universities. *Journal of Medical Internet Research, 17*(7), e170.

Bernstein, M. H., Stein, L. A. R., Neighbors, C., Suffoletto, B., Carey, K. B., Ferszt, G., … Wood, M. D. (2018). A text message intervention to reduce 21st birthday alcohol consumption: Evaluation of a two-group randomized controlled trial. *Psychology of Addictive Behaviors, 32*(2), 149–161.

Bertholet, N., Godinho, A., & Cunningham, J. A. (2019). Smartphone application for unhealthy alcohol use: Pilot randomized controlled trial in the general population. *Drug and Alcohol Dependence, 195*, 101–105.

Bewick, B. M., Mulhern, B., Barkham, M., Trusler, K., Hill, A. J., & Stiles, W. B. (2008). Changes in undergraduate student alcohol consumption as they progress through university. *BMC Public Health, 8*, 163–170.

Bewick, B. M., Trusler, K., Mulhern, B., Barkham, M., & Hill, A. J. (2008). The feasibility and effectiveness of a web-based personalised feedback and social norms alcohol intervention in UK university students: A randomised control trial. *Addictive Behaviors, 33*(9), 1192–1198.

Bewick, B. M., West, R. M., Barkham, M., Mulhern, B., Marlow, R., Traviss, G., & Hill, A. J. (2013). The effectiveness of a web-based personalised feedback and social norms alcohol intervention on United Kingdom university students: Randomized controlled trial. *Journal of Medical Internet Research, 15*(7), e137.

Bewick, B. M., West, R. M., Gill, J., O'May, F., Mulhern, B., Barkham, M., & Hill, A. J. (2010). Providing web-based feedback and social norms information to reduce student alcohol intake: A multisite investigation. *Journal of Medical Internet Research, 12*(5), e59.

Borsari, B., & Carey, K. B. (2000). Effects of a brief motivational intervention with college student drinkers. *Journal of Consulting and Clinical Psychology, 68*(4), 728–733.

Brendryen, H., Johansen, A., Duckert, F., & Nevsvag, S. (2017). A pilot randomised controlled trial of an internet-based alcohol intervention in a workplace setting. *International Journal of Behavioral Medicine, 24*(5), 768–777.

Buckner, J. D., Neighbors, C., Walukevich-Dienst, K., & Young, C. M. (2019). Online personalized normative feedback intervention to reduce event-specific drinking during Mardi Gras. *Experimental and Clinical Psychopharmacology*. https://doi.org/10.1037/pha0000259

Carey, K. B., Carey, M. P., Maisto, S. A., & Henson, J. M. (2006). Brief motivational interventions for heavy college drinkers: A randomized controlled trial. *Journal of Consulting and Clinical Psychology, 74*(5), 943–954. https://doi.org/10.1037/0022-006X.74.5.943

Carey, K. B., Carey, M. P., Maisto, S. A., & Henson, J. M. (2009). Computer versus in-person intervention for students violating campus alcohol policy. *Journal of Consulting and Clinical Psychology, 77*(1), 74–87.

Carey, K. B., Scott-Sheldon, L. A., Carey, M. P., & DeMartini, K. S. (2007). Individual-level interventions to reduce college student drinking: A meta-analysis review. *Addictive Behaviors, 32*(11), 2469–2494.

Crane, D., Garnett, C., Michie, S., West, R., & Brown, J. (2018). A smartphone app to reduce excessive alcohol consumption: Identifying the effectiveness of intervention components in a factorial randomised control trial. *Scientific Reports, 8*(1), 4384.

Cunningham, J. A., Khadjesari, Z., Bewick, B. M., & Riper, H. (2010). Internet-based interventions for problem drinkers: From efficacy trials to implementation. *Drug and Alcohol Review, 29*(6), 617–622.

Cunningham, J. A., Shorter, G. W., Murphy, M., Kushnir, V., Rehm, J., & Hendershot, C. S. (2017). Randomized controlled trial of a brief versus extended internet intervention for problem drinkers. *International Journal of Behavioural Medicine, 24*(5), 760–767.

Cunningham, J. A., & Wong, H. T. A. (2013). Assessing the immediate impact of normative drinking information using an immediate post-test randomized controlled design: Implications for normative feedback interventions. *Addictive Behaviors, 38*, 2252–2256.

Daeppen, J. B., Bertholet, N., Gaume, J., Fortini, C., Faouzi, M., & Gmel, G. (2011). Efficacy of brief motivational intervention in reducing binge drinking in young men: A randomized controlled trial. *Drug and Alcohol Dependence, 13*, 69–75.

Davies, E. L., Lonsdale, A. J., Hennelly, S. E., Winstock, A. R., & Foxcroft, D. R. (2017). Personalized digital interventions showed no impact on risky drinking in Young adults: A pilot randomized controlled trial. *Alcohol and Alcoholism*, 1-6. https://doi.org/10.1093/alcalc/agx051

Davoren, M. P., Demant, J., Shiely, F., & Perry, I. J. (2016). Alcohol consumption among university students in Ireland and the United Kingdom from 2002 to 2014: A systematic review. *BMC Public Health, 16*(1), 173.

Deloitte. (2018). *Global mobile consumer survey: US edition.* Available from: https://www2.deloitte.com/content/dam/Deloitte/us/Documents/technology-media-telecommunications/us-tmt-global-mobile-consumer-survey-exec-summary-2018.pdf. Accessed 16 July 2019.

Dempsey, R. C., McAlaney, J., & Bewick, B. M. (2018). A critical appraisal of the social norms approach as an interventional strategy for health-related behaviour and attitude change. *Frontiers in Psychology, 9*, 2180.

Donovan, D. M., Hatch-Maillette, M. A., Phares, M. S. W., McGarry, E., Peavey, K. M., & Taborsky, J. (2015). Lessons learned from follow-up phone booster counselling calls with substance abusing emergency department patients. *Journal of Substance Abuse Treatment, 50*, 67–75. https://doi.org/10.1016/j.jsat.2014.10.013.

Doumas, D., Esp, S., Flay, B., & Bond, L. (2017). A randomized controlled trial testing the efficacy of a brief online alcohol intervention for high school seniors. *Journal of Studies on Alcohol and Drugs, 78*(5), 706–715.

Doumas, D. M., & Andersen, L. L. (2009). Reducing alcohol use in first-year university students: Evaluation of a web-based personalized feedback program. *Journal of College Counselling, 12*, 18–32.

Doumas, D. M., & Hannah, E. (2008). Preventing high-risk drinking in youth in the workplace: A web-based normative feedback program. *Journal of Substance Abuse Treatment, 34*(3), 263–271.

Doumas, D. M., Haustveit, T., & Coll, K. M. (2010). Reducing heavy drinking among first year intercollegiate athletes: A randomised controlled trial of web-based normative feedback. *Journal of Applied Sport Psychology, 22*(3), 247–261.

Dunn, M. E., Fried-Somerstein, A., Flori, J. N., Hall, T. V., & Dvorak, R. D. (2019). Reducing alcohol use in mandated college students: A comparison of a brief motivational intervention (BMI) and the expectancy challenge alcohol literacy curriculum (ECALC). *Experimental and Clinical Psychopharmacology.* https://doi.org/10.1037/pha0000290

Ferrer, R. A., Dillard, A. J., & Klein, W. M. P. (2012). Projection, conformity, and deviance regulation: A prospective study of alcohol use. *Psychology and Health, 27*(6), 688–703.

Festinger, L. (1954). A theory of social comparison processes. *Human Communications, 7*, 117–140.

Foxcroft, D. R., Moreira, M. T., Almeida Santimano, N. M. L., & Smith, L. A. (2015). Social norms information for alcohol misuse in university and college students. *The Cochrane Database of Systematic Reviews, 1*, CD006748. https://doi.org/10.1002/14651858.CD006748.pub3

Ganz, T., Braun, M., Laging, M., Schermelleh-Engel, K., Michalak, J., & Heidenreich, T. (2018). Effects of a stand-alone web-based electronic screening and brief intervention targeting alcohol use in university students of legal drinking age: A randomized controlled trial. *Addictive Behaviours, 77*, 81–88.

Garnett, C., Crane, D., Brown, J., Kaner, E., Beyer, F., Muirhead, C., … Michie, S. (2018). Reported theory use by digital interventions for hazardous and harmful alcohol consumption, and association with effectiveness: Meta-regression. *Journal of Medical Internet Research, 20*(2), e69.

Guillemont, J., Cogordan, C., Nalpas, B., Nguyen-Thanh, V., Richard, J.-B., & Arwidson, P. (2017). Effectiveness of a web-based intervention to reduce alcohol consumption among French hazardous drinkers: A randomized controlled trial. *Health Education Research, 32*(4), 332–342.

Ingersoll, K., Frederick, C., MacDonnell, K., Ritterband, L., Lord, H., Jones, B., & Truwit, B. S. (2018). A pilot RCT on an internet intervention to reduce the risk of alcohol-exposed pregnancy. *Alcohol Clinical Experimental Research, 42*(6), 1132–1144.

Johnson, N. A., Kypri, K., Latter, J., Dunlop, A., Brown, A., Saitz, R., … McCambridge, J. (2018). Effect of electronic brief intervention on uptake of speciality treatment in hospital outpatients with likely alcohol dependence: Pilot randomized trial and qualitative interviews. *Drug and Alcohol Dependence, 183*, 253–260.

Johnson, N. A., Kypri, K., Saunders, J. B., Saitz, R., Attia, J., Latter, J. L., … McCambridge, J. (2018). Effect of electronic screening and brief intervention on hazardous or harmful drinking among adults in the hospital outpatient setting: A randomized, double-blind, controlled trial. *Drug and Alcohol Dependence, 191*, 78–85.

Kaner, E., Dickinson, H., Beyer, F., Muirhead, C., Campbell, F., Pienaar, E. D., … Burnard, B. (2009). The effectiveness of brief alcohol interventions in primary care settings: A comprehensive review. *Drug Alcohol Review, 28*, 301–323.

Kaner, E. F. S., & Bewick, B. M. (2011). Brief alcohol intervention in young people. In J. B. Saunders & J. M. Rey (Eds.), *Young people and alcohol: Impact, policy, prevention, treatment* (pp. 153–169). West Sussex, UK: Blackwell Publishing.

Kenney, S. R., Napper, L. E., LaBrie, J. W., & Martens, M. P. (2014). Examining the efficacy of a brief group protective behavioral strategies skills training alcohol intervention with college women. *Psychology of Addictive Behaviors, 28*(4), 1041–1051.

Khadjesari, Z., Freemantle, N., Linke, S., Hunter, R., & Murray, E. (2015). Correction: Health on the web: Randomised controlled trial of online screening and brief alcohol intervention delivered in a workplace setting. *PLoS One, 10*(4), e0127371.

Kypri, K., & McAnally, H. M. (2005). Randomized controlled trial of a web-based primary care intervention for multiple health risk behaviors. *Preventive Medicine, 41*(3–4), 761–176.

Kypri, K., Saunders, J. B., & Gallagher, S. (2003). Acceptability of various brief intervention approaches for hazardous drinking among university students. *Alcohol and Alcoholism, 38*(6), 626–628.

LaBrie, J. W., Lewis, M. A., Atkins, D. C., Neighbors, C., Zheng, C., Kenney, S. R., … Larimer, M. E. (2013). RCT of web-based personalized normative feedback for college drinking prevention: Are typical student norms good enough? *Journal of Consulting and Clinical Psychology, 81*, 1074–1086.

Larimer, M. E., Lee, C. M., Kilmer, J. R., Fabiano, P. M., Stark, C. B., Geisner, I. M., et al. (2007). Personalized mailed feedback for college drinking prevention: A randomized clinical trial. *Journal of Consulting and Clinical Psychology, 75*, 285–293.

Liu, S., Wu, S., Chen, S., Huang, H., Sun, F., Fang, C., … Shih, S. (2011). Randomized controlled trial of a brief intervention for unhealthy alcohol use in hospitalized Taiwanese men. *Addiction, 106*, 928–940. https://doi.org/10.1111/j.1360-0443.2010.03330.x

Manthey, J., Shield, K. D., Rylett, M., Hasan, O. S. M., Probst, C., & Rehm, J. (2019). Global alcohol exposure between 1990 and 2017 and forecasts until 2030: A modelling study. *The Lancet, 393*(10190), 2493–2502.

Marley, S., Bekker, H. L., & Bewick, B. M. (2016). Responding to personalised social norms feedback from a web-based alcohol reduction intervention for students: Analysis of think-aloud verbal protocols. *Psychology & Health, 31*(9), 1007–1024.

Marques, A. C., & Formigoni, M. L. (2001). Comparison of individual and group cognitive-behavioral therapy for alcohol and/or drug-dependent patients. *Addiction, 96*, 835–846.

McAlaney, J., Bewick, B., & Hughes, C. (2011). The international development of the 'social norms' approach to drug education and prevention. *Drugs: Education, Prevention, and Policy, 18*(2), 81–89.

Miller, M. B., DiBellow, A. M., Carey, K. B., & Pederson, E. R. (2018). Blackouts as a moderator of young adult veteran response to personalized normative feedback for heavy drinking. *Alcoholism: Clinical and Experimental Research, 42*(6), 1145–1153.

Miller, M. B., Meier, E., Lombardi, N., & Leffingwell, T. R. (2015). Theories of behaviour change and personalised feedback interventions for college student drinking. *Addiction Research and Theory, 23*(4), 322–335.

Monzo. (2018). *Supporting people to self-exclude from gambling*. Available from: https://monzo.com/blog/2018/05/16/gambling-self-exclusion. Accessed 16 July 2019.

National Institute for Health and Care Excellence (NICE). (2014). *Behaviour change: Individual approaches (Public Health Guideline PH49)*. Available from: http://www.nice.org.uk/guidance/ph49/chapter/about-this-guidance. Accessed 28 July 2019.

National Institute on Alcohol Abuse and Alcoholism (NIAAA). (2015). *College AIM: Alcohol intervention matrix*. Available from: https://www.collegedrinkingprevention.gov/CollegeAIM/Default.aspx. Accessed 16 July 2019.

Neighbors, C., DiBello, A. M., Young, C. M., Steers, M.-L. N., Rinker, D. V., Rodriguez, L. M., … Lewis, M. A. (2019). Personalized normative feedback for heavy drinking: An application of deviance regulation theory. *Behaviour Research and Therapy, 115*, 73–82.

Neighbors, C., Dillard, A. J., Lewis, M. A., Bergstrom, R. L., & Neil, T. A. (2006). Normative misperceptions and temporal precedence of perceived norms and drinking. *Journal of Studies on Alcohol, 67*, 290–299.

Neighbors, C., Lewis, M. A., Atkins, D. C., Jensen, M. M., Walter, T., Fossos, N., … Larimer, M. E. (2010). Efficacy of web-based personalized normative feedback: A two-year randomized controlled trial. *Journal of Consulting and Clinical Psychology, 78*(6), 898–911.

Neighbors, C., Rodriguez, L. M., Rinker, D. V., Gonzales, R. G., Agana, M., Tackett, J. L., & Foster, D. W. (2015). Efficacy of personalized normative feedback as a brief intervention for college student gambling: A randomized controlled trial. *Journal of Consulting and Clinical Psychology, 83*(3), 500–511.

Parekh, S., King, D., Boyle, F. M., & Vandelanotte. (2014). Randomized controlled trial of a computer-trailed multiple health behaviour intervention in general practice: 12-month follow-up results. *International Journal of Behavioural Nutrition and Physical Activity, 11*, 41.

Pedersen, E. R., Neighbors, C., Atkins, D. C., Lee, C. M., & Larimer, M. E. (2017). Brief online interventions targeting risk and protective factors for increased and problematic alcohol use among American college students studying abroad. *Psychology of Addictive Behaviors, 31*(2), 220–230.

Pedersen, E. R., Parast, L., Marshall, G. N., Schell, T. L., & Neighbors, C. (2017). A randomized controlled trial of a web-based personalized normative feedback alcohol intervention for young-adult veterans. *Journal of Consulting and Clinical Psychology, 85*(5), 459–470.

Pemberton, M. R., Williams, J., Herman-Stahl, M., Calvin, S. L., Bradshaw, M. R., Bray, R. M., … Mitchell, G. M. (2011). Evaluation of two web-based alcohol interventions in the U.S. military. *Journal of Studies Alcohol and Drugs, 72*(3), 480–489.

Perkins, H. W., & Berkowitz, A. D. (1986). Perceiving the community norms of alcohol use among students: some research implications for campus alcohol education programming. *International Journal of the Addictions, 21*, 243–256.

Platt, L., Melendez-Torres, G. J., O'Donnell, A., Bradley, J., Newbury-Birch, D., Kaner, E., & Aston, C. (2016). How effective are brief interventions in reducing alcohol consumption: Do the setting, practitioner group and content matter? Findings from a systematic review and meta regression analysis. *BMJ Open, 6*, e011473. https://doi.org/10.1136/bmjopen-2016-011473

Prince, M. A., Reid, A., Carey, K. B., & Neighbors, C. (2014). Effects of normative feedback for drinkers who consume less than the norm: Dodging the boomerang. *Psychology of Addictive Behaviours, 28*(2), 538–544.

Prosser, T., Gee, K. A., & Jone, F. (2018). A meta-analysis of effectiveness of e-interventions to reduce alcohol consumption in college and university students. *Journal of American College Health, 66*(4), 292–301.

Ridout, B., & Campbell, A. (2014). Using Facebook to deliver a social norm intervention to reduce problem drinking at university. *Drug & Alcohol Review, 33*, 667–673.

Riper, H., Hoogendoorn, A., Cuijper, P., Karyotaki, E., Boumparis, N., Mira, A., … Smit, J. H. (2018). Effectiveness and treatment moderators of internet interventions for adult problem drinking: An individual patient data meta-analysis of 19 randomised controlled trials. *PLoS Medicine, 15*(12), e1002714.

Riper, H., Spek, V., Boon, B., Conijn, B., Kramer, J., Martin-Abello, K., & Smit, F. (2011). Effectiveness of e-self-help interventions for curbing adult problem drinking: A meta-analysis. *Journal of Medical Internet Research, 13*(2), e42.

Sanchez, Z. M., & Sanudo, A. (2018). Web-based alcohol intervention for nightclub patrons: Opposite effects according to baseline alcohol use disorder classification. *Substance Abuse, 39*(3), 361–370.

Schultz, P. W., Nolan, J. M., Cialdini, R. B., Goldstein, N. J., & Griskevicius, V. (2007). The constructive, destructive, and reconstructive power of social norms. *Psychological Science, 18*(5), 429–434.

Sher, K. J., Bartholow, B. D., & Nanda, S. (2001). Short- and long-term effects of fraternity and sorority membership on heavy drinking: A social norms perspective. *Psychology of Addictive Behaviors, 15*(1), 42–51.

Solomon, R. L. (1949). An extension of control group design. *Psychological Bulletin, 46*, 137–150.

Strohman, A. S., Braje, S. E., Alhassoon, O. M., Shuttleworth, S., Van Slyke, J., & Gandy, S. (2016). Randomized controlled trial of computerized alcohol intervention for college students: Role of class level. *American Journal of Drug and Alcohol Abuse, 42*(1), 15–24.

Suffoletto, B., Callaway, C., Kristan, J., Kraemer, K., & Clark, D. B. (2012). Text-message-based drinking assessments and brief interventions for young adults discharged from theemergency department. *Alcohol Clin Exp Res, 36*, 552–560. https://doi.org/10.1111/j.1530-0277.2011.01646.x.

Suffoletto, B., Kristan, J., Chung, T., Jeong, K., Fabio, M., & P., & Clark, D.B. (2015). An interactive text message intervention to reduce binge drinking in young adults: A randomised controlled trial with 9-month outcomes. *PLoS One, 10*(11), e0142877.

Taylor, C. T., Bomyea, J., & Amir, N. (2010). Attentional bias away from positive social information mediates the link between social anxiety and anxiety vulnerability to a social stressor. *Journal of Anxiety Disorders, 24*(4), 403–408.

Tebb, K. P., Erenrich, R. K., Bradner-Jasik, C., Berna, M. S., Lester, J. C., & Ozer, E. M. (2016). Use of theory in computer-based interventions to reduce alcohol use among adolescents and young adults: A systematic review. *BMC Public Health, 16*, 517.

Teeters, J. B., Soltis, K. E., & Murphy, J. G. (2018). A mobile phone-based brief intervention with personalized feedback and text messaging is associated with reductions in driving after drinking among college drinkers. *Journal of Studies on Alcohol and Drugs, 79*(5), 710–719.

Thompson, K., Burgess, J., & MacNevin, P. D. (2018). An evaluation of e-CHECKUPTOGO in Canada: The mediating role of changes in social norm misperceptions. *Substance Use and Misuse, 53*(11), 1849–1858.

Walsh, C. G., Ribeiro, J. D., & Franklin, J. C. (2017). Predicting risk of suicide attempts over time through machine learning. *Clinical Psychological Science, 5*(3), 457–469.

Wechsler, H., Lee, J. E., Kuo, M., Seibring, M., Nelson, T. F., & Lee, H. (2002). Trends in college binge drinking during a period of increased prevention efforts: Findings from 4 Harvard School of Public Health College alcohol study surveys: 1993–2001. *Journal of American College Health, 50*, 203–217.

Wilke, D. J., Mennicke, A., Howell, R. L., & Magnuson, A. B. (2014). A peer-facilitated intervention to reduce risky drinking among fraternity and sorority members. *Journal of Social Work Practice in the Addictions, 14*(1), 42–63.

World Health Organization. (2018). *Global status report on alcohol and health 2018*. Geneva, Switzerland: WHO. Licence: CC BY-NC-SA 3.0 IGO.

21

Motivational and Self-Regulatory Interventions to Reduce Alcohol Consumption

Richard Cooke, Dominic Conroy, and Martin S. Hagger

Introduction

Excessive alcohol consumption is associated with health risks (e.g., risks of injury, illness), social problems (e.g., social disorder, absenteeism, presenteeism, and reduced productivity), and economic costs (e.g., medical costs of treating injuries associated with alcohol, policing of social disorder; Gell, Ally, Buykx, Hope, & Meyer, 2015). Governments and policymakers have therefore committed to reducing population-level alcohol consumption to

R. Cooke (✉)
Department of Psychology, University of Liverpool, Liverpool, UK

Liverpool Centre for Alcohol Research, Liverpool, UK
e-mail: cooker4@liverpool.ac.uk

D. Conroy
School of Psychology, University of East London, London, UK
e-mail: d.conroy@uel.ac.uk

M. S. Hagger
Department of Psychological Sciences, University of California, Merced, Merced, CA, USA

Faculty of Sport and Health Sciences, University of Jyväskylä, Jyväskylä, Finland
e-mail: mhagger@merced.edu

R. Cooke et al. (eds.), *The Palgrave Handbook of Psychological Perspectives on Alcohol Consumption*, https://doi.org/10.1007/978-3-030-66941-6_21

moderate levels to address these problems and reduce the associated costs (World Health Organization, 2010). Alongside policy measures, such as increasing the price of alcohol, raising the legal purchase age, or restricting the number alcohol outlets, behavioural interventions can be used to promote moderate alcohol consumption. Behavioural and social scientists, including psychologists, can play an integral role in informing the development of such interventions by (1) identifying the determinants of alcohol consumption, (2) developing an evidence base of determinants and potential moderating factors, and (3) using this evidence base to inform the content of interventions targeting a reduction in alcohol consumption.

This chapter provides an overview of how psychological theories of motivation and self-regulation have been applied to inform interventions aimed at reducing alcohol consumption. Such interventions have been developed on the basis that motivation and self-regulation capacity represent broad sets of modifiable determinants of excessive alcohol consumption. Psychological theories have guided identification of these determinants and helped to inform interventions designed to reduce excessive alcohol consumption patterns such as heavy episodic drinking (HED; see Chap. 1) and pre-drinking (see Chap. 13). In the next section, we briefly review theories that have identified determinants of excessive alcohol consumption such as HED and provided targets for interventions. This discussion is limited to providing an overview of how these theories have informed the development of motivational interventions (see Chap. 2 for a more detailed discussion of theories).

Psychological Theories of Motivation

Several psychological theories of motivation have been applied to predict alcohol consumption, including Cox and Klinger's (1988) incentive motivation model, Ajzen's (1991) theory of planned behaviour (TPB), and Gibbons and Gerrard's (1995) prototype willingness model (PWM). They all propose that when faced with the decision to drink alcohol or not, individuals weigh up different factors before deciding whether or not to act—a reasoned, deliberative process. For example, the TPB states that the proximal determinant of any action is a person's intention to act or not. Accordingly, people who intend to drink alcohol should be more likely to do so compared with people who do not intend to drink alcohol. Therefore, one approach to reduce alcohol consumption in an individual with a strong intention to drink is to deliver an intervention that modifies the determinants of their intentions. In the TPB, there are three such determinants: attitudes (i.e., positive or negative evaluations of the focal behaviour), subjective norms (i.e., perceptions of approval or disapproval from significant others if one performed the focal behaviour), and perceived behavioural control (PBC, perceptions of control over performing the behaviour). The TPB posits that these constructs determine intentions which, in turn, determine behaviour. The proposed pattern of model effects has been consistently supported in studies applying the TPB to predict alcohol consumption (Cooke, Dahdah, Norman, & French, 2016; Hagger, Chan, Protogerou, & Chatzisarantis, 2016; Hagger, Polet, & Lintunen, 2018).

Extrapolating from the predictions of the TPB, targeting change in attitudes, subjective norms, and PBC, is central to effecting change in intentions and reducing alcohol consumption (Sheeran, Klein, & Rothman, 2017; Steinmetz, Knappstein, Ajzen, Schmidt, & Kabst, 2016). For example, an intervention might present a persuasive message that emphasises (1) the negative aspects of HED (targeting attitude change), (2) important others' disapproval of HED (targeting subjective norm change), and (3) the extent to which HED can be controlled (targeting PBC change). Consistent with the TPB, effecting change in these constructs should result in a concomitant change in intentions, and changing intentions should ultimately reduce HED. This example illustrates how psychological theories that have been used to identify determinants of HED may be used to inform the development of interventions. In the next section, we provide an overview of the process by which theory-based interventions to reduce alcohol consumption are developed.

Designing Theory-Based Interventions to Reduce Alcohol Consumption

Developing effective interventions to reduce alcohol consumption is a particularly challenging endeavour given that consumption is both culturally entrenched, and socially and bio-chemically reinforced. Changing consumption patterns, therefore, may mean breaking strong bonds between drinking alcohol and the socio-cultural and environmental contexts in which the behaviour is enacted (Hagger, 2020; see Section "Psychological Theories of Motivation"). In addition, as with many appetitive behaviours like eating palatable foods, consuming alcohol is highly reinforced through endogenous reward systems (Gilpin & Koob, 2008). These strong links mean that alcohol consumption is likely to be a habitual and highly automatised behaviour for many social drinkers (Hamilton, Gibbs, Keech, & Hagger, 2020). As a consequence, altering drinking patterns requires individuals to possess considerable motivation and self-regulatory skills that are effective in the face of strong cues to enact habitual behaviours, or requires altering the presentation, pervasiveness, or prevalence of environmental cues linked to behavioural enactment (see Section "Psychological Theories of Motivation"; Gardner, Rebar, & Lally, 2020; Hagger, 2019).

The basic model illustrated in Fig. 21.1 outlines the process of a behaviour change intervention as specified in the motivational theories identified earlier. Behaviour change interventions are often designed to focus on psychological mediators of behaviour (e.g., intention, as described in the previous section). As such, behaviour change interventions are assumed to work by modifying the theory-based constructs which serve, ultimately, to change behaviour itself (Hagger, Cameron, Hamilton, Hankonen, & Lintunen, 2020; Hagger, Moyers, McAnally, & McKinley, 2020; Rothman, Klein, & Sheeran, 2020; Sheeran et al., 2017). Identification of theory-based determinants is a critical first step in developing interventions to reduce excessive patterns of alcohol consumption like HED. Once the determinants of HED have been

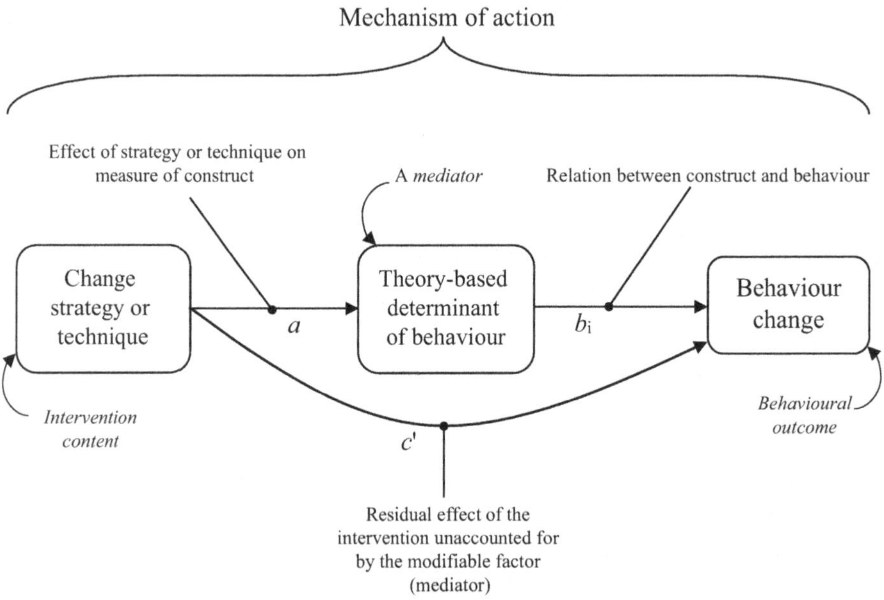

Fig. 21.1 Diagram of a basic model of a behaviour change mechanism of action (Hagger, 2019; Hagger, Moyers, et al., 2020). A behaviour change method or technique is proposed to relate to behaviour change through changes in modifiable theory-based determinants

identified, the next step is to match them with appropriate strategies or techniques, represented by link 'a' in Fig. 21.1.

The emergence of behaviour change taxonomies has provided a common set of definitions and descriptions of the individual behaviour change strategies or *techniques* that make up behavioural interventions. The taxonomies outline the tools necessary to provide clear, consistent, and coherent descriptions of the content of interventions delivered in the field of alcohol research (see Michie et al., 2012, for further discussion). Recently, such work has been extended in efforts to develop an organised network of links between techniques and theory-based determinants, which form the *mechanisms of action* of behaviour change interventions (Carey et al., 2018; Connell et al., 2019; Hagger, Moyers, et al., 2020; Rothman et al., 2020). These advances provide greater understanding of how intervention content links to the determinants of behaviour and can be brought to bear on theory-based behavioural interventions designed to modify behaviours involving alcohol consumption.

Intervention development is based on a basic process model in which behaviour modification is determined by intervention strategies or *techniques* that 'activate' change in key theory-based determinants of the behaviour. Modification of the determinant leads, in turn, to a change in behaviour, represented by link 'b' in Fig. 21.1. The effect of the behaviour change technique on behaviour occurs by modifying the psychological determinant(s), known as a *mechanism of action*. The mechanism represented by links 'a' and 'b' in Fig. 21.1 should, therefore, account for most or all of the effect of the change technique on behaviour, such that the residual effect of the change technique on behaviour (c' in Fig. 21.1) is relatively trivial in size. The mechanism of action for the three motivational interventions that are the focus of this chapter is briefly discussed.

Interventions based on theories like the TPB target change in the belief-based factors shown to relate to behaviour via intentions (see above). Therefore, an attitude-based intervention would be designed to change individuals' beliefs about the potential consequences of HED and their evaluation of them as potentially negative. For example, an intervention might provide a message aimed at bolstering perceptions that HED leads to negative outcomes (e.g., having a hangover, getting into fights). Consistent with the predictions of attitude-based theories such as the theories of reasoned action and planned behaviour, such beliefs are predicted to lead to the formation of negative intentions to engage in HED and a reduction in HED (Ajzen & Schmidt, 2020; Hamilton & Johnson, 2020).

Another example of a theory-based intervention technique that has been used to change HED behavior is mental imagery. Mental imagery requires participants visualise a defined future action/behaviour and then contemplate and/or write about benefits of enacting that behaviour. Two types of mental imagery intervention have been tested in the alcohol literature. First, 'outcome mental simulation' interventions require individuals to imagine positive outcomes linked to behaviour change, for example feeling better as a result of adhering to moderate alcohol consumption guidelines in the next month. Second, 'process mental simulation' interventions require individuals to imagine strategic requirements relevant to the target behaviour, for example, thinking about strategies that might increase the likelihood of successfully drinking alcohol in moderation in the next month, like socialising with friends who support non-drinking (Pham & Taylor, 1999). Consistent with theories such as social cognitive theory (Bandura, 1986), these imagery techniques are predicted to change behaviour by targeting change in perceived self-efficacy by providing a 'self-model' to rehearse successfully performing the behaviour and promote positive emotions for achieving the change (for a full theoretical discussion, see Conroy & Hagger, 2018; Hagger & Conroy, 2020).

Another theory-based intervention technique that has been used to modify alcohol consumption is self-affirmation, derived from Steele's (1988) self-affirmation theory. According to Steele, messages that tell people they need to change their behaviour can challenge an individual's perception of themselves as a 'good' or 'worthy' person by pointing out that current behaviour deviates from health recommendations (i.e., current levels of alcohol consumption exceed government guidelines). By challenging people's perceptions of themselves as moral and competent, such messages may be ignored, or denigrated, because they are perceived as an attack on their sense of self. However, if individuals engage in a self-affirming exercise, like focusing on a valued aspect of their self-concept such as honesty or reliability, prior to presentation of such messages they are more open minded and can make an objective evaluation of the health message which increases motivation to undertake the necessary behavioural changes (Epton, Harris, Kane, van Koningsbruggen, & Sheeran, 2015). The mechanism of action for self-affirmation as an intervention technique is that self-affirming enables individuals to remain open minded about information presented to them and that processing this information leads to changes in intentions that ultimately are associated with changes in behaviour. In the next section, we review the research literature on motivational interventions relevant to the domain of alcohol consumption.

Motivational Interventions Applied to Reduce Alcohol Consumption

In this section we discuss interventions designed to modify excessive alcohol consumption by targeting the motivational drivers of behaviour. Given the large number of interventions that have been tested, we restrict our focus to frequently reported intervention techniques that propose a psychological mechanism of action based on established theories. Examples of these include interventions based on theories like the TPB, social cognitive theory (e.g., mental imagery interventions), and self-affirmation theory. Interventions based on these approaches are proposed to bring about change in behaviour indirectly by changing variables such as intentions or self-efficacy that are assumed to mediate the effects of interventions on behaviour.

TPB-Based Interventions

Norman et al.'s (2018) study is an example of a TPB-based intervention to reduce alcohol consumption. The researchers recruited 892 young people and delivered an intervention to them two weeks before they started university. Participants were presented with messages that targeted key beliefs about HED identified in a pilot study (Epton et al., 2015): that HED is fun, that engaging in HED has a negative effect on studies, and that having friends who engage in HED increases the likelihood of HED. Norman et al. (2018) found that participants presented with these messages reported significantly weaker intentions ($d = 0.27$), consumed fewer alcoholic units ($d = 0.20$), and engaged in fewer HED episodes ($d = 0.17$) six months later compared to participants who did not receive these messages. Additionally, the effect of the intervention on alcohol intake was shown to be mediated by intentions, providing support for the proposed mechanism of action that TPB-based interventions change behaviour by changing intentions.

In contrast, two previous studies of newly enrolled university students produced less equivocal findings for messages based on the TPB on change in alcohol consumption or HED (Cameron et al., 2015; Epton et al., 2014). Epton et al. (2014) recruited over 1000 university students and administered an intervention comprising three intervention techniques: self-affirmation (see 'Self-affirmation interventions'); TPB-based messages; implementation intentions, a self-regulatory intervention defined below (see 'Implementation Intention interventions'). The authors found very few significant differences between intervention and control participants and noted that engagement with the intervention was low: 52% of participants completed the self-affirmation task, 35% viewed the TPB-based messages, and 1% formed an implementation intention. Cameron et al. (2015) ran a replication trial of the methodology used by Epton et al. (2014). They also recruited over 1000 newly enrolled university students and again targeted the same four health behaviours. Although they reported dramatically higher engagement with the intervention tasks—85% of participants completed self-affirmation, 72% viewed health messages, and 41% formed an implementation intention—there was no effect of the intervention on change in any of the health behaviours. A key difference between the studies conducted by Cameron et al. (2015), Epton et al. (2014), and Norman et al. (2018) is that the Cameron et al. and Epton et al. studies targeted change in four health behaviours—alcohol consumption, cigarette smoking, fruit and vegetable consumption, and physical activity—whereas Norman et al. focused only on changing alcohol consumption. In appraising these studies, it is important to acknowledge that targeting change in multiple behaviours within a single intervention may have been asking participants to do too much, and could have led to confusion over the messages, possibly resulted in intervention fatigue (i.e., fatigue due to completing too many intervention elements), or conflicted priorities related to health goals.

The three studies considered above all recruited newly enrolled university students, which may have affected results. A recent study by Norman, Webb, and Millings (2019) compared the effectiveness of TPB-based messages to implementation intentions in university students who had started their university studies. Norman et al. (2019) showed that TPB-based messages did not reduce alcohol consumption despite significantly changing intentions. Overall, evidence for the effectiveness of interventions that use TPB-based messages to reduce alcohol consumption among UK university students is inconclusive.

Mental Imagery Interventions

Most mental imagery alcohol interventions have tested the effectiveness of receiving an outcome mental simulation intervention—that is, visualising what it would be like to drink within alcohol guidelines. For example, Hagger, Lonsdale, and Chatzisarantis (2011) explored the effect of such an intervention on alcohol consumption in a sample of UK employees. Using a randomised controlled design, employees completed a mental imagery exercise requiring them to imagine positive outcomes of moderate drinking in the next month or a control intervention. Results indicated lower levels of self-reported alcohol consumption six weeks after the intervention among employees who had completed the mental imagery intervention compared to those who did not. Subsequent studies (Conroy, Sparks, & de Visser, 2015; Hagger, Lonsdale, & Chatzisarantis, 2012) replicated these effects, although a study by Hagger, Lonsdale, Koka et al. (2012) found no effect of outcome simulation. A meta-analysis of these studies revealed a small average effect size ($d_+ = 0.23$) of outcome imagery techniques on alcohol consumption (Conroy & Hagger, 2018).

Conroy et al. (2015) tested the effectiveness of a 'process mental simulation' intervention, which required individuals to imagine thinking about actions that might increase the likelihood of successfully not drinking alcohol during some social occasions where other peers might themselves be drinking alcohol over the next month. They also tested the effect of an outcome mental simulation and a condition consisting of outcome and process mental simulations. Results revealed a greater decrease in weekly unit consumption among outcome mental simulation intervention participants relative to a control condition. Findings also demonstrated a greater decrease in HED among participants receiving the process mental simulation intervention relative to control condition. However, no differences were found between participants who received both the outcome and process simulation intervention and those in the control condition, meaning that there was no clear benefit in completing both tasks. This finding resonates with discussion above about over-loading participants with multiple interventional exercises.

Much remains unclear in terms of mechanisms of action that may explain the effects of mental imagery alcohol interventions. Studies reported to date have shown that completing mental simulation interventions does not lead to significant changes in TPB variables (Hagger et al., 2011; Hagger, Lonsdale, & Chatzisarantis, 2012; Hagger, Lonsdale, Koka, et al., 2012) or sociability prototypes, that is, how sociable non-drinkers were rated relative to drinkers (Conroy et al., 2015). One possible reason may be that constructs that represent habitual or implicit processes may be more effective in mediating effects of these interventions. For example, imagery interventions may lead to the development of better habits or means to obviate habitual effects. Overall, with three out of four studies testing effects of mental imagery showing significant effects on consumption, this technique offers promise as way to reduce excessive alcohol consumption.

Self-Affirmation Interventions

Harris and Napper (2005) provide an example of a study that tested the impact of self-affirmation on alcohol consumption. Female university students from the UK were randomly allocated to either a self-affirmation condition or a control condition. Participants in the self-affirmation condition completed a manipulation which asked them to choose their most important value (e.g., honesty, reliability) and write about why it was important to them. Control condition participants completed a manipulation which asked them to choose their least important value and write about why it was important to another student. Having completed the respective manipulations, all participants read a short article about the link between alcohol consumption and breast cancer. It was found that although the self-affirmation manipulation produced increased message acceptance and intentions to reduce drinking among participants who exceed weekly alcohol intake guidelines, supporting the proposed mechanism of action, there was no effect on consumption reported one month later. Subsequent studies testing self-affirmation interventions to reduce alcohol consumption in university student samples have generally found similar results (Knight & Norman, 2016; Meier et al., 2015; Norman et al., 2018; Norman & Wrona-Clarke, 2016). In the broader self-affirmation literature, a range of plausible mediators of the effects of self-affirmation have been proposed (e.g., mood, self-esteem, confidence, self-certainty), but no consistent mediators have been found across studies (Harris & Epton, 2009), and there has not been a focus on mediators in the literature applying self-affirmation to alcohol.

In contrast, two studies have shown that self-affirming can reduce alcohol consumption. First, Fox, Harris, and Jessop (2017) showed that a sample of female university students from the UK who self-affirmed prior to viewing a video where a young woman recounted how alcohol had affected her life reported lower alcohol consumption at one week follow-up compared to a peers who did not self-affirm. Second, Armitage, Harris, and Arden (2011) found that self-affirming significantly reduced alcohol consumption reported at one-month follow-up in a UK workplace sample. However, self-affirmation interventions have not been consistently associated with reduced alcohol consumption. In the next section, we outline how self-regulatory interventions are proposed to reduce alcohol consumption and then review the evidence for these interventions.

Self-Regulatory Interventions Applied to Reduce Alcohol Consumption

Self-regulatory processes focus on goal achievement, primarily through planning how to achieve a goal and by checking performance relative to a standard (e.g., 'Have I drunk within government guidelines?'). These processes are thought to underpin behavioural performance. Self-regulatory interventions reflect the fact that changing motivation is rarely sufficient to change behaviour, because people do not always translate their good intentions into action (Heckhausen & Gollwitzer, 1987; Keller, Gollwitzer, & Sheeran, 2020). Research has shown that the link between intentions and behaviour is often modest (Orbell & Sheeran, 1998; Rhodes & de Bruijn, 2013). According to Sheeran (2002), up to 47% of individuals who intend to act in a specific way fail to do so. This phenomenon has been labelled the 'intention-behaviour' gap (Sheeran, 2002; Sheeran & Webb, 2016) and represents a barrier to behaviour change because it means that changing intentions will not necessarily lead to behaviour change. Heckhausen and Gollwitzer's (1987) Model of Action Phases proposes two phases to action: a motivational phase, in which individuals consider their reasons for wanting to act or not, which ends with the formation of an intention to act or not, and a volitional phase, in which individuals plan how to implement their intention. The model predicts that individuals furnishing their intentions with plans identifying when, where, and how to enact the intended behaviour—typically called 'implementation intentions' (Gollwitzer, 1999), or 'action plans' (Schwarzer, 2008)—will be more likely to follow through on their intentions and act. Applied to alcohol, we would expect that individuals asked to reduce their consumption by forming a plan stating when, where, and how they intend to achieve this goal should report drinking less alcohol at follow-up compared to individuals not asked to form such a plan. Thus, planning is the mechanism of action for self-regulatory interventions, although there is variation in the format used to form plans. The next section discusses the evidence base for interventions that focus on application of planning techniques to reduce alcohol consumption.

Implementation Intention Interventions

Murgraff, White, and Phillips (1996) conducted the first experimental test of the effects of planning on reducing alcohol consumption in a sample of UK university students. Half of the students were randomly allocated to a control group that received information on safe drinking limits and health consequences of alcohol consumption. The other half were allocated to an experimental group that was provided with the same information as control participants and was asked to restrict their alcohol intake, to choose a strategy to refuse an alcoholic drink from a set of alternatives (e.g., 'I do not want to get drunk, I would rather have a few tonight'), and to specify a time and place in which this strategy would be implemented. Participants were asked to report how frequently they had engaged in HED in the past two weeks and also how recently they had engaged in HED. Among students engaging in HED in the previous two weeks, those receiving the planning exercise reported a significantly lower frequency of HED at follow-up as well as a significantly greater reduction in HED relative to students in the control condition. Study results support the notion that providing university students with a strategy to reduce their alcohol consumption and asking them to plan when and where to enact that strategy can reduce future HED.

Murgraff, Abraham, and McDermott (2007) reported results of a further experimental study comprising an intervention based on TPB constructs alongside planning. Participants were provided with strategies to boost positive attitudes and self-efficacy to reduce risky drinking. They were asked to form plans for when, where, and on what day they would start to reduce their drinking. Results indicated that participants reduced their alcohol consumption on Friday night when compared to control participants ($d = 0.44$), but that there was no difference between groups for Saturday night drinking. The authors also noted that the intervention was more effective in female compared to male students. However, several limitations of this study—small sample size, insufficient statistical power, high rates of attrition, university student sample—limit the generalisability of these results. In general, results from studies that have delivered implementation intentions to university student samples have been inconsistent: some studies have found significant effects on consumption (Hagger, Lonsdale, Koka, et al., 2012; Norman et al., 2019; Norman & Wrona-Clarke, 2016), but others have not (Cameron et al., 2015; Epton et al., 2014; Hagger, Lonsdale, & Chatzisarantis, 2012; Norman et al., 2018).

Armitage (2009) reported the results of a study testing effects of planning as an intervention to reduce alcohol consumption using a sample of participants recruited from a variety of social settings and working environments (e.g., shopping centres and offices). This approach yielded a sample broadly similar to the English population in terms of qualifications, gender, and ethnicity. Most importantly, the number of people drinking within government guidelines was directly comparable to figures for the English population as a whole. This study extended Murgraff et al.'s (1996, 2007) work by testing additional conditions. There were four groups: (1) a 'passive' control group that received no study measures, (2) an 'active' control group who were asked to plan to reduce their consumption, but not provided with any guidance on how to do this, (3) an experimenter-provided implementation intention group whose members choose implementation intentions from a list provided by the researchers, and (4) a self-generated implementation intention group. This design permitted examination of the effects of self-generated plans as compared to other-generated plans.

Results indicated that individuals in the passive control condition reported the same amount of alcohol consumption at baseline and follow-up, whereas participants in all other conditions reported lower consumption at follow-up. Planned contrasts revealed no significant difference in consumption between the passive and active control conditions, although participants in the experimenter-provided and self-generated implementation intention conditions reported significantly lower alcohol consumption at follow-up compared to both control conditions. These results show that asking individuals to plan on their own is not an effective way to reduce alcohol consumption, with the active control group doing no better than the passive control group at reducing their consumption. Results showed that planning based on principles derived from psychological research can be effective at reducing consumption but that there is not an obvious benefit in asking participants to form their own plans as opposed to choose one from a list of options.

Interestingly, Armitage (2009) reported a compliance analysis which indicated that only 29% of participants in the experimenter-provided planning condition fully complied with intervention instructions to write out one of the three experimenter-provided plans. Thus, 71% of participants did not follow the instructions they were given. Compliance was higher in the self-generated implementation intention condition: 54% of participants complied with instructions to generate an implementation intention, in comparison to 46% who did not. Although compliance did not influence effects of the experimenter-provided plans on alcohol consumption, compliers in the self-generated conditions reported a larger reduction in consumption at follow-up than non-compliers. It should be noted, however, that compliers had higher baseline alcohol consumption than non-compliers, meaning there was more scope for reduction. Overall, Armitage's study has a number of important features such as recruitment of a broad sample, high retention rate (97% of participants completed the study), and demonstrating that unless planning is based on psychological principles, it does not reduce alcohol consumption.

Volitional Help Sheet Interventions

Armitage (2008) created a planning intervention tool called the Volitional Help Sheet (VHS) to assist individuals in linking cues to action. Applied to alcohol, individuals are asked to tick boxes to identify situations in which they engage in consumption, for example 'If I am tempted to engage in HED when I am with others that are drinking a lot', and once they have done this, they are asked to look at the list of solutions provided, for example 'Then I will seek out social situations where people respect the rights of others not to drink' and draw a link between the situation and the solution. The idea is that by linking the cue to the action, individuals will find it easier to enact the desired behaviour.

The efficacy of an intervention using the VHS to reduce alcohol consumption was tested in two experimental studies: one with a sample of university students (Arden & Armitage, 2012) and another with a sample of workplace employees (Armitage & Arden, 2012). Arden and Armitage (2012) found that students using the VHS reported reduced alcohol consumption ($d = 0.58$) and HED frequency ($d = 0.75$) with medium-to-large effect sizes. Similarly, Armitage and Arden's (2012) use of the VHS in the workplace sample led to reduced alcohol consumption ($d = 0.19$) with a small effect size, which was a similar effect size to a group that received a conventional implementation intention exercise ($d = 0.18$). Participants who completed the VHS and were also prompted to make multiple links between conditions and plans reported lower alcohol consumption compared to the control group with a larger effect size than the VHS only and conventional planning exercise ($d = 0.57$). However, it should be noted that high variability in the conditions meant that there were no significant differences between the two planning conditions. To date, only Moody, Tegge, Poe, Koffarnus, and Bickel (2017) have reported a further test of the impact of the VHS on alcohol consumption. In their study, treatment-seeking alcohol drinkers in the USA were randomly allocated to receive either the VHS or the active control condition. Results revealed a small effect of the use of the VHS on consumption ($d = 0.23$). In sum, evidence shows that completing the VHS tends to produce small effects on alcohol consumption.

Overall, results described in this section suggest that self-regulatory interventions involving planning are more effective at changing alcohol consumption in non-student samples, and that even in other samples, there is heterogeneity in effect sizes. In the next section, we review evidence from studies that have tested interventions designed to change behaviour by targeting change in both motivational and self-regulatory processes.

Psychological Interventions that Combine Motivation and Planning Strategies

Given that the Model of Action Phases (Heckhausen & Gollwitzer, 1987) highlights the importance of both motivational and self-regulatory processes in the lead up to intention formation and action, researchers have explored the impact of interventions that target change in both processes as a potentially more effective way to bring about behaviour change. Research adopting this approach has demonstrated that interventions that combine motivational strategies with planning typically bring about larger changes in behaviour than interventions focused on either component alone (Milne, Orbell, & Sheeran, 2002; Prestwich, Lawton, & Conner, 2003; Zhang & Cooke, 2012). In keeping with this approach, several studies have tested the combined effect of motivational and planning interventions as a way to reduce alcohol consumption. We begin by reviewing studies that have combined implementation intentions with mental imagery.

Two studies led by Hagger and colleagues combined implementation intentions with mental imagery, one in a UK university student context (Hagger, Lonsdale, & Chatzisarantis, 2012) and the other drawing on university student samples from Estonia, Finland and the UK (Hagger, Lonsdale, Koka, et al., 2012). Hagger, Lonsdale, and Chatzisarantis (2012) found that although there was no main effect of either intervention component in isolation, there was an effect for the combination of implementation intentions and mental imagery on alcohol consumption at one-month follow-up among participants who had, at baseline, self-reported a high level of consumption. No effect was found for the combination of techniques on HED. In contrast, Hagger, Lonsdale, Koka et al. (2012) found no evidence that completing both the mental simulation and implementation intention interventions together reduced either alcohol consumption or HED at follow-up in any of the three countries.

Armitage et al. (2011) combined a self-affirmation intervention with implementation intentions in an experimental study. Participants from the general population were randomly allocated to one of three conditions: a self-affirmation-only condition, a self-affirmation implementation intention condition, or a no-intervention control condition. Participants assigned to the combined self-affirmation implementation intention condition responded to threatening statements with self-affirming responses using the if-then format recommended for implementation intentions. By doing this, participants combined self-affirmation with formation of an implementation intention, rather than self-affirming *then* forming an implementation intention. Results indicated that participants who completed a self-affirmation implementation intention reported significantly lower alcohol consumption at one-month follow-up compared to participants in the control group. A further study of secondary school children using the same approach indicated that those who completed the self-affirmation implementation intention drank less alcohol compared to control participants at two-month follow-up, although it should be noted that alcohol consumption levels in this sample were low (Armitage, Rowe, Arden, & Harris, 2014).

Armitage and Arden (2016) reported results of two studies in which participants were randomised to read either a standard wine label or a label that included a self-affirmation implementation intention. Participants were then asked to pour the amount of wine they thought it safe to drink and reported their alcohol consumption one month later. Results indicated that the intervention resulted in reduced alcohol consumption compared to controls, with large effect sizes (*d*s = 0.70 and 0.90). Further replication of the effects of self-affirmation implementation intentions in larger sample sizes is required to confirm the efficacy of this technique, particularly given that participants were not actually asked to form implementation intentions in either study.

Two studies tested the effect of interventions combining 'traditional' self-affirmation manipulations with implementation intentions on alcohol consumption (Norman et al., 2018; Norman & Wrona-Clarke, 2016); students in the combined condition completed a self-affirmation intervention prior to reading a health message about the health consequences of HED before forming an implementation intention. Neither study provided evidence that asking participants to self-affirm prior to forming implementation intentions led to a significant reduction in alcohol consumption. To date, Ehret and Sherman's (2018) study is the only one to provide evidence that combining self-affirmation and implementation intentions can reduce alcohol consumption. College students were randomly allocated to one of four conditions using a 2 (self-affirmation, no self-affirmation) by 2 (form implementation intentions, do not form implementation intentions) design; completing both interventions led to higher rates of abstinence one week later.

There are methodological differences between these studies which could explain variation in the effects of the combined interventions. For example, participants in Ehret and Sherman's (2018) study were presented with items from the Protective Behavioural Strategies scale (Martens et al., 2004)—defined as cognitive and behavioural techniques individuals can draw on to limit negative alcohol-related consequences when consuming alcohol. We note here that the self-affirmation intervention described by Ehret and Sherman (2018) may have been more effective compared to other studies because participants were given information on resources that may support their behaviour change (Ferrer & Cohen, 2018). Another difference between studies is the outcome variable used: Ehret and Sherman (2018) used abstinence from drinking as their outcome, as opposed to the volume of consumption, which was used in other studies reviewed in this chapter. Abstinence may be a more accepted health goal in the USA than other countries because the legal age for alcohol consumption is 21 rather than 18, as it is in many other countries. However, drawing definitive conclusions is difficult given the paucity of research in the field. Further research adopting randomised factorial designs is needed to verify the effects of combined self-affirmation and planning interventions. Overall, there is not clear evidence that interventions that combine elements that target motivation and self-regulation are an effective method for reducing alcohol consumption.

Appraising the Evidence

Interventions targeting change in the motivational determinants of alcohol consumption outlined in Section 'Psychological Theories of Motivation' can reduce alcohol consumption. For example, three out of four studies that used outcome mental simulation strategies reported significant reductions in consumption relative to a control group (Conroy et al., 2015; Hagger et al., 2011; Hagger, Lonsdale, & Chatzisarantis, 2012). Furthermore, recent studies have shown that completing a self-affirmation exercise before viewing a video containing a health message can reduce alcohol consumption (Fox et al., 2017) and that presenting newly enrolled university students with messages targeting putative determinants of alcohol intentions (i.e., attitudes, subjective norms, and PBC) can lead to changes in consumption six months later (Norman et al., 2018).

Nevertheless, most interventions using self-affirmation or delivering TPB-based messages have not led to reductions in alcohol consumption. Most of these tests have been evaluated in samples drawn from a high-risk population—university students—who may be more focused on establishing new social networks rather than reducing their alcohol consumption (Ferrer, Dillard, & Klein, 2011). It is therefore possible that motivational interventions are effective at reducing alcohol consumption in other populations, but there is a need for more research to examine this claim.

Relative to interventions that target motivation, there is more evidence for the effectiveness of interventions targeting change in alcohol consumption based on changing self-regulation. This is especially the case in non-student samples where self-regulatory interventions have been consistently shown to lead to significant reductions in alcohol consumption relative to control groups (Armitage, 2009; Armitage et al., 2011; Armitage & Arden, 2012). In contrast, self-regulation interventions using techniques such as planing and implementation intentions delivered to university student samples have been shown to be effective in some studies (Arden & Armitage, 2012; Hagger, Lonsdale, Koka, et al., 2012; Murgraff et al., 2007; Norman et al., 2019; Norman & Wrona-Clarke, 2016), but not others (Cameron et al., 2015; Epton et al., 2014; Hagger, Lonsdale, Koka, et al., 2012; Norman et al., 2018).

Combining motivational and self-regulatory elements in interventions does not appear to be a particularly effective approach to reduce alcohol consumption, especially when contrasted with results for other health behaviours such as fruit and vegetable consumption or physical activity. An explanation for this lack of synergy is that for dietary behaviours and physical activity we want individuals to form goals that encourage increased performance of behaviour (i.e., an approach goal): planning when, where, and how to eat more portions of fruit and vegetables or to engage in more physical activity. Conversely, alcohol consumption interventions focus on reducing performance of behaviour (i.e., an avoidance goal). Research has provided some evidence that asking participants to form avoidance goals for health risk behaviours is less effective than forming approach goals (Sullivan & Rothman, 2008). Most alcohol interventions focus on avoidance goals (e.g., 'Don't drink more than government guidelines'): it is unclear whether asking participants to form approach goals (e.g., 'Drink more non-alcoholic drinks') would be more effective. Future studies should seek to compare the effectiveness of goals focused on different types of non-alcoholic drinks (i.e., non-alcoholic drinks, soft drinks, low-strength alcoholic drinks), based on participant preference. Individuals may be more willing to form approach goals because they encourage the behaviour of drinking non-alcoholic drinks, as opposed limiting or abstaining from drinking alcoholic drinks. However, there is some evidence that temporary abstinence from alcohol consumption, by following the *Dry January* or *Hello Sunday Morning* programmes, is associated short- and long-term effects on alcohol consumption (de Visser & Nicholls, 2020; de Visser & Piper, 2020; de Visser, Robinson, & Bond, 2016; Tait, Paz Castro, Kirkman, Moore, & Schaub, 2019).

An additional point that could account for the lack of synergy between motivational and self-regulatory interventions for alcohol is linked to drawbacks of requesting completion of multiple intervention components. For example, Norman et al. (2018) found that attrition was higher among participants allocated to complete implementation intentions after other interventions (e.g., self-affirmation, TPB messages), compared to participants asked to complete only implementation intentions, so there may be an element of participant fatigue involved when asking people to complete multi-component interventions. It is also important to note the lack of engagement reported in the multi-component, multi-behaviour interventions (Cameron et al., 2015; Epton et al., 2014). Striking a balance between having 'too little' intervention content to change behaviour versus 'too much' content that leads to disengagement or attrition is a key issue for intervention developers to consider. As discussed in the next section, one approach that may assist with this issue is to trial intervention components in digital interventions, where it is potentially quicker and easier to make changes to interventions.

Routes Forward: Extending the Evidence Base

Based on our review, we wish to draw the reader's attention to studies that provide useful leads in terms of extending the evidence base for motivational and self-regulatory interventions to promote moderate alcohol consumption. Taken together, results from Norman et al.'s (2018) study, which found that health messages led to reduced alcohol consumption when received before starting university, and results from Norman et al.'s (2019) study, which found forming implementation intentions reduced alcohol consumption among university students, there seems to be merit in testing the effectiveness of delivering interventions at different times. Delivering motivational interventions *before* young people have experience of university might be an opportune time for them to receive messages on alcohol reduction. It would also be valuable to expand this approach to other groups, such as adolescents and young adults who do not attend university, to see if this approach is similarly effective. Equally, asking university students to form implementation intentions *after* they have started university would allow them to form plans based on recent drinking experiences. It is also worth noting that a challenge for any alcohol intervention is that people's alcohol consumption tends to fluctuate over time (Ferrer et al., 2011; Giese, Stok, & Renner, 2019), so identifying the best time for the delivery of interventions is likely to be critical. Longitudinal intervention studies that deliver interventions at different times in an order that is responsive to temporal changes in alcohol consumption patterns would be a welcome addition to the literature.

There has been increasing interest in delivering interventions using digital channels and in particular via Smartphone applications ('apps'). In developed nations, smartphone ownership ranges from 95% in South Korea to 59% in Greece and Russia, with a median ownership of 76% (Pew Research Center, 2019). This means that device-based apps are a potentially advantageous medium for behaviour change interventions in developed nations; most Smartphone owners often take them everywhere they go, meaning that the app can be used to provide immediate advice or support. For example, the *Drink Less* app was developed on the basis of systematic searches of the research literature (Garnett et al., 2016) and in consultation with experts in behaviour change (Garnett, Crane, West, Brown, & Michie, 2015). This app contains five intervention components: self-monitoring and feedback, normative feedback, action plans, identity change, and cognitive bias re-training. Action plans (Sniehotta, Scholz, & Schwarzer, 2005) are similar to implementation intentions, in that they ask individuals to specify when, where, and how to change their behaviour. Crane, Garnett, Brown, West, and Michie (2017) extensively tested the usability of the app prior to it being made available as a resource. Participants were presented with a prototype version of the app and commented that they needed more guidance on what to do and how the app would work to help them reduce their alcohol consumption. Having made changes to the app to address these concerns, Crane, Garnett, Michie, West, and Brown (2018) reported an evaluation of the app using a fully factorial design with 32 conditions (i.e., a 2 x 2 x 2 x 2 x 2 experimental design), to reflect the fact that each individual either received or did not receive each of the five interventions. Such a design allows the research team to narrow down the more effective intervention components; however, this does require recruitment of a very large sample of participants to provide sufficient power. Although Crane et al. (2018) found a significant main effect of time on consumption, with consumption lower at the end of the study, no main effects were found for any of the intervention components. Although this study provides no evidence that using a digital intervention designed using theories of motivation and self-regulation can reduce alcohol consumption, it provides a useful starting point for researchers in this area. Repeated tests of the effectiveness of digital apps are required given the potential for cost-effectiveness using this mode of delivery.

Finally, as part of our discussion, we acknowledge that intra-individual variables (e.g., individual motivation and self-regulatory capacity) are only one influence on why people engage in excessive alcohol conumption such as HED and that a multitude of external contextual (e.g., drinking at home vs. in licensed premises), environmental (e.g., alcohol advertisements), and social (e.g., friends drinking) influences affect drinking decisions and consumption (see Section 'Psychological Theories of Motivation'). Interventions seeking to reduce individual consumption by targeting intra-individual variables should be considered alongside interventions that target these additional influences.

Conclusion

Intervention research adopting techniques based on psychological determinants of alcohol consumption informed by theories of motivation and self-regulation have been moderately successful in reducing harmful alcohol consumption, with stronger evidence for effectiveness in workplace samples relative to university student samples. Future studies that test these techniques in a broader range of populations, and over longer time periods, are needed to clarify the impact of these types of intervention on alcohol consumption.

References

Ajzen, I. (1991). The theory of planned behavior. *Organizational Behavior and Human Decision Processes, 50,* 179–211. https://doi.org/10.1016/0749-5978(91)90020-T

Ajzen, I., & Schmidt, P. (2020). Changing behavior using the theory of planned behavior. In M. S. Hagger, L. D. Cameron, K. Hamilton, N. Hankonen, & T. Lintunen (Eds.), *The handbook of behavior change* (pp. 17–31). Cambridge, UK: Cambridge University Press. https://doi.org/10.1017/9781108677318.002

Arden, M. A., & Armitage, C. J. (2012). A volitional help sheet to reduce binge drinking in students: A randomized exploratory trial. *Alcohol and Alcoholism, 47,* 156–159. https://doi.org/10.1093/alcalc/agr164

Armitage, C. J. (2008). A volitional help sheet to encourage smoking cessation: A randomized exploratory trial. *Health Psychology: Official Journal of the Division of Health Psychology, American Psychological Association, 27,* 557–566. https://doi.org/10.1037/0278-6133.27.5.557

Armitage, C. J. (2009). Effectiveness of experimenter-provided and self-generated implementation intentions to reduce alcohol consumption in a sample of the general population: A randomized exploratory trial. *Health Psychology, 28,* 545–553. https://doi.org/10.1037/a0015984

Armitage, C. J., & Arden, M. A. (2012). A volitional help sheet to reduce alcohol consumption in the general population: A field experiment. *Prevention Science, 13*, 635–643. https://doi.org/10.1007/s11121-012-0291-4

Armitage, C. J., & Arden, M. A. (2016). Enhancing the effectiveness of alcohol warning labels with a self-affirming implementation intention. *Health Psychology, 35*(10), 1159–1163. https://doi.org/10.1037/hea0000376

Armitage, C. J., Harris, P. R., & Arden, M. A. (2011). Evidence that self-affirmation reduces alcohol consumption: Randomized exploratory trial with a new, brief means of self-affirming. *Health Psychology, 30*, 633–641. https://doi.org/10.1037/a0023738

Armitage, C. J., Rowe, R., Arden, M. A., & Harris, P. R. (2014). A brief psychological intervention that reduces adolescent alcohol consumption. *Journal of Consulting and Clinical Psychology, 82*, 546–550. https://doi.org/10.1037/a0035802

Bandura, A. (1986). *Social foundations of thought and action: A social-cognitive theory*. Upper Saddle River, NJ: Prentice-Hall.

Cameron, D., Epton, T., Norman, P., Sheeran, P., Harris, P. R., Webb, T. L., … Shah, I. (2015). A theory-based online health behaviour intervention for new university students (U@Uni:LifeGuide): Results from a repeat randomized controlled trial. *Trials, 16*. https://doi.org/10.1186/s13063-015-1092-4

Carey, R. N., Connell, L. E., Johnston, M., Rothman, A. J., de Bruin, M., Kelly, M. P., & Michie, S. (2018). Behavior change techniques and their mechanisms of action: A synthesis of links described in published intervention literature. *Annals of Behavioral Medicine*. https://doi.org/10.1093/abm/kay078

Connell, L. E., Carey, R. N., de Bruin, M., Rothman, A. J., Johnston, M., Kelly, M. P., & Michie, S. (2019). Links between behavior change techniques and mechanisms of action: An expert consensus study. *Annals of Behavioral Medicine, 53*(8), 708–720. https://doi.org/10.1093/abm/kay082

Conroy, D., & Hagger, M. S. (2018). Imagery interventions in health behavior: A meta-analysis. *Health Psychology, 37*(7), 668–679. https://doi.org/10.1037/hea0000625

Conroy, D., Sparks, P., & de Visser, R. (2015). Efficacy of a non-drinking mental simulation intervention for reducing student alcohol consumption. *British Journal of Health Psychology, 20*(4), 688–707. https://doi.org/10.1111/bjhp.12133

Cooke, R., Dahdah, M., Norman, P., & French, D. P. (2016). How well does the theory of planned behaviour predict alcohol consumption? A systematic review and meta-analysis. *Health Psychology Review, 10*, 148–167. https://doi.org/10.1080/17437199.2014.947547

Cox, W. M., & Klinger, E. (1988). A motivational model of alcohol use. *Journal of Abnormal Psychology, 97*(2), 168–180.

Crane, D., Garnett, C., Brown, J., West, R., & Michie, S. (2017). Factors influencing usability of a smartphone app to reduce excessive alcohol consumption: Think aloud and interview studies. *Frontiers in Public Health, 5*. https://doi.org/10.3389/fpubh.2017.00039

Crane, D., Garnett, C., Michie, S., West, R., & Brown, J. (2018). A smartphone app to reduce excessive alcohol consumption: Identifying the effectiveness of intervention components in a factorial randomised control trial. *Scientific Reports, 8*(1), 4384. https://doi.org/10.1038/s41598-018-22420-8

de Visser, R. O., & Nicholls, J. (2020). Temporary abstinence during dry January: Predictors of success; impact on Well-being and self-efficacy. *Psychology & Health, 35*, 1–13. https://doi.org/10.1080/08870446.2020.1743840

de Visser, R. O., & Piper, R. (2020). Short- and longer-term benefits of temporary alcohol abstinence during 'dry January' are not also observed among adult drinkers in the general population: Prospective cohort study. *Alcohol and Alcoholism, 55*, 433–438. doi:https://doi.org/10.1093/alcalc/agaa025.

de Visser, R. O., Robinson, E., & Bond, R. (2016). Voluntary temporary abstinence from alcohol during "dry January" and subsequent alcohol use. *Health Psychology, 35*(3), 281–289. https://doi.org/10.1037/hea0000297

Ehret, P. J., & Sherman, D. K. (2018). Integrating self-affirmation and implementation intentions: Effects on college student drinking. *Annals of Behavioral Medicine., 52*, 633. https://doi.org/10.1093/abm/kax032

Epton, T., Harris, P. R., Kane, R., van Koningsbruggen, G. M., & Sheeran, P. (2015). The impact of self-affirmation on health-behavior change: A meta-analysis. *Health Psychology, 34*(3), 187–196. https://doi.org/10.1037/hea0000116

Epton, T., Norman, P., Dadzie, A.-S., Harris, P. R., Webb, T. L., Sheeran, P., … Shah, I. (2014). A theory-based online health behaviour intervention for new university students (U@Uni): Results from a randomised controlled trial. *BMC Public Health, 14*. https://doi.org/10.1186/1471-2458-14-563

Epton, T., Norman, P., Harris, P., Webb, T., Snowsill, F. A., & Sheeran, P. (2015). Development of theory-based health messages: Three-phase programme of formative research. *Health Promotion International, 30*(3), 756–768. https://doi.org/10.1093/heapro/dau005

Ferrer, R. A., & Cohen, G. L. (2018). Reconceptualizing self-affirmation with the trigger and channel framework: Lessons from the health domain. *Personality and Social Psychology Review, 108886831879703*, 285. https://doi.org/10.1177/1088868318797036

Ferrer, R. A., Dillard, A. J., & Klein, W. M. P. (2011). Projection, conformity and deviance regulation: A prospective study of alcohol use. *Psychology & Health*, 1–16. https://doi.org/10.1080/08870446.2011.620106

Fox, K. J., Harris, P. R., & Jessop, D. C. (2017). Experimentally manipulated self-affirmation promotes reduced alcohol consumption in response to narrative information. *Annals of Behavioral Medicine, 51*(6), 931–935. https://doi.org/10.1007/s12160-017-9912-2

Gardner, B., Rebar, A. L., & Lally, P. (2020). 'Habitually deciding' or 'habitually doing'? A response to Hagger (2019). *Psychology of Sport and Exercise, 47*, 101539. https://doi.org/10.1016/j.psychsport.2019.05.008

Garnett, C., Crane, D., West, R., Brown, J., & Michie, S. (2015). Identification of behavior change techniques and engagement strategies to design a smartphone app to reduce alcohol consumption using a formal consensus method. *JMIR mHealth and uHealth, 3*(2), e73. https://doi.org/10.2196/mhealth.3895

Garnett, C., Jamie, B., David, C., Eileen, K., Fiona, B., Colin, M., … Susan, M. (2016). Theory content of digital interventions for reducing alcohol consumption: A systematic review. *Frontiers in Public Health, 4*. https://doi.org/10.3389/conf.FPUBH.2016.01.00062

Gell, L., Ally, A., Buykx, P., Hope, A., & Meyer, P. (2015). *Alcohol's harm to others*. Institute of Alcohol Studies.

Gibbons, F. X., & Gerrard, M. (1995). Predicting young adults' health risk behavior. *Journal of Personality and Social Psychology, 69*(3), 505–517.

Giese, H., Stok, F. M., & Renner, B. (2019). Perceiving college peers' alcohol consumption: Temporal patterns and individual differences in overestimation. *Psychology & Health, 34*(2), 147–161. https://doi.org/10.1080/08870446.2018.1514118

Gilpin, N. W., & Koob, G. F. (2008). Neurobiology of alcohol dependence: Focus on motivational mechanisms. *Alcohol Research & Health: The Journal of the National Institute on Alcohol Abuse and Alcoholism, 31*(3), 185–195.

Gollwitzer, P. M. (1999). Implementation intentions: Strong effects of simple plans. *American Psychologist, 54*(7), 493–503. https://doi.org/10.1037/0003-066X.54.7.493

Hagger, M. S. (2019). Habit and physical activity: Theoretical advances, practical implications, and agenda for future research. *Psychology of Sport and Exercise, 42*, 118–129. https://doi.org/10.1016/j.psychsport.2018.12.007

Hagger, M. S. (2020). Redefining habits and linking habits with other implicit processes. *Psychology of Sport and Exercise, 46*, 101606. https://doi.org/10.1016/j.psychsport.2019.101606

Hagger, M. S., Polet, J., & Lintunen, T. (2018). The reasoned action approach applied to health behavior: Role of past behavior and test of some key moderators using meta-analytic structural equation modeling. *Social Science & Medicine, 213*, 85–94. https://doi.org/10.1016/j.socscimed.2018.07.038

Hagger, M. S., Cameron, L. D., Hamilton, K., Hankonen, N., & Lintunen, T. (2020). Changing behavior: A theory- and evidence-based approach. In M. S. Hagger, L. D. Cameron, K. Hamilton, N. Hankonen, & T. Lintunen (Eds.), *The handbook of behavior change* (pp. 1–14). Cambridge, UK: Cambridge University Press.

Hagger, M. S., Chan, D. K. C., Protogerou, C., & Chatzisarantis, N. L. D. (2016). Using meta-analytic path analysis to test theoretical predictions in health behavior: An illustration based on meta-analyses of the theory of planned behavior. *Preventive Medicine, 89*, 154–161. https://doi.org/10.1016/j.ypmed.2016.05.020

Hagger, M. S., & Conroy, D. (2020). Imagery, visualization, and mental simulation interventions. In M. S. Hagger, L. D. Cameron, K. Hamilton, N. Hankonen, &

T. Lintunen (Eds.), *The handbook of behavior change* (pp. 479–494). Cambridge, UK: Cambridge University Press.
Hagger, M. S., Lonsdale, A., & Chatzisarantis, N. L. D. (2011). Effectiveness of a brief intervention using mental simulations in reducing alcohol consumption in corporate employees. *Psychology, Health & Medicine, 16*(4), 375–392. https://doi.org/10.1080/13548506.2011.554568
Hagger, M. S., Lonsdale, A., & Chatzisarantis, N. L. D. (2012). A theory-based intervention to reduce alcohol drinking in excess of guideline limits among undergraduate students: Undergraduate alcohol intervention. *British Journal of Health Psychology, 17*, 18–43. https://doi.org/10.1111/j.2044-8287.2010.02011.x
Hagger, M. S., Lonsdale, A., Koka, A., Hein, V., Pasi, H., Lintunen, T., & Chatzisarantis, N. L. D. (2012). An intervention to reduce alcohol consumption in undergraduate students using implementation intentions and mental simulations: A cross-National Study. *International Journal of Behavioral Medicine, 19*, 82–96. https://doi.org/10.1007/s12529-011-9163-8
Hagger, M. S., Moyers, S., McAnally, K., & McKinley, L. E. (2020). Known knowns and known unknowns on behavior change interventions and mechanisms of action. *Health Psychology Review, 14*(1), 199–212. https://doi.org/10.1080/17437199.2020.1719184
Hamilton, K., & Johnson, B. T. (2020). Attitude and persuasive communication interventions. In M. S. Hagger, L. D. Cameron, K. Hamilton, N. Hankonen, & T. Lintunen (Eds.), *The handbook of behavior change* (pp. 445–460). Cambridge, UK: Cambridge University Press. https://doi.org/10.1017/97811086773180.031
Hamilton, K., Gibbs, I., Keech, J. J., & Hagger, M. S. (2020). Reasoned and implicit processes in heavy episodic drinking: An integrated dual-process model. *British Journal of Health Psychology, 25*(1), 189–209. https://doi.org/10.1111/bjhp.12401
Harris, P. R., & Epton, T. (2009). The impact of self-affirmation on health cognition, health behaviour and other health-related responses: A narrative review. *Social and Personality Psychology Compass, 3*(6), 962–978. https://doi.org/10.1111/j.1751-9004.2009.00233.x
Harris, P. R., & Napper, L. (2005). Self-affirmation and the biased processing of threatening health-risk information. *Personality & Social Psychology Bulletin, 31*(9), 1250–1263. https://doi.org/10.1177/0146167205274694
Heckhausen, H., & Gollwitzer, P. M. (1987). Thought contents and cognitive functioning in motivational versus volitional states of mind. *Motivation and Emotion, 11*, 101–120.
Keller, L., Gollwitzer, P. M., & Sheeran, P. (2020). Changing behavior using the model of action phases. In M. S. Hagger, L. D. Cameron, K. Hamilton, N. Hankonen, & T. Lintunen (Eds.), *The handbook of behavior change* (pp. 77–103). Cambridge, UK: Cambridge University Press.
Knight, R., & Norman, P. (2016). Impact of brief self-affirmation manipulations on university students' reactions to risk information about binge drinking. *British Journal of Health Psychology, 21*(3), 570–583. https://doi.org/10.1111/bjhp.12186

Martens, M. P., Taylor, K. K., Damann, K. M., Page, J. C., Mowry, E. S., & Cimini, M. D. (2004). Protective behavioral strategies when drinking alcohol and their relationship to negative alcohol-related consequences in college students. *Psychology of Addictive Behaviors: Journal of the Society of Psychologists in Addictive Behaviors, 18*(4), 390–393. https://doi.org/10.1037/0893-164X.18.4.390

Meier, E., Miller, M. B., Lechner, W. V., Lombardi, N., Claborn, K. R., & Leffingwell, T. R. (2015). The inability of self-affirmations to decrease defensive Bias toward an alcohol-related risk message among high-risk college students. *Journal of American College Health, 63*(5), 324–329. https://doi.org/10.1080/07448481.2014.1003377

Michie, S., Whittington, C., Hamoudi, Z., Zarnani, F., Tober, G., & West, R. (2012). Identification of behaviour change techniques to reduce excessive alcohol consumption: Behaviour change and excessive alcohol use. *Addiction, 107*(8), 1431–1440. https://doi.org/10.1111/j.1360-0443.2012.03845.x

Milne, S., Orbell, S., & Sheeran, P. (2002). Combining motivational and volitional interventions to promote exercise participation: Protection motivation theory and implementation intentions. *British Journal of Health Psychology, 7*(Pt 2), 163–184. https://doi.org/10.1348/135910702169420

Moody, L. N., Tegge, A. N., Poe, L. M., Koffarnus, M. N., & Bickel, W. K. (2017). To drink or to drink less? Distinguishing between effects of implementation intentions on decisions to drink and how much to drink in treatment-seeking individuals with alcohol use disorder. *Addictive Behaviors, 83*, 64. https://doi.org/10.1016/j.addbeh.2017.11.010

Murgraff, V., Abraham, C., & McDermott, M. (2007). Reducing friday alcohol consumption among moderate, women drinkers: Evaluation of a brief evidence-based intervention. *Alcohol and Alcoholism (Oxford, Oxfordshire), 42*, 37–41. https://doi.org/10.1093/alcalc/agl083

Murgraff, V., White, D., & Phillips, K. (1996). Moderating binge drinking: It is possible to change behaviour if you plan it in advance. *Alcohol and Alcoholism (Oxford, Oxfordshire), 31*, 577–582.

Norman, P., Cameron, D., Epton, T., Webb, T. L., Harris, P. R., Millings, A., & Sheeran, P. (2018). A randomized controlled trial of a brief online intervention to reduce alcohol consumption in new university students: Combining self-affirmation, theory of planned behaviour messages, and implementation intentions. *British Journal of Health Psychology, 23*(1), 108–127. https://doi.org/10.1111/bjhp.12277

Norman, P., Webb, T. L., & Millings, A. (2019). Using the theory of planned behaviour and implementation intentions to reduce binge drinking in new university students. *Psychology & Health, 34*, 1–19. https://doi.org/10.1080/08870446.2018.1544369

Norman, P., & Wrona-Clarke, A. (2016). Combining self-affirmation and implementation intentions to reduce heavy episodic drinking in university students.

Psychology of Addictive Behaviors: Journal of the Society of Psychologists in Addictive Behaviors, 30, 434–441. https://doi.org/10.1037/adb0000144

Orbell, S., & Sheeran, P. (1998). "Inclined abstainers": A problem for predicting health-related behaviour. *British Journal of Social Psychology, 37*, 151–165.

Pew Research Center. (2019). *Smartphone ownership is growing rapidly around the world, but not always equally*. Pew Research Center. https://www.pewresearch.org/global/2019/02/05/smartphone-ownership-is-growing-rapidly-around-the-world-but-not-always-equally/

Pham, L. B., & Taylor, S. E. (1999). From thought to action: Effects of process-versus outcome-based mental simulations on performance. *Personality and Social Psychology Bulletin, 25*(2), 250–260. https://doi.org/10.1177/0146167299025002010

Prestwich, A., Lawton, R., & Conner, M. (2003). The use of implementation intentions and the decision balance sheet in promoting exercise behaviour. *Psychology & Health, 18*(6), 707–721. https://doi.org/10.1080/0887044031000159449 3

Rhodes, R. E., & de Bruijn, G.-J. (2013). How big is the physical activity intention-behaviour gap? A meta-analysis using the action control framework. *British Journal of Health Psychology, 18*, 296–309.

Rothman, A. J., Klein, W. M. P., & Sheeran, P. (2020). Moving from theoretical principles to intervention strategies: Applying the experimental medicine approach. In M. S. Hagger, L. D. Cameron, K. Hamilton, N. Hankonen, & T. Lintunen (Eds.), *The handbook of behavior change*. Cambridge, UK: Cambridge University Press.

Schwarzer, R. (2008). Modelling health behavior change: How to predict and modify the adoption and maintenance of health Behaviors. *Applied Psychology, 57*(1), 1–29. https://doi.org/10.1111/j.1464-0597.2007.00325.x

Sheeran, P., Klein, W. M. P., & Rothman, A. J. (2017). Health behavior change: Moving from observation to intervention. *Annual Review of Psychology, 68*(1), 573–600. https://doi.org/10.1146/annurev-psych-010416-044007

Sheeran, P., & Webb, T. L. (2016). The intention-behavior gap: The intention-behavior gap. *Social and Personality Psychology Compass, 10*(9), 503–518. https://doi.org/10.1111/spc3.12265

Sheeran, P. (2002). Intention—Behavior relations: A conceptual and empirical review. *European Review of Social Psychology, 12*, 1–36. https://doi.org/10.1080/14792772143000003

Sniehotta, F. F., Scholz, U., & Schwarzer, R. (2005). Bridging the intention–behaviour gap: Planning, self-efficacy, and action control in the adoption and maintenance of physical exercise. *Psychology & Health, 20*(2), 143–160. https://doi.org/10.1080/08870440512331317670

Steele, C. M. (1988). The psychology of self-affirmation: Sustaining the integrity of the self. In *Advances in experimental social psychology* (Vol. 21, pp. 261–302). Elsevier. http://linkinghub.elsevier.com/retrieve/pii/S0065260108602294

Steinmetz, H., Knappstein, M., Ajzen, I., Schmidt, P., & Kabst, R. (2016). How effective are behavior change interventions based on the theory of planned behavior?: A three-level meta-analysis. *Zeitschrift für Psychologie, 224*(3), 216–233. https://doi.org/10.1027/2151-2604/a000255

Sullivan, H. W., & Rothman, A. J. (2008). When planning is needed: Implementation intentions and attainment of approach versus avoidance health goals. *Health Psychology, 27*(4), 438–444. https://doi.org/10.1037/0278-6133.27.4.438

Tait, R. J., Paz Castro, R., Kirkman, J. J. L., Moore, J. C., & Schaub, M. P. (2019). A digital intervention addressing alcohol use problems (the "daybreak" program): Quasi-experimental randomized controlled trial. *Journal of Medical Internet Research, 21*(9), e14967. https://doi.org/10.2196/14967

World Health Organization (Ed.). (2010). *Global strategy to reduce the harmful use of alcohol.* Geneva, Switzerland: World Health Organization.

Zhang, Y., & Cooke, R. (2012). Using a combined motivational and volitional intervention to promote exercise and healthy dietary behaviour among undergraduates. *Diabetes Research and Clinical Practice, 95*(2), 215–223. https://doi.org/10.1016/j.diabres.2011.10.006

22

Does Cognitive Bias Modification Reduce Alcohol Consumption?

Andrew Jones and Matt Field

Introduction

Regular alcohol consumption is associated with the development of cognitive biases that guide attention to alcohol cues, such as the sight or smell of alcohol in the environment, facilitate appetitive responses to alcohol cues, and disrupt cognitive control processes (such as behavioural self-control and goal-directed action) when in the presence of alcohol cues. Cognitive bias modification (CBM) is an overarching term for a collection of interventions that aim to change cognitive biases to alcohol-related cues and thereby reduce the risk of excessive alcohol consumption and/or (re)lapse. The aim of this chapter is to introduce these cognitive biases and explore how they contribute to the development and maintenance of alcohol consumption, before examining the effectiveness of different types of CBM interventions. Our focus will be on the most commonly researched types of biases and their modification: attentional, approach, inhibition, and interpretation. Where possible we interpret research in the context of the experimental medicine approach, which involves (1) observing the relationship between a cognitive bias and drinking

A. Jones (✉)
Department of Psychology, University of Liverpool, Liverpool, UK
e-mail: ajj@liverpool.ac.uk

M. Field
Department of Psychology, University of Sheffield, Sheffield, UK
e-mail: matt.field@shef.ac.uk

R. Cooke et al. (eds.), *The Palgrave Handbook of Psychological Perspectives on Alcohol Consumption*, https://doi.org/10.1007/978-3-030-66941-6_22

behaviour, (2) manipulating biases to establish causal relationships, often in laboratory settings, as a precursor to (3) investigating whether CBM changes cognitive biases and alcohol consumption in naturalistic settings. We conclude that current evidence for CBM is mixed and that improving the quality of research in this area will help provide consensus as to whether CBM approaches will lead to effective treatments in future.

What Are Cognitive Biases and How Do They Originate?

Dual-process theories of alcohol consumption (see Chap. 3) suggest consumption is driven by a combination of two distinct but related cognitive processes: associative (also known as automatic or impulsive) and reflective (Wiers et al., 2007). Associative processes are the outcome of learned associations between alcohol-related cues (e.g. the sight and/or smell of alcohol) and the rewarding effects of consumption. According to dual-process theories, over the course of a person's drinking history, associative links between alcohol cues and rewarding effects of consumption will be reinforced and strengthened, to the extent that alcohol-related cues will eventually trigger and guide consumption with minimal conscious, top-down influence (*drinking without thinking*). It is these fast, associative processes that form the basis of cognitive biases (discussed below).

By contrast, reflective processes are slower, rational, deliberative decision making schema, which are based on appraisals of the feasibility and value of actions. These processes have been shown to have both a direct influence on alcohol consumption, as well as also regulating the influence of associative processes on consumption (see Chaps. 2 and 4). Reflective processes are associated with increased intelligence (Arffa, 2007), academic achievement (Best, Miller, & Naglieri, 2011) and self-regulation in general (Hofmann, Schmeichel, & Baddeley, 2012). Specific behaviours might include the ability to adapt responses based on variable environmental contingencies (shifting), retain and update information in memory (working memory), and inhibit inappropriate actions (inhibition) (Miyake & Friedman, 2012).

According to dual-process models, reflective processes moderate the influence of associative processes on consumption, such that people are able to behave in accordance with their longer-term goals rather than succumb to transient temptations. For example, exposure to an alcohol-related advert on the TV might trigger the association between alcohol consumption and its rewarding properties (Stautz, Frings, Albery, Moss, & Marteau, 2017), which would in turn evoke an implicit approach behaviour towards a bottle of wine in the kitchen. However, a person might *remember* that their current goal is to avoid drinking today (linked to awareness of an important meeting the next day), which would in turn *inhibit* cognitive biases that influence drinking behaviour, with the consequence being that the person stops approaching the bottle of wine. Of course, not everybody that drinks alcohol does so at a harmful level, and population variability in alcohol consumption might be explained by the relative strength of associative and reflective processes *within* individuals. A person in whom associative processes are strong but reflective processes are weak might be more driven by alcohol-related cues and less likely to be able to regulate their behaviour, whereas a person for whom associative processes are weak but reflective processes are strong would be better able to resist temptation in their environment in pursuit of their longer-term goals (Friese, Hofmann, & Wiers, 2011).

Types of Cognitive Bias and How They Are Measured

The identification of cognitive biases originated through pioneering research into the processing of emotionally threatening information in anxiety. In a seminal study, Colin MacLeod and colleagues (1986) developed the dot-probe task (discussed below) using a computer to measure biases in attention in people with anxiety. Computerised assessment permits direct measurement of cognitive biases, which are difficult to directly observe and may be difficult to capture by self-report. This study is often referenced as the beginning of cognitive bias research. Since this time, different types of bias have been identified and operationalised using a variety of computer tasks. Here we focus on the four tasks most commonly researched with regard to alcohol use: attentional bias, approach bias, inhibitory bias, and interpretation bias. To aid understanding we provide a visual overview of the types of tasks that can be used to measure cognitive biases in Fig. 22.1A–D.

Attentional Biases

Attentional bias is defined as the *'tendency for alcohol-related stimuli to capture and/or hold the attention'* (Field et al., 2016). This selective attention is thought to occur through *sensitisation* of activity in brain regions and neurotransmitters (e.g. dopamine in the mesolimbic pathway) which attribute motivational

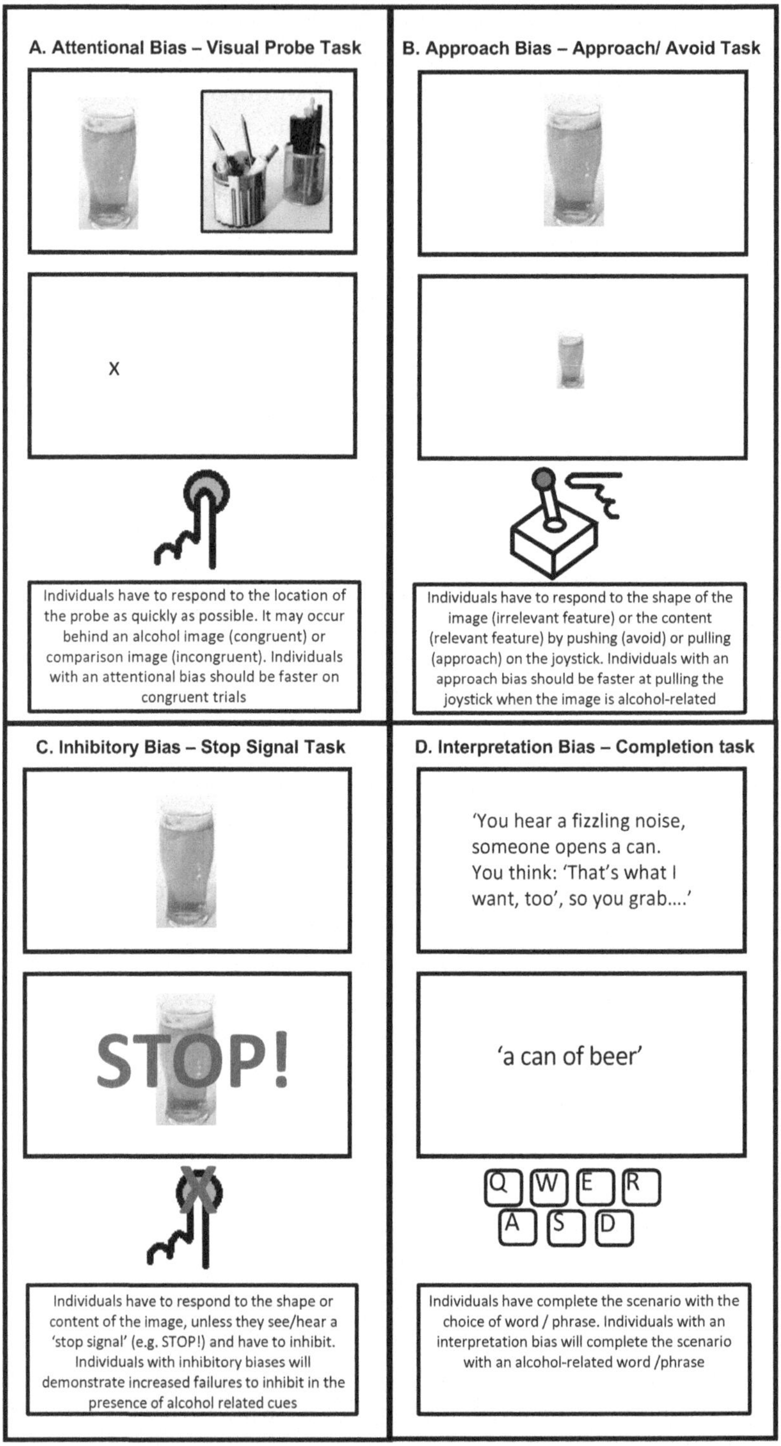

Fig. 22.1 A schematic representing typical trials for different cognitive bias tasks

salience to alcohol-related cues (Robinson & Berridge, 2000). Over time and through associative links (alcohol-related cues –> pleasurable effects) attention is guided towards alcohol-related cues, and the motivation ('wanting') to obtain alcohol is triggered by these cues. Importantly, the sensitisation of this system means that these associations and subsequent biases are persistent and they continue to influence behaviour after long periods of abstinence, thereby increasing the risk of (re)lapse (Garland, Franken, & Howard, 2012).

Most studies measure attentional bias using a variation of the Stroop task or a dot-probe task (see Field & Cox, 2008). The conventional Stroop task presents colour words in different colours (e.g. the word 'red' in blue text), with participants instructed to state the colour of the word. To measure attentional biases for alcohol, words related to alcohol (e.g. 'bottle', 'vodka') and non-alcohol-related control words (e.g. 'candle', 'books') are presented in different colours and participants have to quickly identify their colour. If participants are slower to name the colours for alcohol words, it is inferred that the content of the alcohol words attracted their attention and impaired colour-naming performance (Cox, Fadardi, & Pothos, 2006).

Alternatively, the dot-probe task presents an alcohol and control image side by side on a computer screen. After a brief period (typically 50–3000 milliseconds), both images disappear and a probe appears in the spatial location that was previously occupied by one of the images. Participants have to respond to the probe as quickly as possible by identifying its location or content (e.g. pressing a left key if the probe appeared on the left). If participants were previously attending to the alcohol-related image and the probe were to appear in the location that had previously been occupied by the alcohol image, then they should be faster to respond to the location or content of the probe (see Fig. 22.1: Panel A). Attention is a complex behaviour which involves initially orientating to a cue (the cue 'grabbing; your attention), maintaining your attention on the cue, and disengaging from the cue (to look elsewhere), and attentional biases are thought to be present across each (discussed in Field, Munafò, & Franken (2009)).

Approach Biases

Approach biases represent an automatic tendency to move towards or bring alcohol-related stimuli closer in order to obtain alcohol. They are triggered by exposure to alcohol-related cues and arise from underlying appetitive associations between those cues and positive valence or arousal (Wiers, Van Woerden, Smulders, & De Jong, 2002). These biases are distinct from attentional biases as they represent a behavioural response, rather than a shift in attentional allocation, to alcohol-related cues. Most studies measure approach biases by using the Stimulus Response Compatibility task or the approach/avoid task. In the Stimulus Response Compatibility task participants have to press a key to move an on-screen manikin towards or away from alcohol or control images (Field, Kiernan, Eastwood, & Child, 2008). If they are faster to move the manikin towards alcohol-related images this is indicative of an approach bias. In the approach/avoid task participants are asked to use a joystick to exert a pulling ('approach') or pushing ('avoid') motion in response to images (Wiers, Rinck, Kordts, Houben, & Strack, 2010). If participants are faster to pull the joystick when they see an alcohol-related cue, this suggests an approach bias (see Fig. 22.1: Panel B).

Inhibitory Biases

Inhibitory biases are the inability to effectively inhibit learned (pre-potent) behaviours in the presence of alcohol-related cues in the environment. These biases are likely a consequence of the automatic action tendency biases evoked by alcohol-related cues (see above), which subsequently make inhibition more difficult given the incompatibility of approaching something and inhibiting behaviour simultaneously. To measure inhibitory biases, researchers use tasks that involve stopping, changing, or delaying an inappropriate response, such as the Stop Signal or Go/No-Go tasks (Verbruggen & Logan, 2008). During these tasks participants are required to make a rapid motor response to alcohol-related cues until these responses become fast, efficient, and require little conscious effort. On a minority of trials a 'Stop Signal' or a 'No-Go cue', a prompt to refrain from responding on that trial, will be presented. Failure to inhibit the motor response when in the presence of an alcohol-related cue is indicative of inhibitory biases to alcohol (see Fig. 22.1: Panel C).

Interpretation Biases

Interpretation biases are another aspect of alcohol-related, learned associations. They can be measured without directly mentioning the target behaviour by providing participants with a variety of ambiguous cues (e.g. words or phrases) that *could* be interpreted as alcohol related, but also have other interpretations (Woud et al., 2014). Participants' task is to complete an ambiguous scenario, for example '*You are lying on a large blanket and you are having a jolly and cheerful time. You hear a fizzling noise, someone opens a can. You think: 'That's what I want, too', so you grab'*. Here the participant could say an alcohol beverage (e.g. '*a can of beer*') or a non-alcohol beverage (e.g. '*a can of lemonade*'). These sentence continuations are coded for their alcohol content, with the proportion of alcohol-related responses indicative of the strength of the underlying interpretation bias (see Fig. 22.1: Panel D).

It is worth noting that the biases covered above are generally unobservable without the use of computer-administered tasks. In addition, biases do not act in isolation and may interact with each other to drive behaviour, for example, *a bottle of beer in the environment might grab your attention … you may then automatically approach it to obtain it … which in turn will make it difficult to inhibit any responses towards it.* It is unlikely that any one of these biases is better or worse than any other in predicting behaviour, and in isolation they may predict only small amounts of variance (if any) in alcohol use which we discuss below.

Are Cognitive Biases Associated with Alcohol Use?

Considerable research effort has been devoted to studying the role of cognitive biases in the development and maintenance of regular drinking and alcohol use disorders. In this section we consider the robustness and strength of the association between cognitive biases and individual differences in alcohol consumption. We then consider if cognitive biases have a *causal* influence on alcohol consumption. In line with the experimental medicine framework (paths A and B, Fig. 22.2), identification of a causal influence of cognitive biases on alcohol consumption would establish those cognitive biases as plausible targets for behavioural interventions to reduce alcohol consumption (Sheeran et al., 2017).

Attentional Biases

Narrative reviews suggested that attentional biases were an important characteristic of regular drinkers and people with alcohol use disorders (Field & Cox, 2008). However, as the evidence base has expanded, questions were raised about the robustness of this association (Field, Marhe, & Franken, 2014) and about the replicability of findings that attentional biases could predict treatment outcome in patients with alcohol use disorders (Christiansen,

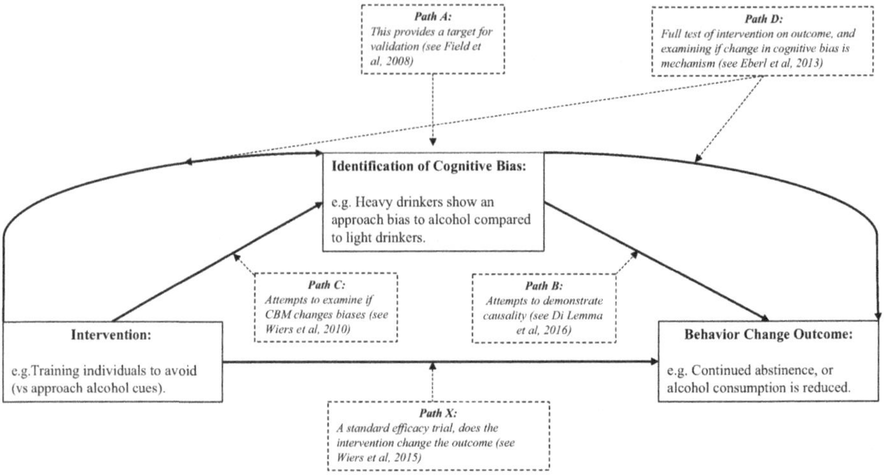

Fig. 22.2 The experimental medicine framework as applied to approach bias modification. (adapted from Sheeran, Klein, & Rothman, 2017). Notes. Path A represents the laboratory studies which examine whether there is an association between cognitive biases and alcohol use (e.g. are biases greater in heavy vs. light drinkers). Path B represents laboratory studies which manipulate cognitive biases before measuring immediate alcohol consumption in an attempt to demonstrate causality. Path C represents studies which examine whether CBM directly changes cognitive biases. Path X represents a standard trial in which CBM is used to change alcohol consumption/(re)lapse in the real world, but the mechanisms of action are not investigated. Path D represents a trial in which CBM is used to change alcohol consumption/(re)lapse in the real world and whether the mechanism of action is a change in the underlying cognitive bias. Dashed arrows and boxes present examples of studies for each pathway)

Schoenmakers, & Field, 2015). In a recent theoretical model, Field et al. (2016) concluded that the role of attentional bias in addiction, including alcohol use disorders, may be overstated. Instead, attentional bias may be the output of underlying evaluative processes (i.e. are substance cues perceived positively or negatively in the current circumstances) that guide behaviour, with attentional biases having *limited* direct causal influence on drinking behaviour.

Attempts to establish causality require the training of attention towards/away from alcohol-related cues, before examining subsequent alcohol consumption. For example, participants might complete a dot-probe task in which the probe infrequently appears in the spatial location that had been occupied by an alcohol-related image ('avoid alcohol group') or frequently appears in the spatial location that had been occupied by an alcohol image ('attend alcohol group'). In principle, if the probe infrequently replaces the alcohol-related image, participants should learn to direct their attention away from alcohol-related images. Wiers, Boffo, and Field (2018) reviewed five relevant studies and found inconsistent evidence that training attention away from alcohol-related cues influences attentional biases or subsequent alcohol consumption in the laboratory. As is often the case, promising initial findings failed to replicate when studied in more robust designs (Field et al., 2007; Schoenmakers, Wiers, Jones, Bruce, & Jansen, 2007).

Approach Biases

The existence of approach biases for alcohol has been widely documented according to a recent systematic review (Kakoschke, Kemps, & Tiggemann, 2016). However, it is worth noting that there are also numerous failures to replicate studies or find an association between approach biases and alcohol use (e.g. Field, Di Lemma, Christiansen, & Dickson, 2017).

To examine potential causal relationships approach biases can be trained in a similar way to attentional biases, by altering the response contingencies during an approach/avoid task. To train participants to avoid alcohol, they push the joystick away from all or the majority of alcohol images (an avoidance movement) whilst approaching (pulling the joystick towards themselves) control or neutral images. These contingencies are reversed in a comparison group, who are required to approach alcohol and avoid control images. Wiers et al.'s (2018) narrative review suggests strong evidence for a causal link between approach biases and alcohol use/(re)lapse, in that approach bias training reduces approach biases for alcohol, but also reduces ad-libitum alcohol consumption. However, these apparently robust findings are not always observed, for example in the first laboratory study of approach bias training Wiers et al. (2010) demonstrated no significant reduction in ad-libitum alcohol consumption following 'alcohol avoid' training compared to 'alcohol approach' training across the whole sample. The hypothesised significant reduction in alcohol consumption, following approach bias training, was however observed in participants in whom the training changed their biases in the predicted direction, according to a *post-hoc* analysis. This is a key aspect of path D in the experimental medicine approach, and we revisit this pattern of findings (drinking behaviour changes only if the cognitive bias does) below.

Inhibitory Bias

A meta-analysis has demonstrated a small but significant inhibitory bias to alcohol-related cues in heavy/hazardous drinkers and alcohol-dependent patients, compared to light drinkers/controls (Jones, Robinson et al., 2018). Individual studies have demonstrated that these biases can predict variance in hazardous drinking behaviour (Petit, Kornreich, Noël, Verbanck, & Campanella, 2012), as well as ad-libitum alcohol consumption in non-dependent drinkers (Field & Jones, 2017). In dependent samples, the magnitude of inhibitory bias may predict likelihood of relapse following treatment (Czapla et al., 2015). However, it is worth noting that several individual studies have failed to replicate the effect of alcohol cues on inhibitory control (e.g. Baines, Field, Christiansen, & Jones, 2019).

Numerous studies have examined the causal relationship between inhibitory biases to alcohol-related cues and ad-libitum alcohol consumption. Jones and Field (2012) manipulated the contingencies for inhibition to alcohol-related cues on a Stop Signal task, so that one group inhibited to the majority of alcohol-related cues (90%), another group inhibited to the majority of neutral cues (90%), and one group did not inhibit at all. They demonstrated that the group that inhibited to the majority of alcohol-related cues consumed less alcohol than the group that inhibited to neutral cues and the group that did not inhibit at all. Similar findings have been demonstrated by other groups using variations of this design (Bowley et al., 2013), and meta-analyses have confirmed small, robust effects (d ~ 0.43: Allom, Mullan, & Hagger, 2015; Jones, Di Lemma, et al., 2016). Taken together, these findings suggest a causal role of inhibitory biases in alcohol consumption.

Interpretation Bias

Relatively few studies have investigated interpretation biases for alcohol. For example, Woud, Fitzgerald, Wiers, Rinck, and Becker (2012) compared heavy and light drinking students and demonstrated that heavy drinking students generated a greater number of alcohol-related continuations to ambiguous scenarios. They also demonstrated that the number of continuations was significantly correlated with self-reported alcohol consumption and problematic consumption. The same research group also demonstrated that the number of alcohol-related continuations made by alcohol-dependent patients was significantly higher than control patients (individuals with a mood or anxiety disorder) and also associated with problematic drinking (Woud et al., 2014). van Duijvenbode, Didden, Korzilius, and Engels (2016) replicated these findings and demonstrated interpretation biases in problem drinkers with and without mild-to-borderline intellectual disability.

Studies have attempted to manipulate the likelihood of an alcohol continuation of a scenario (e.g. Salemink, Woud, Roos, Wiers, & Lindgren, 2019), to manipulate these interpretation biases and test causality. To do this they provided 32 scenarios and asked participants to complete a word fragment. This fragment had only one possible solution and produced a word consistent with an alcohol- or non-alcohol-related interpretation. For example, the scenario could be '*You are going to the theatre with your partner, and you buy a refreshing drink. You buy a glass of*', and the fragments would be '*W_NE*' (WINE) or '*C_KE*' (COKE). In an alcohol-training condition these scenarios would always end with an alcohol-related fragment, and in a control condition they would end in a neutral fragment. Following training participants were presented with novel ambiguous scenarios, and individuals in the alcohol-training group interpreted these as more alcohol related, compared to the control condition. However, these differences did not translate to differences in subsequent ad-libitum alcohol consumption (Salemink et al., 2019; Woud, Hutschemaekers, Rinck, & Becker, 2015). These findings suggest that interpretation biases may be present in people with alcohol use disorders, although a causal influence on drinking behaviour has not been established.

Evidence for the Effectiveness of Cognitive Bias Modification Outside of the Laboratory

Laboratory manipulations of cognitive biases are essential for demonstrating the causal relationship between those biases and subsequent alcohol consumption, and those CBM interventions provide the basis of an intervention that might be applied outside of the laboratory. The strength of the experimental medicine approach is that it allows researchers both to test the efficacy of an intervention and to determine *why* it was effective (see Fig. 22.2 and legend for examples specifically related to approach biases). Therefore, many studies have attempted to (1) manipulate biases in the laboratory and examine alcohol consumption in the 'real world' or (2) manipulate biases and examine alcohol consumption in the real world. It is also worth noting that the types of studies below can be demarcated into those which (1) examine CBM (as a treatment adjunct) in clinical settings in RCTs with alcohol-dependent patients and (2) examine CBM online in problem drinkers (Wiers et al., 2018), and these studies may have different outcomes.

Attentional Bias Modification

Several studies have examined the effects of attentional bias modification on 'real-world' alcohol consumption. For example, McGeary, Meadows, Amir, and Gibb (2014) created a training programme which required heavy drinking students in the USA to complete two sessions per week of attentional bias modification in their own home for one month, compared to a control condition. They demonstrated that students in the training group reduced their alcohol consumption over the course of the training compared to students in the control group. In a sample of social, heavy, and harmful drinkers, Fadardi and Cox (2009) trained attention away from alcohol cues using a modified Stroop task in the laboratory. Compared to social drinkers (individuals who consumed alcohol at lower risk levels; see Chap. 1) and heavy drinkers (males who consumed 22–50 units of alcohol per week/females who consumed 15–35 units of alcohol per week), harmful drinkers (males who consumed 50+ units of alcohol per week/females who consumed 35+ units of alcohol per week) demonstrated a reduction in attentional bias to alcohol and a reduction in their alcohol consumption following training. This effect was maintained at three-month follow-up. However, a major limitation of this study was a lack of control group, who did not receive training. In a later study by Cox, Fadardi, Hosier, and Pothos (2015) attentional bias modification was combined with a different intervention (life advancement motivational training, which focused on individuals' strategising to lead a satisfying life without using alcohol excessively) in heavy drinkers using a 2 × 2 cross-over design (attentional bias modification present or absent and motivational training present or absent). Participants were required to complete training once per week for four weeks, and alcohol consumption was followed up at three and six months post training. This study demonstrated that attentional bias modification led to reductions in alcohol consumption at three-month follow-up, but not immediately following training or at six-month follow-up. The life advancement motivational training was similarly effective; however, when attentional bias modification was combined with life advancement motivational training, there was little additional benefit. Wiers et al. (2015) incorporated Fadardi and Cox's training paradigm into an entirely online intervention over a month-long period and compared it to three variations of approach bias training and a control group. They recruited a community sample and demonstrated reduced alcohol consumption in all groups (even the control group). This study also had a considerable dropout rate (56%), suggesting CBM studies conducted entirely online without face-to-face contact may not be so effective. To summarise, in non-clinical samples attentional bias modification may reduce alcohol consumption, at least in the short term, but only when delivered face to face.

In clinical samples, Schoenmakers et al. (2010) randomised abstinent alcohol-dependent patients to five sessions of attentional bias medication or control over a three-week period. They showed that active training reduced the difficulty in disengaging attention away from alcohol-related cues but did not significantly reduce craving or time taken to relapse. Clerkin, Magee, Wells, Beard, and Barnett (2016) examined attentional bias modification for both alcohol and negative emotional faces in socially anxious alcohol-dependent samples and demonstrated little convincing evidence of changes in attentional bias or alcohol-related outcomes which could be attributed to training. Finally, Rinck, Wiers, Becker, and Lindenmeyer (2018) examined the effects of attentional bias (and approach bias) modification for relapse prevention in abstinent alcoholics. In a randomised controlled trial (RCT) 1405 patients were randomly allocated to one of four conditions: (1) six sessions of approach bias retraining, (2) six sessions of attentional bias retraining, (3) three sessions of each training, (4) six sessions of sham training or no training at all, over a two-week period. Rinck et al. demonstrated that compared to the sham and no-training groups, the three active CBM groups had greater percentages of treatment success (defined as no relapse, or a single relapse shorter than three days with no negative consequences) after one year. They also demonstrated that three conditions were equally effective, suggesting that there is no specific advantage to approach bias modification, attentional bias modification, or their combination. In an exploratory analysis, there was no evidence that changes in cognitive biases as a result of treatment mediated the treatment effects. As such, this study found no support for path D in the experimental medicine framework (Fig. 22.2).

Approach Bias Modification

Only one study has tested approach bias modification in a non-clinical sample. Wiers et al. (2015) demonstrated no beneficial effects of approach bias training delivered online, compared to attentional retraining or a control group for problem drinkers. In clinical samples, there is some evidence that approach bias modification can reduce relapse. Wiers, Eberl, Rinck, Becker, and Lindenmeyer (2011) assigned 214 detoxified alcohol-dependent patients to avoid alcohol or control groups. The control groups either were given no training at all or completed sham training in which the contingencies to approach and avoid alcohol were 50%. Participants completed four sessions over consecutive days. Following training, patients who were trained to avoid alcohol demonstrated significant avoid-alcohol biases (having previously demonstrated approach-alcohol biases). Most importantly, when compared to the control groups there were fewer instances of relapse in the 'avoid alcohol' training groups at 1-year follow-up.

Eberl et al. (2013) attempted to replicate these promising findings using a group of 509 patients, who were asked to complete 12 sessions of training over a three-month period. Approach bias training led to increased avoidance bias in the trained group, but not the no-training control. They also demonstrated significantly improved treatment effects (reduction in relapse) compared to the control group. Importantly, they found that the change in approach/avoidance bias to alcohol following training significantly mediated the effects on treatment outcome, suggesting that the greater the effect of training on bias, the better the treatment outcome. Finally, as discussed above Rinck et al. (2018) have demonstrated that approach bias alone or in combination with attentional bias led to reduced relapse rates in abstinent alcoholics over a one-year period.

Inhibitory Control Training

Three studies examined whether manipulating inhibitory control in the laboratory could have a sustained influence on self-reported alcohol consumption over a week-long period. While Houben, Nederkoorn, Wiers, and Jansen (2011) demonstrated reductions in self-reported alcohol consumption, neither Jones and Field (2012) nor Bowley et al. (2013) were able to replicate these findings. It is notable that these studies were conducted using samples of heavy drinking students, who were unlikely to be motivated to reduce their alcohol consumption (an issue with many studies, see Chap. 21, Wiers et al., 2018).

Jones, McGrath, et al. (2018) examined the effects of inhibitory control training delivered via the internet over a four-week period, in a pre-registered study design using a sample of heavy drinkers who explicitly reported motivation to reduce their consumption. Participants were randomised to one of three inhibitory control training interventions or a control group who received sham training, and asked participants to complete up to 14 sessions of training. They observed a marked reduction in alcohol consumption during the training period that was maintained at six-week follow-up; however, this was a non-specific reduction that was seen in all groups, including the control group (cf. Cox et al., 2015). Furthermore, they found no evidence that inhibitory control training changed inhibitory bias to alcohol-related cues, failing to support path B of the experimental medicine framework.

Strickland, Hill, Stoops, and Rush (2019) compared inhibitory control training, against training to improve working memory and a control group who completed simple arithmetic, in a group of patients with alcohol disorder. Each condition completed the training (or control) sessions daily for two weeks, followed by a two-week follow-up. The study was conducted entirely online and used crowdsourcing to recruit participants. Individuals who were trained to improve their inhibitory control to alcohol-related cues demonstrated an improvement in inhibitory control on the training task during the test period. They also demonstrated a reduction in the number of drinking days (any alcohol consumed) and heavy drinking days at follow-up compared to baseline. However, these findings are difficult to interpret, as they also observed increases in drinking days in the control group.

Interpretation Bias Training

Two studies delivered interpretive bias training in the laboratory to heavy drinking university students from the Netherlands and examined alcohol consumption over a one-week period following training. Neither study demonstrated any beneficial effects of receiving this training (Salemink et al., 2019; Woud et al., 2015).

Summarising the Evidence for Cognitive Bias Modification

Whilst results from some studies (e.g. Rinck et al., 2018; Wiers et al., 2011) suggest that CBM may be a promising treatment for problematic drinking or alcohol use disorder, the narrative is often more convincing than the data. In 2016, Cristea, Kok, and Cuijpers (2016) in a meta-analysis dampened much of the enthusiasm for the effect of CBM. They meta-analysed published CBM studies alone or in combination with other treatments, for any type of addictive substance (smoking and alcohol consumption), including 25 studies, 18 of which focused on alcohol and 7 focused on smoking. Cristea et al. concluded that there was no overall effect of CBM on alcohol use or craving (g = 0.10, 95% CI -0.01 to 0.22), in the studies focused on alcohol. Furthermore, they identified considerable risk of bias in these studies, such as unclear allocation concealment and attrition, suggesting that most studies were of poor methodological quality. The conclusion from this analysis was that there are 'serious doubts on the clinical utility of CBM interventions (for addiction (pg. 2))'.

Rigorous meta-analyses are thought to provide a higher standard of evidence than individual studies (Fagerland, 2015). However, this meta-analysis was criticised for several reasons. Included studies comprised a range of methodologies, including RCTs, laboratory studies, and online studies, which vary in their internal validity. This makes it hard to compare results across studies. Studies also varied in samples that were recruited, with some studies recruiting problematic drinkers and others recruiting clinical samples. As shown above, results for CBM were not consistent across samples. Clearly these types of studies are not homogeneous; they have different aims (abstinence vs. reductions in consumption), recruit different participants (patients vs. heavy/problem drinkers), in different settings (clinic vs. online with no personal contact): see Wiers et al. (2018) for more detail. A look-back at the studies discussed above suggests that CBM administered in the clinic to reduce relapse often has positive results, whereas online studies in heavy drinkers often lead to non-specific treatment effects (reduced drinking irrespective of CBM condition). This suggests that the effectiveness of CBM may be moderated by the sample it is delivered to.

Proponents of CBM also suggest that the effects on alcohol consumption and abstinence outcomes should only be observed if the training reliably changes cognitive biases. Otherwise, the intervention is not working as intended and proposed in the experimental medicine approach (path D). Grafton et al. (2017) argued that researchers have begun to confuse process and procedure: the term 'cognitive bias modification' has been used to refer to both the *process* of cognitive bias change and the *procedure* of attempting to change cognitive bias; Grafton et al. argue that the term 'cognitive bias modification' should be used to describe only the process rather than the procedure.

In response to these points, a recent meta-analysis examined individual participant data within a Bayesian statistical framework (Boffo et al., 2019). In this analysis they included individuals with a clinical diagnosis of substance use, who were suffering from substance-related problems or were aware they were part of an intervention to change their behaviour (more appropriately representing the typical conditions and inclusion criteria of an RCT, rather than a study establishing causality). These analyses demonstrated evidence for CBM directly influencing (reducing) cognitive biases both in the same task (near-transfer: path C in the experimental medicine approach) and in related tasks (far-transfer). Most importantly, there was no evidence that CBM reduced relapse (−0.27, 95% credible interval = −0.68 to 0.22) or alcohol use behaviour (0.19, 95% credible interval - 0.23 to 0.58; tests of path X). Again, these findings suggest limited evidence for CBM as a psychological intervention for alcohol use disorders. Using a Bayesian framework allows us to draw evidence directly for the null hypothesis, rather than only the alternative hypothesis.

Other Limitations with CBM Studies

Below we discuss some of the main limitations with existing CBM studies which impact the interpretation, reliability, and replicability of CBM research for alcohol.

Power and Experimental Design Issues in CBM Laboratory Studies

Perhaps the most obvious limitation with the existing CBM literature is that many studies lack statistical power to reliably detect the effects of CBM on outcomes. It is common for laboratory-based studies examining the causal mechanisms of cognitive biases to be underpowered, given the effects identified in studies are generally small (Cristea et al., 2016; Jones, Di Lemma, et al., 2016). Indeed in the parallel literature of CBM for food intake, estimates of statistical power range from 24 to 41% (Jones, Hardman, Lawrence, & Field, 2017) and we have little reason to suggest they are improved in alcohol-related studies. Therefore, there may be a considerable and unacceptable risk of type II error in these studies. While concerns about statistical power appear to be endemic throughout psychological research (Szucs & Ioannidis, 2017), such concerns have particular salience in CBM studies because results from these studies are used to inform interventions; power calculations for translational research are often based on an effect size generated in laboratory studies. With this in mind, there are some studies that serve as notable exceptions by recruiting larger samples (Rinck et al., 2018) or providing justification for statistical power (Jones, McGrath, et al., 2018).

Two experimental design issues with CBM laboratory studies have the potential to limit the translatability of findings to clinical trials. First, laboratory studies often have a comparison group which trains bias *towards* alcohol to establish causality, which will likely inflate any effect size estimates. Of course, it would be unethical to have such a comparison group in clinical trials. Second, the outcome used to generate an effect size is often the effects of receiving CBM training on ad-libitum consumption. It is debatable whether this outcome adequately reflects real-world drinking, as research has suggested ad-libitum consumption predicts only a small amount of variance in real-world drinking (Jones et al., 2016).

Reliability of Tasks Used in CBM Training

A further issue when interpreting and implementing CBM findings is the potential unreliability of the task(s) used. Most CBM studies adapt a task originally designed to *measure* cognitive biases and alter the contingencies in order to change the underlying cognitive biases. The reliability of these tasks following this adaptation process is rarely considered, however. Existing research has demonstrated that tasks used to measure cognitive biases have less than adequate internal reliability (Jones, Christiansen, & Field, 2018). One potential reason for this is that outcomes from these tasks rely on 'difference' scores to create biases. For example, attentional bias on the dot-probe task is inferred from the difference between reaction times when the probe occurs behind the alcohol image (congruent trial) to when it appears behind the neutral image (incongruent trial) [Attentional Bias = Incongruent RT – Congruent RT]. This method is thought to provide some control over an individual's general reaction time. However, subtracting two variables which are correlated with each other reduces their shared variance and increases error in the measurement (Draheim, Mashburn, Martin, & Engle, 2019). One example of this can be seen in the study of Rinck et al. (2018), who report extremely poor reliabilities of their assessment tasks for approach bias (ranging from α 0.00 to 0.58). Measurements with poor reliability may not reflect their latent variable (i.e. they are inseparable from random noise) and have a considerable impact on reproducibility/replicability (Kanyongo, Brook, Kyei-Blankson, & Gocmen, 2007). If we cannot adequately measure these target variables, it can make these approaches unfalsifiable, and without adequate reliability, any attempt to examine mediation effects (the all-important path D in the experimental medicine approach: Fig. 22.2) will yield meaningless estimates (Rodebaugh et al., 2016). Therefore, it is essential that efforts are made to improve the psychometric properties of the tasks used to implement CBM or replace them with more reliable tasks.

Should Researchers Persevere with CBM Approaches?

Despite two meta-analyses demonstrating CBM has no effect on alcohol use behaviours or relapse (Boffo et al., 2019; Cristea et al., 2016), CBM retains many proponents who suggest that it should be prioritised in future research (particularly changes in cognitive biases as a mechanism of treatment action (Holmes et al., 2018)). Others however suggest that cognitive biases are nothing more than an interesting artefact of alcohol use; their clinical utility is negligible and further obscured by attempts to explain away failed studies with potential 'boundary conditions or hidden moderators' (Cristea, 2018). It is important for the field to arrive at some consensus for the efficacy of CBM, ideally through well-powered and designed RCTs, using tasks with demonstrable reliability. Data from studies employing such designs will clarify the potential of CBM as an intervention for alcohol outcomes. However, if after conducting such studies the consensus is that there is no evidence that CBM training has a significant effect on alcohol use, we should be willing to abandon its implementation in favour of more effective alternatives, which will reduce research waste.

Conclusion

At first glance CBM is seemingly an attractive treatment based on easily understood theories, which might overcome treatment barriers and have long-lasting effects. However despite considerable attempts to change the cognitive biases which may lead people to consume alcohol or (re)lapse, it is impossible to provide a consensus statement for the effectiveness of CBM for alcohol, given the substantial heterogeneity of study designs and findings, in combination with important but largely overlooked methodological issues. In order to provide more definitive answers about the clinical utility of CBM for alcohol use, the development of reliable tasks and high-powered, pre-registered RCTs are required.

References

Allom, V., Mullan, B., & Hagger, M. S. (2015). Does inhibitory control training improve health behaviour? A meta-analysis. *Health Psychology Review, 10*, 168–186.

Arffa, S. (2007). The relationship of intelligence to executive function and non-executive function measures in a sample of average, above average, and gifted youth. *Archives of Clinical Neuropsychology, 22*, 969–978.

Baines, L., Field, M., Christiansen, P., & Jones, A. (2019). The effect of alcohol cue exposure and acute intoxication on inhibitory control processes and ad libitum alcohol consumption. *Psychopharmacology, 236*, 2187–2199.

Best, J. R., Miller, P. H., & Naglieri, J. A. (2011). Relations between executive function and academic achievement from ages 5 to 17 in a large, representative national sample. *Learning and Individual Differences, 21*, 327–336.

Boffo, M., Zerhouni, O., Gronau, Q. F., van Beek, R. J. J., Nikolaou, K., Marsman, M., & Wiers, R. W. (2019). Cognitive Bias modification for behavior change in alcohol and smoking addiction: Bayesian meta-analysis of individual participant data. *Neuropsychology Review, 29*, 52–78.

Bowley, C., Faricy, C., Hegarty, B., Johnstone, S. J., Smith, J., Kelly, P., & Rushby, J. (2013). The effects of inhibitory control training on alcohol consumption, implicit alcohol-related cognitions and brain electrical activity. *International Journal of Psychophysiology, 89*, 342–348.

Christiansen, P., Schoenmakers, T. M., & Field, M. (2015). Less than meets the eye: Reappraising the clinical relevance of attentional bias in addiction. *Addictive Behaviors, 44*, 43–50.

Clerkin, E. M., Magee, J. C., Wells, T. T., Beard, C., & Barnett, N. P. (2016). Randomized controlled trial of attention bias modification in a racially diverse, socially anxious, alcohol dependent sample. *Behaviour Research and Therapy, 87*, 58–69.

Cox, W. M., Fadardi, J. S., Hosier, S. G., & Pothos, E. M. (2015). Differential effects and temporal course of attentional and motivational training on excessive drinking. *Experimental and Clinical Psychopharmacology, 23*, 445–454.

Cox, W. M., Fadardi, J. S., & Pothos, E. M. (2006). The addiction-stroop test: Theoretical considerations and procedural recommendations. *Psychological Bulletin, 132*, 443–476.

Cristea, I. A. (2018). Experimental psychopathology should not be examined with rose-tinted glasses. *Lancet Psychiatry, 5*, 465–466.

Cristea, I. A., Kok, R. N., & Cuijpers, P. (2016). The effectiveness of cognitive bias modification interventions for substance addictions: A meta-analysis. *PLoS One, 11*(9), e0162226.

Czapla, M., Simon, J. J., Richter, B., Kluge, M., Friederich, H. C., Herpertz, S., … Loeber, S. (2015). The impact of cognitive impairment and impulsivity on relapse of alcohol-dependent patients: Implications for psychotherapeutic treatment. *Addiction Biology, 21*, 873–884.

Draheim, C., Mashburn, C. A., Martin, J. D., & Engle, R. W. (2019). Reaction time in differential and developmental research: A review and commentary on the problems and alternatives. *Psychological Bulletin, 145*, 508–535.

Eberl, C., Wiers, R. W., Pawelczack, S., Rinck, M., Becker, E. S., & Lindenmeyer, J. (2013). Approach bias modification in alcohol dependence: Do clinical effects replicate and for whom does it work best? *Developmental Cognitive Neuroscience, 4*, 38–51.

Fadardi, J. S., & Cox, W. M. (2009). Reversing the sequence: Reducing alcohol consumption by overcoming alcohol attentional bias. *Drug and Alcohol Dependence, 101*, 137–145.

Fagerland, M. W. (2015). Chapter 12 – evidence-based medicine and systematic reviews. In P. Laake, H. B. Benestad, & B. R. Olsen (Eds.), *Research in medical and biological sciences* (2nd ed., pp. 431–461). Amsterdam, Netherlands: Academic Press.

Field, M., & Cox, W. M. (2008). Attentional bias in addictive behaviors: A review of its development, causes, and consequences. *Drug and Alcohol Dependence, 97*, 1–20.

Field, M., Di Lemma, L., Christiansen, P., & Dickson, J. (2017). Automatic avoidance tendencies for alcohol cues predict drinking after detoxification treatment in alcohol dependence. *Psychology of Addictive Behaviors, 31*, 171–179.

Field, M., Duka, T., Eastwood, B., Child, R., Santarcangelo, M., & Gayton, M. (2007). Experimental manipulation of attentional biases in heavy drinkers: Do the effects generalise? *Psychopharmacology, 192*, 593–608.

Field, M., & Jones, A. (2017). Elevated alcohol consumption following alcohol cue exposure is partially mediated by reduced inhibitory control and increased craving. *Psychopharmacology, 234*(19), 2979–2988.

Field, M., Kiernan, A., Eastwood, B., & Child, R. (2008). Rapid approach responses to alcohol cues in heavy drinkers. *Journal of Behavior Therapy and Experimental Psychiatry, 39*, 209–218.

Field, M., Marhe, R., & Franken, I. H. A. (2014). The clinical relevance of attentional bias in substance use disorders. *CNS Spectrums, 19*, 225–230.

Field, M., Munafò, M. R., & Franken, I. H. A. (2009). A meta-analytic investigation of the relationship between Attentional Bias and subjective craving in substance abuse. *Psychological Bulletin, 135*, 589–607.

Field, M., Werthmann, J., Franken, I. H., Hofmann, W., Hogarth, L., & Roefs, A. (2016). The role of attentional bias in obesity and addiction. *Health Psychology, 35*, 767–780.

Friese, M., Hofmann, W., & Wiers, R. W. (2011). On taming horses and strengthening riders: Recent developments in research on interventions to improve self-control in health behaviors. *Self and Identity, 10*, 336–351.

Garland, E. L., Franken, I. H. A., & Howard, M. O. (2012). Cue-elicited heart rate variability and attentional bias predict alcohol relapse following treatment. *Psychopharmacology, 222*, 17–26.

Grafton, B., MacLeod, C., Rudaizky, D., Holmes, E. A., Salemink, E., Fox, E., & Notebaert, L. (2017). Confusing procedures with process when appraising the impact of cognitive bias modification on emotional vulnerability(dagger). *The British Journal of Psychiatry, 211*, 266–271.

Hofmann, W., Schmeichel, B. J., & Baddeley, A. D. (2012). Executive functions and self-regulation. *Trends in Cognitive Sciences, 16*, 174–180.

Holmes, E. A., Ghaderi, A., Harmer, C. J., Ramchandani, P. G., Cuijpers, P., Morrison, A. P., … Craske, M. G. (2018). The lancet psychiatry commission on psychological treatments research in tomorrow's science. *Lancet Psychiatry, 5*, 237–286.

Houben, K., Nederkoorn, C., Wiers, R. W., & Jansen, A. (2011). Resisting temptation: Decreasing alcohol-related affect and drinking behavior by training response inhibition. *Drug and Alcohol Dependence, 116*, 132–136.

Jones, A., Button, E., Rose, A. K., Robinson, E., Christiansen, P., Di Lemma, L., & Field, M. (2016). The ad-libitum alcohol 'taste test': Secondary analyses of potential confounds and construct validity. *Psychopharmacology, 233*, 917–924.

Jones, A., Christiansen, P., & Field, M. (2018). Failed attempts to improve the reliability of the alcohol visual probe task following empirical recommendations. *Psychology of Addictive Behaviors, 32*, 922–932.

Jones, A., Di Lemma, L. C. G., Robinson, E., Christiansen, P., Nolan, S., Tudur-Smith, C., & Field, M. (2016). Inhibitory control training for appetitive behaviour change: A meta-analytic investigation of mechanisms of action and moderators of effectiveness. *Appetite, 97*, 16–28.

Jones, A., & Field, M. (2012). The effects of cue-specific inhibition training on alcohol consumption in heavy social drinkers. *Experimental and Clinical Psychopharmacology, 21*, 8–16.

Jones, A., Hardman, C. A., Lawrence, N., & Field, M. (2017). Cognitive training as a potential treatment for overweight and obesity: A critical review of the evidence. *Appetite, 124*, 50–67.

Jones, A., McGrath, E., Robinson, E., Houben, K., Nederkoorn, C., & Field, M. (2018). A randomised controlled trial of inhibitory control training for the reduction of alcohol consumption in problem drinkers. *Journal of Consulting and Clinical Psychology, 86*(12), 991–1004.

Jones, A., Robinson, E., Duckworth, J., Kersbergen, I., Clarke, N., & Field, M. (2018). The effects of exposure to appetitive cues on inhibitory control: A meta-analytic investigation. *Appetite, 128*, 271–282.

Kakoschke, N., Kemps, E., & Tiggemann, M. (2016). Approach bias modification training and consumption: A review of the literature. *Addictive Behaviors, 64*, 21–28.

Kanyongo, G. Y., Brook, G. P., Kyei-Blankson, L., & Gocmen, G. (2007). Reliability and statistical power: How measurement fallibility affects power and required sample sizes for several parametric and nonparametric statistics. *Journal of Modern Applied Statistical Methods, 6*, 81–90.

MacLeod, C., Mathews, A., Tata, P (1986). Attentional bias in emotional disorders. *Journal of Abnormal Psychology, 95*, 15–20.

McGeary, J. E., Meadows, S. P., Amir, N., & Gibb, B. E. (2014). Computer-delivered, home-based, attentional retraining reduces drinking behavior in heavy drinkers. *Psychology of Addictive Behaviors, 28*, 559–562.

Miyake, A., & Friedman, N. P. (2012). The nature and organization of individual differences in executive functions: Four general conclusions. *Current Directions in Psychological Science, 21*, 8–14.

Petit, G., Kornreich, C., Noël, X., Verbanck, P., & Campanella, S. (2012). Alcohol-related context modulates performance of social drinkers in a visual go/no-go task: A preliminary assessment of event-related potentials. *PLoS One, 7*, e37466.

Rinck, M., Wiers, R. W., Becker, E. S., & Lindenmeyer, J. (2018). Relapse prevention in abstinent alcoholics by cognitive bias modification: Clinical effects of combining approach bias modification and attention bias modification. *Journal of Consulting and Clinical Psychology, 86*, 1005–1016.

Robinson, T. E., & Berridge, K. C. (2000). The psychology and neurobiology of addiction: An incentive-sensitization view. *Addiction, 95*, 91–117.

Rodebaugh, T. L., Scullin, R. B., Langer, J. K., Dixon, D. J., Huppert, J. D., Bernstein, A., … Lenze, E. J. (2016). Unreliability as a threat to understanding psychopathology: The cautionary tale of Attentional Bias. *Journal of Abnormal Psychology, 125*, 840–851.

Salemink, E., Woud, M. L., Roos, M., Wiers, R., & Lindgren, K. P. (2019). Reducing alcohol-related interpretive bias in negative affect situations: Using a scenario-based cognitive Bias modification training paradigm. *Addictive Behaviors, 88*, 106–113.

Schoenmakers, T., Wiers, R. W., Jones, B. T., Bruce, G., & Jansen, A. T. M. (2007). Attentional re-training decreases attentional bias in heavy drinkers without generalization. *Addiction, 102*, 399–405.

Schoenmakers, T. M., de Bruin, M., Lux, I. F. M., Goertz, A. G., Van Kerkhof, D. H. A. T., & Wiers, R. W. (2010). Clinical effectiveness of attentional bias modification training in abstinent alcoholic patients. *Drug and Alcohol Dependence, 109*, 30–36.

Sheeran, P., Klein, W. M. P., & Rothman, A. J. (2017). Health behavior change: Moving from observation to intervention. *Annual Review of Psychology, 68*, 573–600.

Stautz, K., Frings, D., Albery, I. P., Moss, A. C., & Marteau, T. M. (2017). Impact of alcohol-promoting and alcohol-warning advertisements on alcohol consumption, affect, and implicit cognition in heavy-drinking young adults: A laboratory-based randomized controlled trial. *British Journal of Health Psychology, 22*, 128–150.

Strickland, J. C., Hill, J. C., Stoops, W. W., & Rush, C. R. (2019). Feasibility, acceptability, and initial efficacy of delivering alcohol use cognitive interventions via crowdsourcing. *Alcoholism: Clinical and Experimental Research, 43*, 888–899.

Szucs, D., & Ioannidis, J. P. A. (2017). Empirical assessment of published effect sizes and power in the recent cognitive neuroscience and psychology literature. *PLoS Biology, 15*, e2000797.

van Duijvenbode, N., Didden, R., Korzilius, H. P. L. M., & Engels, R. C. M. E. (2016). Everybody is…drinking! Interpretation Bias in problematic drinkers with and without mild to borderline intellectual disability. *Journal of Mental Health Research in Intellectual Disabilities, 9*, 101–117.

Verbruggen, F., & Logan, G. D. (2008). Automatic and controlled response inhibition: Associative learning in the go/no-go and stop-signal paradigms. *Journal of Experimental Psychology: General, 137*, 649–672.

Wiers, R. W., Bartholow, B. D., van den Wildenberg, E., Thush, C., Engels, R. C. M. E., Sher, K. J., … Stacy, A. W. (2007). Automatic and controlled processes and the development of addictive behaviors in adolescents: A review and a model. *Pharmacology Biochemistry and Behavior, 86*, 263–283.

Wiers, R. W., Boffo, M., & Field, M. (2018). What's in a trial? On the importance of distinguishing between experimental lab studies and randomized controlled trials: The case of cognitive Bias modification and alcohol use disorders. *Journal of Studies on Alcohol and Drugs, 79*, 333–343.

Wiers, R. W., Eberl, C., Rinck, M., Becker, E. S., & Lindenmeyer, J. (2011). Retraining automatic action tendencies changes alcoholic patients' approach bias for alcohol and improves treatment outcome. *Psychological Science, 22*, 490–497.

Wiers, R. W., Houben, K., Fadardi, J. S., van Beek, P., Rhemtulla, M., & Cox, W. M. (2015). Alcohol cognitive bias modification training for problem drinkers over the web. *Addictive Behaviors, 40*, 21–26.

Wiers, R. W., Rinck, M., Kordts, R., Houben, K., & Strack, F. (2010). Retraining automatic action-tendencies to approach alcohol in hazardous drinkers. *Addiction (Abingdon, England), 105*, 279–287.

Wiers, R. W., Van Woerden, N., Smulders, F. T. Y., & De Jong, P. J. (2002). Implicit and explicit alcohol-related cognitions in heavy and light drinkers. *Journal of Abnormal Psychology, 111*, 648–658.

Woud, M. L., Fitzgerald, D. A., Wiers, R. W., Rinck, M., & Becker, E. S. (2012). 'Getting into the spirit': Alcohol-related interpretation bias in heavy-drinking students. *Psychology of Addictive Behaviors, 26*, 627–632.

Woud, M. L., Hutschemaekers, M. H., Rinck, M., & Becker, E. S. (2015). The manipulation of alcohol-related interpretation biases by means of cognitive Bias modification--interpretation (CBM-I). *Journal of Behavior Therapy and Experimental Psychiatry, 49*, 61–68.

Woud, M. L., Pawelczak, S., Rinck, M., Lindenmeyer, J., Souren, P., Wiers, R. W., & Becker, E. S. (2014). Alcohol-related interpretation Bias in alcohol-dependent patients. *Alcoholism: Clinical and Experimental Research, 38*, 1151–1159.

23

Psychological Perspectives on Alcohol: Visions for the Future

Emma Louise Davies, Dominic Conroy, Martin S. Hagger, Richard O. de Visser, and Richard Cooke

Introduction

The *Handbook of Psychological Perspectives on Alcohol* provides a wide-ranging treatment of psychological research applied to alcohol consumption in multiple social contexts authored by an eminent cast of contemporary international researchers. This chapter summarises the main messages arising from the Handbook, reflects on what is currently known derived from psychological enquiry, considers where the gaps in knowledge lie, and sets out an agenda for future research to assist in filling these gaps. Specifically, four broad themes

E. L. Davies (✉)
Department of Psychology, Health and Professional Development, Oxford Brookes University, Oxford, UK
e-mail: edavies@brookes.ac.uk

D. Conroy
School of Psychology, University of East London, London, UK
e-mail: d.conroy@uel.ac.uk

M. S. Hagger
Department of Psychological Sciences, University of California, Merced, Merced, CA, USA

Faculty of Sport and Health Sciences, University of Jyväskylä, Jyväskylä, Finland
e-mail: mhagger@merced.edu

R. Cooke et al. (eds.), *The Palgrave Handbook of Psychological Perspectives on Alcohol Consumption*, https://doi.org/10.1007/978-3-030-66941-6_23

arising from the research presented in this Handbook are identified, and the state of the research and avenues for future research under each are outlined: *samples*, *methods*, *theories*, and *applications*.

Section I: Psychological Theories and Predictors

Psychological theories play an important role in identifying the key determinants of outcomes, particularly behaviour, and can aid intervention development by identifying which determinants to target using behaviour change techniques (Hagger, Cameron, Hamilton, Hankonen, & Lintunen, 2020; Kok et al., 2016; Michie et al., 2013). In the first section of the Handbook, the application of a range of psychological theories to predict alcohol consumption was summarised (Chaps. 2 and 3). These chapters identified a range of individual determinants—such as enhancement motives, drinking intentions, drinking refusal self-efficacy—that were consistently related to alcohol consumption (Chap. 4). However, studies testing these determinants often fail to capture them all because they tend to be confined to separate models; when theories are integrated, the factors that are uniquely effective in predicting consumption can be identified. Unfortunately, few studies have taken an integrated approach—by including predictors from multiple theories or models—and more comprehensive and systematic application of integrated theories is needed to identify the unique, independent determinants of alcohol consumption going forward.

It is said that the road to hell is paved with good intentions, and nowhere is this more clearly symbolised than in research exploring people's drinking behaviours. For example, individuals may form plans to avoid or limit drinking, but when these are tested by friends and family (e.g., friends applying social pressure to visit the pub or bar for a drink, offering to pay for drinks, or refusing to take no for an answer when faced with a drink being refused),

R. O. de Visser
Brighton and Sussex Medical School, University of Sussex, Falmer, UK
e-mail: r.o.devisser@bsms.ac.uk

R. Cooke
Department of Psychology, University of Liverpool, Liverpool, UK

Liverpool Centre for Alcohol Research, Liverpool, UK
e-mail: cooker4@liverpool.ac.uk

such plans often fall by the wayside. Recognising that individuals' plans about controlling consumption can be overridden in drinking contexts, often resulting in them drinking more than they intend to, researchers have started to explore other influences on drinking behaviour. For instance, research on dual-process models highlights the importance of 'implicit' constructs that reflect non-conscious processes that can also influence consumption (Chap. 3; Hamilton, Gibbs, Keech, & Hagger, 2020). To date, large-scale studies incorporating these constructs alongside social cognition constructs are rare; one reason for this is that measuring implicit constructs often involves collecting reaction time data, which is harder to do within a survey. Theories also fail to account for individual differences, such as personality, that can predict drinking behaviour. In their comprehensive overview of personality factors and consumption, Mezquita et al. (Chap. 5) consider research on how specific traits link to alcohol consumption and also how to harness these traits in interventions. They conclude that while the role of personality in predicting alcohol consumption may be small, it is an important factor to consider when encouraging people to drink less.

The theories presented in Section I of the Handbook have provided alcohol researchers with the means to examine determinants of drinking in a great deal of detail, but these theories leave a considerable amount of variance in consumption unaccounted for, highlighting their insufficiency as accounts of individuals' drinking behaviour. As these chapters have shown, there are numerous weaknesses in methods and applications in existing research into theories, and there is no single ideal theory that can predict alcohol consumption in all segments of the population, particularly as much of the existing research draws on student populations. In addition, research findings regarding theories are difficult to generalise due to studies varying in how they define drinking behaviours. Although theories provide a means to make sense of complexity, as Crossley (2001) suggests, such theories have limitations and boundary conditions such that they can never fully capture the determinants of behaviour and often neglect other important influences such as factors in the external environment. Furthermore, theories tend to focus on individual factors, albeit those that are social determined, which may not encompass the influence of the social context in which drinking tends to occur.

Section II: Social and Contextual Factors

de Visser (Chap. 6) opens this section by clearly framing the ways in which drinking alcohol should always be regarded as an inherently social behaviour; social and cultural factors shape drinking behaviours, whether or not drinking takes place with other people in social contexts. However, as Aresi and Bloomfield (Chap. 7) point out, trying to identify nation-specific drinking cultures results in an oversimplification of the drinking behaviours of people in different countries, and there are within-person differences that can help explain why and how an individual might drink in different ways on different occasions. Clapp and Madden (Chap. 8) raised important points on the methods that should be adopted to understand the interacting external environmental, physiological, and social processes that influence drinking behaviour. They advocate the use of innovative research methods to study alcohol consumption in ecologically valid real-world settings, such as research participants wearing a transdermal sensor during a trip to the pub. Use of such methods may make it challenging to recruit participants, but Monk and Heim (Chap. 9) also make a strong case for more research to be conducted in settings that closely mirror 'real-world' settings. For example, more research should be conducted in 'bar labs', as well as in situ in bars and pubs, house parties, or pre-drinking sessions, and other under-researched real-world settings. This is something that Vasiljevic and Pechey (Chap. 10) explored in their chapter about choice architecture, which involves changing the features of small-scale physical environments, such as within bars and restaurants. Changing these features, for example by altering glass size or shape, impact behaviour through automatic processes; for example, individuals are prompted to drink faster or slower depending on whether their glass has straight or curved edges, due to perceptual biases. However, as Vasiljevic and Pechey demonstrated, findings to date have been inconclusive regarding the impact of changes to features of the micro-environment, and it is challenging to conduct ecologically valid studies when changes in glassware may impact on sales. Taken together, the chapters in Section II show that an array of contextual features—ranging from the broad social context, through to the specific drinking context and the characteristics of a specific serving of alcohol—which can influence individuals' alcohol consumption. Theories described in Section I are rarely able to account for these contextual factors in a satisfactory way for a number of reasons including (1) failure to assess these factors in studies alongside measures of theory constructs, (2) a near-exclusive focus on conducting studies in non-drinking contexts, and (3) adoption of theories that focus on how individuals self-report influences on their behaviour. The chapters presented in this section should provide impetus to researchers to modify theory and research practices to encompass a wider range of determinants in research on alcohol consumption.

Section III: Drinking Identities

The inherently social nature of drinking means that a closer look at social influence can reveal a great deal about people's drinking identities. Section III provides various perspectives on processes of social influences, which can take place online, as well as face to face. Lyons and Goodwin (Chap. 11) review research on alcohol identities, which they point out has generally focused on gender. Their chapter discusses research suggesting that historically men's drinking was seen as a way to demonstrate hegemonic masculinity, whereas women's drinking was considered unfeminine. However, a wide variety of cultural, social, and economic changes mean that psychological research has to move beyond simple binaries to make sense of how gender identity interacts with alcohol consumption. Nowhere have traditional notions of identity been more visible than within the world of social media, where people carefully curate idealised versions of their lives. Alcohol marketing combined with an airbrushed representation of drinking cultures contributes to the notion that drinking is always positive, fun, and enjoyable.

Although taking part in sports is often considered health promoting, the prototypical heavy drinking student is often inextricably linked to membership of student sports teams. The alcohol–sports paradox is the focus of Partington and Partington's (Chap. 12) chapter, illustrating the juxtaposition between 'healthy' and 'unhealthy' behaviours in this population. University students often engage in pre-drinking, which is the focus of Caudwell and Hagger's (Chap. 13) chapter. However, despite knowing that pre-drinking is associated with negative outcomes, very few interventions have targeted this specific pattern of drinking behaviour, and doing so presents unique difficulties given the inherently strong social pressure to pre-drink. This point is addressed by Conroy and de Visser (Chap. 14), who illustrate the challenges of managing or refusing alcohol, which requires a high level of knowledge, skills, and motivation.

Section III of the Handbook illustrates how specific aspects of identity—from gendered expectations and how individuals present themselves online, sports team membership, social practices associated with pre-drinking, the ways in which individuals try to moderate their drinking—all contribute to understanding drinking behaviour. These identities vary within and between cultures—as illustrated in Section II—and it is clear that more cross-cultural work is needed in this sphere.

Returning to the theories as outlined in Section I, the emphasis on identity is often missing in psychological research. Whilst the prototype willingness model (Gibbons, Gerrard, Ouellette, & Burzette, 1998) promotes consideration of social images of drinkers and how individuals might take on aspects of these images if they too drink in similar ways, Section III demonstrates that these social images are likely to be markedly different depending on what aspect of identity is salient at the time when the individual is asked to reflect on them.

Section IV: Developmental Trajectories for Alcohol Use

Early experiences within home are responsible for shaping aspects of individuals' identities and behaviours, and Cook et al. (Chap. 15) argue that alcohol should not be treated differently from any other formative experience. They point out that although adolescence is the focus of most alcohol research conducted with young people, early representations of alcohol experienced in childhood can have an important influence on later cognitions and behaviour. A further limit to understanding young people's drinking, according to Rolando and Beccaria (Chap. 16), is the relative lack of research adopting qualitative methods compared to research using quantitative research methods. In comparative research with Finnish and Italian adolescents, they illustrate the potential of qualitative studies to provide rich data. Early representations of drinking are strongly influenced not only by culture but also by parents' beliefs and behaviour regarding alcohol. Sawyer et al. (Chap. 17) exemplify the important role of parental communication, which in some cases can be a very effective means of reducing alcohol harms, but also has the potential to increase consumption. Two-way, open dialogue is critical, and it is important to avoid lecturing young people. Furthermore, as they get older, young people are increasingly influenced by peers, rather than parents. Modecki et al. (Chap. 18) provide a comprehensive account of the role of peers and social and school environments as both risk and protective factors for alcohol misuse. Chapters in Section IV provide a stark reminder of the likely disproportionate influence of alcohol on the behaviour of those who, in most regions, are not old enough to legally drink. With such a powerful influence on very early cognitions, it is unsurprising that interventions aimed at reducing alcohol consumption in young people is a priority for researchers as well as governments and organisations interested in the health and welfare of young people.

Section V: Interventions to Reduce Alcohol Consumption

Efforts to help people reduce or manage their drinking may be targeted at the population level or targeted at specific groups, such as young people (Perman-Howe, Davies, & Foxcroft, 2018). Product labelling is an example of a population-level intervention, universally communicating alcohol health information, such as drinking guidelines (see Chap. 1) to all consumers. However, as Blackwell et al. (Chap. 19) note, despite a wealth of experimental work on the impacts of labelling, there is a lack of information on alcohol products about guidelines on low-risk drinking or the possible health effects of consumption, including information on calories that is provided on other drink products. In many jurisdictions it is difficult to combat alcohol industry resistance to the inclusion of such information, even if it only has an impact on knowledge rather than behaviour (Wilkinson & Room, 2009), and so individual targeted interventions are needed.

Digital interventions offer advantages over face-to-face interventions because of their potential to engage people outside clinical settings and to reach large numbers of people relatively cheaply (Kaner et al., 2015). However, Bewick et al. (Chap. 20) argue that at present, the potential of electronic personalised feedback interventions is underutilised. Such interventions provide people with tailored advice based on information they provide. In this domain, there are several studies based on student samples, which Cooke et al. (Chap. 21) suggest may be best served by motivational interventions that are delivered before young people go to university, or self-regulatory interventions, such as forming 'if-then' plans, after young people have started university. Motivational interventions often target beliefs that underlie consumption (according to theories covered in Section I), whereas self-regulatory interventions can be used to address social situational pressures to drink, outlined in Sections II and III. Finally, in this section, Jones and Field (Chap. 22) look at the role of cognitive bias modification (CBM) in reducing alcohol consumption. CBM attempts to regulate implicit associations that drive alcohol consumption and which mean that habitual behaviours are enacted regardless of good intentions to avoid alcohol. Despite the appeal of CBM as a means of overcoming these powerful cues to drinking, Jones and Field caution that this field of research is fraught with failed attempts at replication. Their concluding comments remind us that the field of alcohol research as a whole needs to conduct more high-powered, pre-registered studies, and engage in transparent publishing practices that allow null results to be made available to the research community.

What is clear from each chapter in Section V is that available interventions are not universally effective, and each technique has limitations and boundary conditions. This signals the need for more systematic evaluation of interventions aimed at reducing alcohol consumption in different populations and contexts, particularly through registered replications, which will assist in identifying which strategies are most effective for particular groups and what interpersonal and contextual factors moderate their effects. It also suggests that people may vary in the intervention type that best suits their needs, and so intervention studies where participants are allowed a choice of intervention type could also be explored in future studies. Such an approach may prove more acceptable to individuals and reduce the sample attrition that can bedevil alcohol intervention studies (Radtke, Ostergaard, Cooke, & Scholz, 2017) and is consistent with the notion of personalised medicine that is increasingly emphasised in health psychology (Davidson & Cheung, 2017).

Limitations in the Field of Alcohol Research

Before considering research recommendations for the field, the limitations inherent in research methods and evidence used in psychological enquiry into alcohol consumption should be carefully considered. Some of the limitations have already been noted within the section summaries. These limitations are shared across the topics covered in the volume and can be divided into four key categories: samples, methods, theories and determinants, and applications of findings.

Limitations Linked to Sampling in Alcohol Research

Many of the studies cited in this Handbook rely on university student participants. Although students are a legitimate population for the study of alcohol consumption because they tend to engage in 'binge' drinking frequently (Davoren, Demant, Shiely, & Perry, 2016), this overreliance on student samples means that there is limited evidence about the generalisability of research findings and interventions aimed at reducing alcohol consumption to other populations. In particular, theories have been mostly tested on student samples and in samples often composed of more women than men. This approach is a concern because many cross-sectional and population-level surveys show that men drink more than women and men are at greater risk from short-term harms such as violence (Bellis et al., 2015; Davies, Cooke, Maier, Winstock,

& Ferris, 2020; NHS Digital, 2020). There is a need to confirm that variables shown to predict women's drinking also predict men's drinking because this should not be assumed. For example, Barratt and Cooke (2018) compared prediction of heavy episodic drinking (HED) among men and women using theoretical variables and past HED. Although drinking intentions predicted HED alongside past HED in women, the only factor that predicted HED in men was past HED. Such findings have implications for the application of theories; because theories inform interventions designed to reduce drinking, if they are not based on actual determinants of drinking for men or women, they may not be effective. For example, Murgraff, Abraham, and McDermott (2007) reported that their implementation intention reduced alcohol consumption in women but not men (see Chap. 21).

Linked to this, it has been noted that alcohol research beyond the gender binary is rare (Flentje et al., 2020; Flentje, Bacca, & Cochran, 2015). Many researchers fail to collect information beyond biological sex (e.g., male/female), which means that the experiences of trans and non-binary people are rarely represented in alcohol research (Connolly & Gilchrist, 2020). Those studies which do identify trans participants frequently fail to present analysis that disaggregates gender minority from sexual minority participants (Cochran, Peavy, & Santa, 2007; Talley et al., 2016). Although researchers may argue that they lack sufficient numbers of trans or non-binary participants to make statistical comparisons, this is not a compelling reason to overlook the experiences of a sub-group who, evidence has suggested, may typically consume alcohol in higher rates and experience higher levels of alcohol-related harms than cisgender individuals (Connolly et al., under review; Hughes, Wilsnack, & Kantor, 2016).

Alcohol research is also largely based on racially and ethnically homogeneous samples. Much of the research is conducted on white participants and conducted by white researchers, indicating that research in psychology applied to alcohol consumption lacks diversity. For example, samples in the Global Drug Survey are often around 85% white (Davies, Conroy, Winstock, & Ferris, 2017; Davies et al., 2021). While research suggests that white population groups drink more than other ethnic groups (Hurcombe, Bayley, & Goodman, 2010; Wade, 2020), there is a need for more research to determine the reasons, motives, and determinants for these differences. Furthermore, minority groups such as indigenous populations in Australia and New Zealand tend to experience a greater burden of alcohol problems (Kypri et al., 2013) suggesting the need to consider greater diversity. There is, therefore, a need for more research into the reasons, motives, and determinants of alcohol drinking in non-white populations. Oei and Jardim (2007) showed that psychological variables accounted for a greater amount of variance in alcohol consumption in a sample of white Australian university students compared to variance in consumption in a sample of Asian Australian university students.

In addition, adolescents and young adults tend to drink less alcohol than in the past (Livingston & Vashishtha, 2019; Vashishtha et al., 2020). Growing interest in non-drinking, lighter drinking, the fluidity, and transitioning nature of drinking 'styles' in recent discussion (Banister, Conroy, & Piacentini, 2019; Conroy & Measham, 2019; Davies, Smith, Johansson, Hill, & Brown, 2019) has drawn attention to the tendency to focus on alcohol consumption in unhelpful and inaccurate binaries (e.g., 'social' vs. 'problem' drinking). Addressing these limitations will involve greater acknowledgement of the diversity of drinking styles (and transition between styles), and this, in turn, can help produce a more accurate, meaningful, and measured discussion of theories of alcohol consumption and practical measures involved in promoting moderate drinking. According to recent UK data (NHS Digital, 2020) alcohol consumption is actually more prevalent in older age groups, such as adults aged 45–54 years. There is very little psychological research on the determinants of drinking in people in this, or older age groups, which means that interventions delivered to this population are likely to be based on drivers of drinking among younger populations that may be less relevant. There is also a real lack of research on alcohol among young people who do not pursue higher education, even though members of such groups may also engage in heavy alcohol consumption and may lack the support services accessible on university campuses.

Limitations Linked to Design and Methods

The preponderance of cross-sectional designs used in psychological research studies limits inferences of causality. Given that a key feature of a 'strong' or 'good' theory is that it provides causal explanation of relations between constructs and outcomes (Davis, Campbell, Hildon, Hobbs, & Michie, 2015), this is problematic as it limits the extent to which theories can be considered as effective in determining consumption. Furthermore, the lack of panel designs and experimental or intervention research of theory effects also means that there is little evidence that theories can effectively account for change in alcohol behaviour (Hagger, Moyers, McAnally, & McKinley, 2020). In turn, this limits the utility of theories in informing interventions aimed at curbing alcohol consumption.

Further to this, as authors in Section II have highlighted, there is a need to conduct alcohol research within the settings that alcohol consumption takes place. There are inherent problems with recall—alongside social desirability and self-concept preservation—that influence the completion of questionnaire measures when a participant is sober and when these measures are completed a long time after a drinking occasion.

Authors such as Rolando and Beccaria (Chap. 16) propose that one of the reasons that important gaps exist in the understanding of the psychology of alcohol consumption is that there is a relative lack of qualitative research compared to quantitative in the field. They argue that the complexity of alcohol use is better understood by engaging with individuals and giving them a voice within carefully designed qualitative studies. This is a compelling argument, and in recent years there are a great many examples where qualitative research has enabled a more nuanced understanding of people's views and experiences related to alcohol behaviours than a quantitative approach would allow. For example, quantitative surveys have shown that alcohol units are not well known or understood (Cooke, French, & Sniehotta, 2010; De Visser & Birch, 2012), but qualitative studies have revealed a range of reasons for this lack of knowledge and understanding (Furtwängler & de Visser, 2017; Lovatt et al., 2015). However, as well as increasing the use of qualitative methods, it would be beneficial to see more researchers using mixed methods to address research questions about the psychology of alcohol consumption and to see more engagement in systematic integration of the findings of quantitative and qualitative elements of research studies.

Limitations Linked to Theories and Determinants

Alongside the methodological issues within the current body of research on theories of alcohol consumption, there is a need to consider the fixation of researchers on testing hypotheses derived from a narrow set of theories or constructs in research on alcohol. The problems of repeated application of similar theories with little progression and variation still remain, and may be hindering progress in theory development and, in turn, the development of effective interventions. One of the key problems with these theories is that often the variance they explain in alcohol consumption is relatively small. It is rare for researchers to use an integrated approach to explore the merit of theoretical constructs drawn from multiple theories or varied perspectives, but this could help move the field forward and focus attention on additional determinants and processes that relate to alcohol consumption. For example, Atwell,

Abraham, and Duka (2011) combined constructs from multiple theories discussed in Section I, such as drinking motives, self-efficacy, and prototype perceptions, and examined the relative importance of each as well as how they interacted. They found that sensation seeking and age of initiation were better able to account for alcohol consumption in students than many of the theoretical constructs. More research using integrated theories is needed, and researchers need to move away from testing theories in isolation. The focus on individual theories is articulated in Sniehotta et al.'s (2014) critique of the use the theory of planned behaviour, and researchers have advocated the augmenting, extending, and modification of the theory to provide more comprehensive predictions of behaviour (Armitage, 2015; Caudwell & Hagger, 2015; Caudwell, Keech, Hamilton, Mullan, & Hagger, 2019; Conner, 2015; Hamilton et al., 2020), including drinking behaviour (Caudwell et al., 2019; Caudwell & Hagger, 2015; Hamilton et al., 2020). Such models signpost potential avenues for future research that are not confined to individual theories and focus, instead on key constructs and associated process derived from multiple theories. As with all theory testing, it is important that such theories are subjected to systematic rigorous tests to provide robust data to confirm or disconfirm their predictions, with subsequent revision or modification where necessary.

Limitations in the Application of Findings and Their Impact

It is important that scientific enquiry into the psychological determinants of alcohol consumption and associated processes is sufficiently translatable so that it can be used to improve and extend people's lives. However, as the chapters in Section V illustrate, relatively little is known about how to effectively help people who are motivated to reduce their drinking before it becomes a serious problem. The development and implementation of preventive interventions based on sound psychological research has the potential to reduce the number of people who become alcohol dependent, as well as making significant savings in health services and the broader economy. For example, Blackwell et al. (Chap. 19) outline how improving the features and content of alcohol product labelling could make them have more impact. However, this research will only have promise if these research findings are implemented into policy to replace the currently mandated messaging such as 'drink responsibly' that is strategically ambiguous, vague, and with little basis on evidence

(Smith, Atkin, & Roznowski, 2006). Nevertheless, the introduction of such messaging may only improve people's knowledge and may not lead to behaviour change (Wilkinson & Room, 2009). The key challenge when it comes to translation is to engage stakeholders and those in leadership positions, such as those working in government, policy, and public health, and advocate the implementation of these messages where they will have most effect. Although awareness of health effects and drinking guidelines is necessary in order to encourage 'low-risk' drinking, messages need to actively provide strategies that help people improve their motivation and behavioural skills to manage situations where they might drink to excess or over guideline limits, like refusing the offer of a drink (see Chap. 14). Turning to interventions that focus on personalised feedback and motivational strategies to promote alcohol reduction, why are these interventions not demonstrating optimal effectiveness? Intervention designers often strongly advocate for theory (Michie et al., 2016), so one hypothesis for the lack of effectiveness may be because many current interventions lack a theoretical basis. There is some evidence to suggest that this is the case. For example, a review of research on digital interventions to reduce alcohol consumption found that few of the apps used to mention a theoretical basis or adopt known behaviour change techniques (Crane, Garnett, Brown, West, & Michie, 2015). However, as noted above, basis in theory and adoption of identified behaviour change techniques alone is not the sole consideration when developing an effective intervention; one must also consider whether the adopted theory is fit for purpose.

There has also been a tendency for publication bias towards positive results in intervention studies, and there is a need to encourage publication of null findings. This provides a more balanced literature to identify what intervention strategies may work, for whom, and when, and, importantly, identify what interventions may *not* work, or the contexts or populations in which they may be ineffective (Davies, Lonsdale, Hennelly, Winstock, & Foxcroft, 2017).

Setting an Agenda for Future Research on the Psychology of Alcohol Consumption

Having considered the limitations of the current body of research on the psychology of alcohol consumption, this section sets out an agenda for future psychological enquiry into alcohol, with specific focus on samples, methods, theories, and applications.

Those interested in the psychology of alcohol consumption are urged to conduct research *with* underrepresented communities

The vast majority of psychological studies concerning alcohol consumption have been conducted with samples that are primarily white in ethnicity, with university students over-represented. Alcohol consumption and its harms hold the potential to affect *all* members of society. The authors of chapters in this Handbook highlight the need to proactively favour research on samples that are adequately representative of the diversity of populations affected by alcohol, including young people who do not attend university, middle-aged, and older adults, people from non-white and ethnic minority populations, and people from diverse sexual orientation and gender minorities.

This suggested shift in research focus is important to reflect the diversity of populations in the world, which will provide better evidence of the generalisability of psychological theories applied to alcohol, but is also important because some underrepresented groups, such as trans people (Connolly et al., 2020), may be at greater risk of harm from alcohol consumption and may benefit from tailored forms of intervention and support (Connolly et al., 2020). In addition, research on diverse groups is important for the direction and framing of interventions. For example, where minority group identity intersects, for example in terms of race and gender, then greater care and attention may be needed to address alcohol issues with the population in a sensitive way (Wilkerson, Di Paola, McCurdy, & Schick, 2020).

It is also important that psychological research on alcohol in diverse populations is mindful to engage those communities in the design, implementation, and dissemination of the research. Engaging members of these communities, such as patients, and members of target groups from the general public has been a commitment health care research for some time (Brett et al., 2014; Staniszewska et al., 2017) but psychology researchers have been less inclined to do so and could do more to ensure that underrepresented groups are involved in the research process. Such involvement is important in order to ensure that research methods, including intervention content, are culturally sensitive and account for perspectives of the target population.

In addition to a commitment to pursuing more diverse samples in psychological research applied to alcohol, there is also a need to diversify those that conduct the research. Promoting greater diversity among those tasked with conducting and producing research evidence may increase the breadth of perspectives and methods used and promote research that is more sensitive and responsive to cultural and ethnic issues. Means to promote greater diversity in researchers in the field would be to promote diversity in recruitment and access to high-quality education and training in research. The onus is on the providers of research training from universities to learned societies to create opportunities and policies to encourage and promote those from minority backgrounds to engage in research in the field of psychology applied to alcohol.

Greater methodological diversity can enhance psychological perspectives on alcohol consumption

As Aresi and Bloomfield note in Chap. 7, mixed methods can provide a contextualised account of drinking cultures, which is often needed to understand the complexity of behaviours such as pre-drinking, as illustrated by Caudwell and Hagger (Chap. 13). Research examining determinants of drinking behaviours over time using longitudinal or cross-lagged panel designs, as well as experimental and intervention designs, needs to become more commonplace in order to make inferences of temporal stability, direction, and causality in social psychological theories applied to alcohol consumption. Greater use of ecological momentary assessment methods would also benefit psychological research on alcohol consumption. In a traditional survey, participants are asked to recall how much alcohol they consumed over the past week, fortnight, or month. Completing this task is contingent on memory that may well be influenced by drinking alcohol. As an alternative, researchers should consider asking participants to complete surveys in the moment, or as near as possible to performance of consumption as is feasible. The rapid development of smartphone technology and other portable devices (e.g., smartwatches, tablets), and the reduction in their cost, allows for easy delivery of surveys and collection of behavioural data, so researchers should be making greater use of such methods in future research.

Studies using longitudinal methods are also needed including cohort studies that do more than just measure alcohol consumption. Intervention studies are one potential vehicle for addressing this issue as they typically include longer-term follow-up measurement than traditional survey studies. By encouraging intervention researchers to measure predictors of consumption as secondary outcomes, such studies will achieve two complementary goals. First, they will afford researchers the opportunity to determine how their intervention works through observation of whether changes in secondary outcomes mediate effects of the intervention. Second, they will allow researchers to determine the extent to which predictors remain stable over time, and whether current theories are able to predict about alcohol consumption over long time periods.

A more integrated theoretical approach to the psychology of alcohol consumption is needed

As with many other areas of psychology, researchers tend to confine their perspectives on exploring phenomena to a single theoretical approach, focusing on testing a narrow set of predictions afforded by such an approach. Given that there are a vast number of theories in psychology (Davis et al., 2015), usually with considerable overlap in the content of their constructs and predictions, this approach can lead to considerable redundancy across theories and stall progress in theory development. In many cases, theories include constructs with almost identical focus, but different names, presenting considerable challenges to those attempting to make sense of trends in determinants and processes (Hagger, 2014). As the chapters in the current volume attest, this phenomenon is highly prevalent in alcohol research studies. This hinders scientific progress and can make it difficult for practitioners to make sense of research trends and identify the key constructs and processes relevant to determining alcohol consumption. A more integrated theoretical approach (Hagger, 2009) for alcohol is needed. It can be argued that alcohol use requires a specific model because it differs from other health behaviours in terms of its importance to identity and social influences, and as an intoxicant, it impacts people's beliefs and decision making the more they drink. Such an approach will help identify the core constructs and process that are consistently and reliably related to alcohol consumption and, therefore, serve as strong candidates to target in interventions. In addition, research is needed to match these determinants to key behaviour change techniques that are effective in bringing about behaviour change and testing their mechanisms of action through the mediation of the determinants (Connell et al., 2019; Rothman, Klein, & Sheeran, 2020).

Additionally, more research is needed to compare socio-structural determinants of alcohol consumption with psychological determinants, including considering the role of ethnicity as a mediator and moderator of effects of theory constructs like attitudes and intentions (Godin et al., 2010; Hagger & Hamilton, 2020; Schüz, Brick, Wilding, & Conner, 2020; Schüz, Li, Hardinge, McEachan, & Conner, 2017). Theoretical research also needs to do more to acknowledge how macro-environmental factors, such as availability of alcohol, local cost of alcohol, and density of bars and pubs within living areas, influence individuals' alcohol consumption. These factors meaningfully affect consumption (Anderson, Chisholm, & Fuhr, 2009; Babor et al., 2010; Radaev, 2019), and so their exclusion will likely lead to a shortfall in the variance explained in alcohol consumption as they may not be fully accounted for by psychological constructs such as beliefs about control, and individuals' behaviour may be influenced by factors and processes beyond their awareness, such as environmental cues. Related to this, research on dual-process models suggests a role for 'implicit' constructs that reflect non-conscious processes as determinants of alcohol consumption (e.g., Chap. 13; Hamilton et al., 2020). However, large-scale studies incorporating these constructs alongside motivational and social cognition constructs are rare, and collecting data on implicit measures may be difficult or lack reliability in large population representative studies.

This move towards using integrated theories needs to happen in both theory and intervention research and needs to provide more stringent tests of predictions using experimental and other designs. For example, with sufficient sample sizes, researchers can test the effectiveness of different components of their interventions (Bedendo et al., 2020; Collins, Murphy, Nair, & Strecher, 2005).

There is also a need for theoretical research to take place in situ more as a way to account for contextual/environmental/social influences on drinking beliefs and behaviour. Although it is convenient to send people a link to a survey, this approach assumes that the responses expressed at that point in time are unlikely to change when in a drinking context, and this is a risky assumption when it comes to alcohol. As mentioned in the previous section, ecological momentary assessment could allow the measurement of theoretical constructs in situ, as could field experiments.

Research on the psychology of alcohol consumption needs to make more impact

As the chapters in this book have demonstrated, research applying psychological theory and methods to alcohol use has provided important theoretical insights as well as potentially translatable findings important to inform practice. However, translation and implementation into practice have hitherto not been as effective as they need to be in order for policy and campaigns introduced by policymakers, governments, and organisations to be evidence based and highly effective. So, how can insights derived from psychological research be more effectively translated? A worked example may provide an illustration.

Consider the use of unit-based alcohol guidelines adopted by the UK government with similar systems used by many other national health authorities to highlight limits considered safe for health. Various studies have indicated that people lack awareness of the guidelines, are not aware of what constitutes a unit of alcohol, and do not consider unit-based guidelines to be relevant to everyday experiences of drinking (e.g., Davies et al., 2020; De Visser & Birch, 2012; Furtwängler & de Visser, 2017). These findings needs to be communicated to policy makers and public health bodies who have the power to make changes to guidelines to make them more relevant to the general public. Although there *is* a need for standardised units of alcohol measurement for drinkers, clinicians, and researchers, if they are to be used as a basis for guidelines used to inform the general public, they must be framed in ways that make them easily translatable and have utility in everyday contexts.

A further example can be seen in research on warning labels on alcohol product packaging. There is good evidence to suggest that warning labels comprising images accompanied by clear, specific messages are likely to have more of an impact (Chap. 19), although it seems that governments would need to mandate the use of health warning labels in order for them to become commonplace. However, a substantive barrier to their introduction is lobbying from the vastly powerful alcohol industry. For example, when Canadian researchers attempted to test the effectiveness of alcohol health warnings in a real-world setting, the alcohol industry quickly realised this affected sales and demanded the study be modified (Vallance et al., 2020). Furthermore, as mentioned previously, voluntary alcohol labelling initiatives with cooperation from the alcohol industry have resulted in labels on alcohol product packaging that contain vague messaging (e.g., 'drink responsibly'), which may be relatively impotent instruments of behaviour change.

Concluding Comments

The five sections of this Handbook have explored and critiqued psychological perspectives on alcohol consumption regarding theories and predictors, social contextual factors, drinking identities, developmental trajectories, and interventions to reduce alcohol consumption. By reviewing the content of these sections, this final chapter has outlined limitations within the field as a whole, relating to samples, design and methods, theories and determinants, and the application of findings to improve people's lives. This chapter has set out four key areas of change within the proposed agenda for the future of research on the psychology of alcohol consumption. First, the need to diversify participant samples and work in collaboration with underrepresented communities will broaden generalisability of theories and interventions. Second, a greater methodological diversity was called for, including further recourse to such methods and technologies that allow data to be collected nearer to the time of consumption. Third, it is clear that an integrated theoretical approach, which includes socio-structural determinants of behaviour, will enable researchers to better understand the complexities of alcohol consumption. Fourth, the translation and implementation of findings into policy must be improved for this valuable field of research to have the desired impact on people's health. Greater collaboration across disciplinary and national boundaries, together with careful and considered involvement of people with lived experience of alcohol and its impacts, will enable this exciting field of research to continue to flourish.

References

Anderson, P., Chisholm, D., & Fuhr, D. C. (2009). Effectiveness and cost-effectiveness of policies and programmes to reduce the harm caused by alcohol. *The Lancet, 373*(9682), 2234–2246. https://doi.org/10.1016/S0140-6736(09)60744-3

Armitage, C. J. (2015). Time to retire the theory of planned behaviour? A commentary on Sniehotta, Presseau and Araújo-Soares. *Health Psychology Review, 9*(2), 151–155. https://doi.org/10.1080/17437199.2014.892148

Atwell, K., Abraham, C., & Duka, T. (2011). A parsimonious, integrative model of key psychological correlates of UK University Students' alcohol consumption. *Alcohol and Alcoholism, 46*(3), 253–260. https://doi.org/10.1093/alcalc/agr016

Babor, T., Caetano, R., Casswell, S., Edwards, G., Giesbrecht, N., Graham, K., Grube, J. W., Hill, L., Holder, H., Homel, R., Livingston, M., Österberg, E., Rehm, J., & Room, R., Ingeborg. (2010). *Alcohol: No ordinary commodity: Research and public policy*. Oxford, UK: Oxford University Press. https://doi.org/10.1111/j.1360-0443.2010.02945.x

Banister, E., Conroy, D., & Piacentini, M. (2019). Non-drinkers and non-drinking: A review, a critique and pathways to policy. In D. Conroy & F. Measham (Eds.), *Young adult drinking styles: Current perspectives on research, policy and practice* (pp. 213–232). Springer International Publishing. https://doi.org/10.1007/978-3-030-28607-1_11

Barratt, J. M., & Cooke, R. (2018). Do gender and year of study affect the ability of the theory of planned behaviour to predict binge-drinking intentions and episodes? *Drugs: Education, Prevention and Policy, 25*(2), 181–188. https://doi.org/10.1080/09687637.2016.1257564

Bedendo, A., McCambridge, J., Gaume, J., Souza, A. A. L., Formigoni, M. L. O. S., & Noto, A. R. (2020). Components evaluation of a web-based personalized normative feedback intervention for alcohol use among college students: A pragmatic randomized controlled trial with a dismantling design. *Addiction, 115*(6), 1063–1074. https://doi.org/10.1111/add.14923

Bellis, M. A., Quigg, Z., Hughes, K., Ashton, K., Ferris, J. A., & Winstock, A. (2015). Harms from other people's drinking: An international survey of their occurrence, impacts on feeling safe and legislation relating to their control. *BMJ Open, 5*(12). https://doi.org/10.1136/bmjopen-2015-010112

Brett, J., Staniszewska, S., Mockford, C., Herron-Marx, S., Hughes, J., Tysall, C., & Suleman, R. (2014). Mapping the impact of patient and public involvement on health and social care research: A systematic review. *Health Expectations, 17*(5), 637–650. https://doi.org/10.1111/j.1369-7625.2012.00795.x

Caudwell, K. M., & Hagger, M. S. (2015). Predicting alcohol pre-drinking in Australian undergraduate students using an integrated theoretical model [article]. *Applied Psychology-Health and Well Being, 7*(2), 188–213. https://doi.org/10.1111/aphw.12044

Caudwell, K. M., Keech, J. J., Hamilton, K., Mullan, B. A., & Hagger, M. S. (2019). Reducing alcohol consumption during pre-drinking sessions: Testing an integrated behaviour-change model. *Psychology & Health, 34*(1), 106–127. https://doi.org/10.1080/08870446.2018.1518527

Cochran, B. N., Peavy, K. M., & Santa, A. F. (2007). Differentiating LGBT individuals in substance abuse treatment: Analyses based on sexuality and drug preference. *Journal of LGBT Health Research, 3*(2), 63–75. https://doi.org/10.1300/J463v03n02_07

Collins, L. M., Murphy, S. A., Nair, V. N., & Strecher, V. J. (2005). A strategy for optimizing and evaluating behavioral interventions. *Annals of Behavioral Medicine, 30*(1), 65–73. https://doi.org/10.1207/s15324796abm3001_8

Connell, L. E., Carey, R. N., de Bruin, M., Rothman, A. J., Johnston, M., Kelly, M. P., & Michie, S. (2019). Links between behavior change techniques and mechanisms of action: An expert consensus study. *Annals of Behavioral Medicine, 53*(8), 708–720. https://doi.org/10.1093/abm/kay082

Conner, M. (2015). Extending not retiring the theory of planned behaviour: A commentary on Sniehotta, Presseau and Araújo-Soares. *Health Psychology Review, 9*(2), 141–145. https://doi.org/10.1080/17437199.2014.899060

Connolly, D., Davies, E. L., Lynskey, M., Barratt, M. J., Maier, L., Ferris, J., … Gilchrist, G. (2020). Comparing intentions to reduce substance use and willingness to seek help among transgender and cisgender participants from the global drug survey. *Journal of Substance Abuse Treatment, 112*, 86–91. https://doi.org/10.1016/j.jsat.2020.03.001

Connolly, D., Davies, E. L., Lynskey, M., Maier, L. J., Ferris, J., Winstock, A., & Gilchrist, G. (under review). *Differences in alcohol and other drug use and dependence between transgender and cisgender participants from the 2018 global drug survey.*

Connolly, D., & Gilchrist, G. (2020). Prevalence and correlates of substance use among transgender adults: A systematic review. *Addictive Behaviors*, 106544. https://doi.org/10.1016/j.addbeh.2020.106544

Conroy, D., & Measham, F. (2019). Book introduction: Young adult drinking styles. In D. Conroy & F. Measham (Eds.), *Young adult drinking styles: Current perspectives on research, policy and practice* (pp. 1–17). Springer International Publishing. https://doi.org/10.1007/978-3-030-28607-1_1

Cooke, R., French, D. P., & Sniehotta, F. F. (2010). Wide variation in understanding about what constitutes 'binge-drinking' [Article]. *Drugs-Education Prevention and Policy, 17*(6), 762–775. https://doi.org/10.3109/09687630903246457

Crane, D., Garnett, C., Brown, J., West, R., & Michie, S. (2015). Behavior change techniques in popular alcohol reduction apps: Content analysis. *Journal of Medical Internet Research, 17*(5) Art e118. https://doi.org/10.2196/jmir.4060

Crossley, M. L. (2001). Rethinking psychological approaches towards health promotion [article]. *Psychology & Health, 16*(2), 161–177. https://doi.org/10.1080/08870440108405497

Davidson, K. W., & Cheung, Y. K. (2017). Envisioning a future for precision health psychology: Innovative applied statistical approaches to N-of-1 studies. *Health Psychology Review, 11*(3), 292–294. https://doi.org/10.1080/17437199.2017.1347514

Davies, E. L., Conroy, D., Winstock, A. R., & Ferris, J. A. (2017). Motivations for reducing alcohol consumption: An international survey exploring experiences that may lead to a change in drinking habits. *Addictive Behaviors, 75*, 40–46. https://doi.org/10.1016/j.addbeh.2017.06.019

Davies, E. L., Cooke, R., Maier, L. J., Winstock, A. R., & Ferris, J. A. (2020). Drinking to excess and the tipping point: An international study of alcohol intoxication in 61,000 people. *International Journal of Drug Policy, 83*, 102867. https://doi.org/10.1016/j.drugpo.2020.102867

Davies, E. L., Puljevic, C., Connolly, D., Zhuparris, A., Ferris, J. A., & Winstock, A. R. (2021). The world's favorite drug: What we have learned about alcohol from over 500,000 respondents to the Global Drug Survey. In D. Frings & I. P. Albery (Eds.), The Handbook of Alcohol Use (pp. 17–47). Academic Press. https://doi.org/10.1016/B978-0-12-816720-5.00022-0

Davies, E. L., Lonsdale, A. J., Hennelly, S. E., Winstock, A. R., & Foxcroft, D. R. (2017). Personalized digital interventions showed no impact on risky drinking in young adults: A pilot randomized controlled trial. *Alcohol and Alcoholism*, 1–6. https://doi.org/10.1093/alcalc/agx051

Davies, E. L., Smith, J., Johansson, M., Hill, K., & Brown, K. (2019). Can't dance without being drunk? Exploring the enjoyment and acceptability of conscious clubbing in young people. In D. Conroy & F. Measham (Eds.), *Young adult drinking styles: Current perspectives on research, policy and practice* (pp. 233–252). Springer International Publishing. https://doi.org/10.1007/978-3-030-28607-1_12

Davis, R., Campbell, R., Hildon, Z., Hobbs, L., & Michie, S. (2015). Theories of behaviour and behaviour change across the social and behavioural sciences: A scoping review. *Health Psychology Review, 9*(3), 323–344. https://doi.org/10.1080/17437199.2014.941722

Davoren, M. P., Demant, J., Shiely, F., & Perry, I. J. (2016). Alcohol consumption among university students in Ireland and the United Kingdom from 2002 to 2014: A systematic review. *BMC Public Health, 16*(1), 1–13. https://doi.org/10.1186/s12889-016-2843-1

De Visser, R. O., & Birch, J. D. (2012). My cup runneth over: Young people's lack of knowledge of low-risk drinking guidelines. *Drug and Alcohol Review, 31*(2), 206–212. https://doi.org/10.1111/j.1465-3362.2011.00371.x

Flentje, A., Bacca, C. L., & Cochran, B. N. (2015). Missing data in substance abuse research? Researchers' reporting practices of sexual orientation and gender identity. *Drug and Alcohol Dependence, 147*, 280–284. https://doi.org/10.1016/j.drugalcdep.2014.11.012

Flentje, A., Barger, B., Capriotti, M., Lubensky, M., Tierney, M., Obedin-Maliver, J., & Lunn, M. (2020). Screening gender minority people for harmful alcohol use. *PLoS One, 15*, e0231022. https://doi.org/10.1371/journal.pone.0231022

Furtwängler, N. A. F., & de Visser, R. O. (2017). University students' beliefs about unit-based guidelines: A qualitative study. *Journal of Health Psychology, 22*(13), 1701–1711. https://doi.org/10.1177/1359105316634449

Gibbons, F. X., Gerrard, M., Ouellette, J. A., & Burzette, R. (1998). Cognitive antecedents to adolescent health risk: Discriminating between behavioral intention and behavioral willingness. *Psychology & Health, 13*(2), 319–339. https://doi.org/10.1080/08870449808406754

Godin, G., Sheeran, P., Conner, M., Bélanger-Gravel, A., Gallani, M. C. B. J., & Nolin, B. (2010). Social structure, social cognition, and physical activity: A test of four models. *British Journal of Health Psychology, 15*(1), 79–95. https://doi.org/10.1348/135910709X429901

Hagger, M. (2014). Avoiding the "déjà-variable" phenomenon: Social psychology needs more guides to constructs [general commentary]. *Frontiers in Psychology, 5*(52). https://doi.org/10.3389/fpsyg.2014.00052

Hagger, M. S. (2009). Theoretical integration in health psychology: Unifying ideas and complementary explanations [editorial material]. *British Journal of Health Psychology, 14*, 189–194. https://doi.org/10.1348/135910708x397034

Hagger, M. S., Cameron, L. D., Hamilton, K., Hankonen, N., & Lintunen, T. (2020). *The handbook of behavior change* (M. S. Hagger, L. D. Cameron, K. Hamilton, N. Hankonen, & T. Lintunen, Eds.). Cambridge, UK: Cambridge University Press. https://doi.org/10.1017/9781108677318.

Hagger, M. S., & Hamilton, K. (2020). Effects of socio-structural variables in the theory of planned behavior: A mediation model in multiple samples and behaviors. *Psychology & Health*, 1–27. https://doi.org/10.1080/08870446.2020.1784420

Hagger, M. S., Moyers, S., McAnally, K., & McKinley, L. E. (2020). Known knowns and known unknowns on behavior change interventions and mechanisms of action. *Health Psychology Review, 14*(1), 199–212. https://doi.org/10.1080/17437199.2020.1719184

Hamilton, K., Gibbs, I., Keech, J. J., & Hagger, M. S. (2020). Reasoned and implicit processes in heavy episodic drinking: An integrated dual-process model. *British Journal of Health Psychology, 25*(1), 189–209. https://doi.org/10.1111/bjhp.12401

Hughes, T. L., Wilsnack, S. C., & Kantor, L. W. (2016). The influence of gender and sexual orientation on alcohol use and alcohol-related problems: Toward a global perspective. *Alcohol Research: Current Reviews, 38*(1), 121–132. https://pubmed.ncbi.nlm.nih.gov/27159819; https://www.ncbi.nlm.nih.gov/pmc/articles/PMC4872607/

Hurcombe, R., Bayley, M., & Goodman, A. (2010). *Ethnicity and alcohol: A review of the UK literature*. London, UK: J. R Foundation.

Kaner, E. F. S., Beyer, F. R., Brown, J., Crane, D., Garnett, C., Hickman, M., Muirhead, C., Redmore, J., Michie, S., & de Vocht, F. (2015). Personalised digital interventions for reducing hazardous and harmful alcohol consumption in community-dwellin g populations. *Cochrane Database of Systematic Reviews* (1). https://doi.org/10.1002/14651858.cd011479

Kok, G., Gottlieb, N. H., Peters, G. J., Mullen, P. D., Parcel, G. S., Ruiter, R. A., … Bartholomew, L. K. (2016). A taxonomy of behaviour change methods: An intervention mapping approach. *Health Psychology Review, 10*(3), 297–312. https://doi.org/10.1080/17437199.2015.1077155

Kypri, K., McCambridge, J., Vater, T., Bowe, S. J., Saunders, J. B., Cunningham, J. A., & Horton, N. J. (2013). Web-based alcohol intervention for Māori university students: Double-blind, multi-site randomized controlled trial. *Addiction, 108*(2), 331–338. https://doi.org/10.1111/j.1360-0443.2012.04067.x

Livingston, M., & Vashishtha, R. (2019). Have recent declines in adolescent drinking continued into young adulthood? In D. Conroy & F. Measham (Eds.), *Young adult drinking styles: Current perspectives on research, policy and practice* (pp. 21–46). Springer International Publishing. https://doi.org/10.1007/978-3-030-28607-1_2

Lovatt, M., Eadie, D., Meier, P. S., Li, J., Bauld, L., Hastings, G., & Holmes, J. (2015). Lay epidemiology and the interpretation of low-risk drinking guidelines by adults in the United Kingdom. *Addiction, 110*(12), 1912–1919. https://doi.org/10.1111/add.13072

Michie, S., Carey, R. N., Johnston, M., Rothman, A. J., de Bruin, M., Kelly, M. P., & Connell, L. E. (2016). From theory-inspired to theory-based Interventions: A protocol for developing and testing a methodology for linking behaviour change techniques to theoretical mechanisms of action. *Annals of Behavioral Medicine*. https://doi.org/10.1007/s12160-016-9816-6

Michie, S., Richardson, M., Johnston, M., Abraham, C., Francis, J., Hardeman, W., … Wood, C. (2013). The behavior change technique taxonomy (v1) of 93 hierarchically clustered techniques: Building an international consensus for the reporting of behavior change interventions. *Annals of Behavioral Medicine, 46*(1), 81–95. https://doi.org/10.1007/s12160-013-9486-6

Murgraff, V., Abraham, C., & McDermott, M. (2007). Reducing friday alcohol consumption among moderate, women drinkers: Evaluation of a brief evidence-based intervention. *Alcohol and Alcoholism, 42*(1), 37–41. https://doi.org/10.1093/alcalc/agl083

NHS Digital. (2020). *Statistics on alcohol, England 2020.* https://digital.nhs.uk/data-and-information/publications/statistical/statistics-on-alcohol/2020

Oei, T. P., & Jardim, C. L. (2007). Alcohol expectancies, drinking refusal self-efficacy and drinking behaviour in Asian and Australian students. *Drug and Alcohol Dependence, 87*(2–3), 281–287. https://doi.org/10.1016/j.drugalcdep.2006.08.019

Perman-Howe, P. R., Davies, E. L., & Foxcroft, D. R. (2018). The classification and organisation of alcohol misuse prevention with a focus on environmental prevention. *Current Addiction Reports, 5*(1), 87–92. https://doi.org/10.1007/s40429-018-0190-2

Radaev, V. (2019). Making sense of alcohol consumption among Russian young adults in the context of Post-2009 policy initiatives. In D. Conroy & F. Measham (Eds.), *Young adult drinking styles: Current perspectives on research, policy and practice* (pp. 313–332). Springer International Publishing. https://doi.org/10.1007/978-3-030-28607-1_16

Radtke, T., Ostergaard, M., Cooke, R., & Scholz, U. (2017). Web-based alcohol intervention: Study of systematic attrition of heavy drinkers. *Journal of Medical Internet Research, 19*(6), e217. https://doi.org/10.2196/jmir.6780

Rothman, A. J., Klein, W. M. P., & Sheeran, P. (2020). Moving from theoretical principles to intervention strategies: Applying the experimental medicine approach. In M. S. Hagger, L. D. Cameron, K. Hamilton, H. N, & T. Lintonen (Eds.), *The handbook of behavior change* (pp. 285–299). Cambridge, UK: Cambridge University Press.

Schüz, B., Brick, C., Wilding, S., & Conner, M. (2020). Socioeconomic status moderates the effects of health cognitions on health behaviors within participants: Two multibehavior studies. *Annals of Behavioral Medicine, 54*(1), 36–48. https://doi.org/10.1093/abm/kaz023

Schüz, B., Li, A. S.-W., Hardinge, A., McEachan, R. R. C., & Conner, M. (2017). Socioeconomic status as a moderator between social cognitions and physical activity: Systematic review and meta-analysis based on the theory of planned behavior. *Psychology of Sport and Exercise, 30,* 186–195. https://doi.org/10.1016/j.psychsport.2017.03.004

Smith, S. W., Atkin, C. K., & Roznowski, J. (2006). Are "drink responsibly" alcohol campaigns strategically ambiguous? *Health Communication, 20*(1), 1–11. https://doi.org/10.1207/s15327027hc2001_1

Staniszewska, S., Brett, J., Simera, I., Seers, K., Mockford, C., Goodlad, S., … Tysall, C. (2017). GRIPP2 reporting checklists: Tools to improve reporting of patient and public involvement in research. *BMJ, 358*, j3453. https://doi.org/10.1136/bmj.j3453

Talley, A. E., Gilbert, P. A., Mitchell, J., Goldbach, J., Marshall, B. D., & Kaysen, D. (2016). Addressing gaps on risk and resilience factors for alcohol use outcomes in sexual and gender minority populations. *Drug and Alcohol Review, 35*(4), 484–493. https://doi.org/10.1111/dar.12387

Vallance, K., Stockwell, T., Hammond, D., Shokar, S., Schoueri-Mychasiw, N., Greenfield, T., … Hobin, E. (2020). Testing the effectiveness of enhanced alcohol warning labels and modifications resulting from alcohol industry interference in Yukon, Canada: Protocol for a quasi-experimental study [protocol]. *JMIR Research Protocols, 9*(1), e16320. https://doi.org/10.2196/16320

Vashishtha, R., Livingston, M., Pennay, A., Dietze, P., MacLean, S., Holmes, J., … Lubman, D. I. (2020). Why is adolescent drinking declining? A systematic review and narrative synthesis. *Addiction Research & Theory, 28*(4), 275–288. https://doi.org/10.1080/16066359.2019.1663831

Wade, J. M. (2020). Is it race, sex, gender or all three? Predicting risk for alcohol consumption in emerging adulthood. *Journal of Child and Family Studies*. https://doi.org/10.1007/s10826-020-01780-8

Wilkerson, J. M., Di Paola, A., McCurdy, S., & Schick, V. (2020). Covariates of hazardous alcohol use among sexual and gender minorities in Texas: Identifying the most vulnerable [article]. *Addictive Behaviors, 105*, 7, Article 106327. https://doi.org/10.1016/j.addbeh.2020.106327

Wilkinson, C., & Room, R. (2009). Warnings on alcohol containers and advertisements: International experience and evidence on effects. *Drug and Alcohol Review, 28*(4), 426–435. https://doi.org/10.1111/j.1465-3362.2009.00055.x

Index[1]

A

Abstinence, 2, 13, 15, 147, 151, 152, 193, 196, 288, 339, 340, 378, 514–516, 531, 542
Action anticipated regret, 81
Adolescence, 16, 57, 58, 62, 108, 114, 115, 117, 351, 357, 361, 364, 367, 380, 383, 385, 393, 401, 406, 410, 427, 428n1, 430–432, 435, 440, 556
Alcohol control, 1, 6, 7, 139–140, 378, 452
Alcohol expectancies, 14, 26–31, 37, 39–42, 44, 45, 80, 84, 89–93, 96, 276, 280–281, 287, 354–358, 404, 405, 432, 463
Alcohol Expectancy Theory, 25–27, 31, 37, 44
Alcohol experimentation, 433
Alcohol identity, 311, 314, 555
Alcohol industry, 7, 246, 406n3, 453, 455, 464, 465, 557, 568
Alcoholism typologies, 106–109, 124
Alcohol policies, 7, 12, 141, 170, 175, 256, 376
Alcohol-related harm, 6, 8, 15, 61, 235, 274, 276, 287, 299, 301, 304, 311–313, 316, 326–327, 420, 429, 438, 457–459, 465–467, 477, 483, 490, 559
Alcohol use disorder (AUD), 105, 106, 109, 114, 115, 117, 119, 120, 123, 124, 186, 196, 198, 333, 379, 380, 433, 533, 534, 537, 541, 543
Alcohol Use Disorder Identification Test (AUDIT), 8, 30, 40, 41
Anticipated regret, 80–81, 89, 90, 92
Attitudes, 34, 35, 37, 39, 44, 52, 57, 58, 60, 66, 67, 84, 135–137, 162, 168, 172, 175, 209, 276, 283, 286, 310, 352, 354, 359, 375, 380, 382, 391–394, 405, 411, 412, 421, 432, 436, 452, 453, 458, 461, 464–466, 478, 479, 482–484, 500, 501, 510, 515, 566
Automatic, 14, 46, 52–54, 65, 66, 68, 230, 343, 433, 456, 528, 531, 532, 554

[1] Note: Page numbers followed by 'n' refer to notes.

R. Cooke et al. (eds.), *The Palgrave Handbook of Psychological Perspectives on Alcohol Consumption*, https://doi.org/10.1007/978-3-030-66941-6

B

Big Five model of personality, 111, 113
Binge drinking, 3, 4, 25, 27–31, 37, 40, 41, 44, 46, 63, 299, 300, 314–316, 558
Blackouts, 5, 9

C

Cognitive biases, 518, 527–545
Cognitive bias modification (CBM), 17, 527, 528, 537–545, 557
Cognitive model of binge drinking, 25, 27–31, 37, 40, 41, 44, 46
Cognitive processes, 208, 230, 528
College students, 44, 59, 116, 188, 194, 261, 273, 275, 285, 303, 305, 313, 335, 481, 485, 514
Conformity, 32, 33, 38, 41, 45, 82, 83, 89, 92, 93, 278, 281, 282, 302, 306–308, 404
Conformity motives, 32, 33, 38, 41, 45, 83, 89, 93, 281, 404
Context, 2, 15, 57, 60, 61, 64–68, 85, 94–95, 135–138, 140–143, 145–147, 150–152, 160–163, 170–172, 177, 187–189, 193–196, 198, 207–211, 213, 214, 216, 217, 240, 241, 243–245, 284, 285, 288, 304, 313, 315, 316, 328, 333–335, 339, 343, 344, 352, 359, 365, 366, 383, 384, 387, 391–393, 402, 413, 414, 428, 430–437, 440, 458, 464, 465, 467, 501, 513, 527, 551, 553, 554, 558, 563, 567, 568
Contextual factors, 12, 14, 15, 18, 95, 136, 138, 207, 208, 213, 214, 220, 308, 315, 553–554, 558, 568
Coping motives, 32, 33, 38, 82, 89, 114, 119, 120, 404
Cross-cultural, 40, 68, 97, 163, 164, 167, 169, 171, 176, 378–381, 383, 386, 555
Cross-sectional design, 30, 31, 33, 40, 43, 83, 89, 168, 311, 560
Cultural factors, 15, 160, 161, 174, 262, 377, 553

D

Declines in drinking, 463
Descriptive norms, 40, 81–82, 89, 90, 92, 94, 138–140, 148, 283–285, 287, 435, 436, 482
Drink, 2–5, 8, 10–12, 14–16, 25–27, 30, 32, 33, 35–39, 44, 54, 55, 57, 58, 61, 62, 64, 66–68, 80, 82–84, 87, 91, 93, 97, 106–108, 124, 138–140, 143–152, 162, 165, 176, 186, 187, 192, 194, 209, 210, 212, 214, 215, 217–219, 230–237, 239, 242–245, 256, 258, 265, 273, 275, 281–283, 288, 289, 303, 304, 316, 325–341, 343, 344, 353, 357, 360, 362, 363, 365, 380, 383–390, 393, 402–405, 407–409, 411–413, 415–421, 428, 429, 433, 451–460, 462, 463, 465, 467, 479, 482, 485, 500, 506, 510, 512, 514, 516, 529, 537, 552–554, 556–560, 563, 566
Drinkers, 3–7, 9, 11, 13, 27, 28, 30, 34, 36, 38, 41, 56, 58, 59, 61–64, 86, 92, 106, 107, 114, 118, 120, 121, 138, 139, 150, 152, 187, 189–193, 196, 233–235, 240, 245, 256, 262, 264, 280, 282, 286, 312, 326, 327, 329, 330, 333, 335, 338, 353, 355, 362, 386–388, 390, 393, 403, 412, 413, 433, 434, 454–458, 462, 463, 465, 467, 483–485, 487, 502, 507, 512, 533, 536–540, 542, 556, 568

Drinking, 2, 5–10, 25, 27–31, 53, 77, 105, 135, 148–150, 159, 162, 185–191, 207, 234, 236–244, 255, 285, 299, 325, 329–333, 375–377, 388–393, 402, 427, 451, 480, 501, 528, 552, 555–556
Drinking behaviour, 2, 3, 7, 10–14, 16, 17, 25, 26, 32, 43, 54, 57, 61, 62, 64, 66, 77, 78, 90, 91, 141, 148–150, 162, 168, 169, 185, 187–189, 191, 193, 194, 196, 197, 211, 236–242, 245, 273, 275–277, 280, 283, 284, 286–289, 331, 335, 343, 352, 361, 362, 367, 402, 406, 409, 413, 421, 433, 435, 436, 453, 454, 467, 480, 482, 483, 485, 487, 527–529, 534–537, 552–555, 562, 565
Drinking culture, 15, 17, 136, 139–141, 148, 151, 152, 159, 160, 162–166, 168–178, 189, 256, 259–264, 266, 277, 375, 377, 378, 380, 385, 389, 391, 392, 394, 554, 555, 565
Drinking intentions, 35, 62, 78, 79, 84, 460, 486, 552, 559
Drinking norms, 140, 175, 276, 286, 385, 386, 391, 392
Drinking patterns, 1, 3, 5, 8–10, 16, 27, 36, 38, 41, 61, 106, 118, 164–166, 170–172, 176–178, 187, 256, 299, 300, 363, 366, 379, 389, 404, 462, 502
Drinking practices, 2, 7, 162, 168, 171, 173, 176, 177, 210, 212, 221, 255, 259, 261, 262, 264, 265, 336, 338, 375, 376, 385, 389–391, 394
Drinking refusal self-efficacy (DRSE), 26–31, 37, 39–41, 44, 45, 79, 80, 83–84, 89–93, 96, 97, 209, 289, 315, 316, 335, 336, 339–342, 393, 552
Drinking trajectories, 390, 440
Drinking typologies, 27
Drunk as I want to be, 9
Drunkenness, 140, 148, 163, 164, 169, 171, 176, 196, 256, 306, 314, 330, 363, 378–380, 384–388, 390–393, 402, 403, 412, 415, 416, 483, 490
Dry January, 13, 151, 152, 339, 340, 516

E

Economic, 1, 107, 123, 301, 316, 402, 458, 499, 555
Emerging adulthood, 115, 116, 393
Enhancement motives, 32, 33, 38, 39, 44, 45, 82, 83, 87, 89, 90, 92, 97, 118, 120, 215, 281, 282, 303, 305, 307, 308, 314, 404, 552
Ethnicity, 161, 255, 260, 262, 275, 403, 482, 510, 564, 566
Experimental research, 44, 435

F

Feel the effects, 9
Femininity, 146, 260–264
Friendships, 145, 146, 152, 216, 256, 259, 261, 263, 285, 338, 430
Fun, 2, 3, 9, 26, 118, 124, 143, 144, 150, 187, 233, 256, 260, 263–265, 305–308, 382, 386, 388, 404, 418, 505, 555

G

Gender, 5, 15, 33, 78, 140, 146, 148, 149, 168, 170–173, 188, 189, 192, 207, 208, 213–215, 219, 220, 255, 258, 260–263, 275, 280, 282, 305–307, 353, 362, 381, 408, 417, 434, 462, 479, 510, 555, 559, 564

Gender role, 146
Generations, 161, 172, 193, 384, 385, 390, 391, 393
Global positioning system (GPS), 193, 197
Government, 2, 3, 5–8, 13, 138, 229, 231, 316, 326–328, 331, 332, 405, 406n3, 455, 464, 465, 499, 504, 509, 510, 516, 556, 563, 567, 568
Government guidelines, 13, 138, 327, 331, 405, 504, 509, 510, 516

H

Habits, 41, 46, 53, 78, 97, 106, 123, 170, 175, 178, 343, 359, 385, 387, 389, 390, 467, 507
Hangover, 5, 9, 57, 142, 145, 149, 328, 407, 503
Heavy drinking, 63, 97, 116, 118, 119, 148, 172, 175, 191, 194, 256, 276, 282, 287, 328, 362, 380, 382, 388, 390, 404, 428n1, 487, 536, 538, 540, 541, 555
Heavy Episodic Drinking (HED), 3–5, 8, 11, 16, 25, 32, 33, 38, 41, 43, 77, 81, 84, 85, 92, 93, 97, 114, 115, 118, 123, 189, 273–275, 280, 283, 285, 289, 300, 301, 314–316, 330, 339, 356, 362, 375, 379, 380, 387, 388, 390, 407, 409, 429, 430, 436, 438, 440, 466, 500–503, 505, 507, 510, 512–514, 519, 559
Hello Sunday Morning, 13

I

Identity, 2, 13, 15–18, 138, 144, 148–150, 163, 168, 171, 172, 255, 256, 259–266, 277–280, 287–289, 311, 314, 336, 428, 430–434, 436, 438, 518, 555–556, 564, 566
Implementation intention interventions, 505, 509–511, 513
Implementation intentions, 64, 312, 313, 505, 506, 509–514, 517, 518, 559
Implicit, 17, 25, 32, 46, 60, 66–68, 160, 189, 220, 236, 284, 311, 314, 354, 433, 434, 436, 484, 507, 529, 553, 557, 567
Implicit attitudes, 66, 67
Implicit processes, 17, 32, 236, 434, 507
Impulsivity, 78, 108, 109, 112, 114, 116, 120, 121, 136, 276
Inaction anticipated regret, 81
Incentive motivation model, 25, 31–33, 38, 40, 41, 44, 46, 82, 281, 302, 303, 307, 500
Information-Motivation-Behavioural Skills (IMB) model, 327, 331
Injunctive norms, 81, 139, 140, 148, 210, 283, 482, 483
Intentions, 14, 15, 25, 33–41, 44, 45, 52, 54, 56–62, 64, 67, 68, 78, 79, 84–90, 92–97, 137, 139, 283, 287, 310–313, 330, 338, 435, 436, 454, 456, 458–461, 464, 486, 500–506, 508–511, 513–515, 552, 557, 559, 566
Interventions, 11, 39, 51, 62–65, 77, 96, 105, 121–123, 144, 163, 185, 208, 230–244, 273, 285–287, 300, 311–314, 331, 338–340, 428, 457, 477–489, 500–506, 508–515, 527, 552, 557–558

J

Just-in-time adaptive interventions (JITAI), 195, 196

L

Labelling, 17, 231–236, 244–246, 332, 451–459, 461, 462, 464–467, 557, 562, 568
Labelling interventions, 453, 464–467
Longitudinal design, 29, 39, 40, 44, 98, 113, 117, 168
Low-risk drinking, 5–8, 36, 325, 326, 329–333, 557, 563
Low-risk drinking guidelines, 5–7, 331, 451, 454–457

M

Macro, 190
Macro element, 190
Macro-environmental factors, 566
Macro-social, 136, 140, 144, 146, 150, 152
Masculinity, 172, 260–264, 555
Mental health, 29, 122, 145, 256, 407, 432, 477
Mental imagery, 338, 339, 503, 506, 507, 513
Mental imagery interventions, 339, 504–507
Methodological issues, 26, 31, 42–46, 78, 91–96, 545, 561
Mezzo element, 190
Micro element, 190
Micro-environment, 212, 230, 554
Model of Action Phases (MAP), 17, 311, 509, 513
Motivation, 6, 14, 25, 31–33, 38, 40, 41, 44, 46, 61, 69, 82, 108, 118, 122, 193, 195, 217, 277, 281, 302, 303, 307, 310, 312, 314, 316, 325, 328–332, 334, 338–340, 343, 344, 355, 435, 436, 439, 456, 457, 460, 462, 467, 500–502, 504, 509, 513–516, 518, 519, 531, 540, 555, 563
Motivational interventions, 500, 503–508, 515–517, 557
Motivational phase, 311, 509

N

National Institute for Alcohol Abuse and Alcoholism (NIAAA), 4, 5, 428–430, 479
Nausea, 5
Non-drinkers, 27, 56, 62, 139, 147, 148, 150, 151, 171, 327, 337, 338, 362, 402, 507
Non-drinking, 65, 94, 95, 135, 138, 144, 147, 152, 342, 465, 504, 554, 560

O

Observation, 27, 37–39, 168, 171, 186, 191–193, 209, 210, 212, 359, 360, 362, 363, 391, 393, 565
Operationalise, 4, 138, 139, 334

P

Parental influence, 360–363, 411
Parenting, 145, 161, 360, 402, 405, 406
Peer influence, 189, 304, 311, 328, 402, 430, 431, 434, 435, 437
Peers, 17, 55, 63, 64, 82, 96, 120–122, 136, 138, 148, 149, 151, 191, 192, 260, 265, 277, 283, 284, 289, 301, 336, 338, 355, 359, 363, 364, 384, 385, 388, 393, 413, 421, 427, 428, 430–436, 440, 480, 482–484, 508, 556
Perceived behavioural control (PBC), 34–41, 44, 45, 52, 85, 86, 89, 92, 97, 137, 209, 310, 311, 501, 515

Personalised feedback interventions, 17, 480–490, 557
Personality, 14, 40, 78, 105–124, 135, 137, 138, 277, 285, 335, 336, 355, 392, 553
Pleasure, 256, 264, 386
Pre-drinkers, 187, 301, 303, 311, 315
Pre-drinking, 16, 275, 299–317, 500, 555
Pre-gaming, 186, 189, 300n1, 307
Pre-loading, 16, 300
Prospective design, 30, 33, 43, 83, 113, 311
Prototype evaluation, 55, 86, 92
Prototypes, 14, 41, 46, 55–69, 86, 87, 89, 90, 92, 93, 97, 139, 507, 518, 562
Prototype similarity, 55, 58–61, 86, 92
Prototype Willingness Model (PWM), 14, 51, 54–69, 86, 209, 500, 556

Q

Questionnaire, 65–69, 80–83, 111–113, 168, 302, 306–307, 331, 354, 357, 365, 408, 409, 561

R

Rational, 25, 343, 528
Reasoned actor, 2, 14
Reasoned processes, 343, 434
Reducing alcohol consumption, 197, 311, 316, 501, 509, 515, 516, 556–558
Relax, 2, 14, 26, 119, 124
Risk, 3, 5–8, 41, 52, 54–64, 68, 91, 115, 121, 136, 148, 163, 186, 189, 192, 194, 195, 197, 229, 232, 243, 273–280, 284–285, 287, 289, 299–301, 311–314, 326, 327, 334, 351, 353, 362, 365, 375, 376, 378, 382, 383, 385–388, 393, 404, 409, 416, 427–429, 431–433, 435, 436, 438, 439, 451, 452, 456–461, 463–467, 480, 481, 487, 499, 516, 527, 531, 538, 542, 543, 556–558, 564

S

SCRAM, 11
Secure Continuous Remote Alcohol Monitoring (SCRAM), 11, 218, 219
Selective testing of variables, 42–43, 91–93
Self-affirmation, 504–506, 508, 513–515, 517
Self-affirmation implementation intention, 513, 514
Self-affirmation interventions, 505, 508, 513, 515
Self-Determination Theory (SDT), 308, 310, 311
Self-regulation, 334, 500, 515, 516, 518, 519, 528
Self-regulatory interventions, 17, 480, 505, 508–513, 516, 517, 557
Self-report, 10, 41, 65, 69, 191, 193, 197, 211, 215, 216, 219, 220, 337, 354, 433, 488–490, 529, 554
Sensation seeking, 40–42, 78, 111, 112, 114–116, 122, 136, 138, 277, 336, 431, 562
Sociability, 111, 113, 114, 139, 507
Social, 1, 27, 51, 77, 105, 135, 160, 185, 207, 230, 255, 277, 300, 328, 353, 375, 402, 427, 456, 478, 499, 538, 551
Social drinkers, 27, 28, 62, 502, 538
Social drinking norms, 385, 386
Social factors, 12, 136, 141, 186, 213–215, 359
Social harms, 353

Social media, 15, 16, 142, 149–151, 177, 255, 256, 258–266, 364, 414, 440, 555
Social motives, 32, 33, 38, 40, 87, 93, 94, 282, 302, 303, 404
Social norms, 17, 82, 91, 137, 150–152, 162, 209, 243, 260, 263, 283–287, 389, 390, 392, 428, 437, 482, 484
Socioeconomic, 141, 243, 457
Study design, 43–44, 46, 97, 165, 166, 237, 364, 540, 545
Subjective norms, 34, 35, 37, 44, 52, 57, 60, 81, 94, 137, 310, 435, 501, 515
Surveys, 9–11, 44, 63, 64, 92, 94, 168, 186, 191, 192, 234, 256, 304, 331, 332, 376, 380, 383, 388, 402–404, 407, 408, 411, 412, 428, 454, 456, 480, 553, 558, 561, 565, 567

T

Technology, 15, 16, 84, 193, 194, 196, 197, 210, 216–220, 258, 259, 489, 490, 565, 569
Temporary abstinence, 13, 339, 340, 516
Theory-based determinants, 502, 503
Theory-based interventions, 63, 501–504
Theory of Planned Behaviour (TPB), 34, 37–41, 44–46, 52, 58–60, 69, 94, 137–139, 209, 308, 311, 435, 500, 501, 503, 505, 507, 510, 517, 562
Theory of Reasoned Action (TRA), 33, 34, 38, 52
Timeframe, 5, 8, 10, 39, 43, 95–96
The Tipping Point, 9, 36
Transdermal Sensors, 11, 554
Transition, 115, 117, 143, 147, 343, 357, 361, 366, 433, 560
Transtheoretical Model (TTM), 137, 150, 151, 341–343
Trends, 16, 44, 96, 173, 176, 198, 231, 278, 378, 380, 463, 566

U

Underrepresented groups, 564
University students, 3, 28–30, 37, 40, 46, 67, 80–84, 86, 87, 90–95, 138, 139, 143, 149, 150, 168, 169, 213, 261, 275, 276, 289, 301, 304, 305, 330, 334, 339, 454, 455, 480, 481, 485, 488, 490, 505, 506, 508–510, 512, 513, 515–517, 519, 541, 555, 558, 560, 564
Urgency Perseverance Premeditation and Sensation Seeking (UPPS) model, 112

V

Violence, 140, 187, 194, 197, 278, 326, 378, 382, 403, 558
Volitional Help Sheet (VHS), 512–513
Volitional phase, 311, 312, 341, 509
Vomiting, 5, 9, 460

W

Willingness, 56–69, 78, 79, 86, 87, 89–94, 97, 230, 438

Y

Young adult drinkers, 192
Young adults, 6, 7, 15, 16, 33, 45, 51, 57, 59, 114, 141, 149, 152, 255–260, 262–265, 329–330, 337, 375, 381, 389, 433, 437, 455, 463, 486, 517, 560
Youth, 146, 172, 177, 255, 256, 375–377, 379, 380, 383, 386, 388–394, 403, 428, 430–432, 434–437, 440

The manufacturer's authorised representative in the EU is Springer Nature Customer Service Centre GmbH, Europaplatz 3, 69115 Heidelberg, Germany. If you have any concerns regarding our products, please contact ProductSafety@springernature.com

Printed and bound by CPI Group (UK) Ltd, Croydon, CR0 4YY
30/09/2026
02225701-0019